Non-secret Formulas: A Collection Of Over Four Thousand Formulas And One Thousand Prize Prescriptions For The Use Of Physicians And Druggists

Thomas Michael Griffiths

Nabu Public Domain Reprints:

You are holding a reproduction of an original work published before 1923 that is in the public domain in the United States of America, and possibly other countries. You may freely copy and distribute this work as no entity (individual or corporate) has a copyright on the body of the work. This book may contain prior copyright references, and library stamps (as most of these works were scanned from library copies). These have been scanned and retained as part of the historical artifact.

This book may have occasional imperfections such as missing or blurred pages, poor pictures, errant marks, etc. that were either part of the original artifact, or were introduced by the scanning process. We believe this work is culturally important, and despite the imperfections, have elected to bring it back into print as part of our continuing commitment to the preservation of printed works worldwide. We appreciate your understanding of the imperfections in the preservation process, and hope you enjoy this valuable book.

Non-Secret Formulas......

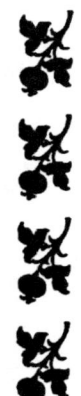

A collection of over four thousand formulas and one thousand prize prescriptions for the use of Physicians and Druggists, to which has been added a selection of articles from standard authorities on Photography, Tablet Triturates, Compressed Tablets, Elixirs, Proprietaries, and original formulas for toilet articles, perfumery and articles of household use, making a valuable book of reference on subjects appertaining to the business of an up-to-date pharmacist.

FIRST EDITION, PRICE $5.00 PER COPY.

BY

T. M. GRIFFITHS,

3818 Laclede Avenue,   ST. LOUIS.

——— ——— 1897 ——— ———

Buxton & Skinner Sta. Co., Printers,
215-221 Chestnut Street.

Entered according to Act of Congress in the year 1897, by T. M. Griffiths, in the office of the Librarian of Congress at Washington, D. C.
All rights reserved.

LANE LIBRARY

PREFACE.

The necessity of a thoroughly reliable formula book for ready reference will be apparent to everyone engaged in the drug business or in any of its kindred branches. Especially useful will be a formula book written and compiled by one who has had thirty years practical experience in the laboratory.

It contains valuable recipes used by well-known firms engaged in the manufacture of Pharmaceuticals and Druggists' Specialties. The formulas given for perfumeries, toilet articles and flavoring extracts, are those used by one of the largest firms in the United States, modified to suit the requirements of the retail trade.

The physicians' formulas are principally the prescriptions offered in competition for prizes given by a well-known journal. They are revised, corrected and commented upon by a distinguished physician, and are selected with the view of being useful to the busy medical practitioner.

The formulae of the New York Hospital and the London Children's Hospital, will, it is hoped, be found a useful addition to the medical library.

Full instructions and a complete line of formulas are given for preparing compressed tablets, tablet triturates and granular effervescent salts, medicinal lozenges, unofficinal pills, elixirs, solutions, emulsions, chlorodynes, anodynes, anaesthetics, liniments, insecticides, garden and lawn fertilizers, cements, glues and mucilages, marking, writing, copying and hektograph inks and pads, Infants' food, teething, soothing and cooling powders, the various remedies for infantile diseases are fully treated of. Recipes are also given for cleansing and scouring, and cleansing preparations, furniture creams and polishes, metal cleaning and polishing preparations, soap and soap making (on a small scale), deodorants and disinfectants. To these are added a complete formulary of curry powders, sausage and meat flavorings, Worcestershire sauces, digestive relishes, baking powder of every variety, including alum, acid phosphate, cream of tartar and tartaric acid, slow and quick rising, as well as flavoring extracts of standard and superior grades, soluble lemon, soluble ginger, ginger ale and soluble tincture of tolu, fruit flavors from the ethers and from pure fruit juices, syrups, root beer and root beer extracts, shoe dressings and polishes, stove and grate enamels, beverages and liqueurs, tasteless syrup of quinine, and formulas for making goods similar to many of the leading proprietaries.

The formulas for the home treatment of Dipsomania are written by a physician who has had several years of practical experience as house physician in the Keeley Institute in Dwight, Illinois.

Of especial interest to retail druggists and to photographic amateurs, are the articles on "How to do the photographic trade," and the way to make it pay, the material to keep in stock, how to make the various chemical solutions and developers, to take, print and mount photographs, how to prepare the dark room, etc., etc., being a complete guide to the details of the photographic art.

The veterinary part of the work is very complete indeed, and embraces valuable formulas for stock foods, condition powders, hog cholera remedies, poultry powders, poultry tonics and bird remedies; to which is added a treatise on the diseases of domestic animals and pets, horses, cattle, sheep, pigs, goats, dogs, poultry, turkeys, geese, rabbits, pigeons and canaries, their treatment and cure.

The article on perfumery is a practical guide for the manufacture of everything connected with the perfumers' art, and written with especial care to meet the wants of those who, with a very small outlay of capital desire to engage in a pleasant, profitable business, and who do not desire to invest much money in the venture until assured of success. Full instructions are given for preparing the higher grades of handkerchief extracts usually sold at $3.50 to $4.00 per pound; also a full line of formulas for making the cheaper kind of goods from essential oils and tinctures. The latter formulas will be found valuable in enabling the manufacturer to compete successfully with the grade of goods offered at a low price by department stores. In this part of the book are also added reliable formulas for colognes, cologne mixtures, bay rums and bay rum mixtures, Florida waters, Florida water mixtures, lavender water, violet waters, verbena and other toilet waters of pronounced excellence; sachet powders, fumigating pastilles, solid or frozen perfumes, toilet powders, infant powders, toilet creams, enamels, cold creams, camphor ices, freckle creams, arsenical and other face lotions, milk of roses, cream of roses, frostilline, shampoos, dandruff pomades, brilliantine, lip salve, shaving creams, stick pomades, cocoanut cream, and many other toilet preparations that command a ready sale.

The part devoted to preparations for the hair contains formulae for hair colorers, hair dyes, quinine and jaborandi hair tonics, with explicit directions for their manufacture.

The article on dental preparations comprises tooth powders, tooth pastes, antiseptic tooth washes and dental obtundents, together with many other formulas useful to the dental profession.

In the keen competition of these days there is an urgent demand for reliable formulas to compete with the great number of proprietary remedies in the market. Substitution by unscrupulous parties of worthless preparations to replace articles of acknowledged merit, is dishonest first, last and all the time; but surely the druggist has a perfect right to compete with advertised remedies by offering, praising and pushing the sale of his own preparations when he makes them of good material and by a meritorious formula. Furthermore, should he take pains to convince the physicians in his neighborhood of the excellence of the goods of his own manufacture, and succeed in having them prescribed, it surely comes under the head of fair business competition, and cannot be objected to, unless by those who are so blinded by avarice that they are unwilling to acknowledge any virtue in a preparation, unless they are pecuniarily interested in the profits.

In the determined fight the druggists are making against monopolies, a book of reliable formulas will be of benefit in evening up profits. Bearing this in mind, there is a good line of formulae inserted for the production of goods similar to and in many cases superior to such well-known articles as acid phosphate, ammonol, antikamnia, aristol, Ayer's sarsaparilla, Baby's quinine, beef, celery and sarsaparilla, bismuth hair dye, blackberry brandy, blood and kidney tea,

PREFACE.

brilliantine, bromidia, buchu (Wayne's), butter coloring, cascara cordial, celery compound, chill tonic (tasteless), chlorides compound (elixir of, 1, 2, 3, 4, 5 and 6), coca kola, cod liver oil and malt, cologne (Hoyt's), consumption cure (Piso's), copying pads (hektograph), dioviburnum elixir, fig syrup, fluid lightning, Frey's vermifuge, gold cure for Dipsomania, Helonias cordial, household ammonia, home treatment (Keeley Cure), iodides compound (elixir of, 6), iodide of iron syrup (rapid method of making), kamnafuga, kidney and liver cure, kola champagne essence, lactated pepsin elixir, listerine (will stand the tr. chlor. iron test), lithiated hydrangea, magic neuralgic drops, mead syrup, mistura gonorrhoea, nervina, odontundor, phosphorus paste (never changing, easily made), pepsin ferro. mang., pepsin powder, purgative effervescing salts, Roback's bitters, rough on rats, rubifoam, saline fruit salt (Eno's), syrup of hypophosphites haematic, syrup of iodide of iron (tasteless), syrup of white pine (new method), tasteless chill powder, Vance's chilblain cream, viburnum compound, vin mariani, wild cherry bitters, wine of pepsin, wine of cod liver oil, wire fence liniment, wizard oil, worm cakes, worm powders, Worcestershire sauce (genuine), and hundreds of others that are money makers and well adapted to the requirements of those who desire to push a few well-paying specialties of merit. While expressing my thanks and obligations to all sources from which I quote, I am especially indebted to the Scientific American Encyclopedia for some of its admirable articles on cleaning, scouring, photography, cements and insecticides; to the Standard Formulary for its article on Elixirs; to the Pharmaceutical Era, The Western Druggist, The London Chemist and Druggist, The Druggists' Circular and to Scoville's Art of Dispensing, for many useful articles and formulae.

I trust that it is not necessary to insist upon any claim to the average degree of originality, for if the book does not bear the evidence of honest and independent work by one familiar with the pestle and mortar, it is a defect not likely to be removed by the ———— and argumentative of prefaces.

March 17th, 1897.

1 **Drams** instead of Ounces of Iron —.

Change 2644 and 2645 to read **12** ounces of Cinchonine Alkaloid instead of 1½ ounces.

I have had numerous enquiries as to the quantity of Iron by hydrogen required to be added to Formulas Nos. 2644 and 2645 to produce tasteless Syrup of Quinine with Iron. The usual amount is one grain to the teaspoonful. Weigh out the Iron and place in the bottle before filling with the Syrup.

T. M. GRIFFITHS.

PART I.

NON-SECRET FORMULAS.

BLOOD PURIFIERS AND ALTERATIVES.

1. Syrup of Sarsaparilla with Iodide of Potash. A

106 gallons sugar house syrup.
51 gallons spirits, 188 per cent.
60 pounds iodide of potash.
34½ gallons distilled water.
5 gallons fluid extract sarsap. co.
2 gallons fluid extract dandelion.
2 gallons fluid extract senna.
2 gallons fluid extract columbo.
7½ ounces oil sassafras.
3¾ ounces oil anise.
1¾ ounces oil wintergreen.
64 ounces burnt sugar coloring.
M. S. A.

2. Syrup of Sarsaparilla with Iodide of Potash. B

100 gallons sugar house syrup.
60 gallons spirits, 188 per cent.
76 gallons distilled water.
32 pounds iodide of potash.
5 gallons fluid extract sarsap co.
2 gallons fluid extract dandelion.
2 gallons fluid extract senna.
2 gallons fluid extract stillingia.
2 gallons fluid extract yellow dock.
1 gallon fluid extract rhubarb.
12 ounces oil sassafras.
6 ounces oil anise.
3 ounces oil wintergreen.
64 ounces burnt sugar coloring.
M. S. A.

3. Syrup of Sarsaparilla with Iodide of Potash. C

62½ gallons sugar house syrup.
19 gallons spirits, 188 per cent.
15 pounds iodide of potash.
65½ gallons distilled water.
3½ gallons fluid extract sarsap co.
1 9-16 gallons fluid extract dandelion.
1 9-16 gallons fluid extract senna.
1 9-16 gallons fluid extract yellow dock.
8 ounces oil sassafras.
4 ounces oil anise.
4 ounces oil wintergreen.
40 ounces burnt sugar coloring.

4. Indian Alterative Medicine.

5 pounds ground sarsaparilla.
5 pounds ground prickly ash.
5 pounds ground burdock.
2 pounds ground poke root.
5 pounds ground stillingia.
2½ pounds iodide potash.

Percolate the drugs with proof spirits until five gallons extract is obtained; dissolve the iodide of potash in the extract.

This is a powerful alterative medicine.

5. Compound Extract Sarsaparilla with Iodide of Potash.

2 pounds ground stillingia.
1 pound ground may apple.
1 pound ground poke root.
1 pound ground prickly ash.
1 pound iodide of potash.

Percolate the drugs with proof spirits until five gallons extract is obtained; dissolve the iodide of potash in the extract and add
5 gallons syrup of sarsaparilla with Iodide of potash, formula "A."

6. Compound Extract Red Clover.

5 pounds ground red clover.
2½ pounds ground stillingia.
1¼ pounds ground poke root.
1 pound iodide of potash.

Percolate the drugs with dilute alcohol until five gallons extract is obtained; dissolve the iodide of potash in one gallon of distilled water and add—make up to 10 gallons with syrup of sarsaparilla and iodide of potash formula "A."

7. Syrup of Trifolium Compound.

24 pints fluid extract licorice root.
24 pints fluid extract red clover.
12 pints fluid extract stillingia.
12 pints fluid extract burdock.
6 pints fluid extract poke root.
3 pints fluid extract prickly ash bark.
12 pints fluid ext. berberis aquifolium.
12 pints fluid extract cascara bitterless.
20 pints glycerine.
20 pints alcohol, 188 per cent.
60 pints water.
120 pounds granulated sugar.
5½ pounds iodide of potash.
2 ounces oil sassafras.
1 ounce oil wintergreen.
½ ounce oil anise.

M. S. A.

8. Sarsaparilla Blood Purifier

Indorsed by the Illinois Pharmaceutical Association.

Potassium iodide	240 grains.
Water	2 fl. ounces.
Fld. ext. burdock	2 fl. ounces.
Syr. sarsaparilla comp.	8 fl. ounces.
Syrup (dextrin or sugar) enough to make	16 fl. ounces.

Dose: One to four teaspoonfuls according to age.

9. Blood Cleanser.

Potassium iodide	64 grains.
Liquor potassa	4 drams.
Tincture cardamon co.	6 drams.
Fld. ext. sarsaparilla	1 ounce.
Tincture capsicum	20 minims.
Syrup of orange	1 ounce.
Salicylate of soda	128 grains.
Cinnamon water enough to make	16 ounces.

Dose: One or two tablespoonfuls to be taken three times a day. Children, 1 to 3 teaspoonfuls in a little water twice a day. This medicine should be continued for at least 14 days.

10. Blood Mixture without Iodide of Potassium.

Liquor arsenicalis	32 minims.
Potassium chlorat	32 grains.
Fl. ext. sarsap. co.	2 ounces.
Spirits chlorof	2 drams.
Aqua ad	8 ounces.

Dose: One tablespoonful to be taken three times a day after meals.

11. Robson's Blood Purifier.

Potash iodide	32 grains.
Soda sulphate	32 grains.
Potash liquor	4 drams.
Syrup sarsap. co.	10 drams.
Spirits of wintergreen, 1 to 16	1 ounce.
Iron sulphate	4 drams.
Chloroform water to make	8 ounces.

Dose: One or two tablespoonfuls.

12. Blood Remedy.

Citrate iron and ammonia	2 drams.
Iodide potash	2 scruples.
Liq. hydrarg. perchlor.	1 ounce.
Syrup simple	1 ounce.
Water	6 ounces.

Dose: One tablespoonful three times a day.

13. Blood Remedy for Scrofulous Disorders of the Blood.

Potassium iodide	64 grains.
Soda sulph	1 ounce.
Liquor potassa	½ ounce.
Fld. ext. stillingia co.	2 ounces.
Fl. ext. sarsap. co.	2 ounces.
Cinnamon water	3½ ounces.

Dose: One tablespoonful three times a day.

14. Clarke's Blood Mixture.

Clarke's Blood Mixture.—In 1875 a bottle of this was submitted by Dr. Wm. O'Neil to Dr. A. S. Taylor for analysis. According to the report of the latter, which was sent by Dr. O'Neil to the "Lancet":

"The quantity of the liquid contained in the bottle was 8 ounces. It had a dark-brown color, but was clear and free from any sediment. It had the smell of chloric ether (a compound of alcohol and chloroform), and a sweetish saline taste, which was not unpleasant. Its reaction on test paper was alkaline. On shaking it, it formed a brown-colored froth. When evaporated to dryness it left a thick dark saccharine extract, weighing, for the ½ ounce, about 29 grains. When this extract was incinerated it left a white saline residue, which proved to be iodide of potassium. The brown coloring matter had the usual properties of burnt sugar (caramel). In addition the mixture contained a small quantity of solution of potash, just sufficient to correct the acidity of the burnt sugar. Alcohol and chloroform (as chloric ether) were detected in it. Arsenic, antimony, lead, copper, and other metallic poisons were sought for, but the mixture was found to be quite free from any metallic impregnation.

"The composition of the mixture was found to be as follows in 8 ounces:

Potassium iodide .... 64 grains.
Chloric ether, B. P....... 4 drams.
Liquor potassae, B. P..... 30 minims
Water, colored with burnt
 sugar to the requisite tint 7½ ounces.

It is, nevertheless, the general opinion that decoction of hemidesmus, or sarsaparilla, is used in place of burnt sugar."

15. For Eczema, Patches on the Face, &c.

Liq. arsenicalis .... 32 minims.
Tr. ferri perch........... 1 dram.
Magnesia sulph.......... 1 ounce.
Glycerine .... ½ ounce.
Water enough for......... 8 ounces.

Dose: One tablespoonful three times a day.

16. For Hives or any Simple Cutaneous Disorder.

Magnesia sulph........... ½ ounce.
Magnesia carb. powd...... 2 scruples.
Potassium nitrate .... 2 scruples.
Tinct. ginger............. 30 minims.
Tinct. cardamon co....... 40 minims.
Peppermint water enough
 to make................ 2 ounces.

Dose: Two tablespoonfuls to be taken at bedtime, and the remainder to be taken in the morning, if necessary.

17. Blood Purifying Mixture.

Potass. iodid. ....1 dram.
Potass. bicarb. ....1½ drams.
Liq. arsenicalis ....1½ drams.
Spt. chloroformi .... ½ dram.
Ext. sarsae co. conc......2 ounces.
Aq. ad....................8 ounces.
M.

Dose: A dessertspoonful in a little water thrice daily, immediately after food.

The arsenic in it clears the skin, while as a tonic it is not inferior to quinine.

18. Blood Purifying Herbs.

Rad. sarsae inciss.........1½ ounces.
Chiratae .... ½ ounce.
Rad. sassafras ....3 drams.
Succ. glycyrrhiz. contus.... ½ ounce.
Rad. zingib. contus.........2 drams.
Sem. coriand. contus......2 drams.
Sodae bicarb. ....1 dram.
Potassii iodid. ....1 dram.
M.

Directions: Boil the contents of the packet with a quart of water for half an hour, stirring now and then. Strain the decoction through a piece of flannel into a scalded jug, and set aside to cool. Add a glass of whisky to preserve the decoction, and put it up in pint bottles. Take half a wineglassful before food three times a day.

19. Mixture for Purifying the Blood.

Potass. iodid. ....1 scruple.
Liq. taraxaci ....2 drams.
Dec. sarsae co...........6½ ounces.
Ol. sassafras ....1 minim.
Liq. potass. ....½ dram.
Mist. gent. co. conc........1½ ounces.
M. S. A.

Dose: One tablespoonful.

20. Cheap Blood Purifier.

Sugar house syrup......... 10 gallons.
Chloric ether .... 2½ gallons.
Burnt sugar coloring...... ½ gallon.
Water distilled .... 27½ gallons.
Iodide of potash......... 5½ pounds.
Liquor potassa .... 40 ounces.
Oil sassafras .... 3 ounces.
Oil anise .... 1 ounce.
Oil wintergreen .... 1 ounce.

Dissolve the iodide in the water, the oils in the chloric ether, and add to the syrup and coloring. Dose, one tablespoonful.

21. Alterative Juice Formula.

From the British Medical Journal as that given by J. Marion Sims.

Fld. ext. smilax sarsap....	2 ounces.
Fld. ext. stillingia.........	2 ounces.
Fld. ext. burdock..........	2 ounces.
Fld. ext. poke root........	2 ounces.
Tincture prickly ash.......	1 ounce.

22. Sarsaparilla Purgative Mixture.

Fl. ext. sarsaparilla.......	1 ounce.
Fl. ext. licorice...........	1 ounce.
Fl. ext. senna.............	3 ounces.
Fl. ext. mandrake	1 ounce.
Glycerine	2 ounces.
Iodide of potash...........	64 grains.

Dose: One tablespoonful in water.

23. Extract Beef, Celery and Sarsaparilla.

Syrup sarsaparilla formula No. 3	1 gallon.
Cudahy, Swift or Armour's fluid beef	4 ounces.
Celery seed ground........	1 ounce.
Percolated with alcohol....	4 ounces.
And water	8 ounces.

M. S. A.

24. Mexican Extract Sarsaparilla.

Mexican sarsaparilla......	5 pounds.
Yellow dock	5 pounds.
Stillingia	5 pounds.
Mandrake	7 pounds.
Senna leaves	7 pounds.
Licorice root	7 pounds.
Iodide potash	2 pounds.
Sugar house syrup........	5 gallons.
Alcohol	8 gallons.
Water q. s. to make......	42 gallons.

Macerate the drugs for 3 days, and percolate.

25. Blood and Liver Syrup, with Iron.

Iodide of potash..........	256 grains.
Citrate of iron and ammonia	256 grains.
Fluid extract senna.......	2 ounces.
Fluid extract licorice......	2 ounces.
Water	1 ounce.
Co. syrup of sarsaparilla..	11 ounces.

M. S. A.

Dose: One to two teaspoonfuls in half tumbler of cold water, three times a day after meals.

TONICS, BITTERS, WINES, &c.

26. Iron Tonic Bitters.

Cinchona bark	1 pound.
Coca leaves	1 pound.
Soluble citrate iron.......	½ pound.
Caraway seed	1 pound.
Gentian root	½ pound.
Orange peel recent........	3 pounds.
Red saunders	¼ pound.
Water	15 gallons.
Simple syrup	2 gallons.
Cologne spirits 188 per cent	7 gallons.

Percolate the drugs with the spirits and water; add the simple syrup, and add enough California Port Wine to make the product measure 30 gallons.

27. Glover's Iron Tonic Cordial.

Fl. ext. casc. sag. bark....	2 pounds.
Fl. ext. gentian root.......	1 pound.
Fl. ext. chamomile flowers..	1 pound.
Am. cit. iron.............	1 pound.
Oil orange	4 ounces.
Gran. sugar	30 pounds.
Alcohol	9½ gallons.
Sherry wine	2 gallons.
Water	30 gallons.

28. Glover's Iron Tonic Bitters.

Cinchonidia	3½ ounces.
Cinchonine	3½ ounces.
Quinine	1 ounce.
Sherry wine	25 gallons.
White sugar	105 pounds.
Oil orange	8 ounces.
Alcohol	15 gallons.

Water q. s. to make product 100 gallons, finally add 2 pounds am. cit. iron.

29. Wine of Iron (Bitter.)

Cit. iron and ammonia....	128 grains.
Simple elixir	2 ounces.
Sherry wine	13 ounces.
Hot water	1 ounce.

Isinglass (q. s. to detannate wine).

30. German Herb Bitters.

Orange peel ground.......	8 ounces.
Coriander seed ground....	1 ounce.
Gentian root ground......	¼ ounce.
Ginger root	1 ounce.
Alcohol, 188 per cent.....	2 gallons.
Water	3 gallons.
Simple syrup	½ gallon.

Macerate the drugs for three days in a portion of the alcohol and water; percolate with the remainder of the alcohol and water, and run enough water through the percolator, until in all five gallons of the percolate is obtained; filter and add the simple syrup.

31.   Roback's Bitters.

Orange peel ground.......	80 ounces.
Cassia bark ground........	22 ounces.
Cloves ground	6 ounces.
Coriander ground	30 ounces.
Caraway seed ground.....	6 ounces.
Red saunders and caramel..	q. s.
Proof spirits, 100°.........	18 gallons.
Water	12 gallons.
Sugar	4 pounds.

Macerate the drugs 7 days with a portion of the spirits and water, then percolate with the remainder; add the sugar and filter.

32.   Walton's Bitters.

Orange peel	20	ounces.
Virg. snake root..........	14	ounces.
Cinchona bark, yellow.....	8	ounces.
Coriander seed	6	ounces.
Anise seed	5	ounces.
Gentian root	5	ounces.
Wormwood herb	2	ounces.
Proof spirits, 100°........	31	gallons.
Water	8½	gallons.
Simple syrup	2	gallons.

Macerate the drugs 7 days, and filter.

33.   Samson's Bitters.

Cloves ground	3 ounces.
Cassia bark ground........	5 ounces.
Licorice root ground.......	4 ounces.
Orange peel ground.......	22 ounces.
Coriander seed ground.....	14 ounces.
Grains of paradise ground.	1 ounce.
Wormwood herb ground...	2 ounces.
Proof spirits, 100°.........	32 gallons.
Water	18 gallons.
Simple syrup	3 gallons.

Macerate the drugs with a portion of the spirits and water, q. s. to cover the drugs; in seven days percolate with the remainder of the spirits and water, filter, and add the simple syrup

34.   Wood's Wine of Iron Bitters.

Orange peel recent ground.	10 ounces.
Coriander seed recent grd..	2 ounces.
Cardamon seed recent grd.	1 ounce.
California port wine.......	10 gallons.
Cinchonidia sulphate	2 drams.
Aromatic sulph. acid......	2 drams.
Water	2 pints.
Spirits, 188 per cent.......	1 pint.
Simple syrup	2 pints.
Am. Cit. Iron.............	4 ounces.

M. S. A.

35.   Stoughton Bitters.

Orange peel ground.......	16 ounces.
Angostura bark ground....	10 ounces.
Licorice root ground.......	16 ounces.
Virg. snake root ground...	5 ounces.
Galangal root ground......	5 ounces.
Nutmegs ground	2 ounces.
Cassia bark ground........	5 ounces.
Powdered catechu	2 ounces.
Spanish saffron ground....	2 ounces.
Jamaica ginger ground....	2 ounces.
Cardamon seed ground....	2 ounces.
Red saunders ground......	2 ounces.
Coriander seed	10 ounces.
Caraway seed	1 ounce.

Macerate the drugs for fourteen days with five gallons of proof spirits. Then percolate with proof spirits, until fifteen gallons of percolate is obtained. Run water through the percolator until two gallons of water has passed through; mix this with three gallons of heavy simple syrup, and add to the fifteen gallons, making the total product twenty gallons.

36.   Wild Cherry Bitters.

Wild cherry bark ground..	16	ounces.
Orange peel ground.......	8	ounces.
Cardamon seed ground....	2	ounces.
Coriander seed ground.....	4	ounces.
Grains of paradise.........	2	ounces.
Cologne spirits proof......	16	gallons.
Water	9	gallons.
Simple syrup	1½	gallon.

Macerate the drugs with a portion of the spirits and water, q. s. to cover the drugs, in seven days percolate with the remainder of the spirits and water, filter, and add the simple syrup. Color with burnt sugar coloring, if a darker color is desired.

37.   Orange Bitters.   A

Orange peel recent ground.	5 pounds.
Coriander seed ground.....	2 pounds.
Lemon peel recent ground.	1 pound.
Saccharine (1 to 300)......	¼ ounce.
Cologne spirits 188 per cent	8 gallons.
Distilled water	12 gallons.

Dissolve the saccharin in the cologne spirits, macerate the drugs with a portion of the spirits and water, q. s. to cover the drugs, let stand for fourteen days, keeping well covered, then percolate with the remainder of the spirits and water; filter if necessary.

38. Orange Bitters. B

Orange peel recent ground.	2 pounds.
Coriander seed ground.....	½ pound.
Cinchonidia sulphate	½ ounce.
Orange flower water.......	32 ounces.
Saccharin	⅛ ounce.
Salicylic acid	⅛ ounce.
Cologne spirits 188 per cent	1½ gallons.
Water	7½ gallons.

Dissolve the saccharin, cinchonidia, and salicylic acid in two pints of the spirits, and set aside until needed. Macerate the drugs with six pints of spirits and six pints of water for seven days. Then place in a percolator and percolate with the remainder of the spirits and water; when percolation is finished, add the spirits containing the salicylic acid, saccharin and cinchonidia, filter if necessary, using blotting or filtering paper, beaten into a pulp, and a canton flannel filtering bag, made so as to have the soft woolen nap on the inside of the bag. These directions for filtering are for large quantities and for rapid work. For smaller quantities the ordinary paper filter and glass funnel will do. Avoid any alkaline matter in filtering this preparation.

39. Blackberry Brandy or Cordial.

German cherry juice......	½ gallon.
Soluble essence of ginger..	⅛ gallon.
Spirits proof	½ gallon.
Simple syrup	1 gallon.
Water	¾ gallon.
Tincture of orris root.....	4 ounces.
Caramel	1 ounce.

M. S. A.

40. Hop Tonic Bitters.

Hops ground	1 pound.
Buchu leaves ground......	¼ pound.
Orange peel ground.......	½ pound.
Gentian root ground......	¼ pound.
Cardamon seed ground....	⅛ pound.
Boiling water	3 gallons.
Cologne spirits 188 per cent	1 gallon.
Saccharine (1 to 300).......	⅛ ounce.

Pour the boiling water on the drugs. Let stand for five hours, and strain. Dissolve the saccharin in the spirits, add the cologne spirits and saccharin and filter.

41. Nerve Tonic in Debility.

Liq. strychniae	5 minims.
Liq. arsenicalis	3 minims.
Tinc. aurantii	20 minims.
Tinc. zingiberis	10 minims.
Sp. chloroformi	10 minims.
Aq. destill. ad............	1 ounce.

M.

For one dose: Twice daily after meals.

42. Calisaya Tonic.

Orange peel ground.......	5 ounces.
Cinchona bark ground.....	5 ounces.
Cardamon seed ground....	1 ounce.
Coriander seed ground.....	1 ounce.
Cologne spirits 188 per cent	32 ounces.
Water	16 ounces.
Syrup simple	32 ounces.

Percolate the drugs with the spirits and water, add the simple syrup and color with cochineal coloring, q. s.

43. Iron and Quinine Tonic. A

Citrate of iron and quinine	128 grains.
Am. Citrate of iron.........	128 grains.
Glycerine	2 ounces.
Orange bitters, B. (formula 38)	14 ounces.

Dose: One teaspoonful.

44. Iron and Quinine Tonic. B

Tinc. citro chloride of iron	1 ounce.
Acid phosph. dilute........	1 ounce.
Hydrochlorate of quinine..	1 scruple.
Glycerine	4 ounces.
Orange bitters, B. (formula 38)	14 ounces.

Dose: One to two teaspoonfuls in water.

45. Tonic for Nervous Debility. A

Acid hydrobromic dil......	1 ounce.
Acid phosphoric dil........	1 ounce.
Tinct. nux vomica.........	½ ounce.
Tinct. jam. ginger........	½ ounce.
Glycerine	1 ounce.
Orange bitters, B. (formula 38)	12 ounces.

Dose: One tablespoonful three times a day before meals.

46. Aromatic Bitters.

Curacoa orange peel grd...	1 pound.
Cinnamon bark true grd...	¼ pound.
Gentian root ground.......	⅛ pound.
Nutmegs ground	1-16 pound.
Cloves ground	1-16 pound.
Cardamon seed ground....	1-16 pound.
Cologne spirits 188 per cent	3 gallons
Water	5¼ gallons.
Simple syrup	½ gallon.

Macerate the drugs for seven days with a portion of the spirits and water, then percolate with remainder; filter and add the syrup.

47. Tonic Blood Mixture.

Tincture nux vomica......	½ ounce.
Fl. extract stillingia.......	2½ ounces.
Liquor arsenicalis	36 minims.
Bichlor. hydrarg.	1 grain.
Potassium iodide	30 grains.
Alcohol	1 dram.
Saccharin	5 grains.
Cinnamon water to make.	12 ounces.

M. S. A.

Dose: One to two tablespoonfuls three times a day after meals. This is a powerful alterative and tonic and very valuable in scrofulous and syphilitic affections.

48. Spring Blood Renovator.

Sulphate magnesia	8 ounces.
Hyposulphite soda	4 ounces.
Iodine resublimed	60 grains.
Simple syrup	10 ounces.
Alcohol, 188 per cent......	10 ounces.
Tincture capsicum	30 minims.
Oil sassafras	10 minims.
Oil wintergreen	5 minims.
Caramel	1 ounce.
Liquor potassa	1 dram.
Water q. s. to make.......	60 ounces.

49. Tonic for Nervous Debility.   B

Hypophosphite potash	1 ounce.
Water	4 ounces.
Fl. ext. coca leaves........	4 ounces.
Fl. ext. damiana	4 ounces.
Fl. ext. nux vomica.......	¼ ounce.
Acid hydrobromic dil......	4 ounces.
Simple elixir, red, q. s. to make	60 ounces.

Dose: One to two dessertspoonfuls three times a day before meals.

50. Mist. Acid Tonic.

Charing Cross Hospital.

Acidi nitrici diluti.........	7 minims.
Acidi hydrochlorici diluti..	8 minims.
Aquae chloroformi	2 drams.
Inf. gentianae ad..........	1 ounce.

M. Ft. haust.

51. Tonic Mixture Alkaline.   A

Ammonia carb	4 grains.
Soda bicarb	10 grains.
Infusion gentian co........	1 ounce.

For one dose.

52. Tonic Mixture Alkaline.   B

Cit. iron am..............	2 drams.
Soda bicarb	1 dram.
Spirits ammonia arom.....	3 drams.
Tinct. nux vomica	1½ dram.
Aqua chlorof. to make.....	6 ounces.

Dose: One tablespoonful three times a day after meals.

53. Calisaya Bark and Iron Cordial.

Sulphate quinine	90 grains.
Sulphate cinchonia	60 grains.
Citric acid	20 grains.
Simple elixir, red..........	½ gallon.
Sol. citrate iron...........	2½ ounces.

M. S. A.

54. Coca Leaves Cordial.

Proof spirits	44 ounces.
Simple syrup	64 ounces.
Fluid extract coca leaves..	8 ounces.
Tincture orange peel......	8 ounces.
Water	4 ounces.
Citric acid	½ ounce.

M. S. A.

55. Coca Wine.

Coca leaves ground........	1 pound.
Cologne spirits 188 per cent	32 ounces.
Water	32 ounces.
Oil orange	64 minims.
Oil lemon	16 minims.
Oil coriander	4 minims.
Oil anise	2 minims.
California muscatel wine..	4 gallons.
Sugar	2 pounds.

M. S. A.

56. Orange Wine. Artificial.

Water	9 gallons.
Granulated sugar	5 pounds.
Tartaric acid	8 ounces.
Oil of orange..............	2 ounces.
Alcohol	1 gallon.
Orange flower water......	1 pint.
Salicylic acid	20 grains.

Dissolve the oil of orange and salicylic acid in the alcohol. Dissolve the tartaric acid and sugar in the water, and mix with the alcohol. Color with caramel one ounce.

57. Cascara Cordial.

Cascara sagrada ground...	1 pound.
Senna leaves ground......	½ pound.
Licorice root ground......	½ pound.
Sal soda powdered........	⅛ pound.
Water	48 ounces.

Mix the drugs thoroughly, and macerate with the water for twelve hours, place in a percolator and percolate with a mixture of

| Alcohol .... | 32 ounces. |
| Water .... | 16 ounces. |

to the percolate obtained add

Oil cardamon	30 minims.
Oil anise	15 minims.
Oil orange	15 minims.
Oil angelica German......	15 minims.
Saccharin	30 grains.
Dissolved in alcohol.......	8 ounces.

Continue the percolation of the drugs with water until seven pints in all are obtained; in this dissolve granulated sugar 3 pounds, and strain.

58 Viburnum Compound.

Cramp. bark, powdered...	6 ounces.
Scull cap., powdered......	3 ounces.
Wild yam powdered.......	6 ounces.
Cloves, powdered	6 ounces.
Cinnamon, powdered	3 ounces.
Alcohol, 188 per cent......	90 ounces.
Water	24 ounces.
Syrup simple	9 ounces.

Percolate the drugs with the spirits and water, and add the syrup to the percolate.

59. Dioviburnum Mixture.

Cramp. bark, powdered...	4 ounces.
Helonias, powdered	4 ounces.
Blue cohosh, powdered	4 ounces.
Squaw vine, powdered....	4 ounces.
Oil anise	20 drops.
Oil wintergreen	16 drops.
Alcohol, 188 per cent......	10 ounces.
Water	50 ounces.
Caramel	1 ounce.
Angelica wine, sweet.....	16 ounces.

60. Quinine and Iron Mixture.

Quininae sulph...........	1½ drams.
*Acid. nitric. dil..........	2 drams.
Tr. ferri perchlor.........	2 ounces.
Glycerini	1 ounce.
Aq. chloroform ad........	20 ounces.

M.

Dose: A dessertspoonful in a wineglassful of water thrice daily.

This mixture keeps well, the nitric acid counteracting the reducing effect of glycerine and light upon the ferric salt.

61. Kola Coca Wine.

Kola nuts ground............	2 ounces.
Coca leaves ground..........	2 ounces.
Spirits, 188 per cent.........	6 ounces.
Water	4 ounces.

Muscatel, angelica, sherry, port or claret or a mixture of half port and half claret wines as may be preferred; q. s. to make 32 ounces.

Macerate the coca and kola with the spirits and water for seven days; percolate and run enough wine though the percolator to make 32 ounces.

Aromatics—such as cardamom, coriander and orange can be added if considered desirable.

62. Coca Wine.

Coca leaves ground.........	4 ounces.
Spirits, 188 per cent........	6 ounces.
Water	4 ounces.
Hydrobromic acid dil......	½ ounce.

Muscatel, angelica, sherry, port or claret or a mixture of one-third port to two-thirds of claret wine as may be preferred; q. s. to make 32 ounces.

The latter mixture is preferable if desired to replace Vin Mariani.

63. Pepsin Wine. A

Pepsin scales	256 grains.
Hydrochloric acid..........	60 minims.
Distilled water	2 ounces.
Glycerine	2 ounces.
Sweet muscatel wine	12 ounces.

Dissolve the pepsin in the water and acid, let it stand with occasional agitation for three days, add the wine and glycerine, strain, or filter if desired.

64. Pepsin Wine. B

Pepsin saccharated	256 grains.
Hydrochloric acid	60 minims.
Distilled water	2 ounces.
Simple elixir white........	2 ounces.
Sweet muscatel, sweet angelica or sherry wine....	12 ounces.

Dissolve the pepsin in the water and acid, let it stand with occasional agitation for three days, add the wine and filter, then add the simple elixir. An additional two ounces of wine may be substituted for the simple elixir if preferred.

65. Wine of Damiana.

Fl. ext. of damiana	2 ounces.
Simple elixir white	2 ounces.
Sherry, sweet angelica or sweet muscatel wine	12 ounces.

Mix.

66. Wine of Damiana Compound.

Hypophosphite of potash	640 grains.
Distilled water	2 ounces.
Fl. ext. of damiana	2 ounces.
Fl. ext. of nux vomica	30 minims.
Fl. ext. of coca leaves	½ ounce.
Acid hydrobromic dil	2 ounces.
Dry sherry wine	8 ounces.
Glycerine enough to make	16 ounces.

67. Wine of Beef.

Extract of beef	1 ounce troy.
Simple elixir white	2 ounces.
Sherry or port wine enough to measure	16 ounces.

68. Wine of Beef and Iron. A

Extract of beef	1 ounce troy.
Cit. iron am. or	
Phosphate iron, scales	64 grains.
Hot water	1 ounce.
Simple elixir white	2 ounces.
Detannated port or sherry wine enough to measure	16 ounces.

Port wine is preferable to sherry in this preparation.

Rub the extract of beef with the elixir, add the wine, dissolve the iron in the ounce of hot water, and mix; let stand for at least four weeks and filter.

This is an excellent preparation. A tablespoonful represents one ounce of fresh beef and two grains of iron.

69. Wine of Beef and Iron. B

Extract of beef	½ ounce troy
Cit. iron am. or	
Phosphate iron, scales	64 grains.
Hot water	1 ounce.
Simple elixir white	2 ounces.
Detannated port or sherry wine enough to measure	16 ounces.

Prepare in the same manner as formula A.

70. Celery Compound.

Celery seed ground	16 ounces.
Sulphate of cinchonidia	½ ounce.
Orange peel ground	8 ounces.
Coriander seed ground	8 ounces.
Citric acid	4 ounces.
Alcohol	4 gallons.
Water	12 gallons.
Syrup	2 gallons.

Macerate for seven days; percolate and filter. Color with caramel 14 ounces.

71. Bitter Wine of Iron. A

Soluble citrate iron and quinine	580 grains.
Tincture sweet orange peel	4 ounces.
Simple syrup	10 ounces.
Sherry wine detannated q. s. to make	2 pints.

Dose: One-half to one tablespoonful.

72. Bitter Wine of Iron. (Mitchell's.) B

Calisaya bark ground	192 grains.
Gentian root ground	128 grains.
Citrate iron soluble	192 grains.
Sherry wine	13 ounces.
Brandy	1 ounce.
Alcohol	1 ounce.
Oil orange	12 minims.
Sugar	2 ounces.
Solution tersulphate of iron	2 ounces.
Water of ammonia q. s.	

Dissolve the oil in the alcohol and mix with the sherry wine and brandy. Percolate with this the ground drugs, recover 15 fluid ounces of tincture by pouring on water. Dilute the iron solution with twice its bulk of water and add ammonia in slight excess. Wash and drain the precipitate thoroughly. Mix this with the tincture, and agitate occasionally until a filtered portion has a light yellow color and does not precipitate with tincture of the chloride of iron. Filter, dissolve the citrate of iron and sugar, and bring up the measure with a little water to 16 fluid ounces; a fluid ounce represents 12 grains of calisaya bark, 8 grains of gentian root, and 12 grains of citrate of iron. Dose, one to three fluid drams

73. Wine of Rhubarb.

Rhubarb powdered	3¼ ounces.
Calamus powdered	140 grains.
Sherry wine, stronger, q. s. to make	2 pints.

Moisten the mixed powders with three ounces of the wine. Place the mixture in a percolator and run through enough wine to make two pints.

Dose: One to four fluid drams.

74. Aromatic Wine.

Lavender oil	10 minims.
Origanum oil	10 minims.
Peppermint oil	10 minims.
Rosemary oil	10 minims.
White thyme oil	10 minims.
Wormwood oil	5 minims.
Alcohol	1 ounce.
Sherry wine	15 ounces.

Dissolve the oils in the alcohol and add the wine. This wine is used as a stimulating lotion for indolent ulcers.

TONICS.

From the Chemist and Druggist, to which the prescriptions were contributed in a competition instituted by that journal, the comments being by a medical practitioner.

GENERAL FERRUGINOUS.

75. For Anæmia.

Ferri et am. cit.	2 drams.
Tr. nuc. vom.	1½ drams.
Spt. am. co.	6 drams.
Syr. aurant	6 drams.
Aq. ad	6 ounces.
M.	

One-half ounce t. d. s. ex aq. p. c.

Pil. aloes et myrrh	5 grains.

Cap. j. h. s. s. om. alt. noct.

76. NERVINE TONICS.

Ferri et quininae citrat.	2 scruples.
Sp. chlorof.	1½ drams.
Acid. hydrobrom. dil.	2 drams.
Tinct. aurant	4 drams.
Syrup	4 drams.
Aq. ad	8 ounces.
M.	

One-eighth ter die sd.

77.

Ferri et quin. cit.	1 dram.
Acid. hydrobrom. dil.	3 drams.
Liquor. strychniae	1½ drams.
Aq. chloroform. ad	8 ounces.

One-half ounce ter in die sd.

78.

Ferri et quiniae cit.	1 dram.
Acid. hydrobrom. dil.	1½ drams.
Tinct. nucis vomic.	1 dram.
Aq. chloroformi	3 ounces.
Aq. ad	6 ounces.
M.	

One-half ounce in water twice or thrice daily.

79.

Fer. et quin. cit.	1 dram.
Tr. nucis vom.	½ dram.
Sp. chlorof.	3 drams.
Syr. aurantii	6 drams.
Aq. ad	6 ounces.
M.	

One-half ounce ter die pro dos.

80.

Ferri et quin. cit.	½ dram.
Sp. chlorof.	½ dram.
T. nucis vom.	½ dram.
Aq. ad	6 ounces.

M. Ft. mist.

One-sixth part 3 times a day, between meals.

81.

Tr. ferri perch.	1 dram.
Glycerin	3 drams.
Aquae ad	6 ounces.

M. Ft. mist.

Sig.: One ounce ter die sumend ex aq. post cibos.

82.

Ferri et quin. cit.	1 dram.
Ferri et ammon. cit.	2 drams.
Spirit. chlorof.	3 drams.
Infus. quass. ad	6 ounces.
M.	

Sig.: A tablespoonful twice or thrice a day.

Some experience is needed to tell when, or when not, iron is required as an integral portion of a tonic. When iron is indicated, the above mixtures would suit the case.

83.

Quin. disulph.	12 grains.
Acid. hydrobrom. dil	2 drams.
Tr. nuc. vom.	1 dram.
Inf. gent. co. ad.	6 ounces.

Sig.: One-half ounce t. d. s. ex cyath. vin. aq.

84.

Quininae hydrochlor.	16 grains.
Acid. hydrochlor. dil.	1½ drams.
Liq. strychninae	24 minims.
Spt. chloroformi	2 drams.
Aq. ad	8 ounces.

M. Ft. mist.

Capiat one-half ounce ter in die ex aqua.

These two mixtures are more suitable as tonics in cases of debility accompanied by neuralgic symptoms.

85. TONIC LAXATIVES.

Ferri sulph.	1½ drams.
Mag. sulph.	4 drams.
Acid. sulph. dil.	2 drams.
Spt. chlorof.	3 drams.
Inf. calumbae ad	8 ounces.

Coch. one mag. ex aq. ter in die sum. post cib.

86.

Pil. ferri (Blaud)	3 grains.
Ext. nuc. vom.	⅛ grain.
Aloes. soc.	¼ grain.

Ft. pil.

One after breakfast and dinner.

Excellent types of an aperient tonic, specially in cases of anaemia.

The first mixture is much used (with some slight modifications) in many large hospitals.

Sodii sulphat. is preferable to mag. sulph. It is quite as active and does not produce such griping as mag. sulph. is apt to do.

87.

Ext. aloes socot.	32 grains.
Boracis	32 grains.
Tinct. card. co.	1 dram.
Ext. glycyrrh. liq.	1 ounce.
Glycerini	1 ounce.
Aquae ad	4 ounces.

M.

Sig.: A teaspoonful three times a day in water after meals.

A little tinct. zingib. or tinct. capsici would improve this recipe.

88.

Sodae sulph.	6 drams.
Acid. nitrohydrochl. dil.	1 dram.
Sp. chloroformi	2 drams.
Sp. aetheris nitris	2 drams.
Syrupi	2 drams.
Infus. gent. co. ad	6 ounces.

M.

Sig.: 1 part ter in die.

89.

Ferri quin. cit.	2 scruples.
Mag. sulph.	1 dram.
Glycerin.	2 drams.
Aq. chlorof. ad	6 ounces.

One-half ounce t. d. s.

90.

Ferri et quiniae cit.	1 dram.
Magnes. sulph.	4 drams.
Syrupi	4 drams.
Aquae chloroform. ad	8 ounces.

M.

Capt. cochl. j. ampl. bis vel ter die.

I would prefer ext. cascara liq. to mag. sulph. in 89 and 90 also some corrigent.

"PICK-ME-UPS."

TYPICAL PRESCRIPTIONS.

91.

Spt. ammon. aromat.	½ dram.
Liq. ammon. acetatis. conc.	½ dram.
Tinct. lavand. co.	½ dram.
Inf. valerian. ad	1 ounce.

Liq. ammon. acetatis should be an ingredient of a "pick-me-up" if caused by drink.

92.

Spt. ammoniae aromat.	½ dram.
Tinct. lavand. co.	½ dram.
Spt. chloroformi	15 minims.
Aquae menth. pip. q. s. ad.	1 ounce.

93.

Tinct. calumb.	1 dram.
Syr. zingib.	1 dram.
Ext. cocae liq.	1 dram.
Magnes. fld. ad	2 ounces.

94.

Sodae bicarb.	15 grains.
Sp. am. co.	30 minims.
Tinct. nuc. vom.	10 minims.
Tinct. capsici.	10 minims.
Spirit. chlorof.	30 minims.
Tinct. card. co.	1 dram.
Aq. ad	1½ ounces.

95.

Sodii bicarb.	10 grains.
Spt. ammon. co.	1 dram.
Tr. nux vomica	10 minims.
Spt. eth. chlor.	15 minims.
Inf. gent. co. ad	1 ounce.

96.
 Spt. ammon. aromat...... 20 minims.
 Tinct. cardam. comp....... 1½ drams.
 Spt. chloroform........... 20 minims.
 Tinct. capsici............ 2 minims.
 Tinct. nux vomicae....... 4 minims.
 Syr. aurantii............. 3 drams.
 Aq. potas. effer. ad....... 1½ ounces.
 M.

97.
 Sp. ammon. co............ 6 drams.
 Tr. capsici............... 24 minims.
 Tr. humuli............... 2 drams.
 Spt. chloroformi.......... 1½ drams.
 Tinct. cinchon. co........ 6 drams.
 Aq. ad................... 6 ounces.
 Ft. mist.
Cap. One ounce p. r. n.

98.
 Sp. ammon. arom.......... ½ ounce.
 Tr. card. co.............. ½ ounce.
 Sp. chloroformi........... 1½ drams.
 Aquae ad................. 8 ounces.
 M. Ft. mist.
One-eighth when necessary.

99.
 Spt. ammon. co........... ½ dram.
 Tinct. card. co........... ½ dram.
 Tinct. cinch. co.......... ½ dram.
 Aq. destill. ad........... 1½ ounces.

100.
 Potas. bromid............ 20 grains.
 Sp. chloroform........... 20 minims.
 Tinct. gent. co........... 10 minims.
 Tinct. card. co........... 10 minims.
 Sp. am. arom............. 10 minims.
 Aq. m. pip. ad........... 2 ounces.
 M.

101.
 Tinct. cinchon. co........ 6 drams.
 Sodae bicarb............. 1½ drams.
 Spt. ammon. arom......... 4 drams.
 Tinct. gent. co........... 6 drams.
 Aq. ad................... 6 ounces.
 M. Ft. mist.
Sig.: One-sixth part every four hours.

102.
 Tr. card. co.............. 1 dram.
 Sodae bicarb............. 10 grains.
 Sp. chlorof............... 10 minims.
 Aq. ad................... 1 ounce.
 T. d. s. Mitte six ounces.

103.
 Euonymin .... ½ grain.
 Podophyllin. res.......... ¼ grain.
 Pil. coloc. et hyos........ 4 grains.
Hora somni sd. p. r. n. Mitte six.

104.   ACIDULOUS.
 Acid. nitric. dil.......... 1½ drams.
 Mist. gentian. co. P. L...: 4 ounces.
 Aq. chloroform. ad........ 8 ounces.
 Fiat mist.
 Sig.: One ounce pro dos.

105.
 Tr. nucis vomicae. 2 drams. 2 scruples.
 Acid. nitrohyd. dil. 2 drams. 2 scruples.
 Tr. gentianae co.......... 2 ounces.
 Syrup. simpl............. 2 ounces.
 Aq. ad................... 8 ounces.
 M. Ft. mist.
 Sig.: One-half ounce ter die sd. ex aq. one-half ounce.

Two excellent examples of an acid tonic.

106.   ALKALINE.
 Ammon. carb............. 4 grains.
 Sodae bicarb............. 10 grains.
 Inf. gent. co............. 1 ounce.
 Sig.: One ounce t. d. in ea. fl. oz.

107.
 Ferri ammon. cit.......... 2 drams.
 Sodae bicarb............. 1 dram.
 Spt. ammon. arom......... 3 drams.
 Tinct. nucis vom.......... 1½ drams.
 Aq. chlorof. ad........... 6 ounces.
One-half ounce t. d. s. ex aquae post cibos.

108.
 Tinct. gentian. co........ 6 drams.
 Tinct. zingib............. 6 drams.
 Spt. am. arom............ 6 drams.
 Tinct. rhei............... 6 drams.
 M.
 Sig.: One dram ex aqua ante cibum p. r. n.
Good types of an alkaline tonic.

GENERAL FERRUGINOUS.

109.   For Anæmia.

Ferri et ammon. cit.	½ dram.
Tinct. nux vom.	½ dram.
Glycerole pepsin (Armour's).	2 drams.
Aqua chlorof. ad.	6 ounces.

Capt. One ounce ter die post cib.

110.

Ferri et ammon. cit.	1 dram.
Tr. nucis vom.	1 dram.
Sp. ammon. aromat.	3 drams.
Sp. chlorof.	2 drams.
Infus. quassiae ad.	6 ounces.

Capt. One-half ounce ter die.

111.

Ferri et ammon. cit.	40 grains.
Sp. am. arom.	3 drams.
Glycerin	6 drams.
Sp. chlorof.	1½ drams.
Inf. quassiae ad.	8 ounces.

M.
One-eighth ter die sd. post cib.

LIVER DISORDERS.

This group of mixtures is very suitable for cases of sluggish or torpid action of the liver caused by deficient exercise, sedentary occupation, or over-eating.

112.

Liq. tarax.	½ ounce.
Inf. gent. co. conc.	½ ounce.
Tinct. nucis vom.	1 dram.
Tinct. capsici.	½ dram.
Ext. cascarae sag. liq. Formula No. 57.	2 drams.
Sp. chloroformi.	2 drams.
Aquae ad.	8 ounces.

Ft. mist.
Sig.: One ounce, bis die, vel p. r. n.
Has been used with great success in chronic constipation, and as a general "pick-me-up." This is a very good type of a liver-mixture.

113.

Acid. nitro-hyd. dil.	1½ drams.
Tr. podophylli.	80 minims.
Succ. taraxaci.	1 ounce.
Tinct. nucis vom.	80 minims.
Syr. zingiberis.	1 ounce.
Aq. chlorof. ad.	8 ounces.

M. Ft. mist.
One-eighth pt. 3 times a day.
For sluggish liver with coated tongue, etc.

114.

Acid. nitro-hydroch. dil.	1½ drams.
Tr. nuc. vom.	3 drams.
Sp. chlorof.	1½ drams.
Succ. taraxaci.	6 drams.
Tr. aurant.	6 drams.
Aq. ad.	6 ounces.

M. Ft. mist.
Sig.: One-half ounce ter die ex aq. one ounce.
Aq. aurant. would do.

115.

Acid. nit. hydroch. d.	2 drams.
Succ. tarax.	½ ounce.
Tr. nuc. vom.	2 drams.
Sp. aeth. nit.	2 drams.
Tr. sennae.	1 ounce.
Inf. gent. co. ad.	8 ounces.

M. Ft. mist.
One-eighth part three times a day.

116.

Acid. nit. mur. dil.	2 drams.
Liq. strych.	1 dram.
Succ. tarax.	6 drams.
Aqua. ad.	6 ounces.

One-half ounce ter die.

117.

Ac. nit. mur. dil.	2 drams.
Tinct. nuc. vom.	1 dram.
Tinct. gent. co.	3 drams.
Syr. aurantii	1 dram.
Aquae ad	6 ounces.

Ft. mist.
Cap. cochl. mag. ter in die. a. c.

118.

Potas. nitrat.	1 dram.
Ol. cajuputi	12 minims.
Sp. chlorof.	1½ drams.
Suc. taraxaci	4 drams.
Dec. aloes co.	1½ ounces.
Inf. gent. co. ad.	8 ounces.

M.
One-eighth part ter die sd.

119.

Acid. hydroch. dil.	10 minims.
Tr. nucis. vom.	10 minims.
Sp. chlorof.	10 minims.
Aq. ad	1 ounce.

T. d. s. Mitte 8 ounces.

120.
    Euonymin .... ½ grain.
    Pil. hydrarg. .... 1 grain.
    Pil. coloc. co. .... 2 grains.
    Ext. hyoscy. .... ¼ grain.
    M. Ft. pil. Mitte 12
2 h. s. s. p. r. n.

121.
    Acidi nitro-hydrochlor. dil. 1½ drams.
    Tincturae gentianae co..... 1 ounce.
    Tincturae cardamomi co... 2 drams.
    Tincturae aurantii .... 2 drams.
    Syrupus zingiberis .... 6 drams.
    Aquae chloroformi ad ..... 6 ounces.
    Misce. Fiat mistura.
Sig.: One tablespoonful three times a day.

122.
    Pil. hydrargyri .... 9 grains.
    Pil. rhei co................. 21 grains.
    Gingerin .... 1 grain.
    Misce. Fiat pil. 6.
Sig.: Two to be taken at bedtime occasionally, followed next morning by a dose of Franz Josef or Rubinat water.

123.
    Acid. nitro mur. dil....... 2 drams.
    Tr. nucis vom. .... 2 drams.
    Inf. gent. co. ad .... 6 ounces.
Sig.: One-half ounce ter die sd.

124.
    Acid. nit. hyd. dil.......... 80 minims.
    Sp. chlorof..... .... 80 minims.
    Inf. gent. co. ad .... 6 drams.
    M.
One-eighth ter die.
As a tonic mixture or for liver complaints; well diluted with water a grateful drink for thirst or feverish symptoms.

125.
    Acid. nitro mur. dil........ 2 drams.
    Infus. gentian. ad .... 6 ounces.
    M.
Sig.: A tablespoonful in a glass of water after dinner.

126.
    Ext. cascar. sag. liq. insip... 1 dram.
    Acid. nitric dil............. 1 dram.
    Tr. capsici. .... 15 minims.
    Tr. chlorof. co. .... 2 drams.
    Aquae ad .... 6 ounces.
Cap. one-sixth ter die ante cib.

CONGESTION OF LIVER.

In congestion of the liver, caused by drink or error of diet, alkalies are generally found to act better than acids, thus:

127. TYPICAL PRESCRIPTION.
    Potass. bicarb. .... 1 dram.
    Sodae bicarb. .... 1 dram.
    Spt. chlorf. .... 1 dram.
    Tinct. nuc. vom. .... 1 dram.
    Tinct. zingib. .... ½ dram.
    Succ. tarax. .... ½ ounce.
    Aquae ad .... 8 ounces.
One ounce at 11 a. m. and 5:30 p. m.

Chloride of ammonium in full doses is much used in the Tropics for congestion of the liver. It is equally valuable here.

128.
    Tr. podoph. ammon. .... 2 drams.
    Potas. bicarb. .... 2 drams.
    Tr. nuc. vomicae .... 30 minims.
    Aqua chlorof. ad .... 7 ounces.
One-half ounce t. d. s.

129.
    Sodae bicarb. .... 2 drams.
    Tinct. nuc. vom. .... 1 dram.
    Infus. gent. co. ad......... 6 ounces.
One tablespoonful to be taken half-an-hour before dinner and supper.

130.
    Resin. podoph. .... 2 grains.
    Spt. ammon. arom.......... 2 drams.
    Succ. tarax. .... 1 ounce.
    Dec. aloes co. ad .... 8 ounces.
    M. Ft. mist.
One ounce bis die.

131. LAXATIVE AND LIVER MIXTURE.
    Extr. cascarae sagrad. liq... 30 minims.
    Glycerini pur. .... 30 minims.
    Extracti byni liq.......... 1 dram.
    M. Ft. mistura.
Two drams ex aquae cyatho vinoso nocte maneque pro re nata sumenda.

FOR BILIOUSNESS, SICKNESS, CONSTIPATION, GIDDINESS, &c.
132.
    Magnes. sulph. .... 6 drams.
    Inf. gent. co. conc.......... 1 ounce.
    Aq. chlorof. ad............. 8 ounces.
    M.
One-eighth ter die at 11, 3 and 7.

133.

Sol. mag. sulph. (1 in 2)	2 ounces.
Mag. carb. pond.	1 dram.
Sodae bicarb.	80 grains.
Tr. zingib.	1 dram.
Aq. menth. pip. ad	8 ounces.

Sig.: One ounce bis die.

134.

Ext. nucis vom.	¼ grain.
Ext. aloes soc. pulv.	1 grain.
Ext. gentianae	2 grains.

M. Ft. pil. sec. art.

Sum. one once or twice a day, one hour before meals, as required.

135.

| Mist. sennae co., B. P. | 2 ounces. |
| Aq. menth. pip. ad | 8 ounces. |

Ft. mist.

One-eighth part ter die sumend.

136.

Pil. hydrarg.	3 grains.
Ext. coloc. co.	8 grains.
Ext. hyoscy.	2 grains.

Ft. Pil. 3—i. h. s. s.

137.

Ac. nit. hyd. dil.	1½ drams.
Tr. nuc. vom.	1 dram.
Aq. chlorof.	2 ounces.
Liq. tarax.	6 drams.
Inf. gent. co. ad	6 ounces.

M. Ft. mist.

One-sixth ter die.

138.

Ammon. carb.	1 dram.
Soda carb.	2 drams.
Mag. carb.	1 dram.
Tr. cardam. co.	½ ounce.
Tr. calumbae	½ ounce.
Sacch. alb.	3 drams.
Ol. menth. pip.	8 drops.
Aquae adde.	8 ounces.

M. Ft. mist.

One-half ounce ter in die ex aqua.

More suited for acidity and gastralgia.

139. LIVER TONICS.

Acid. hydrochlor. dil.	5 minims.
Liq. strychniae	5 minims.
Sp. chlorof.	5 minims.
Glycer. acid. pepsin.	30 minims.
Ess. malti	2 drams.
Aq. ad	½ ounce.

In a wine glass of water 3 times daily before food.

140.

| Pil. rhei co. | 2 grains. |
| Pil. hydrarg. | 2 grains. |

Ft. pil.

One omni nocte si opus sit.

141.

Podophylli resin	6 grains.
Ext. nucis vom.	6 grains.
Pil. colo. et hyoscyami	108 grains.

Ft. mass et divide in pilulae 24.

Sig.: One every second or third night.

142.

Mag. sulph.	3 drams.
Quininae sulph.	12 grains.
Acid. nit. mur. dil.	1½ drams.
Spt. chlorof.	1½ drams.
Tr. lavand. co.	1½ drams.
Aquae ad	8 ounces.

M. Ft. mist.

One ounce. 4tis. horis.

143.

Ferri cit. c. quininae	1 dram.
Sp. chlorof.	1½ drams.
Tr. aurant.	3 drams.
Aq. ad.	6 ounces.

Ft. mist.

One-half ounce in one-half ounce aq. ter die sumend.

144.

Sol. quininae sulph. (12 grs. to 1 ounce.)	1 ounce.
Tr. nucis vom.	1 dram.
Sp. chlorof.	1 dram.
Aq. ad.	6 ounces.

Sig.: One-half ounce bis terve die.

The last three are more general tonics than liver medicines.

145.

Ac. nit. mur. dil.	20 minims.
Succ. taraxaci	1 dram.
Syrup. aurant.	2 drams.
Inf. gent. ad	1½ ounces.

M. Ft.
Haust. sum. ante cibos.

DYSPEPSIA.

ALKALINE MIXTURES FOR DYSPEPSIA.

Alkaline mixtures are best in cases of atonic dyspepsia and ill-health. Alkalies increase the flow of acid in the stomach, and should be taken after meals. They are often of special service in the dyspepsia of young people, who complain of lassitude, backache, and headache.

146.

Potass. bicarb.	1 dram.
Tinct. gent. co.	2 drams.
Tinct. lupuli	2 drams.
Tinct. calumbae	2 drams.
Liq. taraxaci	2 drams.
Aq. distill. ad	6 ounces.

Misce et filtra.
Cap. one-half ounce ter die ex aqua.

Pil. rhei comp.	5 grains.

Cap. i. h. s. s. p. r. n.

147.

Sodii bicarb.	2 drams.
Sp. ammon. ar.	4 drams.
Tinct. capsic.	12 minims.
Inf. aurant. co.	3 ounces.
Aq. menth. pip. ad	6 ounces.

One-twelfth part in water three times a day after food.

148.

Pot. bicarb.	2 drams.
Spt. ammon. aromat.	1 dram.
Tinct. card. co.	2 drams.
Spt. chloroform.	1½ drams.
Tinct. zingiberis	2 drams.
Syrupi	½ ounce.
Aquae ad	6 ounces.

A sixth part to be taken soon after breakfast, dinner, and tea.

149.

Sod. bicarb.	1 dram.
Sp. amm. co.	1½ drams.
Tr. nuc. vom.	1 dram.
Inf. gent. co. con. 1-7	6 drams.
Aq. chlorof. ad	6 ounces.

One-half ounce ter die ante cib.
If with constipation, add—

Ex. cascar. liq.	2 drams.

150.

Potass. citrat.	2 drams.
Sodii bicarb.	1 dram.
Sp. ammon. arom.	2 drams.
Tr. calumbae	2 drams.
Aq. chloroformi	3 ounces.
Aquae ad	6 ounces.

M.
Capt. part. sext. ter in die ante cibos.

151.

Sod. bic.	1 dram.
Pot. bic.	1 dram.
Spt. am. ar.	3 ounces.
Aeth. chlor.	2 ounces.
Aq. ad	8 ounces.

One-sixth part. c. one-half ounce succ. limon. prep. in stat. efferv.

152.

Potass. bicarb.	1½ drams.
Tinct. card. co.	3 drams.
Spt. am. arom.	3 drams.
Inf. gent. ad	6 ounces.

M.
One-sixth ter die sumend.

153.

Potass. bromide	4 scruples.
Potass. bicarb.	4 scruples.
Sp. ammon. co.	1½ drams.
Sp. chloroformi	1 dram.
Inf. gentianae co. ad	8 ounces.

M. Fiat mistura.
Cap. coch. 2, amplum. ter in die inter cibos.

154.

Sod. bicarb.	1½ drams.
Pot. brom.	80 grains.
Sp. am. co.	2 drams.
Tr. card. co.	2 drams.
Spt. chlorof.	1½ drams.
Inf. calumb. ad	8 ounces.

M. Ft. m.
One ounce t. d. s.

BISMUTHIC.

Here are several formulae containing a soluble bismuth salt. Most of these mixtures will do good in cases of dyspepsia accompanied by pain, flatulence, and fullness after eating.

155.

Mist. bismuthi co. (Seller's)	4 drams.
Ext. cascarae sag. liq. (miscible)	2 drams.
Glycerol. pepsin	2 drams.
Glyc. acid. carbol.	12 minims.
Syr. hypophos. co.	1 ounce.
Aq. caryoph. ad	8 ounces.
M. Ft. mist.	

One-eighth part 3 times a day after food.

156.

Sodii bicarb.	1½ drams.
Liq. bismuthi	6 drams.
Spt. ammon. ar.	3 drams.
Acid. hydrocyan. dil.	12 minims.
Syr. zingib.	6 drams.
Inf. gent. co. ad	6 ounces.
M.	

Capt. one-half ounce ter hora ex aqua.

157.

Sodii bicarb.	2 drams.
Liq. bismuthi	6 drams.
Sp. ammon. ar.	3 drams.
Ac. hydrocy. dil.	1 dram.
Inf. gent. co. ad	8 ounces.
M.	

One-half ounce ter die p. c.

158.

Sodae bicarb.	2 drams.
Liq. bismuthi	1 ounce.
Sp. am. co.	2 drams.
Liq. tarax.	1 ounce.
Ex. chlorof.	1½ drams.
Inf. calumbae ad	8 ounces.
M. Ft. mist.	

One-half ounce ter die.

159.

Potass. bicarb.	2 drams.
Mist. bism. coct.	2 drams.
Pepsin (Seller's)	6 ounces.
Aquae chlorofor.	6 ounces.

Capt. one ounce ter die post cibos.

160.

Liq. bismuthi et ammon. citr.	1 ounce.
Sodii bicarb.	2 drams.
Tinct. capsici	1 dram.
Spt. chloroformi	1½ drams.
Infus. calumbae	2 ounces.
Aquae menth. pip. ad	6 ounces.
M. Ft. mist.	

One-half ounce ex one-half ounce aquae ter in die post cibos sumend.

161.

Sodae bicarb.	1 dram.
Liq. bismuthi	1 ounce.
Spt. chlorof.	2 drams.
Spt. ammon. ar.	3 drams.
Ess. zingib.	½ dram.
Aq. calcis ad	4 ounces.

Sig.: One-half ounce thrice daily after food.

162.

Pot. bicarb.	2 drams.
Liq. bismuthi	4 drams.
Tr. capsici	1 dram.
Tr. gent. co.	3 drams.
Spt. chlorof.	1½ drams.
Inf. chirettae ad	6 ounces.
Ft. mist.	

One-half ounce quater in die sumend. post cibos ex aqua.

163.

Liq. bismuthi	2 ounces.
Sodae carb.	3 drams.
Tr. hyosc.	4 drams.
Spt. chlorof.	3 drams.
Acid. hydrocyan. dil.	1 dram.
Inf. calumb. conc.	6 drams.
Aquae ad	8 ounces.
M. Ft. mist.	

Cap. ounce ex aqua ter die post cibos.

164.

Liq. bism. et am. cit.	6 drams.
Sodii bicarb.	80 grains.
Acid. hydrocyan. dil.	24 minims.
Liq. strychniae	40 minims.
Tr. card. co.	2 drams.
Aq. menth. pip. ad	8 ounces.

Cap. one ounce t. d. s.

165.

Potass. bicarb.	15 grains.
Liq. bismuthi	20 minims.
Sp. amm. co.	20 minims.
Sp. chlorof.	10 minims.
Aq. menth. pip. ad	1 ounce.

Misce. Mitte 8 ounces or q. s.
To be taken after meals when required.

166.

Spirit. ammon. arom.	5 drams.
Liq. bismuthi	5 drams.
Spirit. chloroformi	2 drams.
Infus. gentian. ad	4 ounces.

M.

Sig.: A teaspoonful in a wineglassful of water quarter of an hour before meals. Shake the bottle.

167.

Sp. ammon. ar.	5 drams.
Sp. chlorof.	4 drams.
Liq. bismuthi	5 drams.
Infus. gentian. ad	4 ounces.

M.

Sig.: A teaspoonful thrice daily in water before meals.

168.

Soda bicarb.	2 drams.
Liq. bismuth	1 ounce.
Syrup. aurant.	4 drams.
Inf. gent. co. conc.	1 ounce.
Aq. chlorof. ad	8 ounces.

Ft. mist.

One ounce ter die post cibos.

The following mixtures contain an insoluble salt of bismuth, and equally are suitable in cases of dyspepsia accompanied by pain, flatulence, discomfort after eating, etc.

169.

Sodii sulphocarb.	2 drams.
Bismuth. subnit.	2 drams.
P. tragac. co.	1 scruple.
Tr. nucis vom.	2 drams.
Spt. am. arom.	2 drams.
Aq. menth. pip. ad	6 ounces.

M. Ft. mist.

One-half ounce ter in die post cibos.

170.

Bism. subnit.	10 grains.
Sodae bicarb.	10 grains.
Mucil. trag.	q. s.
Aq. chlorof.	10 minims.
Tr. nucis vom.	5 minims.
Aq. ad	1 ounce.

T. d. s. post cib. mitte 8 ounces.

Ext. cascar. sag. liq.	1 ounce.
Ext. glycyrrh. liq.	1 ounce.

M.

One dram primo mane c. aqua pro renata.

171.

Bismuth. carb.	2 drams.
Sodii bicarb.	2 drams.
Pulv. tragac. ver.	20 grains.
Tinct. zingiberis	6 drams.
Tinct. cascarillae	1 ounce.
Aq. menth. pip. ad	8 ounces.

M. Ft. mist.

Signa.: An eighth part to be taken in a little water shortly after meals 2 or 3 times a day.

172.

Bismuthi carb.	4 grains.
Sodii bic. (Howd's)	60 grains.
Am. carb.	2 grains.
Aeth. chlor.	10 minims.
Ess. zingib.	10 minims.
P. tragac.	1 grain.
Tr. calumbae	30 minims.
Inf. gent. conc.	1 dram.
Aq. menth. pip. ad	1 ounce.

M. Ft. mist.

Pro dosis.

173.

Bismuth. carb.	2 drams.
Sodae bicarb.	3 drams.
Ammon. carb.	1 dram.
Pulv. tragac. co.	3 drams.
Tr. zingib. fort.	2 drams.
Tinct. rhei	1 ounce.
Sp. chloroformi	2 drams.
Infus. gent. co. ad	6 ounces.

Sig.: One-half ounce ter die ad. post cibos.

174.

Bismuth. carb.	1 dram.
P. tragac. comp.	½ dram.
Spt. myristicae	3 drams.
Acid. hydrocyan. dil	½ dram.
Inf. gentianae co. ad	6 ounces.

M. Ft. mist.

Capiat one-half ounce ter in die.

175.

    Bismuth. carbon. .... 1 dram.
    Sodii bicarbonatis .... 2 drams.
    Pulv. acaciae .... 1 dram.
    Mag. carb. pond. .... 2 drams.
    Tinct. limonis .... ½ ounce.
    Acid. hydrocyanic. dil..... 6 minims.
    Aqua ad .... 6 ounces.
One-half ounce ex aq. ter in die sumend.

176.

    Bism. carb. .... 3 drams.
    Sod. bicarb. .... 3 drams.
    Muc. trag. .... 1 ounce.
    Tr. lupuli .... 6 drams.
    Aq. ad. .... 6 drams.
    M.
One-half ounce ter die ante cibos.

177.

    Bismuth. carb. .... 1 dram.
    Sodii bicarb. .... 1 dram.
    Spt. chloroform. .... 1 dram.
    Syrup. aurantii .... 1 ounce.
    Aqua ad .... 6 ounces.
    Ft. mist.
Cap. one-half ounce ter in die post cib.

178.

    Bismuth. carb. .... 1 dram.
    Sod. bicarb. .... 1 dram.
    Pulv. acacia .... 1 dram.
    Sp. chlorof. .... 1½ drams.
    Inf. gent. .... 4 ounces.
    Aq. ad. .... 8 ounces.
    M. Ft. mist.
Cap. one ounce ter in die.

179.

    Sod. bicarb. .... 80 grains.
    Inf. gent. co. conc. ...... 1 ounce.
    Aq. menth. pip. ad. .... 8 ounces.
    M.
One-eighth ter die at 11, 3, and 7.

180.

    Sodii bicarb. .... 1 dram.
    Tr. gent. co. .... 4 drams.
    Spt. chloroformi .... 2 drams.
    Aquae ad .... 6 ounces.
Signe.: One-half ounce ter die post cib. hor. j.

181.

    Sp. ammon. ar. .... 15 minims.
    Tinct. chloroformi co. .... 15 minims.
    Tinct. gentianae co. ...... 15 minims.
    Tinct. nucis vom. .... 10 minims.
    Syrupi zingiberis. .... 1 dram.
    Aquae ad .... 1 ounce.
    M. Ft. haust.
Ter die sum. ante cibos.

182.

    Tr. zingib. .... 4 drams.
    Sod. bicarb. .... 4 drams.
    Tr. nuc. vom. .... 40 minims.
    Syrupi .... ½ ounce.
    Aq. menth. pip. ad. .... 12 ounces.
One ounce bis vel ter die post cibos.

183.

    Stomachic and Mild Aperient.

    Magnes. sulph. .... ½ ounce.
    Pulv. rhei. .... 2 drams.
    Magnes. carb. .... 4 drams.
    Aether chlor. .... 1 dram.
    Spt. ammon. co. .... ½ ounce.
    Tr. rhei co. .... 1 ounce.
    Tr. zingib. .... 2 drams.
    Aquae menth. pip. ad. ..... 8 ounces.
    M. Ft.
Capt. one-half ounce ex aqua ter die.

184.

    Magnes. sulph. .... 1½ drams.
    Potash bicarb. .... 1½ drams.
    Tinct. capsici. .... 14 minims.
    Tinct. nucis vom. .... 1 dram.
    Spt. chlorof. .... 1 dram.
    Infus. gent. co. ad. ...... 6 ounces.
One-sixth part. ter die ante cibos.

185.

    Magnes. sulph. .... 4 drams.
    Magnes. carb. .... 1 dram.
    Sodae carb. .... 1½ drams.
    Tinct. chlorof. co. .... 1½ drams.
    Aq. menth. pip. .... 2 ounces.
    Aquae ad. .... 8 ounces.
    M.
One-eighth part ter die 11, 4, and bedtime.

186.

    Mag carb. p. .... 1 dram.
    Mag. sulph. .... 1 ounce.
    Amm. Carb. .... 1 dram.
    Tr. nucis. vom. .... 1 dram.
    Aq. chloroformi ad. .... 8 ounces.
One-half ounce quartis horis.

187.

Sodii bicarb.	1 dram.
Magnes. sulph.	½ ounce.
Tr. nuc. vom.	½ dram.
Inf. gent. co. conc.	2 drams.
Syrup	2 drams.
Aq. chlorf.	3 ounces.
Aquae ad.	6 ounces.

M. Ft. mist.
One-half ounce ter die ante cib.

Mag. sulph. I regard as the least desirable of aperients, unless given for its immediate effects in the form of a draught.

188.

Bismuth. carb.	1 ounce. 2 scruples.
Sodae bicarb.	1 dram. 2 scruples.
Tr. chlor. et morph.	1 dram.
Pulv. rhei.	32 grains.
Pulv. zingib. opt.	32 grains.
Aq. ad.	8 ounces.

F. mist.
Sumat one ounce ter die 1 hora post cibum.

189.

Sodii bicarb.	1 dram.
Pepsin porci.	½ dram.
Spt. ammon. co.	1½ drams.
Liq. bismuthi.	2 drams.
Chlorodyni	24 minims.
Inf. gent. co. ad.	6 ounces.

M. Ft. mist.
Cap. one-half ounce ter die ante cibum.

190.

Pepsin. solubis.	½ dram.
Liq. bismuthi.	4 drams.
Ext. opii liq.	24 minims.
Acid. hydrocy. dil.	12 minims.
Tr. card. co.	1½ drams.
Sp. chlorof.	1 dram.
Aq. ad.	8 ounces.

M Ft. mist.
Sig.: One-half ounce post cibos semihora.

191.

Bismuth. carb.	80 grains.
Magn. carb.	80 grains.
P. tragac. co.	1 dram.
Sp. aetheris.	2 drams.
Tr. nucis vom.	1 dram.
Liq. morph. hyd.	24 minims.
Aquae ad.	8 ounces.

M.
One ounce ter die ante cibos.

192.

Liq. bismuth.	4 drams.
Vin. pepsin.	1 ounce.
Tr. zingib. fort.	80 minims.
Tr. card. co.	4 drams.
Chlorodyni	40 minims.
Aq. menth. pip. ad.	8 ounces.

M. Ft. mist. et. sig.
One ounce ter in die post. cib.

193.

Bism. carb.	2 scruples.
Mag. carb.	1 dram.
P. trag. co.	2 scruples.
Vin. opii.	1 dram.
Aq. chlorof.	4 ounces.
Aq. menth. pip. ad.	8 ounces.

Cap. one ounce ter in die post cibos.

194.

Potass. bicarb.	10 grains.
Liq. bism. et ammon. cit.	½ dram.
Spt. ammon. arom.	15 minims.
Tinct. chlorof. et. morphi.	8 minims.
Inf. gentian. ad.	1 ounce.

M.
Three times a day before meals.

195.

Potass. bicarb.	160 grains.
Liq. bismuthi.	1 ounce.
Pepsin. liquid. (Schacht.).	1 ounce.
Nepenthe	80 minims.
Inf. gentian. co. ad.	8 ounces.

Sig.: One-half ounce ex aq. ter in die p. c.

196.

Sodae bicarb.	8 drams.
Liq. bism. am. cit.	1 ounce.
Chlorodyni	2½ drams.
Tinct. nucis vom.	1½ drams.
Tinct. rhei.	1½ ounces.
Aq. menth. pip. ad.	8 ounces.

M.
One-half ounce ter die sd. post cibos.

197.

Pil. coloc. c. hyoscy.	6 grains.
Pil. hydrarg.	3 grains.

In pil. 2 h. s. s.
Some of these formulae contain opium, and would be indicated in cases where the bowels are relaxed or where there is marked colicky pain.

ACID MIXTURES FOR DYSPEPSIA.

The following is a good formula (ex "Medical Reprints").

198.

Acid. nitro-mur dil.......	3 drams.
Tinct. calumb.............	6 drams.
Pulv. rhei.................	1½ drams.
Lactopeptin	3 drams.
Spt. chlorof...............	3 drams.
Aquae	8 ounces.

One ounce t. d. s. before food.

Acid mixtures are often more lasting in their action in cases of dyspepsia provided they agree. Mineral acids diminish the formation of vegetable acids in the stomach, and are, therefore, indicated in cases of acidity, gouty dyspepsia, and the dyspeptic weakness of old people whose gastric juice is feeble in digesting-power and lacking in hydrochloric acid.

199.

Ex. rham. pursh...........	1 ounce.
Ac. nit. hydro. dil........	5 drams.
Syr. zingib................	1 ounce.
Inf. gent. ad..............	8 ounces.

M.
Sig.: Two drams in aq. p. c.

200.

Pepsin. porci..............	36 grains.
Glycerini	4 drams.
Tr. nucis vom.............	1 dram.
Acid. hydroch. dil.........	2 drams.
Tr. capsici................	12 minims.
Inf. sennae co. conc. 1-7...	2 drams.
Tr. card. co...............	3 drams.
Inf. gent. co. ad...........	6 ounces.

M. Ft. mist.
Sig.: One-half ounce ex aq. 5 minutes a. c.

201.

Aq. nit. hyd. dil...........	2 drams.
Tr. nuc. vom..............	1 dram.
Tr. capsic.................	48 minims.
Syr. aurant................	1 ounce.
Aq. m. p. ad..............	8 ounces.

One-half ounce t. d. s. p. c. ex aq.

202.

Acidi nitromur. dil........	2 drams.
Spt. chloroformi...........	2 drams.
Inf. gent. co. ad...........	6 ounces.

M.
Sig.: One-half ounce ter in die semihorae ante cibos ex aquae.

203.

Acid. hydroch. dil.........	2 drams.
Tinct. capsici.............	1 dram.
Pepsin fluid...............	1 ounce.
Succi tarax................	1 ounce.
Inf. gent. co. ad...........	6 ounces.

M.
Sig.: One-half ounce ter die after food.

204.

Pepsin (B. P.).............	1½ scruples.
Acid. nitro-hydrochlor. dil.	1½ drams.
Tr. nucis. vom.............	1 dram.
Infus. gent. co. ad.........	6 ounces.

Ft. mist.
One ounce ter in dies ante cibos.

205.

Ac. nit. mur. dil...........	2 drams.
Liq. strychninae...........	48 minims.
Tr. card. co...............	4 drams.
Glyc. pepsin (Armour).....	3 drams.
Glycer	6 drams.
Aquae ad..................	8 ounces.

M.
One-half ounce t. d. s. p. c. ex. aq.

206.

Res. podoph...............	8 grains.
Glycerol. pepsini (Armour).	3 drams.
Ac. nit. mur. dil...........	2½ drams.
Tinct. zingib..............	½ ounce.
Aq. cinnam. ad............	8 ounces.

M. Ft. mist.
Sig.: One-half ounce ter in die.

207.

Acidi nitro-hydrochlorici diluti	2 drams.
Aetheris chlorici...........	2 drams.
Glycerini acidi pepsini.....	½ ounce.
Inf. gentianae co. ad.......	8 ounces.

M.
Sig.: A tablespoonful in half a wineglassful of water three times a day, half an hour before meals.

208.

Acidi hydrochlorici diluti..	10 minims.
Tincturae aurantii.........	15 minims.
Pepsin	5 grains.
Ext. Byni fluid............	1 dram.
Aquae q. s. ad.............	1 ounce.

M. Fiat mistura.
Cap. one ounce ter in die post cibos cum carbonis una tabella 5 grains post prandium.

209.

Pepsin solubilis equal to 48 grains, B. P.	
Acid. mur. dil.	2 drams.
Liq. strychniae	1 dram.
Quin. sulph.	6 grains.
Infus. quass. conc.	6 drams.
Aq. chlorof. ad.	6 ounces.

Sig.: One-half ounce ex aq. t. d. s. p. c.
(Note: Ess. m. pip. or chlorodyne can be added q. s. if required.)

210.

Quininae hydrochlor.	16 grains.
Acid. hyd. chlor. dil.	3 drams.
Glycerin. pepsin.	2 ounces.
Tr. nux vom.	3 drams.
Tr. strophanthi.	1 dram.
Aquae ad.	8 ounces.

M. Ft.
Cap. one-half ounce ex aqua ter die post cibum.

211.

Acid. nit. hydrochl. dil.	1½ drams.
Vin. pepsin.	1 ounce.
Succ. tarax.	4 drams.
Inf. quassiae conc.	1 ounce.
Aq. chlorof. ad.	8 ounces.

Ft. mist.
One ounce ter die inter cibos.
Pil. aloin co. no. six.
Two altera omnis nocte.

212.

Liq. pancreat. (Benger's)	2 ounces.
Sodae bicarb. (Howard's).	½ ounce.
Aq. bullientis ad.	8 ounces.

Sig.: One-half ounce after every meal.
A very excellent combination in cases of the deficient power of digesting fats.

213.

Pepsin. porci.	36 grains.
Ext. nuc. vomic.	3 grains.

M. Ft. pil. 12.
One pill every day with dinner.
For feeble action of the gastric juices this pill would be good.
For Fullness after Eating, Bad Taste in the Mouth, Sickness, and General Symptoms of Deranged Stomach, with Acidity, want of Appetite, etc.
To my way of thinking, the old-fashioned dec. aloes co. conc. still holds the field in cases of troublesome dyspepsia.

214. Typical Prescription.

Dec. aloes co. conc. (sine croco)	2 ounces.
Tinct. capsici	1½ drams.
Sodae biborat.	½ dram.
Ext. glycyrrh. liq.	2 drams.
Glycerin	6 drams.
Aquae ad.	6 ounces.

One-half ounce t. d. s.

215.

Sodii. bicarbonatis.	2 ounces.
Pulv. rad. rhei.	2 scruples.
Spt. ammon. aromat.	4 drams.
Spt. chloroformi	1½ drams.
Tinct. nucis vomicae.	80 minims.
Tinct. gentianae co.	4 drams.
Syrup. zingiberis.	1 ounce.
Aq. menthae pip. ad.	8 ounces.

M. Ft. Mist.
Sig.: One ounce ter die ex aq. paulat. ante cibos sem. hori.

216.

Sodii bicarb.	4 scruples.
Succi taraxaci.	1½ ounces.
Ext. cas. sag. liq. (miscible)	1 dram.
Spirit. chlorof.	2 drams.
Infus. gent. comp. ad.	6 ounces.

M.
Cap. one-half ounce ter die post cibos ex aqua.

217.

Sodii bicarb.	64 grains.
Tinct. podophylli.	64 minims.
Tinct. zingiberis.	½ ounce.
Inf. gent. co. ad.	8 ounces.

M.
Cap. one ounce ter in die.

218.

Pepsin porci.	1½ grains.
Pulv. capsici.	½ grain.
Ext. aloes aquos.	½ grain.
Ex. tarax.	1 grain.

M. et ft. pil.
Sig.: Two vel 3 post cibos.

219.

Sodii bicarb.	2 drams.
P. rhei co.	2 drams.
Bismuthi carb.	2 drams.
P. tragac. co.	10 grains.
Inf. gent. ad.	8 ounces.

Misce. Fiat mist.
Cap. one ounce ter in die.

220.
    Sodii bicarb. .... 1 dram.
    Spt. chlorof. .... 2 drams.
    Spt. am. arom. .... 2 drams.
    Tinct. rhei. .... 4 drams.
    Gent. co. conc. .... 1 ounce.
    Aq. ad. .... 8 ounces.
    M. Ft. Mist.
Sig.: Two drams ex aqua post cibum t. d. s.

221.
    Sodii bicarb. .... 3 drams.
    Bism. carb. .... 2 drams.
    Pulv. rhei. .... ½ dram.
    Spt. ammon. a. .... 3 drams.
    Spt. zingib. .... 1 ounce.
    Aq. chlorof. ad. .... 6 ounces.
One-half ounce ter die inter cib. ex aq.

222.
    Pulv. rhei co. .... 1½ dram.
    Pot. bicarb. .... 1 dram.
    Liq. bismuthi. .... ½ ounce.
    Syr. zingiber. .... ½ ounce.
    Inf. gent. ad. .... 6 ounces.
One-half ounce vel one ounce ter in die p. c.

223.
    Pot. bicarb. .... 4 drams.
    Mist. sennae co. .... 2 ounces.
    Sp. aether nit. .... 6 drams.
    Aq. ad. .... 6 ounces.
One-half ounce 4tis. horis. If pain be severe add chlorodyne 1½ ounces.

224.
    Sod. bicarb. .... 2 drams.
    Tinct. rhei. .... 4 drams.
    Tinct. casc. co. .... 4 drams.
    Inf. gent. co. ad. .... 8 ounces.
    M.
Sig.: A small tablespoonful in water three times a day after food.

225.
    Potassii bicarb. .... 1½ drams.
    Infus. rhei. conc. .... 3 drams.
    Tinc. euonymi. .... 24 minims.
    Tinct. juglandin (1 in 10)... 48 minims.
    Infus. gent. co. ad. .... 6 ounces.
    Ft. mist.
Cap. one ounce ter in die semi-hora ante cibos.

226.
    Sodii carb. .... 2 drams.
    Tr. rhei. .... 3 drams.
    Spt. am. co. .... 4 drams.
    Tr. card. co. .... 3 drams.
    Aq. ad. .... 6 ounces.
One-sixth part 3 times daily.

227.
    Pulv. rhei. co. .... 40 grains.
    Tr. rhei. .... 1 dram.
    Sp. am. ar. .... ½ dram.
    Aq. menth. p. ad. .... ½ ounce.
Ft. hst. H. s. s. 1½ ounces.

228.
    Pulv. rhei. .... 2 grains.
    Ammon. carb. .... 5 grains.
    Ess. chlorof. .... 5 minims.
    Ol. menth. pip. .... ¼ minims.
    Inf. gent. co. ad. .... 1 ounce.
    Ft. haust.
T. d. s.

229.
    Liq. bismuthi. .... 1½ ounces.
    Pulv. rhei. co. .... 3 drams.
    Ess. menth. pip. .... 2 drams.
    Aq. ad. .... 8 ounces.
    M.
One-half ounce ter in die.

230.
    Ammon. carb. .... 1 dram.
    Pot. bicarb. .... 2 drams.
    Pot. bromidi. .... 1½ drams.
    Tr. nux vomic. .... 2 drams.
    Inf. rhei. con. .... 6 drams.
    Aquae chlorof. .... 8 ounces.
    M. Ft. Mist.
One-half ounce t. d. s. ante cibos in aquae.

231.
    Sodii bicarb. .... 64 grains.
    Mag. carb. pond. .... 80 grains.
    Pulv. rhei. .... 32 grains.
    Tinct. zingiber. .... 2 drams.
    Aq. chloroform. ad. .... 8 ounces.
    M. Ft. Mist.
Cap. one ounce ter in die.

232.
    Bismuth. trisnit. .... 1½ drams.
    Sodii bicarb. .... 2 drams.
    Magnes. pond. .... ½ dram.
    Pulv. rhei. .... ½ dram.
    Spt. ammon. aromat. .... 2 drams.
    Ess. menthae. pip. .... ½ dram.
    Acid. hydrocyanic. dil. ..... 6 minims.
    Aquae ad. .... 6 ounces.
One-half ounce ter in die.

233.
    Bismuth. carb. .... 2 drams.
    Sod. bicarb. .... ½ ounce.
    P. tragac. co. .... 1 dram.
    Sp. ammon. co. .... 2 drams.
    Pulv. rhei. .... 1 dram.
    Aq. chlor. ad. .... 8 ounces.
    F. m.
One ounce 4tis horis post cib. ex aqua.

In these mixtures an aperient distinctly aids their action.

This group would be effective, but I doubt if their influences would be lasting without proper attention to diet and regimen.

Flatulence is often caused by fermentative changes and then the following is magical:

234. Typical Prescription.

Liq. hydrarg. perchlor.	1 ounce.
Spt. chlorof.	2 drams.
Tinct. cardam. co.	4 drams.
Aquae ad.	8 ounces.

One ounce 4tis horis.

235.

Pot. bicarb.	2 drams.
Dec. aloes co. conc.	1½ ounces.
Aquae chlorof. ad.	8 ounces.

One-eighth part for a dose.

236.

Sod. bic.	1½ drams.
Tinct. rhei.	2 drams.
Tinct. zingib. ft.	1 dram.
Spt. am. arom.	2 drams.
Spt. chlorof.	3 drams.
Aquae ad.	6 ounces.

Ft. mist.

Cap. one-half ounce 4tis horis.

237.

Tr. nuc. vom.	1½ drams.
Tinct. rhei.	1½ ounces.
Glycer. acid. carbolic.	1½ drams.
Ammon. carb.	80 grains.
Sp. zingib.	6 drams.
Aq. ad.	8 ounces.

M.

Dose for adult: one-half ounce c. one-half ounce aquae ter die.

238.

Ext. aloes.	1 grain.
P. rhei.	2 grains.
Ext. nuc. vom.	⅔ grain.

M.

One at bedtime.

239.

Pulv. rhei.	40 grains.
Sodii bicarb.	80 grains.
Ol. menth. pip.	5 minims.
Inf. gent.	4 drams.
Aq. chlorof. ad.	1 ounce.

Adults, one ounce ter die. Children, one-half ounce to two drams.

240.

Pulv. rhei co.	20 grains.
Tinct. card. co.	15 minims.
Spt. chloroformi.	10 minims.
Spt. ammoniae aromat.	10 minims.
Tr. capsici.	2 minims.
Aq. menth. pip. q. s. ad.	1 ounce.

M. Fiat mistura.

Cap. one ounce o. q. h. cum granis v. carbonis salicis in forma tabellae.

241. A

Bism. carb.	2 drams.
Sodii bicarb.	2 drams.
Mucilag. acaciae.	1 ounce.
Tr. chlorof. co.	3 drams.
Aq. menth. pip. ad.	6 ounces.

M. Ft. Mist.

A tablespoonful three times a day in a little water after meals.

Or this powder—

242. B

Bism. carb.	½ ounce.
Sodii bicarb.	½ ounce.
Pulv. cinnam. co.	2 drams.
Ess. m. pip.	1 dram.
Magnes. carb. pond.	6 drams.

M. Ft. pulv.

Sig.: A small teaspoonful three times a day after food, mixed well in a little milk or water.

243. BISMUTHIC MIXTURES.

Sodii bicarb.	2 drams.
Bismuthi trisnit.	1 dram.
Pulv. trag. co.	1 dram.
Sp. ammon. co.	3 drams.
Sp. chloroformi.	1½ drams.
Ess. menth. pip.	20 minims.
Aquae ad.	8 ounces.

M. Fit. mist.

One ounce 4tis. horis.

244.

Bismuthi carb.	2 drams.
Sodae bicarb.	1½ drams.
Pulv. tragacanth. co.	1½ drams.
Tinct. nucis. vom.	1 dram.
Syr. zingib.	2 drams.
Aquae ad.	8 ounces.

M.

Capiat one-half ounce ter hora ex aqua.

245.
>Sodii bicarb. .... 2 drams.
>Bism. subcarb. .... 1 dram.
>Mucil. tragac. .... 1 ounce.
>Aq. chloroformi. .... 4 ounces.
>Aq. ad. .... 8 ounces.
>M.

One-eighth ter die ante cibos.

In addition in some cases following pills:

246.
>Hyd. c. creta. .... 1½ grains.
>Pil. rhei. co. .... 2 grains.
>Ext. hyoscy. .... ½ grain.
>Ft. pill. j.

One alt. nocte. Mitte two.

247.
>Bismuthi carb. .... 1 dram 1 scruple.
>Sodii bicarb. .... 1 dram 1 scruple.
>Pulv. tragac. co. .... 1 dram 1 scruple.
>Spt. ammon. aromat. . 2 drams.
>Spt. chloroformi. .... 1 dram 1 scruple.
>Acid. hydrocyanic. dil 16 minims.
>Aquae ad. .... 8 ounces.
>M. Ft. mist.

Sig.: One ounce ter die sum p. c.

248.
>Sodii bicarb. .... 2 drams.
>Bismuth. subnit. .... 1 dram.
>P. trag. co. .... 1 dram.
>Spt. ammon. co. .... 3 drams.
>Spt. chlorof. .... 1½ drams.
>Ess. menth. pip. .... 20 minims.
>Aquae ad. .... 8 ounces.
>M. Ft. mist.

One ounce ter die post cibos.

249.
>Bismuth. subnit. .... 2 drams.
>Sodae bicarb. .... 2 drams.
>Tinct. cardam. co. .... 4 drams.
>Spt. chloroformi. .... 1½ drams.
>Aq. menthae pip. ad. ...... 6 ounces.
>Ft. mist.

Cap. one ounce ter in dies.

250.
>Sodii bicarb. .... 2 drams.
>Bism. carb. .... 2 drams.
>Acid. hydrocyan. dil. ...... 24 minims.
>Sp. chlorof. .... 80 minims.
>Tr. nucis vom. .... 80 minims.
>Aq. ad. .... 8 ounces.

One ounce t. die a. cib.

251.
>Bismuth. carb. .... 40 grains.
>Sodii bicarb. .... 40 grains.
>Pulv. trag. co. .... 40 grains.
>Tinct. chlorof. co. .... 1½ drams.
>Tinct. nucis vom. .... ½ dram.
>Aq. ad. .... 8 ounces.
>M. Ft. mist.

Cap. one ounce ter die p. c.

252.
>Sod. bicarb. .... 1 dram.
>Bismuth. carb. .... 2 drams.
>Aeth. chlor. .... 1 dram.
>Tr. nuc. vom. .... 1½ drams.
>Tr. aurant. .... 2 drams.
>Aq. ad. .... 8 drams.

One-eighth pt. t. d. s.
Pil. rhei et hyd. gr. lvss.
iv.
2 alt. nocte. sd.

253.
>Bismuth. carb. .... 2 drams.
>Sodae bicarb. .... 2 drams.
>Pulv. trag. co. .... 30 grains.
>Tr. nucis vom. .... 1 dram.
>Tr. aurant. .... 3 drams.
>Aq. anethi ad. .... 6 ounces.

M. Ft. mist. one-twelfth part ¼ hr. before meals three times daily.

254.
>Bismuth. carb. .... 1½ drams.
>Sodae bicarb. .... 1½ drams.
>Tr. nucis vom. .... 1 dram.
>Pulv. pepsin. .... 1 dram.
>Pulv. trag. co. .... 40 grains.
>Sp. chlor. .... 1 dram.
>Aq. ad. .... 6 ounces.

Misce: One-twelfth partis ter die ex aq. pauxillo hora ¼ ante cibos.

255.
>Sodii bicarb. .... 1 dram 20 gr.
>Bism. carb. .... 1 dram 20 gr.
>Mucilage. .... ½ ounce.
>Tr. nucis vom .... 40 minims.
>Inf. calumb. ad. .... 8 ounces.

Cap. one ounce ter die ante cibos.

A further instalment of bismuth-mixtures. Some suspending vehicle, such as pulv. acacae or pulv. trag. co., has evidently been omitted.

256.
>Bism. carb. .... 3 drams.
>Sod. carb. .... 3 drams.
>Ext. cascar. .... 1 dram.
>Tinct. hyosc. .... 2 drams.
>Sp. chlor. .... 2 drams.
>Inf. quas. ad. .... 6 ounces.

Coch. mag. ter in die ante cib.

257.
    Sodae bicarb. .... 2 drams.
    Bismuth. carb. .... 1 dram.
    Sp. ammon. aromat. .... 3 drams.
    " chloroformi. .... 1½ drams.
    Tinct. zingib. fort. .... 1½ drams.
    Inf. gent. co. ad. .... 8 ounces.
    M. Ft. mist.
Cap. one ounce t. d. s. p. c.

258
    Sodae bicarb. .... 1¼ drams.
    Bismuth. carb. .... 1½ drams.
    Acid. hydrocyan. dil. .... 24 minims.
    Tinct. zingiberis. .... 2 drams.
    Aquae chlorof. ad. .... 6 ounces.
Fiat mist.
One tablespoonful in water shortly after meals.

259.
    Bismuthi subnit. .... 2½ drams.
    Tinct. nucis vom. .... 1 dram.
    Succ. tarax. .... 1 ounce.
    Infus. quassiae. ....
    Infus. calumbae. ....
        aa partes aequales ad. .. 8 ounces.
    M. Ft. mist.
Sig.: Coch. mag. sum. ter die ex aqua.

260.
    Sod. bicarb. .... 2 drams.
    Spt. ammon. ar. .... 3 drams.
    Acid. hydrocyan. dil. .... ½ dram.
    Bismuth. carb. .... ½ dram.
    Inf. gent. .... 6 drams.
    Aquae chlorof. ad. .... 6 ounces.
    M. Ft. mist.
One-half ounce ter die post cib.

261.
    Sodae bicarb. .... 1½ drams.
    Bism. carb. .... 2 drams.
    Spt. ammon. arom. .... 3 drams.
    Inf. calumbae. .... 4 ounces.
    Spt. chlorof. .... 1½ drams.
    Inf. gent. co. ad. .... 8 ounces.
    M. One ounce ter die p. c.

262.
    Bismuth. subcarb. .... 1 dram.
    Pulv. sodii bicarb. .... 1 dram.
    Pulv. tragac. .... 6 grains.
    Spt. chloroform. .... 1½ drams.
    Tinct. nucis vom. .... 1 dram.
    Aq. ad. .... 4 ounces.
    Mist. Ft. mist.
One-half ounce ter die half an hour after meals.

MIXTURES FOR NEURALGIA.

263.   **Typical Prescription.**
    Quininae sulph. .... 15 grains.
    Antipyrin .... 1 dram.
    Tinct. cimicifugae .... 2 drams.
    Acid. hydrobrom. dil. ...... 2 drams.
    Tinct. aurantii .... 1½ drams.
    Aquae .... 6 ounces.
One-half ounce pro dose.
          or
    Quin. valerianat. .... 2 grains.
    Ft. pil.
One ter d. s.

264
    Quininae hydrobrom. ...... 3 grains.
    Acidi hydrobrom. dil ...... 20 minims.
    Aquae ad .... 1 ounce.
    M.
Sig.: The draught. Repeat in 3 hours if required.

265.
    Quin. sulph. .... 24 grains.
    Ac. hydrobrom. dil. .... 2 drams.
    Pot. brom. .... 3 drams.
    Tr. gelsem. .... 1½ drams.
    Aq. chlorof. ad .... 6 ounces.
Sig.: One-half ounce every hour until relief comes, afterwards thrice daily.

266.
    Quininae sulph. .... 1 scruple.
    Acid. sulph. dil. .... ½ dram.
    Potass. brom. .... 2 drams.
    Tr. gelsem. .... 1 dram.
    Am. chlor. .... 2 drams.
    Aq. chlorof. ad .... 8 ounces.
One ounce every 3 or 4 hours.

267.
    Quin. sulph. .... 12 grains.
    Ammon. brom. .... 3 drams.
    Acid. sulph. dil. .... 1 dram.
    Tr. belladonnae .... 2 drams.
    Tr. gelsem. .... 1 dram.
    Aq. chlorof. ad .... 6 ounces.
Sig.: One-half ounce every 3 or 4 hours.

268.
    Potass. bromidi .... 2 drams.
    Quin. sulph. .... ½ dram.
    Acid. hydrobrom. dil. ..... 2 drams.
    Tr. cardam. co. .... ½ ounce.
    Aq. chlorof. ad .... 6 ounces.
One-half ounce 3tia vel 4ta hora sd.

269.
>   Quin. sulph. .... 1 scruple.
>   Acid. hydrobrom. dil. ..... 1 dram.
>   Tinct. gelsem. semp. ...... 1½ drams.
>   Tinct. cimicifug. .... 3 drams.
>   Syr. aurant. .... 1 ounce.
>   Aq. chlorof. ad .... 8 ounces.
>   M. Ft. mist.

One-eighth part every 4 hours.

270.
>   Ammon. chlor. .... 1 dram.
>   Quininae sulph. .... 12 grains.
>   Acid. hydrobrom. d. .... 3 drams.
>   Syr. aurantii .... 6 drams.
>   Aquae chlorof. ad .... 6 ounces.

Cap. one-sixth 4tis horis.

271.
>   Quin. sulph. .... 36 grains.
>   Acid. hydrobrom. dil. ..... 2 drams.
>   Tinct. gelsem. .... 1 dram.
>   Sol. sodii sulphat. (1 in 6).. 1½ ounces.
>   Aquae chlorof. ad .... 6 ounces.

One-half ounce for dose.

Excellent if constipation is present.

272.
>   Quin. bromid. .... 9 grains.
>   Amm. bromid. .... 1½ drams.
>   Tinct. gelsem. .... 1½ drams.
>   Ac. hydrobrom. dil. .... ½ dram.
>   Glycerini .... 3 drams.
>   Aq. chlorof. ad .... 6 ounces.

One ounce s. d. s.

273.
>   Tr. gelsem. semp. .... 2 drams.
>   Tr. quin. ammon. .... 1 ounce.
>   Syr. aurantii .... 1 ounce.
>   Aq. ad .... 8 ounces.

One-eighth 4tis horis.

274.
>   Quininae sulph. .... 20 grains.
>   Ammon. bromid. .... 1½ drams.
>   Acid. hydrobrom. dil. ..... 3 drams.
>   Tr. aurant. .... 6 drams.
>   Aq. chlor. ad .... 8 ounces.
>   M.

One-eighth bis vel ter die ex aq.

275.
>   Quininae sulph. .... 12 grains.
>   Ac. hydrobrom. dil. .... 2 drams.
>   Tinct. gelsemii semper. ... 1½ drams.
>   Spt. chlorof. .... 1½ drams.
>   Aquae ad .... 8 ounces.
>   M.

One-sixth 4tis horis sd.

276.
>   Quin. sulph. .... 18 grains.
>   Ac. hydrobrom. dil. .... 2 drams.
>   Tr. gelsem. semp. .... 1 dram.
>   Aq. chlor. ad .... 6 ounces.
>   M. Ft.

Dose: A sixth part every 4 hours till pain is relieved.

277.
>   Quin. sulph. .... 24 grains.
>   Acid. hydrobromic. dil. ... 2 drams.
>   Tinct. gelsemii .... 1 dram.
>   Tinct. opii .... 1 dram.
>   Mist. camphorae ad .... 3 ounces.
>   M. Ft. mist.

Two drams quaque 4tis horis sum.

278.
>   Quin. sulph. .... 36 grains.
>   Tr. gelsemii .... 3 drams.
>   Acid. hydrobrom. dil. ..... 2 drams.
>   Glycerini .... ½ ounce.
>   Inf. quass. ad .... 6 ounces.

Sig.: One-half ounce every 4 hours.

279.
>   Quin. sulph. .... 24 grains.
>   Acid. hydrobrom. dil. ..... ½ ounce.
>   Tinct. gelsemii .... 1½ drams.
>   Aq. chlorof. ad .... 6 ounces.
>   M. Ft. mist.

Sig.: A tablespoonful three times a day in water.

280.
>   Quin. sulph. .... 12 grains.
>   Ac. hydrobrom. dil. .... 2 drams.
>   Ac. sulph. dil. .... 20 minims.
>   Tr. gelsem. .... 1½ drams.
>   Sp. chlorof. .... 2 drams.
>   Aq. ad .... 6 ounces.
>   M.

One-half ounce 4tis horis as long as pain lasts.

281.

Ammon. chlor.	4 scruples.
Quin. sulph.	8 grains.
Acid. hydrobrom. dil.	1 dram.
Tr. aconit. (Flem.)	8 minims.
Tr. gelsem.	80 minims.
Aq. chlorof. ad	8 ounces.

M. Ft. mist.

Sig.: One dram 4tis horis.

282.

Phenazoni	4 scruples.
Quin. sulph.	1 scruple.
Acid. hydrob. dil.	2 drams.
Tr. aconiti	16 minims.
Syr. flor. aurant.	1 ounce.
Aq. chlor. ad	8 ounces.

M.

One-eighth pt. o. 4 h. dum op. sit., diem t. d. s.

283.

Tr. gelsem. semp.	1 dram.
Quin. sulph.	12 grains.
Ac. sulph. dil.	16 minims.
Tr. nucis vom.	1 dram.
Syr. aurant.	6 drams.
Aq. chlor. ad	6 ounces.

Misce.

One-twelfth omni 4tis horis ex aqua cyatho vinar.

284.

Quininae sulph.	20 grains.
Acid. sulph. dil.	20 minims.
Tinct. gelsemii	2 drams.
Liq. strychninae	10 minims.
Aq. ad	6 ounces.

Fiat m.

One ounce ter in die.

285.

Quin. sulph.	18 grains.
Acid. phosph. dil.	2 drams.
Tinct. nucis vom.	1 dram.
Spt. chloroformi	1 dram.
Aq. dest. ad	6 ounces.

M.

One-sixth part every 4 hours.

286.

Ammon. brom.	48 grains.
Tr. aconiti (B. P.)	32 minims.
Tinct. quininae (B. P.)	4 ounces.
Tinct. gelsemii	1½ drams.
Spt. chloroformi	2½ drams.
Aq. ad	8 ounces.

Sig.: One-half ounce 3tis horis.

287.

Quinine sulph.	30 grains.
Tr. aconite	½ dram.
Tr. card. co.	2 drams.
Aq. chloroformi ad	4 ounces.

M. Ft.

Take one tablespoonful every three or four hours until relieved.

288.

Quininae salicyl.	12 grains.
Mucilaginis acaciae	½ ounce.
Tincturae lupuli	1 dram.
Syrupi aurantii	6 drams.
Ammonii bromid.	1 dram.
Aquae chloroformi ad	6 ounces.

M. Ft. mist.

Cap. partem sextam omni tertius horis donec dolor evanuerit.

APERIENT NEURALGIA REMEDIES.

289.

Quin. sulph.	16 grains.
Pot. brom.	8 scruples.
Mag. sulph.	1 ounce.
Acid. sulph. dil.	q. s.
Tr. gelsemii	1½ drams.
Aq. chlorof. ad	8 ounces.

M. Ft. mist.

One-half ounce ter die.

290.

Magnes. sulph.	6 drams.
Quin. sulph.	24 grains.
Ferri sulph.	1 dram.
Acid. sulph. dil.	½ dram.
Tr. gelsemii	1½ drams.
Aq. chlorof. ad	6 ounces.

One-half 4tis horis.

An excellent formula in the neuralgia of anaemia.

291.

Quin. sulph.	16 grains.
Liq. ferri perchl.	3 drams.
Tr. gelsem.	3 drams.
Sp. chloroformi	2 drams.
Mag. sulph.	½ ounce.
Glycerini	1 ounce.
Aq. chlorof. ad	8 ounces.

One-half ounce ter quarterve. in d. ex aq. post cib.

Where constipation is a marked feature of the case, these three mixtures would answer well. Besides quinine normally tends to produce constipation.

292. OPIATE NEURALGIA REMEDIES.

    Ammon. brom. .... 1 dram.
    Tinct. gelsem. .... 2 drams.
    Sp. chlorof. .... 2 drams.
    Ferri ammon. cit. .... 1 dram.
    Aquae ad .... 6 ounces.
One-half ounce every 4 hours.

293.

    Pot. bromid. .... 2 drams.
    Ferri am. cit. .... 2 drams.
    Tr. gelsemii .... 1½ drams.
    Tr. capsici .... 1 dram.
    Sp. chloroform. .... 2 drams.
    Aq. ad. .... 3 ounces.
    Ft. mist.
Two drams secundis horis ex aqua sumendus.

294.

    Ferri quin. cit. .... 1½ drams.
    Amm. brom. .... 3 drams.
    Aq. ad. .... 8 ounces.
One mg. chl. 4tis hrs.

295.

    Ferri et quin. cit. .... 2 drams.
    Sp. chlorof. .... 2 drams.
    Tr. gelsemii .... 1 dram.
    Tr. cimicifugae .... 1 dram.
    Aquae ad .... 6 ounces.
    M. Ft. mist.
Sig.: A tablespoonful three times a day in water.

296.

    Fer. quin. cit. .... ½ dram.
    Tr. gelsemii .... 2 drams.
    Sp. chlorof. .... 2 drams.
    Pot. brom. .... 2 drams.
    Aq. ad .... 6 ounces.
One-half ounce ter die.

297.

    Ferri et quininae cit. ..... 1 dram.
    Tinct. aconiti .... 1 dram.
    Tinct. gelsemii .... 2 drams.
    Spt. gaultheriae (1 ol. to 5 S. V. R.).............. 3 drams.
    Aq. chlorof. ad.......... 8 ounces.
    M. Ft. mist.
Sig.: One-half ounce ter die sumendus post cibos.

298.

    Quin. disulph. .... 16 grains.
    Acid. phosph. dil. .... 1 dram.
    Syr. ferri phosph. co. ..... 2 ounces.
    Aq. ad .... 8 ounces.
One-half ounce ter die ex aqua.

299.

    Quin. sulph. .... 1 scruple.
    Tr. ferri perch. .... 1 dram.
    Pot. brom. .... 1 dram.
    Tr. gelsem. .... 1 dram.
    Sp. chlorof. .... 2 drams.
    Inf. gent. co. ad........... 6 ounces.
    M. Ft. mist.
Sig.: One ounce every 3 hours for three doses, then three times a day.

300.

    Ferri et ammon. cit. ..... 1½ drams.
    Pot. bromidi .... 2 drams.
    Spt. ammon. aromat. ...... 1 dram.
    Spt. chloroformi .... 1½ drams.
    Syrupi .... ½ ounce.
    Aquae ad .... 6 ounces.
A sixth part every 4 hours.

301.

    Quininae sulph. .... 12 grains.
    Liq. ferri perchlor. fort. ... 40 minims.
    Tr. nucis vom. .... 1½ drams.
    Spt. chloroformi .... 1½ drams.
    Aquae ad .... 8 ounces.
    M. Ft. mist.
Dose: One ounce 4tis horis.

302.

    Antipyrin. .... 8 grains.
    Quin. sulph. .... 1½ grains.
    Exalgin. .... ½ grains.
    M. Ft. pulv. tales 12.
Sig.: One every 4 hours.

303. FOR NERVOUS HEADACHE.

    Ferri et quin. cit. .... 1 dram.
    Potass. bromid. .... 1 dram.
    Ammon. bromid. .... 1 dram.
    Sodii bromid. .... 1 dram.
    Syrupi .... 1 ounce.
    Aquae ad .... 6 ounces.
    M.
Sig.: A dessertspoonful thrice daily in water.

Iron is not advisable in cases of severe or recent neuralgia, but it does most good in chronic cases which call for tonics.

NEURALGIA MIXTURES FREE FROM QUININE.

Some people are very intolerant of quinine, and therefore other remedies must be substituted.

304. Typical Prescription.

Croton chloral hyd.	1 dram.
Ammon. bromid.	2 drams.
Tinct. gelsemii	3 drams.
Spt. chloroformi	2 drams.
Aquae ad	6 ounces.

One-half ounce 4tis horis.

305.

Butyl. chloral hydrat.	5 grains.
Ammon. bromid.	20 grains.
Tinct. chloroformi co.	20 minims.
Aquae ad	1 ounce.

M. Fiat haust.
4tis horis sumend.

306.

Tinct. lupuli	3 drams.
Tinct. valerian.	3 drams.
Ammon. mur.	2 drams.
Ammon. carb.	2 scruples.
Ammon. iodid.	1 scruple.
Aquae menth. pip. ad	6 ounces.

One ounce three times daily until pain is relieved.

307.

Tr. gelsemii	1½ drams.
Acid. nit. mur. dil.	2 drams.
Inf. gent. ad	6 ounces.

M.
One-half ounce 2ndis horis.
An excellent general tonic.

308.

Croton chloral.	48 grains.
Tr. gelsem.	2 drams.
Syr. aurant.	½ ounce.
Aq. ad	8 ounces.

M. Ft. mist.
One ounce ter die.

309.

Potass. bromid.	10 grains.
Tinct. gelsem. semp.	10 minims.
Spt. ammon. arom.	15 minims.
Aq. camph. ad	½ ounce.

Mitte six ounces.
Sig.: One-half ounce every 4 hours.

310.

Butyl chloral. hydrat.	1 dram.
Tinct. gelsemii	2 drams.
Sp. vini rect.	4 drams.
Glycerin.	6 drams.
Aq. ad	6 ounces.

One-half ounce 4tis hor. sd.

311.

Ammon. chlor.	2½ drams.
Ammon. brom.	1½ drams.
Tinct. gelsemii	1½ drams.
Ext. glycyrrhizae liq.	4 drams.
Syrupi	4 drams.
Aquae q. s. ad	8 ounces.

M. Ft. mist.
One-half ounce quarta quoque hora sumend.

312.

Ammon. chloridi	2½ drams.
Ammon. bromidi	1½ drams.
Tinct. gelsemii	2½ drams.
Ext. glycyrrh. liq.	3 drams.
Syrupi	6 drams.
Aquae ad	6 ounces.

M.
One tablespoonful in water to be taken every 5 hours.

313.

Pot. bromid.	1 dram.
Tr. aconit.	½ dram.
Sp. ammon. arom.	2 drams.
Aq. chlorof.	3 ounces.
Aq. ad.	6 ounces.

M. Ft.
Cap. one ounce every four hours until relieved.

314.

Ammon. hydrochlor.	3 drams.
Tinct. gelsemin.	1 dram.
Ext. glycyrrh. liq.	3 drams.
Sp. chloroformi	1½ drams.
Aquae ad	6 ounces.

One-sixth 4tis horis.

315.

Calcii hypophos.	5 grains.
Acidi phosph. dilut.	10 minims.
Tinct. aurantii	10 minims.
Aquae chloroformi	½ ounce.
Aquae q. s. ad	1 ounce.

M. Ft. mist.
One ounce ter in die post cibos sumenda.

316.
    Tr. lavand. co. .... 3 drams.
    Spt. aeth. chlor. .... 3 drams.
    Tr. gelsemii .... 2 drams.
    Aq. ad .... 6 ounces.
    M. Ft. mist.
One-half ounce ter die sumend.
    Pil. rhei co. .... 5 grains.
Mitte 12. Cap. one omni nocte.

317.
    Butyl. croton. chloral. ..... 2 grains.
    Ext. gelsemin. .... 1/6 grains.
    Ext. hyoscy. .... q. s.
    M. Ft. pil.
Sumat 4tis horis. Mitte 6.

318.
    Mag. sulph. .... 1 ounce.
    Tr. card. co. .... 2 drams.
    Syr. zingib. .... ½ ounce.
    Aq. ad .... 6 ounces.
    M. Ft. mist.
One ounce pro dosis si opus sit.

NEURALGIA MIXTURES WITH AN OPIATE.

The following mixtures are objectionable from the presence of morphia.

319.
    Potass. bromid. .... 72 grains.
    Tr. gelsemii .... 1½ drams.
    Liq. morph. mur. .... 1 dram.
    Syr. butyl. chlor. hyd. ... 6 drams.
    Aq. ad .... 6 ounces.
One-sixth part 3 vel 4tis hor.

320.
    Potass. brom. .... 1½ drams.
    Tr. gelsem. semper. .... 1½ drams.
    Liq. morph. mur. .... 1 dram.
    Syr. butyl. chlor. hyd. ... 4 drams.
    Aq. ad .... 6 ounces.
Cap. one-sixth part. 4tis horis.

321.
    Ferri quin. cit. .... 1 dram.
    Tr. gelsem. .... 1½ drams.
    Liq. morph. hyd. .... ½ dram.
    Aq. chlorof. .... 3 ounces.
    Aq. ad .... 6 ounces.
    M. Fiat mist.
One-sixth 4tis horis.

322.
    Quininae sulph. .... 15 grains.
    Acid. sulph. dil. .... 20 minims.
    Spt. aether. co. .... ½ ounce.
    Tinct. gelsemii .... 1½ drams.
    Liq. morphinae hydroc. ... 1½ drams.
    Spt. chlorof. .... 1 dram.
    Aquae ad .... 8 ounces.
One-half ounce to one ounce ter die.
Liq. rosae dulc. or sacch. ust. may be used to colour.

323.
    Tr. quin. ammon. .... 1 dram.
    Tr. gelsem. .... 1½ drams.
    Liq. morph. mur. .... 2 drams.
    Syr. aurantii. .... 4 drams.
    Aq. chlorof. ad. .... 6 ounces.
    M.
Sig.: One-half ounce 3tis horis.

324.
    Tr. gelsem. .... 1½ drams.
    Liq. morph. hydrochlor. ... 1 dram.
    Aq. chlorof. ad. .... 2 ounces.
    M.
Sig.: One-half ounce s. o. s.

325.
    Ammon. chlor. .... 1 dram.
    Spt. chlorof. .... 1 dram.
    Tinct. gelsem. .... ½ dram.
    Liq. morph. acet. .... ½ dram.
    Inf. quassiae ad .... 8 ounces.
    M.
One ounce om. tertia hora.

326.
    Quininae sulph. .... 2 grains.
    Acid. sulph. dil. .... 5 minims.
    Mag. sulph. .... ½ dram.
    Chlorodyni .... 10 minims.
    Aquae .... ½ ounce.
Every 4 hours.

327.
    Tr. lupuli .... 10 minims.
    Chlorodyni .... 10 minims.
    Sp. amm. aromat. .... 20 minims.
    Tr. cinchonae co. ad ...... 2 drams.
T. d. e. a. sd.

NEURALGIC HEADACHE MIXTURES.

These formulae are more adapted for headache and migraine.

328.
    Antipyrin .... 5 grains.
    Caffein. cit. .... 5 grains.
    Aquae chloroform. ad ...... 1 ounce.
      M. Ft. haust.
    Si opus sit.

329.
    Antifebrin. .... 5 grains.
    Antipyrin .... 5 grains.
    Phenacetin .... 5 grains.
    Salicin. .... 5 grains.
      M. Ft. pulv.
    Dose: 10 grs. at bedtime, and for influenza in the initial stage or chills 45 grs. divided into 3 doses, one every 4 hours, with a hot gruel at bedtime.

330.
    Phenacetin. .... 12 grains.
      Mitte 3.
    Sig.: One every hour till pain stops.

OUTWARD APPLICATIONS FOR NEURALGIA AND TOOTHACHE.

331.   **Typical Prescription.**
    Chloral ....
    Camphor ....
    Menthol ....
    Equal parts, rubbed up together to form a syrupy liquid.
    To be rubbed on the part affected.

332.
    Ac. carbol. .... 2 drams.
    Camphorae .... 3 drams.
    Menthol .... ½ dram.
    Chloroformi ad .... 1 ounce.

333.
    Ac. carb. .... 15 grains.
    Menthol. .... 10 grains.
    Collodii ad .... 1 dram.
      Ft. gelat.
    Take a little on a match-stalk, and apply to the cavity, dried out with cotton-wool, placing a plug of wool on top.

334.
    Thymol .... 15 grains.
    Menthol .... 15 grains.
    Cocainae .... 1 grain.
    Chloroformi pur. .... ½ ounce.
      Misce. Fiat guttae.
    A few drops on cotton-wool to be inserted in the cavity of the tooth.

335.   B
    Magnesii sulph. .... q. s.
    Nocti si opus sit.

336.
    Menthol. .... 1 dram.
    Spt. aether. ad .... 1 ounce.
      Ft. lotio.
    Sig.: To be applied to the cheek or forehead.

337.
    Lin. camph. co. .... 4 drams.
    Tinct. capsici .... 3 drams.
    Sp. aetheris .... 4 drams.
    S. V. rect. .... 2 ounces.
      M. Ft. lin.
    To be gently rubbed behind the ear and over the brow.

338.
    Tinct. pyrethri .... 3 ounces.
    Sol. sat. camph. (in S. V. R.) 3 ounces.
    Ol. caryoph. .... 2 drams.
    Acid. carbol. pur. .... 2 drams.
    Morph. hydrochl. .... 1 dram.
    Acid. tannici .... 1 ounce.
      M. Ft. applic.
    To be applied on cotton-wool.

339.
    Tinct. aconiti (Fleming's).. } equal
    Tinct. iodi .... } parts.
    Apply to the hollow part of the tooth on cotton-wool.

340.
    Menthol. .... 1 dram.
    Linimenti aconiti .... ½ ounce.
    Linimenti belladonnae ad.. 2 ounces.
      M. Ft. pigmentum.
    Sig.: For external use only. To be painted on the painful parts with a camel's hair brush.
    All these applications would meet the desired end.
    The last three are too poisonous for use for toothache.

NEURALGIC PILLS.

341.
Phosphori .... 1/50 grain.
Stychniae .... 1/32 grain.
Ferri redact. .... 1 grain.
Quinae sulph. .... 1 grain.
Zinci val. .... 1 grain.
Ft. pil. Dose: One 4 ter horis.

HEADACHE.

342.   BILIOUS.
Sodii bicarb. .... 10 grains.
Potassii bicarb. .... 10 grains.
Spt. ammon. co. .... 15 minims.
Tinct. zingiber. .... 5 minims.
Sp. chlorof. .... 10 minims.
Inf. gent. co. ad. ...... 1 ounce.
M. Mitte 8 ounces.
Ter die sumend.

343.
Pulv. rhei. .... 1 ounce.
Pulv. zingiber, jam. .... 1 ounce.
Sodii bicarb. .... 1 ounce.
Sp. am. aromat. .... 2 drams.
Aq. menth. pip. ad. ..... 8 ounces.
M.
One-eighth pt. ter die.

344.
Sodii bicarb. .... 2 drams.
Ammon. carb. .... 2 scruples.
Tr. limonis. .... ½ ounce.
Aquae ad. .... 8 ounces.
One-half ounce t. d. s.

345.
Hyd. c. creta. .... 3 grains.
P. rhei. .... 15 grains.
Sodii bicarb. .... 5 grains.
M. Ft. pulv. Mitte 6.
Sig.: One at bed time.
Rest in a dark room and abstention from all food for a few hours will aid the action of these mixtures.

346.
Acid. nit. mur. dil. .... 2 drams.
Tr. nuc. vom. .... 1½ drams.
Succ. tarax. .... 1 ounce.
Syr. aurant. flor. ...... 1 ounce.
Inf. chiratae ad. .... 6 ounces.
M. Ft. mist.
Sig.: A tablespoonful three times a day in a little water.

347.
Resin. podoph. .... ¼ grain.
Euonymin. .... 1 grain.
Pil. hydrarg. .... ½ grain.
Pil. rhei. co. .... 3 grains.
M. Ft. pil.
Sig.: One to be taken at bed time occasionally, when required.
Blue pill and black draught.
In a decidedly bilious subject I would give 2 gr. of calomel, followed by a draught of eff. sodae sulph. in the morning.

348.
Pil. hydrarg. .... 2 grains.
Ext. coloc. co. .... 2 grains.
Ext. hyoscy. .... 1 grain.
M. Ft. pil.
H. s. s.

349.   COMMON OR SICK.
Sodii sulphatis effervescentis.
                         2 drams—3 drams.
Statim sumend. ex aquae uncis quart.
(Commence one hour after the sodii sulph.)

350.
Antipyrin. .... 5 grains.
Sodii salicyl. .... 5 grains.
Tinct. cardamomi co. .... 10 minims.
Spt. chloroformi. .... 10 minims.
Spt. ammonae aromat. .... 5 minims.
Aquae menthae pip. q. s. ad 1 ounce.
M. Fiat mistura.
One ounce ter horis sumend. donec dolor evanuerit.
This prescription is strikingly good treatment.
I would, however, direct the aperient to be taken in the morning fasting, and give at once—

351.
Antipyrin. .... 40 grains.
Eff. caffein hydrobromate. 6 drams.
Mix, and make into 6 powders.
One hourly in water, if necessary.

352.
Phenacetin. .... 12 grains.
Take now.

353.
Antipyrin. .... 10 grains.
Soda-water. .... 3 ounces.
Ft. haust. s. s.

354.
- Ammon. bromidi. .... 1 dram.
- Spt. ammon. aromat. ..... 1 dram.
- Syrup. aurantii. .... ½ ounce.
- Aquae ad. .... 3 ounces.

Misce.

Two tablespoonfuls for the first dose; then one tablespoonful every four hours until the headache is relieved.

Cures on the spot.

355.
- Pot. bromid. .... ½ dram.
- Spt. ammon. ar. .... ½ dram.
- Aq. camph. ad. .... 1 ounce.

Misce.

Every two hours till easy.

For colds accompanied with "pains all over the body" (as it is described) and sick headache.

356.
- Sodii salicylat. .... 2 drams.
- Tr. card. co. .... 2 drams.
- Tr. camph. co. .... 2 drams.
- Aquae ad. .... 6 ounces.

One-half ounce every 4 hours.

357.
- P. ipecac. c. opii. .... 5 grains.
- Sodae salicylat. .... 10 grains.

Ft. pulv.

To be taken in something hot at bedtime.

358.
- Antifebrin. .... 8 grains.

Ft. pulv.

359.
- Mist. sennae. co. .... 1½ ounces.
- Pot. bicarb. .... 1 dram.
- Aq. menth. pip. ad. ...... 6 ounces.

M. Ft. mist.

Sig.: One ounce ter die sumend. inter cibos.

360.
- Mag. sulph. .... 4 drams.
- Ferri. Sulph. .... 40 grains.
- Acid. sulph. dil. .... 40 minims.
- Liq. tarax. .... 4 drams.
- Aq. chlorof. .... 1½ ounces.
- Aquae .... 6 ounces.

M.

One ounce ter die sd.

All these mixtures would serve their purpose.

APERIENT MEDICINES.

361.
- Acidi nitro-mur. dilut. ..... 1 dram.
- Magnesii sulphatis. .... 3 drams.
  to 6 drams.
- Glycerol. podophylli. ...... 30 minims.
- Succus taraxaci .... 6 drams.
- Misturae ferri aromat. ad.. 6 ounces.

Misce. Ft. mist.

Cujus cap. one ounce ter in die post cibos.

This is undoubtedly a good combination of aperient drugs, but it is unnecessarily complicated. It would have been better to have made one mixture of it.

362.
- Liq. ext. taraxaci. .... 1 ounce.
- Liq. ext. casc. sag. .... 1½ ounces.
- Tinct. nuc. vom. .... 3 drams.
- Glycerin. ad. .... 4 ounces.

M. Ft. mist.

Sig.: A teaspoonful night and morning for two days, then every night.

363.
- Ext. cas. sag. liq. .... 7 minims.
- Dec. al. co. com. .... 10 minims.
- Tr. nuc. vom. .... 5 minims.
- Glycerin .... ½ dram.
- Aq. m. vir. ad. .... 2 drams.

Two drams t. d. s. p. c.

This appears to be a child's mixture, and for this purpose it would do very nicely.

364.
- Pulv. tragacanth. .... 4 grains.
- Syrup. simplicis. .... 2 drams.
- Ol. cassiae. .... 6 minims.
- Ol. ricini. .... 1 ounce.

Ft. emuls. sec. art.

Sig.: Purgative draught.

Pleasant to taste, rapid in action, no griping.

I am not over partial to ol. ricini. It is very certain in its action, but it is hardly consonant with up-to-date elegant pharmacy.

365.
- Liq. ferri dialysati. .... 1 ounce.
- Glycerin. pur. .... 1 ounce.

M. Ft. mist.

One-half dram ex one ounce aquae ter in die post cibos sumenda.

366.
- Liq. rhei. .... 1½ drams.
- Magnes. fl. .... 3 ounces.
- Aeth. chlor. .... 2 drams.
- Aq. m. pip. ad. .... 8 ounces.

M.

One-sixth part for a dose.

With one-half to one ounce of cascara aromatic, Formula No. 57, this mixture would be perfect.

CONSTIPATION.

367. ESPECIALLY FOR FEMALES.

Extracti cascarae sagradae
liq .... 1 dram.
Glycyrrhizae liq............ ½ ounce.
Glycerini pur.............. ½ ounce.
M. Ft. mist.

One dram hora somne sumenda ex aquae cyatho vinoso pro re nata.

LINCTUS FOR A COUGH.

368. Typical Prescription.

Acid. hydrobromic. dil..... 1 dram.
Tinct. cubebae............. 1 dram.
Spt. chloroform............ 1 dram.
Syr. prun. virg............ 4 drams.
Mucilag. ad................ 1½ ounces.

One dram urg. tuss.

369.

Potassii nitratis .... 3 grains.
Vin. ipecac................. 3 minims.
Syr. limonis................ ½ dram.
Aquae ad................... 1 dram.

Q. q. 4h. sd.

370.

Syr. limonis................ ½ ounce.
Vin. ipecac................. 1 dram.
Glycerini pur.............. ½ ounce.
Codeinae .... 4 grains.
Aq. ad..................... 2 ounces.
M. Ft. gtt. tussi.

Cap. one dram omn. nocte et rep. si opus sit.

371.

Oxymel. scillae............ 4 drams.
Tr. cubebae................ 2 drams.
Acet. ipecac............... 3 drams.
Dec. senegae ad........... 3 ounces.
Ft. mist.

Two drams quartis horis sumdum.

372.

Acid. sulph. arom.......... 2 drams.
Tinct. scillae.............. 4 drams.
Syrup. tolu................ 1 ounce.
Aq. ad..................... 3 ounces.
Ft. gutt.

Cap. one dram, p. r. n.

373.

Syr. picis liq.............. 1 uce.
Syr. pruni virgin.......... 1 ounce.
Liq. morphiae............. 1½ drams.
Tr. benzoni co............ 3 drams.
Aquae ad.................. 4 ounces.
M.

Cap. one dram ter horae.

An excellent combination, even without the morphia.

374.

Oxymel. scillae............ 1 ounce.
Vin. ipecac................ 2 drams.
Syr. pruni virg............ ½ ounce.
Ext. glycyrrh. liq......... 1 dram.
Tr. chlorof. and morph. B. P.
(sine morph. and HCN.). 1 dram.

Dose: One dram for adults down to 10 minims for children.

375.

Chlorodyni .... 10 minims.
Syr. ipecac................ 10 minims.
Syr. limonis............... 20 minims.
Syr. pruni virg. ad........ 1 dram.

Cap. ex aqua one-half ounce ter in die vel tussi urgente.

376.

Liq. morphiae hydrochl. .. 48 minims.
Tr. senegae................ 3 drams.
Glycerini .... ½ ounce.
Syr. limonis ad........... 2 ounces.

One dram ter quaterve in die, tusse urgenti, sd.

As a rule, morphia and opium are best eliminated from a cough-linctus, except in those cases of spasmodic teasing cough, violent out of all proportion to the extent of surface involved.

377. COUGH MIXTURES.

Syr. scillae............... 1 ounce.
Ac. hydrobomic. dil....... 6 drams.
Sp. chlorof............... 2 drams.
Aquae ad.................. 8 ounces.
M.

One tablespoonful to be taken every 4 hours.

378.

Am. carb.................. 60 grains.
Vin. ipecac............... 2 drams.
Oxymel. scillae........... 1 ounce.
Ext. glyc. liq. .... 3 drams.
Dec. senegae.............. 1 ounce.
Aq. chlorof. ad........... 8 ounces.
M. Ft. m.

One ounce 4tis horis.

These two mixtures are free from opium, which is a good feature.

379.

Potassae citratis	160 grains.
Acet. ipecac	80 minims.
Tinct. camph. co	2 drams.
Glycerin	4 drams.
Succ. limettae	5 drams.
Syr. scillae	6 drams.
Aquae ad	4 ounces.

M.
St.: C. j. mag. ter die.

380.

Vin. ipecac	2 drams.
Tr. scillae	2 drams.
Tr. opii camph	6 drams.
Spt. chloroform	2 drams.
Glycerini	1 ounce.
Syr. pruni vir	4 drams.
Tr. cocci	1 dram.
Aq. camph. ad	4 ounces.

Dose: Two drams for adults; 1 dram for ten years.

MIXTURES FOR A "COLD" COUGH.

381. Typical Prescription.

Potass. bicarb	2 drams.
Potass. iodid	24 grains.
Tinct. nuc. vom	1½ drams.
Spt. chlorof	1½ drams.
Syr. aurantii	1 ounce.
Aquae ad	6 ounces.

One-half ounce 4tis. horis.

382.

Acid. hydrochl. dil	2 drams.
Vin. ipecac	2 drams.
Liq. opii sed	1 dram.
Ox. scillae	1 ounce.
Syr. pruni virg	1 ounce.
Aq. chlorof. ad	6 ounces.

One-half ounce ter vel quater in die.

383.

Ammonii bromid	10 grains.
Spt. chloroformi	10 minims.
Tinct. camphorae co	10 minims.
Vini Ipecacuanhae	10 minims.
Ext. Byni fluid	2 drams.
Aq. ad	½ ounce.

M. Ft. mistura.
One-half ounce o. q. h. sumenda.

384.

Liq. ammon. acet	2 ounces.
Tinct. scillae	3 drams.
Ext. glycyrrhy. liq	1 ounce.
Succ. conii	½ ounce.
Tinct. camp. co	3 drams.
Inf. senegae ad	6 ounces.

M.
One-half ounce ter die sd.

385.

Syr. rhoeados	40 minims.
Oxy. scillae	½ dram.
Vin. ipecac	15 minims.
Glycerini	½ dram.
Acid. sulph. dil	5 minims.

Sig.: one ounce t. d. in ea. fl. ounce.

386.

Acid. phosph. dil	2 drams.
Vin. ipecac	40 minims.
Glycerine	6 drams.
Tr. camph. co	3 drams.
Tr. scillae	2 drams.
Aq. ad	6 ounces.

M.
One-half ounce 4tis horis ex aquae.

387.

Spt. chlorof	1½ drams.
Tr. camph. co	3 drams.
Vin. ipecac	1 dram.
Liq. ammon. acet	1 ounce.
Syrup. scillae	4 drams.
Mucil. acaciae	4 drams.
Aq. ad	6 ounces.

M. Ft. mist.
White cough-mixture. One tablespoonful three times a day.

388.

Liquor ammon. acet	2 ounces.
Vin. ipecac	1½ drams.
Ox. scillae	6 drams.
Tr. camph. co	2 drams.
Aq. chloroformi ad	8 ounces.

M. Ft. mist.
One ounce 4tis horis, sd.

389.

Pot. citratis	2 drams.
Liq. amm. acet	6 drams.
Tr. camph. co	2 drams.
Vin. ipecac	½ dram.
Oxym. scillae	3 drams.
Inf. cascarill. ad	6 ounces.

M.
One ounce 4tis horis.

390.
>Syr. codeinae............ 3 drams.
>Tr. camph. co............ 3 drams.
>Glycerini .... 6 drams.
>Syr. limonis............. ½ ounce.
>Syr. prun. virg.......... ½ ounce.
>Aquae ad................. 6 ounces.

M.
Sig.: One-half ounce, 2 dis horis sda. ex aqua.

391.
>Oxym. scill.............. 1 ounce.
>Vin. ipec................ 1 dram.
>Tr. camph. co............ 6 drams.
>Glycerini .... 1 ounce.
>Aq. ad................... 8 ounces.

One-half ounce ter die ex aq.

392.
>Vin. antimon............. 2 drams.
>Tr. camph. co............ 4 drams.
>Oxymel. scillae.......... 4 drams.
>Inf. cascarillae ad...... 8 ounces.

M.
One-eighth ter die sd.

393.
>Tr. camph. co............ 4 drams.
>Syrup. tolu.............. 1 ounces.
>Vin. ipecac.............. 4 drams.
>Aq. chloroform. ad....... 8 ounces.

Ft. mist.
St.: One-half ounce c. ½ ounce aquae tussi urgenti.

394.
>Oxy. scillae............. ½ ounce.
>Tinct. camph. co......... ½ ounce.
>Vin. ipecac.............. 2 drams.
>Aq. ad................... 9 ounces.

M.
Cap. one-half ounce 4tis horis.

395.
>Tinct. camph. co......... 4 drams.
>Tinct. scillae........... 3 drams.
>Syr. tolut............... 1 ounce.
>Aquae chloroformi ad..... 8 ounces.

M.
Caplat. one-half ounce tertia hora ex aqua.

396.
>Ammon. carb.............. 1 dram.
>Vin. ipecac.............. 2 drams.
>Chlorodyni .... 2 drams.
>Tinct. stramon........... 2 drams.
>Glycerini .... 1 ounce.
>Inf. senegae ad.......... 6 ounces.

M.
Mixture for spasmodic cough and difficult breathing. One-half ounce ter die sd inter cib.
My objection to all these mixtures is that they contain opium.

CHILDREN'S COUGH SYRUP.

397. **Typical Prescription.**
>Potass. bromidi.......... 24 grains.
>Potass. iodidi........... 6 grains.
>Vin. ipecac.............. 1 dram.
>Spt. chlorof............. 1 dram.
>Liq. ammon. acetatis conc.. 1 dram.
>Syr. aurantii ad......... 1½ ounces.

One dram urg. tuss.

398. For Infantile Bronchial Catarrh (during Dentition).
>Pot. brom................ 20 grains.
>Pot. bicarb.............. 20 grains.
>Vin. ipecac.............. 20 minims.
>Glycer .... 1 dram.
>Syr. simp................ ½ ounce.
>Aq. aneth. ad............ 2 ounces.

M.
Three coch. parv. 3tia 9 hora.

FEVERISHNESS AND COLD IN CHILDREN OVER 1 YEAR AND UNDER 4 YEARS.

399.
>Vin. or acet. ipecac..... 40 minims.
>Liq. am. acet. conc...... 1 dram.
>Spt. aeth. nit........... 1½ drams.
>Syrup. (cold. with liq. cocci) 3 drams.

One coch. min. ter in die.

400.
>Vin. ipecac.............. 1 dram.
>Liq. ammon. acet......... 2 drams.
>Syrup. hemides........... 4 drams.
>Aquae ad................. 3 ounces.

M. Ft. mist.
St.: Coch. med. 4tis horis.

401.
>Sr. tolut................ ½ ounce.
>Vin. ipec................ ½ ounce.
>Sp. am. co............... 1 dram.
>Syr. simp. ad............ 4 ounces.

One dram 3tis horis.

402.
>Potass. citrat........... 1 dram.
>Vin. ipecac.............. 2 drams.
>Syr. tolut............... 6 drams.
>Aq. anisi ad............. 2 ounces.

M.
One dram every 3 or 4 hours.

403.
>Vin. ipecac.............. 2 drams.
>Liq. ammon. acet......... 1 ounce.
>Potas. bicarb............ 1 dram.
>Syrup. tolu.............. ½ ounce.
>Aq. ad................... 4 ounces.

Sig.: A dessertspoonful, etc., according to age.

COUGHS, COLDS, INFLUENZA, ETC.

BRONCHITIS MIXTURES.

404. **Typical Prescription.**

Ammon. carb............	40	grains.
Potass. iodidi............	24	grains.
Tinct. sumbul............	4	drams.
Spt. chloroformi.........	2	drams.
Syr. aurantii.............	6	drams.
Aquae ad................	6	ounces.

One-half ounce 4tis horis.

405.

Ammon. carb..............	3	grains.
Ammon. chlorid...........	1½	grains.
Vini. ipec.................	5	minims.
Glycerin	30	minims.
Syr. pruni virg...........	60	minims.
Aeth. chlor...............	10	minims.
Inf. senegae ad...........	½	ounce.

M. Ft. mist.
Pro dosis.
A good expectorant combination.

406.

Ammon. carb..............	2	scruples.
Tr. camph. co.............	2	drams.
Tr. scillae................	2	drams.
Glycerini	½	ounce.
Inf. senegae ad...........	8	ounces.

M.
One ounce 4tis horis s.

407.

Ammon. carb..............	1	dram.
Spirit. chloroform........	3	drams.
Tinct. scillae.............	3	drams.
Glycerini	6	drams.
Infus. quass. ad..........	6	ounces.

M.
Sig.: A tablespoonful in a glass of water thrice daily.

A smaller dose of ammon. carb. would be better here—say 3 or 4 grains.

408.

Ammon. carb..............	1	dram.
Sp. chloroformi...........	3	drams.
Tinct. scillae.............	3	drams.
Vin. ipecac...............	1	dram.
Ext. glycyrrhizae.........	1	ounce.
Infus. senegae ad.........	6	ounces.

M.
Sig.: A tablespoonful in water thrice daily.

409.

Ammon. carb..............	1	dram.
Vin. ipecac...............	1½	drams.
Tinct. scillae.............	1½	drams.
Spts. chlorof..............	3	drams.
Inf. cascarillae ad........	6	ounces.

Ft. mist.
Cap. one-half ounce 4tis horis.

410.

Amm. carb................	½	dram.
Vin. ipecac...............	1	dram.
Tinct. scillae.............	2	drams.
Sp. chlorof................	2	drams.
Inf. seneg. ad.............	6	ounces.

One-half ounce om. tert. hor.

411.

Ammon. carb..............	½	dram.
Vin. ipecac...............	1½	drams.
Tr. camph. co.............	2	drams.
Spt. chlorof...............	2	drams.
Inf. seneg. ad.............	6	ounces.

Sig.: One-half ounce t. d. s. ex aq. one-half ounce.

412.

Ammon. chlorid...........	1½	drams.
Vin. ipecac...............	2	drams.
Tr. camph. co.............	4	drams.
Ext. glycyrrhiz. liq.......	4	drams.
Aq. ad....................	8	ounces.

One-eighth 4tis horis.

Every one of these eight mixtures would be improved by the addition of 1 to 3 grains of potass. iodidi. I would prefer tinct. serpentariae or tinct. sumbul. to inf. senegae, as the last-mentioned is rather nauseous.

ORDINARY UNCOMPLICATED COLDS.

413. **Typical Prescription.**

Tinct. aconiti.............	1½	drams.
Liq. ammon. acetatis fort..	3	drams.
Spt. aetheris nitrosi.......	3	drams.
Aquae ad.................	6	ounces.

One-half ounce 4tis horis.

414.

Liq. ammon. acet..........	1	ounce.
Sp. aether. nit............	2	drams.
Syr. aurant...............	1	ounce.
Aq. ad....................	8	ounces.

One-half ounce every 4 hours. Smaller doses for children.

415.
    Liq. ammon. acet.......... 3 ounces.
    Sp. aether. nit. .... 2 drams.
    Sp. ammon. arom......... 2 drams.
    Tinct. aconiti............. 24 minims.
    Aq. camph. ad............ 8 ounces.
M. Ft. mist.
One ounce quartis horis.

416.
    Spt. aether. nit............ 1 dram.
    Liq. am. acet. ft.......... 1 dram.
    Mist. sennae co. ad....... 2 ounces.
M. Ft. haust.
H. S. S.
This formula would be excellent in cases complicated with constipation.

417.
    Tinct. aconit.............. 2 minims.
    Potass. nitr............... 5 grains.
    Sp. eth. nit.............. 20 minims.
    Liq. amm. ac. conc........ 10 minims.
    Syr. aurant............... ½ dram.
    Aq. ad.................... 1 ounce.
M.
Ter die sumend.

418.
    Liq. ammon. acet.......... 1½ drams.
    Spt. ammon. arom........ 20 minims.
    Spt. aether. nit........... 20 minims.
    Syr. aurant............... ½ dram.
    Aq. camph. ad............ 1 ounce.
M.
Every 3 or 4 hours.

419.
    Liq. ammon. acet.......... 3 ounces.
    Spt. aeth. nitrosi......... 2 drams.
    Spt. ammon. co. .... 3 drams.
    Potass. bicarb............. 1½ drams.
    Aq. camph. ad............ 8 ounces.
M.
One-sixth part ter die sd.

420.
    Liq. am. acetat............ 1 dram.
    Tinct. carminativ. (B. P. C.) 40 minims.
    Sp. am. aromat........... 40 minims.
    Glycerin .... 2 drams.
    Aq. camph................ 1 ounce.
    Aq. chloroformi ad........ 2 ounces.
M. Ft. haust.
Sumat statim.

421.
    Potass. chlorat............. 1 dram.
    Liq. ammon. acet.......... 2 ounces.
    Spt. aetheris nit........... 4 drams.
    Spt. ammon. aromat....... 2 drams.
    Aquae camph. ad.......... 8 ounces.
Ft. mist.
One-eighth part in water every 3 hours.

422.
    Sp. ammon. co............. ½ ounce.
    Sp. chloroformi........... ½ ounce.
    Liq. ammon. ac. (1-7)..... 3½ drams.
    Sp. camphor.............. 30 minims.
    Syr. tolu. ad............... 2 ounces.
Ft. mist.
For a cold in the head. One dram every 3 or 4 hours in water.

423.
    Pot. nitratis.............. 1 dram.
    Vin. antim................ 1 dram.
    Vin. ipecac................ 1 dram.
    Sp. chlorof................ 2 drams.
    Oxymel scillae............ 1 ounce.
    Aq. ad.................... 8 ounces.
Dose: One-half ounce every 4 hours.

424.
    Spt. aeth. nit.............. 2 drams.
    Liq. amm. conc. .... 2 drams.
    Amm. carb. .... ½ dram.
    Sp. chlorof................ 1½ drams.
    Aq. camph. ad............ 6 ounces.
One ounce 3tus hor.

425.
    Ammon. carb.............. 2 scruples.
    Oxymel scillae............ 6 drams.
    Sp. aether. nit............. 2 drams.
    Aq. camph. ad............ 6 ounces.
For feverish cold. One-sixth part 3 vel 4tis horis.

426.
    Magnes. sulph............ ½ ounce.
    Vin. antim................ ½ dram.
    Spt. aeth. nit.............. 1½ drams.
    Liq. ammon. acet.......... ½ ounce.
    Glycerini .... ½ ounce.
    Aq. ad.................... 8 ounces.
One-eighth part ter die sumend.

427.
 Vin. ipecac.............. 10 minims.
 Sp. aeth. nit.............. 20 minims.
 Liq. ammon. acet.......... 2 drams.
 Syr. tolut................ 1 dram.
 Aquae camph. ad.......... 1 ounce.
 M. Ft. haust.
4tis horis sumd.

428.
 Liq. ammon. acet........ 1½ ounces.
 Sp. aether. nitr........... ½ ounce.
 Vini antimon............. 1 dram.
 Syrupi .... 2 drams.
 Aquae ad................ 6 ounces.
 M.
One ounce 4tis horis.
Spt. aeth. nit. two drams is enough.

429.
 Potass. bicarb............ 1 dram.
 Liq. ammon. acet.......... 1 ounce.
 Sp. aeth. nitr............. 2 drams.
 Vin. ipecac............... 1 dram.
 Spr. chlorof............... 1 dram.
 Aq. camph. ad............ 6 ounces.
 M.
Capt. part. sext. quart. quoq. hor.
The above sixteen mixtures are well adapted for the cure of acute colds.

INFLUENZA COLDS, WITH MUCH ACHING OF LIMBS, ETC.

430.   **Typical Prescription.**
 Ammon. bromidi.......... 2 drams.
 Antipyrin .... 48 grains.
 Syr. aurantii............. 1 ounce.
 Aquae ad................ 6 ounces.
One-half ounce 4tis horis.
Antipyretics of the coal-tar series are particularly useful in colds of an influenza type.

431.
 Salipyrin .... 1½ drams.
 Mucilag. tragac........... 3 drams.
 Syr. aurant.............. 3 drams.
 Aquae ad................ 6 ounces.
 M. Ft. mist.
St.: One ounce 4tis horis.
Found to be very good last winter.

432.
 Liq. ammon. acet......... 1½ ounces.
 Antipyrin .... 1½ drams.
 Syr. simp................. 1 ounce.
 Aq. ad................... 8 ounces.
 M.

Sig.: One-half ounce every 3 hours until pain and fever lessen.
The above two mixtures can often be greatly aided in their action by combining them with bromides.

433.
 Pot. bromid.............. 1½ drams.
 Spt. aether. nit........... 4 drams.
 Tinct. hyoscyami .... 2 drams.
 Vin. ipecac............... 1 dram.
 Liq. ammon. acetatis...... 2 ounces.
 Aquae ad................ 8 ounces.
One ounce 4tis horis.

434.
 Vin. ipecac............... 1½ drams.
 Tr. chlorof. co............ 3 drams.
 Ammon. carb............. 1 dram.
 Ammon. bromidi.......... 2 drams.
 Syr. tolu................. 6 drams.
 Aquae .... 8 ounces.
One-half ounce q. d. s. ex aquae.

435.
 Sodii salicylatis........... 1½ drams.
 Ammon. chloridi .... 1½ drams.
 Potas. nitrat............. 1 dram.
 Tr. aconiti............... 20 minims.
 Tr. hyoscyami............ 1½ drams.
 Ox. scillae............... 1 ounce.
 Aq. camph. ad............ 6 ounces.
One-half ounce om. 2 v. 3 hora ex aq.
Remain indoors; light food.

436.
 Potas. bicarb............. 2 drams.
 Sodae salicylat........... 1½ drams.
 Liq. ammon. acet......... 2 ounces.
 Tinct. camph. co.......... 3 drams.
 Aquae camphorae ad...... 8 ounces.
 M. Ft. mist.
One-eighth part every 4 hours.

The salicylates are also very serviceable, either alone or in combination with coal-tar antipyretics and bromides. Especially is this the case where rheumatism is suspected.

437.
 Tr. quin. ammon.......... 1 ounce.
 Glycerini .... ½ ounce.
 Sp. chlorof............... 1 dram.
 Syr. simpl............... 3 drams.
 M.
One dram every 3 hours.
This is a good type for a "cold" tonic.

438.
    Tr. quininae ammoniatae... 1½ ounces.
    Syr. aurantii............... 1½ ounces.
    M.
    Sig.: A teaspoonful in a glass of water thrice daily.

439.
    Tr. cinchon................ 1 dram.
    Amm. carb................. 4 grains.
    Syr. tolutan............... 1 dram.
    Aq. ad..................... 1 ounce.
    M.
    For incipient cold as evidenced by running at nose.
    To be taken with an equal quantity of water every three hours. Mitte 8 ounces or q. s.

440.
    Spt. amm. co............... ½ ounce.
    Spt. chlorof................ 2 drams.
    Spt. aether. nit............ 2 drams.
    Tr. cinch. co............... ½ ounce.
    Aq. dest. ad............... 8 ounces.
    Cap. one ounce ter in die ex aq.

441.
    Tinct. cinchonae........... ½ ounce.
    Tinct. limonis............. 2 drams.
    Glycerini .... 6 drams.
    Liq. amm. acet............. 1½ ounces.
    Aq. chloroformi............ 3 ounces.
    Aquae ad................... 6 ounces.
    M.
    Cap. one-half ounce 4tis horis ex aqua.

442.
    Potassii citratis........... 1½ drams.
    Liquoris ammonii acetatis
      fortior. .... 3 drams.
    Syrupi limonis............. ½ ounce.
    Aquae chloroformi .... 3 ounces.
    Aquae ad................... 8 ounces.
    Misce. Fiat mistura.
    Sig.: One-sixth part every 6 hours.

443.
    Quininae sulphatis......... 1½ grains.
    Pulveris camphorae........ ½ grain.
    Misce Fiat cachet.
    Sig.: One to be swallowed with each dose of the mixture.
    This is rather too complicated a recipe.

444.
    Spt. ammon. arom.......... 1 dram.
    Spt. aether. nit............ 1 dram.
    Tinct. cinchon. co.......... 2 ounces.
    Aq. camphor............... 2 ounces.
    Aq. chlorof. ad............ 6 ounces.
    One-sixth part in water three times a day.

This group (437 to 444) is of most service to remove the debility of colds, although they are often given with the view of preventing or cutting short influenza and influenza-colds.

I find quinine acts better if combined with antipyrin, ammon bromidi, acid hydrobromic dil., which tend to prevent cinchonism.

In many cases the hypophosphites of lime or soda (with or without cod-liver oil) act better than quinine, especially in the early stages.

CHEST COLDS.

445.
    Vin. ipecac................ 2 drams.
    Spt. amm. aro.............. 2 drams.
    Spt. aetheris .... 2 drams.
    Tinct. senegae .... 2 drams.
    Ox. scillae .... 4 drams.
    Aq. chloroform. ad .... 8 ounces.
    One ounce 4 horis. Bronchitis-kettle to be used, and patients to be kept in one temperature.

446.
    Sp. aether. nit............. 6 drams.
    Sp. ammon. arom.......... 6 drams.
    Sp. chlorof................. 2 drams.
    Ammon. carb. .... 1 dram.
    Infus. senegae ad .... 6 ounces.
    Misce. Fiat mist.
    Cap. One-half ounce ter in die ex aq.

447.
    Tr. aconiti .... 40 minims.
    Oxy. scillae ... . 1½ ounces.
    Tr. camph. co.............. ½ ounce.
    Syr. marubii .... 1 ounce.
    Dec. senegae conc.......... 1 ounce.
    Aquae ad .... 8 ounces.
    M. Ft. mist.
    One-half ounce t. d. s.

448.
    Ammon. carb. .... 32 grains.
    Tinct. scillae .... 80 minims.
    Vin. ipecac................ 80 minims.
    Inf. senegae conc. (1-7).... ½ ounce.
    Syrup. tolu. .... 1 ounce.
    Spt. chlorof............... 2 drams.
    Aq. ad .... 8 ounces.
    M. Ft. mist.
    One ounce ter die.
    The foregoing mixtures would be good in chest colds accompanied by wheezing cough and other bronchial symptoms.

449.
    Sp. am. aromat............. 2 drams.
    Sp. chlorof................. 2 drams.
    Tr. camph. co.............. 4 drams.
    Mist. camph. ad .... 6 ounces.
    One-half ounce 3ts. horis sd.

450.
    Ammon. carb. .... 1 dram.
    Sp. aeth. nit. .... 3 drams.
    Tinct. camph. co. .... 3 drams.
    Sp. chlorof. .... 1 dram.
    Mist. camph. ad .... 6 ounces.
M.
One ounce om. tert. hor. sd.

451.
    Potass. chlorat. .... 5 grains.
    Vin. Ipecac. .... 5 minims.
    Tr. camph. co. .... 15 minims.
    Oxymel. scillae .... 1 dram.
    Liq. ammon. acet. .... 3 drams.
    Aq. anisi ad .... 1 ounce.
Ft. haust. T. d. s.

452.
    Vin. Ipecac. .... ½ dram.
    Liq. amm. acet. .... 2 ounces.
    Tr. camph. co. .... 4 drams.
    Sp. aether. nit. .... 2 drams.
    Syr. tolu. .... ½ ounce.
    Aq. camph. ad .... 8 ounces.
One-eighth part every 3 hours.

453.
    Vin. Ipecac. .... 2 drams.
    Liq. amm. acet. con. .... 3 drams.
    Tinct. camph. co. .... 4 drams.
    Ox. scillae .... 4 drams.
    Inf. senegae conc. .... 1 ounce.
One ounce 4 horis. Linseed poultices every 2 hours.

454.
    Ammon. carb. .... 1 dram.
    Tr. scillae .... 1½ drams.
    Tr. cinchonae co. .... 4 drams.
    Tr. camph. co. .... 2 drams.
    Sp. chlorof. .... 2 drams.
    Aq. ad .... 8 ounces.
M. Ft.
Cap. one ounce ter quaternae die.

455.
    Liquor ammon. acet. .... 1 dram.
    Sp. aether. nit. .... 2 drams.
    Tr. camphor. co. .... 3 drams.
    Vin. antim. tart. .... 1½ drams.
    Syrup tolut. .... 6 drams.
    Aq. camph. ad .... 6 ounces.
M.
One-sixth part 4tis horis.

456.
    Ammon. bicarb. .... ½ dram.
    Tr. camph. co. .... 2 drams.
    Glycerini .... 4 drams.
    Aq. ad .... 6 ounces.
M. Ft. mist.
One-half ounce when the cough is troublesome.

457.
    Liq. ammon. acet. .... 1½ ounces.
    Liq. morph. hydr. .... 1½ drams.
    Aquae chloroformi .... 4 ounces.
    Aquae camph. ad .... 8 ounces.
One-half ounce in forenoon and afternoon. One ounce at bedtime.

458.
    Pot. nit. .... 24 grains.
    Chlorodini .... 2 drams.
    Vin. ant. tart. .... 2 drams.
    Oxymel. scill. .... 1½ ounces.
    Aq. ad .... 6 ounces.
M.
One-half ounce 4tis horis ex. aq.

459.
    Menthol .... 3 grains.
    P. capsic. .... 5 grains.
    P. opii .... ¼ grain.
Ft. pil. 2.
Cap. pil. 2 ter die cum aq. calid.

460.
    Vin. Ipecac. .... 2 drams.
    Liq. morph. hyd. .... 2 drams.
    Syr. scillae .... 1 dram.
    Aq. ad .... 3 ounces.
M.
Sig.: A teaspoonful in water 3 times a day after food.

This group 449 to 460 I regard as objectionable on account of the presence of opium. There are now so many reliable drugs to take its place.

GARGLES.

461.   **Typical Prescription.**
    Acid. sulph. dil. .... 1½ drams.
    Glycerini .... 1 ounce.
    Inf. rosae acid. ad .... 6 ounces.
M.

NON-SECRET FORMULAS.

462.
    Glycer. aluminis .... 1 ounce.
    Glycer. acid. carbol. .... ½ ounce.
    Inf. rosae acid. ad .... 6 ounces.
M. Ft. garg.
    Sig.: A tablespoonful, with an equal quantity of warm water, to be used frequently as a gargle.

463.
    Potassii chlorat. .... 1½ drams.
    Sodii bibor. .... 1½ drams.
    Acid. hydrochlor. dil. ...... 1½ drams.
    Glycerini .... 1 ounce.
    Tinct. capsici .... 10 minims.
    Aquae rosae ad .... 8 ounces.
M. Ft. gargaris.
    Signa.: The gargle to be used frequently as required.

464.
    Pot. chlor. .... 1½ drams.
    Glycer. boracis .... 1 ounce.
    Hazelini .... ½ ounce.
    Tr. hamamelidis .... ½ ounce.
    Aquae ad .... 6 ounces.
M. Ft. garg.
    Sig.: A tablespoonful, with an equal quantity of warm water, to be used frequently as a gargle.

465.
    Acid. tannic. .... 1 scruple.
    Acid. boric. .... 1½ drams.
    Acid. carbolic. liq. .... ½ dram.
    Glycerini .... ½ ounce.
    Aq. rosae ad .... 6 ounces.
Ft. gargar.
Utend one ounce p. r.
    Menthol pastilles .... q. s.
One occasionally.

466.
    Tincturae ferri perch. ...... 1½ drams.
    Potass. chlor. .... 20 grains.
    Glycerini .... ½ ounce.
    Aq. ad .... 2 ounces.
M.
    Sig.: One dram every three hours. Gargle frequently.

467.
    Potass. chlor. .... 1½ drams.
    Glyc. boracis .... ½ ounce.
    Tinct. limonis .... 2 drams.
    Aq. rosae ad .... 8 ounces.
Ft. garg.
Saepe utend.

It is surprising that no u.. is made of sulphur, which is by remedy for sore-throats, especially ated, or with a tendency to diphthe. given early, it will, in nine cases out of arrest the onset of diphtheria.

468.   A Type.
    Sulphur ppt. pur. .... 1½ drams.
    Tinct. aurantii .... 1 dram.
    Glycerini .... 1½ ounces.
    Aquae ad .... 3 ounces.
One dram to be slowly taken hourly.

469.   SORE THROAT MIXTURES.
    Potassii chlorat. .... 1 dram.
    Sodii salicyl. .... 1 dram.
    Antipyrin .... 30 grains.
    Aquae q. s. ad .... 6 ounces.
Misce. Fiat mistura.
Cujus capiat partem sextam quaque quartis horis.
This is a splendid combination for severe sore-throats caused by cold.

470.
    Tinct. ferri perchlor. ...... 1½ drams.
    Mag. sulph. .... *4 drams.
    Pot. chlor. .... ½ dram.
    Glycerini .... 4 drams.
    Aquae ad .... 6 ounces.
Ft. mist.
Cap. one-half ounce 4 hls. (to be swallowed slowly).
*I would prefer sodae sulph.

471.
    Potas. chlorat. .... 2 scruples.
    Potas. nitrat. .... 2 scruples.
    Acid. nit. mur. dil. .... 1½ drams.
    Tr. cinchonae co. .... 4 drams.
    Syr. aurant. .... 1 ounce.
    Aquae ad .... 8 ounces.
M.
One-eighth pt. ter die sd.

472.
    Acid. hydrochlor. dilut. ... 2 drams.
    Tinct. cinchonae comp. .... 4 drams.
    Glycerini .... 1 ounce.
    Tinct. aconiti, B. P. .... 40 minims.
    Spt. chlorof. .... 1½ drams.
    Sol. potassii chlorat. sat. ad. 8 ounces.
M.
    Sig.: One ounce omni quatuor horis. The throat to be slightly gargled before swallowing.

473.

Potassii chloratis	1 dram.
Glycerini acidi carbolici	2 drams.
Liq. ferri perchlor.	2 drams.
Aquae ad	4 ounces.

M.
Sig.: A dessertspoonful in half a wineglassful of water three or four times a day.

474.

Acid. nit. mur. dil.	80 minims.
Tinct. cinchon. co.	1 ounce.
Glycerini	½ ounce.
Aq. chlorof. ad	8 ounces.

M. Ft. mist.
One ounce t. d. s.

475.

Pot. chlor.	10 grains.
Ext. cinch. liq.	10 minims.
Acid. hydroch. dil.	10 minims.
Sp. chlorof.	10 minims.
Aq. ad	1 ounce.

4tis horis sd. Mitte 8 ounce.

476.

Pot. bicarb.	80 grains.
Pot. chlor.	80 grains.
Vin. ipecac.	1 dram.
Liq. morph.	40 minims.
Syr. aurant.	½ ounce.
Aq. ad	8 ounces.

One ounce ter die.
Objectionable from the presence of morphia.

477. Tannin and Rose Gargle.

Acid. tannic.	1 dram.
Pulv. aluminis	½ ounce.
Tr. capsici	1 dram.
Liq. cocci	1 dram.
Syrupi	2 ounces.
Aq. rosae conc.	2 ounces.
Aq. ad	16 ounces.

M. S. A.

CHRONIC RHEUMATISM AND GOUT.

478. Typical Prescription.

Potassae bicarb.	2 drams.
Potass. iodidi	1 dram.
Sodae salicylatis	1 dram.
Vin. colchici	1½ drams.
Inf. buchu ad	6 ounces.

One-half ounce 4tis horis in plenty of water.

The secret of compounding a good mixture for rheumatism consists in having the various ingredients well balanced. Alone, or in unsuitable combination, they might not prove satisfactory.

Many doctors object to the use of colchicum. They do not deny its efficacy in relieving symptoms, but they assert that the disorder returns more readily after its use.

479.

Sodii salicylat.	2 drams.
Pot. iodid.	2 scruples.
Aq. ad.	8 ounces.

M.
Dose for adult: Cap. one ounce 4tis horis.

480.

Potas. bicarb.	2 drams.
Potas. iodidi.	1 dram.
Sp. aeth. nit.	80 minims.
Mag. sulph.	1 ounce.
Vin. colchic.	2 drams.
Aq. chlorof. ad.	8 ounces.

M. Ft. mist.
One ounce ter die sumend.

481.

Pot. iodid.	1½ drams.
Vin. sem. colchici	1½ drams.
Tr. zingib.	1 dram.
Sp. chlorof.	1 dram.
Syrupi	½ dram.
Inf. quassiae ad.	6 ounces.

Dose: One-half ounce ter die.

482.

Potass. iodid.	15 grains.
Potass. nitrat.	½ dram.
Potass. bicarb.	½ dram.
Sp. am. arom.	3 drams.
Aquae ad.	6 ounces.

M.
One ounce 4tis horis.

483.

Salicin	2 drams.
Pot. iod.	1 dram.
Mag. sulph.	½ ounce.
Syr. aurant.	1 ounce.
Aq. ad.	12 ounces.

M.
One ounce bis die.

484.

Sodii salicylat.	3 drams.
Potass. bicarb.	2 drams.
Ess. menth. pip.	10 minims.
Aquae ad.	6 ounces.

M. Ft. mist.
Capiat one-half ounce quaque quarta hora ex aquae.

485.
>Sodii salicylatis............ 10-15 grains.
>Tinct. zingiberis........... 10 minims.
>Aq. ad.................... 1 ounce.
Misce. Ft. mist.
Cujus capiat. one ounce ter quaterve in die.

486.
>Acid salicylic................ 3 drams.
>Soda borat................... 15 grains.
>Aqua menth pip, add......... 4 ounces.
Sig.: One-fourth, to be taken three hours apart.

487.
>Soda salicylate............... 2 drams.
>Potash iodide .... 2 drams.
>Potash carb................... 2 drams.
>Fluid cascara................. 4 ounces.
Formula 57.
Dose: Two teaspoonsful after meals.

488.
>Soda bicarb................... ½ ounce.
>Acid salicylic................ ½ ounce.
>Glycerine .... 2 ounces.
>Water......................... 2 ounces.
S.: Teaspoonful every 3 hours.

489.
>Soda salicylate............... ½ ounce.
>Potash iodide................. ½ ounce.
>Ferri pyrophosphate........... 2 drams.
>Water......................... 6 ounces.
Sig.: One teaspoonful every 8 hours.

490.
>Tr. guaiaci am................ 6 drams.
>Mucilaginis .... 12 drams.
>Lithii cit.................... 1 dram.
>Potass. iod................... 1 scruple.
>Vin. colchic.................. 40 minims.
>Tr. cinch. rub................ 3 drams.
>Aq. ad........................ 8 ounces.
M. Ft. m.
One ounce bis in die.
This is based on an old formula of Sir. A. Garrod. It will cure in many cases when all known remedies fail.

EMBROCATIONS.

491. **Typical Prescription.**
>Chloroform .... 5 drams.
>Tinct. opii................... 4 drams.
>Acid. salicylic............... 4 drams.
>Spt. vini rect. ad............ 12 ounces.
Label "Poison," etc., in blue bottle.

This group is a very weak one. Chloroform, ol. succini rect., ol. cajuput, ol. gaultheriae, etc., might be suggested.

492.
>Ol. sinapis express........... 1 ounce.
>Lin. tereb. acet.............. 2 ounces.
M.

493.
>Vitell. ovi................... 1
>Sp. terebinthae............... 3 ounces.
>Aq. destill................... 3 ounces.
>Acid. acetic. fort............ ½ ounce.
M. Ft. linimentum.
Also for sprains. The parts affected to be well rubbed, night and morning.

494.
>Lin. ammoniae................. 2 ounces.
>Lin. opii..................... 2 ounces.
>Ol. terebinth................. 2 ounces.
M. Ft. lin.
Sig.: To be well rubbed in night and morning.

495.
>Ol. terebinth................. 1 ounce.
>Lin. camph.................... 1 ounce.
>Liquor. ammon................. 1 ounce.
M. Ft. liniment.
Sig.: Rub well the affected parts and bind with flannel.

496.
>Ext. belladonnae alcohol...... ½ ounce.
>Menthol .... 1 dram.
>Acidi oleici.................. ½ ounce.
>Lanolin .... ½ ounce.
>Adipis benz................... ½ ounce.
Misce. Ft. unguentum.
Nocte maneque partibus affectis applicandum.

497. DIURETIC MIXTURE.
>Potas. acet................... 2 drams.
>Sp. ether. nit................ 3 drams.
>Sp. junip..................... 3 drams.
>Acet. scillae................. 2 drams.
>Suc. scoparii................. 6 drams.
>Aq. ad........................ 6 ounces.
M.
One-half ounce ter in die.
This would be a typical diuretic mixture if tinct. digitalis one dram to two drams, or tinct. strophanthus one-half dram to one dram were added thereto.

FOR BACKACHE, THICK URINE AND KIDNEY DISORDERS.

498.
- Pot. bicarb............... 2 drams.
- Tinct. hyoscyami......... 4 drams.
- Pot. nit.................. 1 dram.
- Syrupi .... 1 ounce.
- Inf. buchu ad............. 8 ounces.
- Ft. mist.
- Cap. one-half ounce om. qts. horis.

499. EARACHE.
- Glycerini acidi carbolici.... ½ ounce.

Signetur.: Guttae nocte maneque utendae. This seldom fails to give relief, and is well recommended by several aurists. A little spt. vini rect. would increase its efficacy if any discharge be present.

DIARRHŒA.

500. (FERMENTATIVE.)
- Olei cassiae .... 8 minims.
- Sacchr. alb........ 1 dram. 1 scruple.
- Cretae prep........ 1 dram. 1 scruple.
- Tr. opii........... 1 dram. 1 scruple.
- Sp. ammon. co..... 1 dram. 1 scruple.
- Tr. catechu................ 2 drams.
- Sp. camph................. 12 minims.
- Aq. camphorae ad. .... 6 ounces.
- Ft. mist.

Sig.: One-half ounce to one dram when required.

When, as is sometimes the case, diarrhœa does not yield to mineral acids and opium, such mixtures as the foregoing are good.

501.
- Sodii bicarb............... 2 drams.
- Mucil. acaciae............. 1 ounce.
- Creta prep................. 2 drams.
- Pulv. conf. aromat. P.L.... 1½ drams.
- Ol. cassiae................ 6 minims.
- Ol. menth. pip............. 9 minims.
- Syr. simplic............... ½ ounce.
- Spt. ammon. arom.......... 3 drams.
- Spt. chlorof............... 3 drams.
- Tinct. opii................ 2 drams.
- Aq. ad..................... 6 ounces.
- M.

Adult dose: One-half ounce.

502.
- Tr. opii................... 2½ drams.
- Aether. chlor.............. 1 dram.
- Spt. cinnam................ 2 drams.
- Spt. camphor............... 1 dram.
- Tr. catechu................ 1 dram.
- P. conf. arom.............. 3 drams.
- P. sodii bicarb............ 1 dram.
- P. gum. acac............... 2 drams.
- Aquae ad................... 10 ounces.
- M.

One ounce every two or three hours if required.

503.
- Liq. bismuthi.............. 1 dram.
- Tr. nucis vom.............. 8 minims.
- Spt. chlorof............... 10 minims.
- Acid. hydrocy. dil......... 2 minims.
- Morphinae mur.............. 1/24 grain.
- Pepsin. porci.............. 2 grains.
- Tinct. croci............... q. s.
- Aquae .... ½ ounce.

The last I keep prepared as a stock-mixture, and the quantity named is for one dose—to be given every 3 or 4 hours.

504.
- Tinct. catechu............. ½ ounce.
- Ol. menth. pip............. 6 minims.
- Pulv. cret. aromat. .... 90 grains.
- Mist. cretae ad............ 8 ounces.

Sig.: One-eighth part after each loose motion.

Eight drops tr. opii may be added to each dose.

505.
- Tr. catechu................ 10 minims.
- Tr. opii................... 10 minims.
- Mist. cretae ad............ 1 ounce.
- Ft. mist. 8 ounces.

One ounce every two hours till relieved.

506.
- Bismuth. carb.............. 2 drams.
- Tr. opii................... 40 minims.
- Tr. catechu................ 3 drams.
- Mist. cretae ad............ 4 ounces.

Dose: One-half ounce every three hours.

507.
- Liq. opii sed.............. 20 minims.
- Spt. chlorof............... 1½ drams.
- Tr. cinnamom............... 2 drams.
- Tr. zingiber............... 1½ drams.
- Tr. catechu................ 1 dram.
- Aq. camph. ad.............. 6 ounces.
- M. Ft. mist.

A fourth part to be taken every three hours.

GONORRHŒA MIXTURES.

508.
- Ol. santal. flav. .... 2 drams.
- Pot. bicarb. .... 2 drams.
- P. acaciae. .... q. s.
- Aq. menth. pip. ad. .... 8 ounces.

One ounce t. d. s. p. c.

509.
- Olei santali flav. aug. ...... ½ ounce.
- Olei cubebae. .... 1 dram.
- Olei juniperi. .... 6 minims.
- Syrupi aurantii. .... 1½ ounces.
- Extracti Bynl fluidi. .... 2½ ounces.
- Mucilaginis tragacanth.
  quantum sufficiat ad. .... 6 ounces.

M. Fiat mistura.

Cap. one-half ounce ter in die cum aquae cyatho vinoso decocti hordei.

These are excellently-combined mixtures, but I would prefer to have the ol. santal. given separately in capsule form, on account of taste, etc.

510. IN THE FIRST STAGES.
- Sp. aeth. nit. .... ½ ounce.
- Tinct. hyoscy. .... ½ ounce.
- Potass. bicarb. .... ½ ounce.
- Inf. buchu. ad. .... 8 ounces.

M.

Sig.: One-half ounce three times daily, after food.

Giving the usual directions about food, etc.

RINGWORM.

511.
- Hydrarg. subchlor. .... 20 grains.
- Tinct. iodi. .... ½ ounce.

M.

Sig.: Paint the clear liquid to the part night and morning.

Don't shake the bottle. This remedy is unfailing.

A very good remedy.

512.
- Thymol .... 10 grains.
- Sulph. praecip. .... 30 grains.
- Hydrarg. ammon. .... 20 grains.
- Vaselini .... 1 dram.
- Lanolini ad. .... 1 ounce.

ITCH.

513.
- Liq. arsen. .... 1 dram.
- Mist. albae. .... 4 ounces.
- Aquae menth. pip. ad. ...... 8 ounces.

Ft. mist.

One-half ounce t. d. s. p. c.

Why use a mixture for a purely local affair (unless for the purpose of amusing the sufferer, and keeping his mind off the skin).

514.
- Pot. carb. .... ½ dram.
- Ess. limonis. .... 10 minims.
- Ung. sulph. .... 2 ounces.

Ft. ung.

Circumfrico n. m. que.

This is a very effective ointment.

515. FOR SLEEPLESSNESS.
- Potass. bromid. .... 20 grains.
- Sodii bromid. .... 10 grains.
- Tinct. chloroform. co. ...... 30 minims.
- Aquae ad. .... 1 ounce.

M. Ft. haust.

Hora somni.

Some inf. valerian. would improve this mixture if trouble or worry is the cause of the insomnia.

TENDER FEET.

516.
- Pulv. acid. boracic. .... 8 ounces.
- Carmini .... 5 grains.
- Otto de rosae. .... 2 minims.

Misce bene.

Signe.: The powder to be dusted with a puff on the feet every morning.

A usual formula.

REMEDIES FOR CHILDREN'S AILMENTS.

517. SOOTHING SYRUP.
- Ammon. bromid. .... ½ dram.
- Syr. rhei .... 4 drams.
- Ess. anisi (1-10). .... 10 minims.
- Syrupi .... 4 drams.
- Aq. anethi ad .... 1½ ounces.

M.

One dram 2dis hor.

FOR TEETHING, FEVERISHNESS AND FLATULENCE IN CHILDREN.

518. (Up to 6 months.)
Potass. bicarb. .... 1 grain.
Potass. bromid. .... 1 grain.
Tinct. chloroformi co. ..... 2 minims.
Syr. simplicis .... 20 minims.
Aquae ad .... 1 dram.

519. (Up to 1 year.)
Potass. bicarb. .... 1½ grains.
Potass. bromid. .... 1½ grains.
Tinct. chloroformi co. ..... 3 minims.
Syr. simplicis .... 30 minims.
Aquae ad .... 1 dram.

520. (Up to 2 years.)
Potass. bicarb. .... 2 grains.
Potass. bromid. .... 2 grains.
Tinct. chloroformi co. ..... 4 minims.
Syr. simplicis .... 30 minims.
Aquae ad .... 2 drams.

GRIPE MIXTURE.

521. Typical Prescription.
Sodae bicarb. .... 15 grains.
Pulv. rhei .... 15 grains.
Spt. myrist. .... 15 minims.
Tinct. zingib. .... 5 minims.
Syrupi .... 4 drams.
Aquae ad .... 1½ ounces.
One dram p. r. n. sum.

522.
Pulv. rhei .... 8 grains.
Mag. carb. .... 40 grains.
Syr. zingib. .... 40 minims.
Glycerini .... 2 drams.
Aq. anethi ad .... 2 ounces.
One-half dram vel. one dram when required.

523. THRUSH.
Glyc. ac. borac.
Undoubtedly the best application for thrush.

FOR BED-WETTING IN CHILDREN.
524.
Tinct. belladon. .... 1 dram.
Syr. ferri phosph. comp. ... 1 ounce.
Aquae ad .... 2 ounces.
M.
Sig.: A teaspoonful night and morning.
If not caused by worms, this is a very good mixture.

FOR A CHILD WHO IS FEVERISH AND HAS A LITTLE RASH.
525.
Sod. bicarb. .... 1 scruple.
Spt. aeth. nit. .... 1 dram.
Liq. ammon. acet. .... 3 drams.
Vin. ipecac .... 1 dram.
Aq. ad .... 3 ounces.
M. Ft. mist.
Two drams quartis horis sumend.

526.
Hyd. subchlor. .... 2 grains.
Pulv. jalapae. .... 8 grains.
Sacch. lactis. .... 10 grains.
M. Divid. in pulv. four.
Capt. one omni nocte.
An excellent cooling mixture; but aperients are unadvisable in cases of infectious disease, especially so in measles.

527. FOR THREADWORMS.
Sodii chloridi. .... 2 ounces.
From a teaspoon to a tablespoonful to be dissolved in a small quantity of warm water, and injected into the rectum every or every other night.
Injections perseveringly used almost invariably cure, but they must not be discontinued too soon.

528. (Child 12 years.)
Hyd. subchlor. .... 1½ grains.
Santonin. .... 3 grains.
H. s. s.
Scam. res. .... 2 grains.
Pulv. rhei .... 8 grains.
Santonin only expels round worms. If used for threadworms, its action would probably be but temporary.

DIARRHŒA.
All these remedies will prove excellent in cases of diarrhoea.
Diarrhoea is one of the few diseases which distinctly call for the use of opium.

529.
Acid. sulph. dil. .... 2 drams.
Tr. cardam. co. .... ½ ounce.
Tr. opii .... 1 dram.
Spt. chlorof. .... 2 drams.
Tr. capsici .... 20 minims.
Aq. ad .... 4 ounces.
Sig.: One-half ounce every two hours ex aq. till relieved.

NON-SECRET FORMULAS.

530.
    Tinct. opii .... 1 dram.
    Acid. sulph. dil. .... 1½ drams.
    Tr. lavand. co. .... 1½ drams.
    Aq. menth. pip. ad .... 6 ounces.
M. Ft. mist.
One ounce every 2 hours.

531
    Acid. sulph. dil. .... 10 minims.
    Tinct. opii .... 5 minims.
    Tinct. card. co. .... 1 dram.
    Ess. menth. pip. .... 10 minims.
    Aquae ad .... 1½ ounces.
Pro. dos.
Preceded by a dose of ol. ricini.

532.
    Acidi sulph. dil. .... 2 drams.
    Tr. opii .... 1 dram.
    Syr. gummi rubra. .... 1 ounce.
    Syr. zingiberis .... 1 ounce.
    Aq. cinnam. ad .... 6 ounces.
One-half ounce every three hours, or after each liquid motion.

533.
    Acid. sulph. aromat. ...... 15 minims.
    Tinct. chloroformi et morph 10 minims.
    Aquae chloroform ad .... 1 ounce.
M. Ft. haust.
4tis horis si opus sit.

534.
    Tinct. opii .... 10 minims.
    Ac. sulph. dil. .... 10 minims.
    Aether chlor. (1-10)........ 10 minims.
    Aq. ad .... 1 ounce.
Misce.
Every 4 hours.

535.
    Ac. sulph. arom. .... 2 drams.
    Tinct. opii .... 1½ drams.
    Aquae chlorof. ad .... 6 ounces.
Ft. mist.
Cap. one-half ounce 3 vel 4tis horis ex aquae.

536.
    Acid. sulph. dil. .... 2 drams.
    Spt. chlorof. .... 2 drams.
    Tinct. opii .... 1½ drams.
    Syr. aurant. flor. .... 1 ounce.
    Inf. rosae acid. ad .... 6 ounces.
M. Ft. mist.
Sig.: A tablespoonful every 3 hours in a little water.

537.
    Tinct. opii .... 10 minims.
    Ac. sulph. dil. .... 10 minims.
    Aq. chlorof. ad .... 1 ounce.
M.
Ter die sumend.

538
    Tinct. opii .... 1½ drams.
    Tinct. kino. .... 1 ounce.
    Tinct. catechu ad .... 2 ounces.
M.
Sig.: One dram after every loose motion.

APERIENT REMEDIES.

Aperients are indicated when indigestible food or some irritant is causing disturbance and requires removal.

539.
    Tinct. opii .... 25 minims.
    Ol. ricini .... 3 drams.
    Aq. chlorof. ad .... 1½ ounces.
Ft. haust.
Much used in the Tropics.

540.
    Hyd. c. creta .... 1 grain.
    P. ipec. co. .... 4 grains.
    P. zingib. .... 3 grains.
M. Ft. pulv. Mitte six.
Sig.: One every 3 or 4 hours.
    Olei ricini .... ½ ounce.
Statim sumendus cum lacti.

541.
    Bismuthi carbonatis .... 2 drams.
    Mucilaginis tragacanth. .... 1 ounce.
    Tinct. chloroformi et morphinae .... 1 dram.
    Aquae q. s. ad .... 6 ounces.
Misce. Fiat mistura.
Cujus capiat cochleare amplum una hora post oleum, et repetatur dosis post singulus sedes liquidus.

542. INFANTILE BRONCHITIS.
    Tr. camph. co. .... 1 dram.
    Vin. ipecac. .... 1 dram.
    Sp. aeth. nit. .... 1 dram.
    Sp. ammon. co. .... 1 dram.
    Liq. ammon. acet. .... 6 drams.
    Aquae chlorof. ad .... 2 ounces.
M. Ft. mist.
One dram tertia hors, if necessary.

543.
    Tr. camph. co. .... 4 minims.
    Vin. ipecac. .... 4 minims.
    Glycerini .... 10 minims.
    Liq. amm. acet. .... 10 minims.
    Aq. m. pip. ad .... 1 dram.
    O. 4tis hor.

544.
    Liq. ammon. acet. .... 4 drams.
    Vin. ipecac. .... 1 dram.
    Ol. amygd. dulc. .... 2 ounces.
    Syrup. rhoeados ad .... 4 ounces.
    M. Ft. mist.
    One dram sv. 4 hor.

545.
    Vin. ipecac. ....
    Ol. amygd. dulc. ....
    Syr. papav. ....
    Syr. tolut. ....
    Syr. scillae .... aa. part. aeq.
    M.
    Dose: One-half dram to one and one-half dram 3 or 4 times a day.
    Opium in any form is objectionable.

FEVERISHNESS AND COLD IN CHILDREN
546. OVER 1 AND UNDER 4 YEARS.
    Potass. chlor. .... 32 grains.
    Acid. nit. mur. dil. .... 40 minims.
    Tr. aconit. .... 20 minims.
    Sp. aeth. nit. .... 80 minims.
    Tr. hyoscyami .... 80 minims.
    Glycerin. .... ½ ounce.
    Syrup. .... ½ ounce.
    Aq. ad .... 4 ounces.
    Two drams 2nd horis.
    All the formulae here printed will well answer their purpose.

547.
    Vin. ipecac. .... 1 dram.
    Ammon. carb. .... 10 grains.
    Syr. scillae .... 2 drams.
    Glycerini .... 2 drams.
    Ext. glycyrrh. liq. .... 20 minims.
    Aq. anisi ad .... 2 ounces.
    One dram every 3 or 4 hours for child over 1 year old.

548.
    Vin. ipecac. .... 2 drams.
    Glycerini .... 4 drams.
    Syr. scillae .... 3 drams.
    Inf. senegae ad .... 4 ounces.
    M.
    Sig.: One dram 3 or 4 times a day.

549.
    Pot. nit. .... 24 grains.
    Oxym. scill. .... 3 drams.
    Syr. papav. .... 1 dram.
    Vin. antim. .... 40 minims.
    Aq. ad .... 3 ounces.
    Two drams ter die.

550. DIARRHŒA. (Fermentative.)
    Bismuth. salicyl. .... 2 drams.
    Salol. .... 2 drams.
    P. tragac. co. .... q. s.
    Sodii bicarb. .... 1½ drams.
    Chlorodyni .... 80 minims.
    Aq. cinnam. ad .... 8 ounces.
    M.
    Sig.: One-eighth every two hours till relieved.

This is a good prescription for fermentative changes in the intestines, although liq. hydrarg. perchlor. in ordinary doses usually gives better results.

551.
    Tinct. chlorof. et morph. . 2 drams.
    Tinct. rhei comp. .... 2 drams.
    Aq. menth. pip. ad .... 1 ounce.
    M.
    Sig.: A teaspoonful in three of water when required.

552.
    Pulv. gum acaciae .... 2 drams.
    Creta preparat. .... 2 drams.
    Confect: aromat. .... 2 drams.
    Tinct. opii .... 2 drams.
    Tinct. catechu .... ½ ounce.
    Spt. ammon. arom. .... 2 drams.
    Aquae cinnamom. ad ..... 8 ounces.
    One-half ounce tertiisve quaternis horis.

553.
    Pulv. conf. aromat. .... 1½ drams.
    Pulv. pro. mist. cretae .... 2 drams.
    Potass. bicarb. .... 1½ drams.
    Sp. ammon. ar. .... 1½ drams.
    Liq. opii sed. (Battley). ... 40 minims.
    Tr. cinnam. co., L. P. ..... 6 drams.
    Aether. chlor. .... 1½ drams.
    Aq. ad .... 8 ounces.
    One ounce p. r. n.

554.
    Pulv. cret. arom. .... ½ ounce.
    Tinct. opii .... 2 drams.
    Tinct. catechu .... 1 dram.
    Sp. chlorof. .... 3 drams.
    Aq. menth. pip. ad .... 8 ounces.
    M. Ft. mist.
    One-half ounce ad one ounce tertis horis until relieved.

555.
    Confect. aromat. .... 4 drams.
    Tr. catechu .... 2 drams.
    Tr. krameria .... 2 drams.
    Tr. zingib. .... 2 drams.
    Aq. camph. ad .... 8 ounces.
    Ft. mist.
    St.: One ounce bis vel ter die.

556.
    Sodii bicarb. .... 3 drams.
    Pulv. conf. arom. .... 4 drams.
    Tr. rhei .... 1½ ounces.
    Tr. card. co. .... 1½ ounces.
    Sp. ammon. co. .... ½ ounce.
    Chlorodyni .... 3 drams.
    Tr. krameriae .... 3 drams.
    Tr. catechu .... 6 drams.
    Ol. menth. pip. .... 10 minims.
    Aquae ad .... 16 ounces.
    Adult dose: One-half ounce to one ounce ter die.
    This is for stock bottle. Supply six ounces bottles when required.

557.
    P. cret. aromat. .... 2 drams.
    P. cret. praep. .... 2 drams.
    Chlorodyni .... 1½ drams.
    Tr. catechu .... 2½ drams.
    Sp. ammon. co. .... 2½ drams.
    Sp. chloroformi .... 1 dram.
    Glycerini .... ½ ounce.
    Aq. meth. pip. ad .... 8 ounces.
    One ounce om. 3 vel 4tis hor. vel p. r. n.

558. WHOOPING COUGH.
    Pot. bromid. .... 1 dram.
    Acid. carbolic. .... 16 minims.
    Tr. belladon. .... 1 dram.
    Vin. ipecac. .... 1½ drams.
    Syr. tolu. .... 6 drams.
    Aquae ad .... 4 ounces.
    Coch. one med. 3tis horis.
    (For children from 2-5 years of age.)

559.
    Ac. carbol. .... 15 grains.
    Tr. bellad. .... 40 minims.
    Vin. ipecac. .... 2 drams.
    Glycerini .... 4 drams.
    Aquae ad .... 3 ounces.
    Ft. mist.
    Cap. one dram 4tis horis.

560.
    Syrup. rhoeados. .... 2 ounces.
    Syrup. simplicis .... 2 ounces.
    Vin. ipecac. .... 6 drams, 24 minims.
    Tr. belladonnae .... 3 drams, 12 minims.
    Tr. lobeliae .... 6 drams, 24 minims.
    Ammon. bromid. .... 3 drams, 12 grains.
    Aquae ad .... 8 ounces.

Dose: One-half dram to two drams, according to age.

These formulae are excellent for whooping-cough, the first being, to my idea, the best.

The value of these remedies would be enhanced by frequent chest-frictions of Roche's embrocation and the burning of cresolene in the sick-room.

561. Teething Powder for Child 1 year.
    Mag. carb. pond. .... 4 grains.
    Pot. brom. pulv. .... 1 grain.
    Hyd. subchlor. .... 1/3 grain.
    Sacch. lact. .... 5 grains.
    Ft. pulv. one.

562.   (Under 6 months.)
    Hyd. c. creta .... ¼ grain.
    Mag. carb. pond. .... 1 grain.
    Pulv. sacchar. alb. .... ¾ grain.

563.   (6 months to 1 year.)
    Hyd. c. creta .... ½ grain.
    Mag. carb. pond. .... 1½ grains.
    Pulv. sacchar. alb. .... 1 grain.

564.   (1 to 2 years.)
    Hyd. c. creta .... 1 grain.
    Mag. carb. pond. .... 2 grains.
    Pulv. sacchar. alb. .... 1 grain.
    The usual form of teething-powder. Mothers should be warned not to give them too frequently, as the free dosing of children with mercurials tends to impair the vitality of their teeth.

565.   Soothing Syrup.
    Potass. bromid. .... 6 grains.
    Sodae bicarb. .... 1 dram.
    Glycerini .... 2 dram.
    Sacch. ust. .... q. s.
    Aq. anethi ad .... 1½ ounces.
    Average dose one dram.
    Rather more bromide would be better here, and more glycerine and flavouring added to disguise its saline taste.

566. Diarrhœa Mixture for Children.
    Bismuth. subnitrat. .... ½ dram.
    Tr. camph. comp. .... 1 dram.
    Liq. hydrarg. perchlor. ..... 15 minims.
    Syrupi .... ½ ounce.
    Aq. ad .... 2 ounces.
    Triturate the bismuth for three minutes before adding the water and other ingredients.
    Doses: For children of one to two years, half a teaspoonful; two to five, a small teaspoonful; above five, a whole teaspoonful every three hours.

CHILDREN'S MEDICINES.

The staff of the Evelina Hospital for Sick Children, Southwark, London, have recently published a second edition of the Pharmacopoeia of the hospital, through Messrs. J. & A. Churchill, 7 Great Marlborough Street, W. The little book contains a large number of good prescriptions for children, and as this is a department of knowledge which it takes the general practitioner a long time to master, we are not surprised to hear that the first edition of the work was quickly exhausted. Perhaps the best way to convey an idea of the Pharmacopoeia is to quote a few of the prescriptions, which we accordingly subjoin.—"Chemist and Druggist, London."

567. Linctus Infantilis.
Take of—
- Compound tincture of camph. 2½ minims.
- Ipecacuanha wine .... 2½ minims.
- Glycerine .... 20 minims.
- Peppermint-water to ...... 1 fl. dram.

Mix.
Dose: One fluid dram.

568. Mistura Bismuthi Sedativa.
Take of—
- Carbonate of bismuth ...... 3 grains.
- Carbonate of sodium .... 3 grains.
- Solution of hydrochlorate of morphine .... 1½ minims.
- Compound powder of tragacanth .... 1¼ grains.
- Dill-water to .... 1 fl. dram.

Mix.
Dose: One fluid dram.

569. Mistura Carminativa.
Take of—
- Aromatic spirit of ammonia 2 minims.
- Tincture of ginger .... 1 minim.
- Compound tincture of cardamoms .... 3 minims.
- Dill-water to .... 1 fl. dram.

Mix.
Dose: One fluid dram.

570. Mistura Stomachica.
Take of—
- Carbonate of sodium .... 2 grains.
- Syrup of ginger .... 2½ minims.
- Aromatic spirit of ammonia 4 minims.
- Infusion of rhubarb .... 30 minims.
- Compound infusion of gentian to .... 1 fl. dram.

Mix.
Dose: One fluid dram.

571. Pulvis Acidi Borici Compositus.
Take of—
- Powdered boric acid ....
- Powdered starch .... } equal parts.
- Powdered oxide of zinc ....

Mix.
For local application.

572. Pulvis Santonini Compositus.
Take of—
- Santonin .... 1 grain.
- Compound powder of scammony .... 2½ grains.
- Calomel .... ½ grain.

Mix.
Dose: Four grains.

The dose in each case is for a child six months old. It is a pity that brief notes on the uses of the preparations are not added.

573. Cough Mixture for Children.
- Ammon. carb. .... 15 grains.
- Vin. ipecac. .... 2 drams.
- Syr. scillae .... 3 drams.
- Syr. limonis .... 1 ounce.
- Tr. croci .... 10 minims.
- Aq. ad .... 3 ounces.

M.
Sig.: For children of one year and upwards a teaspoonful to a dessertspoonful, according to age, thrice daily.

574. Whooping Cough Mixture.
- Codeinae .... 1 grain.
- Acid. phosphoric. dil. .... ½ dram.

Dissolve and add—
- Acid. hydrocyan. dil. .... 8 minims.
- Syr. tolutan. .... 1 ounce.
- Aq. ad .... 4 ounces.

M.
Dose: A teaspoonful every four hours.

COUGHS, COLDS, ETC.

575. Adam's Cough Cure.
- Syrup wild cherry .... 24 ounces.
- Syrup tar .... 16 ounces.
- Syrup squills .... 12 ounces.
- Syrup ipecac. .... 4 ounces.
- Tinct. opium camphorated.. 4 ounces.
- Tinct. sanguinaria .... 2 ounces.
- Chloroform .... ½ ounce.
- Arom. spts. ammonia ...... 1 ounce.
- Caramel .... ½ ounce.

576. Standard Cough Syrup.

Syrup squills	1 gallon.
Syrup tolu	1 gallon.
Syrup ipecac	1 gallon.
Paregoric	1 gallon.
Chlorodyne	8 ounces.
Muriate ammonia	32 ounces.

Add the chlorodyne to the syrups. Dissolve the muriate of ammonia in as little water as possible and mix altogether.

577. Brompton Hospital Cough Specific.

Brompton Hospital Cough-specific, copied from the original recipe of the late Charles Hardy, Fulham Road, London:

Treacle	64 pounds.
Water	3½ gallons.
Chloroform	2 ounces.
Essence of lemon	2¼ ounces.
Laudanum	40 ounces.
Dilute sulphuric acid	40 ounces.

Mix.

578. Bronchelixir.

Tinct. opium camphorated.	4 ounces.
Spirits nitrous ether	2½ ounces.
Spirits am. arom.	1½ ounces.
Tinct. senega	1½ ounces.
Wine of antimony	1 ounce.
Spirits of chloroform	1 ounce.
Spirits of camphor	¾ ounce.
Glycerine	3¾ ounces.

Mix the above in order printed; let stand for 48 hours, then filter. Dose: Adults one teaspoonful to be taken in a wineglass of water two or three times a day.

Children from ¼ to ½ a teaspoonful, according to age.

579. Balsam of Honey and Aniseed.

Tincture balsam, tolu, soluble	16 ounces.
Honey	32 ounces.
Syrup simple	24 ounces.
Water	16 ounces.
Alcohol	8 ounces.
Oil anise	¼ ounce.
Muriate of ammonia	4 ounces.
Tartar emetic	48 grains.
Sulphate of morphia	48 grains.
Caramel	¼ ounce.

M. S. A.

Adult dose: One teaspoonful.

580. Rock Candy, Hoarhound and Tolu.

Rock candy syrup	8 gallons.
Hoarhound	½ pound.
Tincture balsam, tolu, soluble	½ gallon.
Chloroform	4 ounces.
Muriate of ammonia	8 ounces.
Tartar emetic	320 grains.
Sulphate of morphia	320 grains.
Oil bitter almonds	320 minims.
Alcohol	1 gallon.
Caramel to color	4 ounces.
Water q. s. to make	10 gallons.

Make an infusion of the hoarhound with 3 pints of the water, and add to the syrup then add the soluble tolu.

Dissolve the muriate of ammonia, tartar emetic and sulphate of morphia in another portion of the water. Dissolve the oil of bitter almonds and chloroform in the alcohol. Mix and add enough water to measure ten gallons. Color with caramel.

Adult dose one teaspoonful.

581. Tar, Tolu and Wild Cherry.

Syrup simple	6 gallons.
Syrup of wild cherry	1 gallon.
Pine tar	1 ounce.
Carb. magnesia	2 ounces.
Sweet spirits nitre	16 ounces.
Tinct. balsam tolu, soluble	½ gallon.
Muriate of ammonia	8 ounces.
Tartar emetic	320 grains.
Sulphate of morphia	320 grains.
Oil of bitter almonds	160 minims.
Alcohol, 188 per cent	1 gallon.
Caramel	4 ounces.
Vinegar of squills	32 ounces.
Water q. s. to make	10 gallons.

Rub the pine tar with carb. magnesia in mortar; add one quart of boiling water; agitate well and let stand for twelve hours; filter and add to the syrups. Add vinegar of squills, tinct. balsam tolu and caramel, separately. Add the sweet spirits nitre and oil of bitter almonds to the alcohol and mix with the syrups.

Dissolve the muriate of ammonia, morphine and tartar emetic in the remainder of the water and add; stir well and strain. Let stand for twenty-four hours before bottling.

Adult dose one teaspoonful.

582. Tar and Wild Cherry.

Sugar house syrup	6 gallons.
Syrup of wild cherry	1 gallon.
Pine tar	1 ounce.
Carb. magnesia	2 ounces.
Laudanum	½ gallon.
Tartar emetic	480 grains.

Muriate of ammonia	8	ounces.
Oil of bitter almonds	160	minims.
Alcohol, 188 per cent	½	gallon.
Vinegar of squills	32	ounces.
Caramel	10	ounces.
Water, q. s. to make	10	gallons.

Rub the pine tar with carb. magnesia in mortar, add one quart of boiling water, agitate well and let stand for twelve hours; filter and add to syrup, then add laudanum, caramel and vinegar of squills, separately; dissolve the oil of bitter almond in the alcohol and mix with the syrups. Dissolve the muriate of ammonia and tartar emetic in the remainder of the water and strain.

Adult dose one teaspoonful.

583. White Pine Expectorant.

First make tinct. white pine and balm of Gilead.

Liquor potassa	2	ounces.
Oil of turpentine	2	ounces.
Liquid styrax	2	ounces.
Balsam tolu	2	ounces.
Carb. magnesia	6	ounces.
Alcohol, 188 per cent	9	ounces.
Boiling water	1	quart.

Mix the liquor potassa and oil of turpentine with the liquid styrax; dissolve the balsam tolu in the alcohol by the aid of a water bath. Place the carbonate of magnesia in a mortar and pour on the styrax, turpentine and liquor potassa, rub the solution thoroughly with the carbonate of magnesia, add the tolu dissolved in the alcohol. After rubbing to a smooth consistency, gradually add to the mixture the boiling water, stirring them well together, set aside for twelve hours, then filter; adding through the filter sufficient water to make the product measure a quart.

584. White Pine Expectorant.

Tinct. white pine and balm of gilead	2	pints.
Rock candy syrup	7	gallons.
Syrup of wild cherry	1	gallon.
Chloroform	5¼ fl.	ounces.
Acetate of morphia	320	grains.
Tincture of bloodroot	10	ounces.
Oil of sassafras	30	minims.
Oil of bitter almonds	60	minims.
Oil of cloves	60	minims.
Alcohol, 188 per cent	1	gallon.
Tartar emetic	320	grains.
Muriate of ammonia	8	ounces.
Caramel	8	ounces.
Water, q. s. to measure	10	gallons.

Add the tinct. white pine, tinct of blood root and caramel to the syrups and mix well, dissolve the oils and chloroform in the alcohol and add. Dissolve the morphia, tartar emetic and muriate of ammonia in the remainder of the water, and mix thoroughly and strain.

Adult dose one teaspoonful.

585. Vegetable Cough Syrup.

Simple syrup	7	gallons.
Syrup of squills	¼	gallon.
Wine of ipecac	16	ounces.
Wine of antimony	16	ounces.
Tinct. of bloodroot	10	ounces.
Alcohol, 188 p. c.	1	gallon.
Oil bitter almonds	60	minims.
Sulphate of morphia	320	grains.
Sweet spirits of nitre	16	ounces.
Caramel	4	ounces.
Water, q. s. to make	10	gallons.

Mix the syrups, wines and tincture of blood root together. Mix the oil of bitter almonds and sweet spirits of nitre with the alcohol and add. Dissolve the sulphate of morphia and caramel in the water and mix all thoroughly—strain.

586. Balsam of Aniseed.

Oil of aniseed	30	minims.
Oil of cinnamon	10	minims.
Oil of coriander	5	minims.
Paregoric	1	ounce.
Tinct. benzoni co.	1	ounce.
Syrup of squills	4	ounces.
Wine of antimony	1	ounce.
Alcohol	1	ounce.
Simple syrup to measure	16	ounces.

Dissolve the oils in the alcohol and add the tinct. benzoni co. and paregoric; add the wine of antimony to the syrups and mix well with the other ingredients.

Adult dose one teaspoonful.

587. Compound Syrup of Flaxseed.

Mistura chloroformi et opii N. F.	640	minims.
Tincture of tolu soluble	1	ounce.
Oil of anise	15	minims.
Fl. extract senega	192	minims.
Syrup of squills	8	ounces.
Alcohol	1	ounce.
Infusion of linseed to measure	16	ounces.

Dissolve the oil of aniseed in the alcohol, add the mistura chloroformi et. opii, tincture of tolu soluble and fl. extract senega to the syrup of squills, and mix all the ingredients together thoroughly.

Adult dose, one teaspoonful.

NON-SECRET FORMULAS.

588. Bronchitis Mixture.
Chloral hydrate............ 128 grains.
Ammon. carb.............. 128 grains.
Tinct. digitalis............ 128 minims.
Syrup of orange............ 4 ounces.
Water, q. s. to measure... 16 ounces.
Dose: A tablespoonful every four hours.

589. Codeine Cough Syrup.
Codeine .... 16 grains.
Powd. ammonium chloride. 1 ounce.
Ipecac wine................ 10 drams.
Spirit of nitrous ether..... 10 drams.
Syrup of squill............ 10 drams.
Syrup of wild cherry to... 16 ounces.

Dissolve the codeine in about two drams of water with the aid of a small quantity of dilute hydrochloric acid; then dissolve the ammonium chloride in the syrup of wild cherry, and add the other ingredients, finally the codeine solution, and mix well.

Dose: A teaspoonful every three or four hours.

590. Pectoral Elixir.
Pulv. glycyrrhiz........... ½ ounce.
Pulv. acaciae.............. ½ ounce.
Tinct. camph. co.......... 2 ounces.
Vin. antimon.............. 1 ounce.
Spt. aether. nitros......... 2 ounces.
Aquae .... 4 ounces.
Ext. pruni virg............ 1 ounce.
Elixir. aromatic. ad....... 16 ounces.

Rub the liquorice and acacia with the water, add the other ingredients gradually, and strain through absorbent cotton.

Dose: A teaspoonful.

591. Cough Balsam.
Ammon. mur.............. 128 grains.
Chlorodyne .... 128 drops.
Syr. ipecac................ 1 ounce.
Syr. squills................ 1 ounce.
Tinct. opium camph....... 1 ounce.
Syr. wild cherry........... 1 ounce.

592. Cherry and Hoarhound.
Syr. marrubii.............. 1 ounce.
Vin. ipecac................ 2 drams.
Spt. aether. nit............ 2 drams.
Oxy. scillae............... 4 drams.
Tr. pruni virg............. 1½ drams.
Tr. lobel................... 2 drams.
Ext. glycyrrhiz. liq........ 4 drams.
Molasses (thinned with water) ad................. 6 ounces.
Dose: One to two teaspoonfuls.

593. Cherry Cough Cure.
Syrup squills.............. 20 ounces.
Syrup of wild cherry....... 20 ounces.
Acetate of morphia........ 20 grains.
Wine of antimony .... 3 ounces.
Paregoric .... 3 ounces.
Sweet spirits of nitre...... 2 ounces.
M. S. A.
Adult dose, one teaspoonful.

594. Influenza Syrup.
Spirits of chloroform...... 1 ounce.
Tinct. of aconite.......... 1 dram.
Paregoric .... 1 ounce.
Spirits of nitrous ether.... ½ ounce.
Liq. ammon. acet. fort..... 1½ ounces.
Bicarb. potassa........... ½ ounce.
Water .... 4 ounces.
Syrup of orange, enough to measure .... 16 ounces.
Adult dose, one tablespoonful three times a day.

595. Cough Remedy without Opium.
Bromide of potassium..... 1 ounce.
Tincture of sanguinaria (blood root)............. 3 fl. drams.
Tincture of hyoscyamus... 2 fl. ounces.
Ether (sulphuric) .... ½ fl. ounce.
Syrup of ipecac........... 2 fl. ounces.
Syrup of tolu.............. 7 fl. ounces.
Alcohol .... 1 fl. ounce.
Water .... 3 fl. ounces.

Dissolve the bromide of potassium in the water and mix the solution with the syrups. Mix the alcohol with the ether and tinctures, then add the mixture to the syrups and mix.

Dose, the same as other cough remedies, but may be given freely without injury.—The Formulary.

596. Cough Mixture for Adults.
Succ. solazzi .... 2 drams.
Gum. acaciae.............. 2 drams.
Aq. bullient............... 4 ounces.
Strain and add—
Vini ipecac................ 2 drams.
Tinct. camph. comp....... 2 drams.
M.
A tablespoonful to be taken occasionally in catarrhal affections.

597. North of England Cough Syrup.
Bromide ammon.......... 320 grains.
Paregoric .... 2½ ounces.
Fl. ext. licorice............ 1 ounce.
Tinct. digitalis............ 3 drams.
Syrup squills.............. 2 ounces.
Simple syrup.............. 4 ounces.
Water, q. s. to measure... 16 ounces.
Adult dose, one to two teaspoonfuls.

COUGH MIXTURES FOR CHILDREN.

The following formulas are found in the Hospital Formulary, of the Department of Public Charities and Correction of New York City. They are the prescriptions of good physicians, and may be used without hesitation in the doses named.

598. Cough Mixture for Infants.
R. Tinct. opii camph.........
   Spts. ammon. arom.....aa fl. 1 ounce.
   Ext. Ipecac fl............ fl. ½ dram.
   Syr. pruni virgin......... fl. 1 ounce.
   Aquae ....q. s. ad fl. 3 ounces.
Mix. Dose: a teaspoonful.

599. Mistura Ammonii Carbonatis.
(Dr. Bosley.)
R. Ammonii carbonat........ ½ dram.
   Syr. senegae.............. fl. 4 drams.
   Syr. ipecac................ fl. 2 drams.
   Syr. tolut................. fl. 4 drams.
   Ext. glycyrrhizae......... ½ dram.
   Aquae cinnamom..q. s. ad fl. 4 ounces.
Mix. Dose: a teaspoonful for children.

600. Mistura Ammonii Chloridi.
(Dr. Bosley.)
R. Ammonii chloridi........ ½ dram.
   Potassii chlorat. .... 40 grains.
   Syr. senegae.............. fl. 4 drams.
   Syr. ipecac................ fl. 3 drams.
   Syr. tolu................. fl. 5 drams.
   Ext. glycyrrhizae......... 1 dram.
   Aquae cinnamomi..q. s. ad fl. 4 ounces.
Mix Dose: a teaspoonful for children.

601. Cough Mixture for Children.
(Without Opium.)
   Vin. ipecac................ 2 drams.
   Oxymel scillae............ 6 drams.
   Tr. belladon.............. 1 dram.
   Spt. aether. nit........... 1½ drams.
   Aq. camph. ad............. 6 ounces.

Dose: Under one year, one teaspoonful; under four years, two teaspoonfuls; under eight years, three teaspoonfuls; under fourteen years, one tablespoonful—every three or four hours in each instance.

602. Palatable Cough Mixture.
The following is good for general use:
   Sodii benzoat.............. ½ dram.
   Tr. chlorof. et morphinae.. 1½ drams.
   Vin. ipecacuanhae .... 2½ drams.
   Syrupi limonis............. 1 ounce.
   Aq. ad.................... 6 ounces.
M.

A dessertspoonful for a dose.

The following is an efficient remedy for the distressing cough which follows a recent cold:

603.
   Vin. ipecac............... ¼ ounce.
   Tr. camph. co............. ½ ounce.
   Spt. chloroformi.......... 2 drams.
   Syrup. scillae ad.......... 2 ounces.
M.

Dose: A teaspoonful every four hours.
For children above four years the prescription should be modified as follows:
   Vin. ipecac............... 2 drams.
   Tr. camph. co............. 2 drams.
   Spt. chloroformi.......... 1 dram.
   Syrup. tolutan............ ½ ounce.
   Syrupi ad................. 2 ounces.
M.

Dose: A half to a whole teaspoonful every three or four hours.

The mixture can in each case be given to stop a severe paroxysm of coughing. The dose is followed in a few minutes by a most grateful feeling of warmth in the chest. If there is much secretion the ipecacuanha should be omitted and ammonium bromide be given instead.

604. Pleasant Cough Syrup. (Ch. & Dr.)
   Oxymel of squills .... 6 ounces.
   Wine of ipecac. .... 1 ounce.
   Fl. ext. licorice........... 2 ounces.
   Essence of peppermint.... 1 ounce.
   Water q. s. to make up to 16 ounces.

Adult dose: One or two teaspoonfuls three times a day.

605. Dr. Wheelock's Cough Mixture. (Era.)
   Sulphuric ether .... 3 fl. drams.
   Tincture of hyoscyamus ... 1 fl. ounce.
   Syrup of wild cherry...... 1 fl. ounce.
   Syrup of tolu .... 1 fl. ounce.
   Water to make .... 4 fl. ounces.
Mix.

606. Cough Syrup. (Old Times.)

Fl. extract licorice	1 ounce.
Liq. morph. acet.	6 fl. drams.
Tinct. quassia	3 fl. drams.
Fl. ext. senega	1 fl. ounce.
Oil of anise	20 drops.
Chloroform	1 fl. dram.
Alcohol	1 fl. ounce.
Molasses	4 fl. ounces.
Syrup of squills q. s. to make up to	16 fl. ounces.

Dose: Two to four teaspoonfuls.

607. Compound Lobelia Mixture.
(Edinburg Infirmary.)

Iodide potassium	2 drams.
Carbonate ammonium	1 dram.
Ethereal tincture lobelia	4 drams.
Spirit chloroform	4 drams.
Ipecacuanha wine	1 dram.
Infusion senega up to	6 ounces.

Dissolve and mix.

A tablespoonful in a wine-glassful of water every four hours.

Useful in bronchitic asthma.

608. Expectorant Mixture. (Era)

Tartar emetic	8 grains.
Fl. ext. ipecac	8 minims.
Tincture opium	4 fl. drams.
Tincture lobelia	2 fl. drams.
Tincture digitalis	2 fl. drams.
Syrup tolu	3 fl. ounces.
Syrup squill, enough to make	8 fl. ounces.

Dose: One teaspoonful.

609. Essence of Linseed. (Ch. & Dr.)

Chlorodyne	45 minims.
Oil of anise	4 minims.
Tincture tolu	½ ounce.
Tincture senega	½ ounce.
Vinegar squills	1½ ounces.
Infusion linseed, enough to make	3 ounces.

Add the oil of anise in the tincture of tolu, to the vinegar of squills and mix the other ingredients by shaking. Dose: One to two drams.

610. Excelsior Cough Syrup. (Ch. & Dr.)

Morphine sulphate	8 grains.
Tartar emetic	4 grains.
Fluid extract ipecac	90 minims.
Tincture bloodroot	1 ounce.
Water	6 ounces.
Syrup, enough to make	2 pints.

Heat the water, add the morphine sulphate and tartar emetic; stir until dissolved and add the syrup cold; shake, and to this mixture add fluid extract ipecac, and the tincture of bloodroot; shake and fill into bottles of size to suit. Dose for adults, one teaspoonful three times daily and after each severe fit of coughing; for children, in proportion to age.

611. Inhalant for Cough of Consumptives.

Joseph Adolphus (Amer. Med. Jour.) recommends the following as a good inhalation that will allay cough, procure rest and often lower temperature in pulmonary consumption, chronic bronchitis, etc.:

Oil of turpentine	2 fl. ounces.
Oil of eucalyptus	4 fl. drams.
Iodoform	1½ fl. drams.
Creosote	3 fl. drams.
Ether	1 fl. ounce.

Direct the patient to put ten or twelve drops on a piece of fine sponge and drop in a wide-mouthed tin vessel containing a little boiling water; cover his head with a cloth large enough to enclose the vessel and inhale the fumes. The effect is often magical.

612. Shiloh's Consumption Cure.
(Fenner's Formulary.)

Muriate of morphine	3 grains.
Muriatic acid	3 minims.
Fluid extract henbane	2 drams.
Fluid extract ginger	3 drams.
Fluid extract wild cherry	3 drams.
Diluted alcohol	3 drams.
Chloroform	1 dram.
Essence peppermint	30 minims.
Syrup of tar	3 ounces.
Simple syrup to make	8 ounces.

Mix.

613. Piso's Consumption Cure. (Era.)

Tincture of tolu	½ ounce.
Fluid extract of lobelia	2 drops.
Fluid extract of cannabis indica	2 drops.
Chloroform	1 dram.
Morphine sulphate	4 grains.
Tartar emetic	4 grains.
Essence spearmint	10 drops.
Water	8 ounces.
Sugar	14 ounces.

Mix the fluid extracts, tincture of tolu, chloroform, and essence spearmint, and shake with some sugar in a bottle. Dissolve the morphine sulphate and tartar emetic in hot water, and add to the sugar, shake until dissolved and filter if necessary.

614. Children's Cough Mixture.

For selling to small shopkeepers. (Ch. and Dr.)

Acet. ipecac.	1 ounce.
Acet. scillae	1 ounce.
Spt. ammon. arom.	1½ ounces.
Ol. anisi	6 drops.
Theriac.	10 ounces.
Aq. chloroformi ad	1 pint.

Dissolve the oil in the spirit, and add to the vinegars; then mix with the treacle, make up to a pint, set aside for three days, and decant.

Dose: Half to a whole teaspoonful thrice daily.

615. Sedative Cough Syrup.

Tr. opii co.	4 ounces.
Syrup. scillae	4 ounces.
Tr. cimicifugae	3 ounces.
Tr. sanguinariae	1½ ounces.
Tr. benzoin. simp.	1½ ounces.
Vin. ipecac.	2 ounces.
Syr. tolutan.	16 ounces.

M.

Dose: A half to a whole teaspoonful, according to age.

616. Cubeb Cough Syrup.

Tinct. cubebs.	2 ounces.
Tinct. tolu soluble	1 ounce.
Tinct. opium co.	1 ounce.
Tartar emetic	8 grains.
Peppermint water	2 ounces.
Simple syrup q. s. to measure	16 ounces.

Dose: One teaspoonful.

617 Coltsfoot Rock Candy. (Nat. Druggist.)

The following is an English recipe: One pound Spanish licorice dissolved in three-fourths pint of water, two ounces gum tragacanth dissolved in one and one-half pints water, twenty-eight pounds finest confectioner's sugar, one ounce essence of lemon, two ounces extract of poppies. Color with Spanish brown—a kind of prepared brown ochre. Make into a paste. By means of a piston and screw, force through a metal tube having star-shaped holes at the bottom. Cut into lengths and dry.

618. Cough Lozenges.

The following recipe makes a good cough lozenge:

Pulv. scillae	1 ounce.
Pulv. ipecac.	6 drams.
Morph. acet.	1 dram.
Acid. benzoic.	1 dram.
Ext. papav. alb.	2 ounces.
Ext. hyoscy.	2 ounces.
Ol. amygd. ess.	10 drops.
Ext. glycyrrh. (mol)	1 vel. q. s. lb.
Pulv. gum acaciae	1 pound.
Antim. tart.	1 scruple.

M. S. A. and form into troches.

COUGH DROP FORMULAS.

The following, appearing in the Confectioners' Union, have been found satisfactory:

619. Montpelier Cough Drops.

Brown sugar	10 pounds.
Tartaric acid	2 ounces.
Cream of tartar	½ ounce.
Water	1½ quarts.
Anise seed flavoring	q. s.

Melt the sugar in the water, and when at a sharp boil add the cream of tartar. Cover the pan for five minutes. Remove the lid and let the sugar boil up to crack degree. Turn out the batch on an oiled slab, and when cool enough to handle mold in the acid and flavoring. Pass it through the acid drop rollers, and when the drops are chipped up, and before sifting, rub some icing with them.

620. Medicated Cough Drops.

Light brown sugar	14 pounds.
Tartaric acid	1¼ ounces.
Cream of tartar	½ ounce.
Water	2 quarts.
Anise seed, cayenne, clove and peppermint flavorings	A few drops of each.

Proceed as before prescribed, but when sufficiently cool, pass the batch through the acid tablet rollers and dust with sugar.

621. Hoarhound Candy

Dutch crushed sugar	10 pounds.
Dried hoarhound leaves	2 ounces.
Cream of tartar	¾ ounce.
Water	2 quarts.
Anise seed flavoring	q. s.

Pour the water on the leaves and let it gently simmer till reduced to three pints; then strain the infusion through muslin, and add the liquid to the sugar. Put the pan containing the syrup on the fire, and when at a sharp boil add the cream of tartar. Put the lid on the pan for five minutes; then remove it, and let the sugar boil to stiff boil degree. Take the pan off the fire and rub portions of the sugar against the side until it produces a creamy appearance; then add the flavoring. Stir all well, and pour into square tin frames, previously well oiled.

INFLUENZA TRADE. (Ch. & Dr.)

The influenza has violated tradition in one respect only. It was clearly understood last year that, in sympathy with what is said of it in history, it had worn itself out by its attacks upon long suffering man, and had retired. It was not expected to return again until towards the middle of the twentieth century; but here it is once more, vigorous and fatal. The mild cases of a fortnight ago are succeeded by others of a more severe type, as in past times, this phenomenon being characteristic of epidemic diseases due to bacillary influence. Given man or woman just now with aching limbs, intense headache, occasional sickness, bloodshot eyes, haggard appearance, shivering, pulse 90 to 100 and feeble, and temperature from 100° to 104°, that man or woman should be told to go home to bed. This is a measure of precaution which must not be avoided. The treatment may take the following course:

622. To Relieve the Headache.

Phenacetin .... 6 grains.

To be taken every four hours in warm water.

623. To Produce Diaphoresis.

Potassae bicarb. .... 15 grains.
Ammon. carb. .... 6 grains.
Tr. aconiti .... 2 minims.
Spt. aether nit. .... 1 dram.
Vin. ipecac. .... ½ dram.
Aq. chloroformi ad .... 2 ounces.
M.
Acid citric .... 20 grains.
Div. in pulv. two.

Half of the mixture to be taken with a powder on going to bed, and to be followed by hot tea or coffee, hot gruel, or hot spirits and water. The second half of the mixture to be taken two hours later.

This mixture is excellent at the onset of the complaint and it generally suffices to produce sufficient diaphoresis, so that the next morning the more severe symptoms, such as headache and aching limbs, have subsided. If not, it should be repeated and the phenacetin powders continued. By giving 6 ounce bottles of the mixture the circumstances of the majority of cases will be met; but after the second dose, the mixture should not be taken oftener than every four hours. It is quite essential to maintain the patient's strength from the first—a not altogether easy thing to do for food is repugnant. However, occasional spoonfuls of beef-tea made from meat-extract, chicken-broth, port wine (coca and cinchona wines are particularly serviceable), and soda and milk are refused by few, and suffice for the purpose. When the feverish symptoms subside—and that happens from two to four days after the onset—the following mixture should be given:

624.

Quininae sulph. .... 6 grains.
Acid. hydrobrom. dil. ..... 1 dram.
Tr. nucis vom. .... 20 minims.
Tr. cardam. co. .... 2 drams.
Aq. ad .... 6 ounces.
M.

A sixth part thrice a day immediately before food.

Of course any good tonic will suit the purpose equally well, but the tendency is to overdose—for example, teaspoonful doses of Easton's syrup, and corresponding quantities of hypophosphite and hypobromate syrups, may really do as much harm as good. Twenty-minim doses are quite sufficient in most cases. In the weakness following influenza the use of mild stimulants is of great benefit, and this is specially true of medicated wines. If cough and other bronchial symptoms supervene, the greatest care must be exercised by the patient, as pneumonia is responsible for many, if not most of the deaths.

Children affected by the disease should be treated in the same manner as adults, and the diaphoretic mixture mentioned above may be given in half-doses for those between 14 and 18. For children under 14 the following is a reliable mixture:

625.

Potass. chlorat. .... ½ dram.
Potass. bicarb. .... 1 dram.
Liq. ammon. acet. .... 6 drams.
Vin. ipecac. .... 2 drams.
Syr. aurantii .... ½ ounce.
Aq. ad .... 6 ounces.
M.

A teaspoonful to a tablespoonful (according to age) every three hours.

626. Bronchitis. (Potter.)

Antimony and potassium
  tartrate ... . 2 grains.
Solution acetate ammonium 4 ounces.
Spirit nitrous ether....... 1 ounce.
Tincture aconite .... ½ dram.
Syrup, enough to make.... 6 ounces.

A teaspoonful every two or three hours.

627.
　Solution acetate ammonium 4 drams.
　Spirit nitrous ether ......
　Syrup ipecac. ... of each 1½ drams.
　Syrup senega .... 1 dram.
　Syrup lemon .... 1 ounce.

A teaspoonful every three hours for children.

628. Pills for Chronic Bronchitis.
　Ammonii chloridi .... 15 grains.
　Ammon. carb. .... 15 grains.
　Pulv. ipecac. .... 3 grains.
　Morph. hydrochloratis .... 1 grain.
　Glycer. tragacanth. ...... q. s.
　Pulv. glycyrrhiz. .... q. s.

Mass, and divide into ten pills. One to be taken night and morning.—Medical Press.

629. Dick's Asthma Cure.
　Tinct. valerian .... 12 ounces.
　Iodide of potash .... ½ ounce.
　Water .... 1 ounce.
　Tinct. hyosciamus .... 6 drams.
　Tinct. tolu .... 6 drams.
　Tinct. opium co. .... 1 dram.
　Simple syrup .... 1 ounce.
　Mix.

Dose: One tablespoonful three times a day half an hour after meals.

630. Asthma Syrup.
　Hydrate of chloral .... 64 grains.
　Iodide of potash .... 64 grains.
　Syrup of orange .... 2 ounces.
　Distilled water .... 14 ounces.

Dose: One tablespoonful three to four times a day.

631. Asthma Mixture. (Potter.)
　Fluid extract grindelia ... ½ ounce.
　Fluid extract lobelia ..... 2 drams.
　Fluid extract belladonna.. 1 dram.
　Potassium iodide .... 3 drams.
　Glycerin .... 3 ounces.

A dessertspoonful as required.

632. Asthma Mixture.
　Tinct. lobelia .... 40 minims.
　Tinct. squills .... 96 minims.
　Iodide of potash .... 32 grains.
　Glycerine .... ½ ounce.
　Camphor water q. s. to
　　make up to .... 8 ounces.

Dose: One tablespoonful three to four times a day.

633. Asthma Inhalant.
Asthma.—The most popular remedies for this disorder are those used by inhalation, and experience demonstrates them the most effective. The following formula has no superior:
　Grindelia .... 8 drams.
　Jaborandi .... 8 drams.
　Eucalyptus .... 4 drams.
　Digitalis .... 4 drams.
　Cubebs .... 4 drams.
　Stramonium .... 16 drams.
　Nitrate of potash .... 12 drams.
　Cascarilla bark .... 1 dram.

The ingredients should be in fine powder, and thoroughly dry before mixing. The composition is used by burning from one-fourth to one-half teaspoonful, and inhaling the smoke. The nitrate of potash is dissolved in water, and the powder moistened with it and dried.

634. Asthma Cigarettes.
　Tobacco .... 90 drams.
　Extract of stramonium ..... 5 drams.
　Iodide of potassium .... 5 drams.
　Nitrate of potassium ...... 5 drams.
　Alcohol .... 45 drams.

Mix, dry, and make a hundred cigarettes.

635. Asthma Powder. A
　Lobelia herb .... 1 ounce.
　Black tea .... 1 ounce.
　Stramonium .... 1 ounce.
　Potassium nitrate .... 1 ounce.
　Powdered anise .... 1 dram.
　Powdered fennel .... 1 dram.
　Mix.

636. Asthma Powder. B
　Grindelia .... 8 drams.
　Jaborandi .... 8 drams.
　Eucalyptus .... 4 drams.
　Digitalis .... 4 drams.
　Cubebs .... 4 drams.
　Stramonium .... 16 drams.
　Potassium nitrate .... 12 drams.
　Cascarilla bark .... 1 dram.
　Mix.

637. Asthma Powder. C
　Pulv. stramonii .... 1 ounce.
　Pulv. pot. nitrat. .... ½ ounce.
　Pulv. lobeliae .... ½ ounce.
　Pulv. sem. anisi .... 2 drams.
　M.

The ingredients should be in fine powder, and thoroughly dry before mixing. The composition is used by burning one-fourth to one-half teaspoonful and inhaling the smoke, which is most conveniently done by using the cover of a tin box.

CATARRH CURES.

638. Catarrh Cure. (For use with Atomizer.)
Sulph. carbolate of zinc.... 480 grains.
Sulphate of hydrastia ..... 480 grains.
Sulphate of zinc .... 240 grains.
Sulphate of morphia ...... 120 grains.
Antisepticina .... 32 ounces.
Distilled ext. of witch hazel 1 gallon.
Distilled water .... 1 gallon.

Filter; use the solution warmed; spray with an atomizer four times a day and for internal use take Catarrh Cure, Formula No. 639.

639. Catarrh Cure. (For internal use.)
Iodide of potash .... 384 grains.
Syrup of orange .... 2 ounces.
Tincture of cardamon co... 2 drams.
Tincture of quassia .... 2 drams.
Dilute alcohol .... 3½ ounces.
Water to make .... 16 ounces.

Dose: One to two teaspoonfuls three times a day in a little water. While taking this mixture internally, the Catarrh Mixture for atomizer or douche, Formula No. 638 should also be used.

640. Bergoline Oil Spray.
Acid camphoric .... 8 grains.
Menthol .... 20 grains.
Oil eucalytol. .... 3 drams.
Bergoline, albolene, glymol or any other inodorous liquid-petrolatum enough to make .... 4 fl. ounces.

Directions: Spray the throat and nose with the above, using a Devilbis No. 9 atomizer for oil or any other good oil atomizer will do.

641. Catarrh Cure. (For use with Douche.)
Carbolic acid crystals...... 1 ounce.
Glycerine .... 1 pint.
Fl. ext. stramonium ...... 2 pints.
Antisepticina .... 2 pints.
Rose water q. s. to make.. 2 gallons.
Filter.

Use the solution warmed; spray with an atomizer three to four times a day.

642. Catarrh Snuff.
Bismuth carbonate .... 10 grains.
Orris root, powdered..... 3 grains.
Thymol, powd. .... 1 grain.
Cocaine hydrochlor. ..... 4 grains.
Sugar of milk .... 20 grains.
Gum arabic, powdered.... 10 grains.
Soda bicarb. .... 2 grains.
Quinine sulphate .... 10 grains.
M.

Sniff up the nostrils several times a day.

643. Sage's Catarrh Snuff.
(Druggist's Circular.)

Dr. Sage of "catarrh snuff" notoriety practiced in this neighborhood. Let your readers, report if they can detect any difference between this and the advertised snuff:

Quinia sulph. ....
Ferri per. sulph. ....aa 6 grains.
Pulv. opii .... 4 grains.
Potassae chloras .... 8 grains.
Lycopodium .... 3 drams.
M.

Sig.: Use as a snuff 3 or 4 times daily.

644. Cream Anodyne for Catarrh.
Bismuth carbonate .... 15 grains.
Thymol .... 2 grains.
Cocaine .... 2 grains.
Quinine sulphate .... 5 grains.
Bergoline or albolene oil.. 2 drams.
White vaseline .... 6 drams.
Mix.

645. Cream Balsam for Catarrh.
Bismuth carbonate .... 30 grains.
Iodide of potash .... 10 grains.
Morphine sulphate .... 2 grains.
Water q. s. or .... 1 dram.
Benzoic acid. .... 10 grains.
Lanoline q. s. to make.... 1 ounce.

Dissolve the iodide of potash and the morphine in the water and mix thoroughly with the other ingredients.

646. Fluid Lightning for Inhalation.
Essential oil of mustard... 30 minims.
Chloroform .... 4 drams.
Tincture of iodine .... 2 drams.
Carbolic acid crystals..... 2 drams.
Spirits ammon. arom. .... 4 drams.
Glycerine q. s. to make.... 4 fl. ounces.

Dissolve the oil of mustard in the chloroform. Mix the tincture of iodine with one ounce of the glycerine and add the spirits ammonia aromatic.

Dissolve the carbolic acid in another ounce of glycerine, and mix altogether.

Directions: Saturate pieces of sponge with the mixture and place in two ounce wide-mouth vials, and inhale. Keep well stoppered.

Label Fluid Electricity for Catarrh, Nervous Headache, Colds in the Head, etc.

DYSPEPSIA AND INDIGESTION REMEDIES.

647. Digestive Syrup.
Cascara sag. formula No. 57 .... 2 pints.
Tinct. cardamom co. ...... 4 ounces.
Tinct. rhubarb arom. ..... 4 ounces.
Tinct. ginger U. S. P. ...... 4 ounces.
Glycerine .... 16 ounces.
Simple syrup .... 20 ounces.
Dose: One to two dessertspoonfuls.

648. Digestive Tonic.
Liquor bismuth .... 2 ounces.
Glycerite of pepsin N. F... 2 ounces.
Cascara sag. formula No. 57 .... 2 ounces.
Tinct. of rhubarb arom. .. 1 ounce.
Tinct. of cardamom ...... 1 ounce.
Water q. s. to make....... 16 ounces.
Dose: One tablespoonful after meals.

649. Dyspepsia Tonic.
Rhubarb .... 6 ounces.
Golden seal .... 1½ ounces.
Cape aloes .... ¼ ounce.
Sal. tartar .... 2 ounces.
Capsicum .... 30 grains.
Ess. peppermint .... 3 drams.
Alcohol .... 2 pints.
Sugar house syrup .... 2 pints.
Water .... 4 pints.

650. Dyspepsia Remedy.
Soda carbonate .... 2 ounces.
Soda phosphate .... 2 ounces.
Hot water .... 1 pint.
Sugar house syrup .... ½ pint.
Essence peppermint ...... 1 ounce.
Tinct. ginger U. S. P. ...... 2 ounces.
Chloroform .... 1 dram.
Alcohol, 188 per cent..... 7 drams.
Caramel .... ½ ounce.
Water q. s. to make....... 32 ounces.
M.
Dose: One tablespoonful three times a day after meals.

651. Pepsin Mixture for Dyspepsia and Indigestion. (Ch. & Dr.)
Pepsin, B. P............... 1 dram.
Acid. hydrochlor. dil. ..... 2 drams.
Glycerini .... 6 drams.
Tr. card. co. .... 4 drams.
Inf. gent. ad .... 8 ounces.

Put the pepsin in a mortar, add the acid and triturate well, then add the glycerine and other ingredients in their order.
Label "Shake the bottle."
Should a stock remedy be required, macerate for a fortnight and strain, or filter, when a clear mixture will be obtained.
Dose: A tablespoonful.

652. Flatulent Dyspepsia. (Ch. & Dr.)
Magnes. sulph. .... 2 drams.
Potass. bicarb. .... 1½ drams.
Spt. chlorof. .... 1 dram.
Tinct. nucis vom. .... 1 dram.
Tinct. capsici .... 14 minims.
Inf. gent. co. ad.......... 6 ounces.
Capt. sext. part ter die ante cibos.

653. Indigestion Mixture.
Liquor bismuth .... 640 minims.
Cascara sag. formula No. 57 .... 640 minims.
Glycerine .... 2 ounces.
Syrup of orange .... 2 ounces.
Water q. s. to make....... 16 ounces.
M.
Dose: One tablespoonful.

654. For Indigestion, accompanied by Vomiting.
Acid. carbolic .... 4 drops.
Subnitrate of bismuth .... 150 grains.
Powdered pepsin .... 60 grains.
Powdered acacia q. s. ....
Tinct. ginger .... 3 drams.
Simple syrup .... 2 drams.
Cinnamon water q. s. to make .... 2 ounces.
Dose: One teaspoonful three times a day; put a shake well label on the bottle.

655. Mixture for Flatulency.
Spirits nitrous ether ..... 2¼ ounces.
Spirits camphor .... ¾ ounce.
Dose: One teaspoonful in a little warm water.

656. Flatulence Mixture.
Sodii bicarb. .... 1 dram.
Spt. ammon. arom. ...... 1 dram.
Tr. gent. co. .... 3 drams.
Tr. card. co. .... 2 drams.
Aq. chlorof. ad .... 2 ounces.
M.
Dose: One tablespoonful.

657. Digestive Powder.
- Pulv. sacch. lact. .... 14 drms.
- Pulv. pepsin .... 140 grains.
- Pancreatini .... 124 grains.
- Veg. diastase .... 10 grains.
- Acid. lact. conc. .... 15 minims.
- Acid. hydrochlor. .... 13 minims.

Dose: One teaspoonful in a wineglass of wine or water between meals.

658. Laxative Digestive Powder.
- Pulv. rhei .... 2½ drams.
- Sodii bicarb. .... 6 drams, 15 grains.
- Pulv. calumba ...... 1 dram, 40 grains.
- Pulv. cinnam. ...... 1 dram, 15 grains.

M. Ft. pulv.

Dose: One teaspoonful in a wineglass of wine or water between meals.

659. Stomachic Powder.
- Bismuth. subnit. .... 5 ounces.
- Potassae bicarbonat. ...... 6 ounces.
- Mag. carb. levis. .... 4 ounces.
- Pulv. cinnam. co. .... 3 ounces.

Mix and sift three times.

From half to a whole teaspoonful an hour after food.

This is a very good preparation for heartburn, flatulence, and other symptoms of dyspepsia. To be put up in 2-ounce W. M. bottles which will admit a teaspoon.

RHEUMATISM, GOUT, ETC.

660. Thomas' Rheumatic and Gout Cure. A
- Potash bicarb. .... 5 ounces.
- Potash iodide .... 2½ ounces.
- Soda salicylate .... 2½ ounces.
- Wine of colchicum .... 3¾ ounces.
- Infusion of buchu q. s. to make .... 1 gallon.

Dose: One tablespoonful four times a day.

661. Rheumatic and Gout Cure. B
- Potash iodide .... 3 drams.
- Fl. ext. hemlock .... 3 drams.
- Fl. ext. senna .... 8 drams.
- Tinct. colch. root .... 3 drams.
- Tinct. guiac. am. .... 4 drams.
- Syrup of sarsaparilla co. q. s. to make up to .... 16 ounces.

662. Gout and Rheumatic Mixture.
- Lith. benz. .... 4 scruples.
- Pot. iod. .... ½ dram.
- Tinct. serpent. .... 2 drams.
- Vin. colch. .... 1 dram.
- Ext. manacae liq. .... 1½ drams.
- Aq. chlorof. ad .... 8 ounces.

Adult dose: Two tablespoonfuls twice a day.

663. Gout and Rheumatic Mixture.
- Sodii salicyl. .... 1½ drams.
- Pot. cit. .... 1 dram.
- Vin. colch. .... 1½ drams.
- Tr. gent. co. .... 2 drams.
- Aq. chlorof. ad .... 2 ounces.

M.

Dose: One tablespoonful.

664. Mixture for Rheumatism.
Mixture for Rheumatism recommended by the late Sir Andrew Clark.
- Potassii iodidi .... ½ dram.
- Potassii bicarb. .... 2 drams.
- Liq. arsenicalis .... 1 dram.
- Inf. gentianae ad .... 8 ounces.

M.

Dose: A tablespoonful three times a day.

665. Salicylic Acid Compound.
- Salicylic acid. .... 640 grains.
- Iodide of potash.......... 320 grains.
- Potash bicarb. .... ½ ounce.
- Fl. ext. buchu .... 2 drams.
- Fl. ext. gelsemium ...... 2 drams.
- Fl. ext. cimcifuga .... 4 drams.
- Fl. ext. pareira brava .... 2 drams.
- Alcohol .... 2 ounces.
- Glycerine .... 2 ounces.
- Syrup of orange q. s. to make up to............. 16 fl. ounces.

666. Rheumatic Mixture. (Ch. & Dr.)
- Quinine sulphate .... 80 grains.
- Potassium iodide .... 2 drams.
- Colchicum wine .... 1 ounce.
- Tincture orange. .... ½ ounce.
- Chloroform water to. .... 8 ounces.

Rub the quinine with the wine, adding a few drops of dilute sulphuric acid to assist solution; then add the tincture, water, and finally the iodide of potassium.

667. Rheumatism.
- Pot. Bromide. .... 2 drams.
- Ferri quinia cit. .... 2 drams.
- Spts. Chloroform. .... 3 drams.
- Tinct. senna co. .... 1 ounce.
- Aqua ad. .... 8 ounces.

Ft. mist. Take a tablespoonful in water twice a day and at bed time.

668. Rheumatic Powders.

Lac. sulphur. .... 1 dram.
Resin guiac powd. .... 1 dram.
Nitrate of potash. .... 40 grains.

Make into four powders.

Dose: One to be taken at bedtime.

669.

A safe and efficient pill for gout and rheumatism.

Ext. colchici. .... 1 dram.
Pulv. ipecac. co. .... 2 drams.
Pil. hydrarg. .... 1 dram.
Sodae carb. exsic. .... 2 drams.

Mix and mass with extract of gentian, make into 3-grain pills, and direct one or two to be given as a dose, night and morning, according to the urgency of the symptoms.

A laxative should be taken once or twice a week to prevent accumulation of colchicum.

670. Gout Pills. (Ch. & Dr.)

Extract colchicum acet. .. 3 grains.
Aloes socotrine. .... 3 grains.
Calomel. .... 3 grains.
Pow'd ipecac. .... 3 grains.

Make into twelve pills.

Dose: Two pills three times a day.

671. Rheumatic Liniments.

Aq. ammoniae .... 2 ounces.
Ol. olivae. .... 2 ounces.
Tinct. opii. .... 2 ounces.
Ol. cinnamom. .... 3 drams.
Ol. sassafras. .... 3 drams.

M.

672

Tr. capsici .... 1 ounce.
Ol. origani. .... 1 dram.
Ol. conii. .... 2 drams.
Lin. saponis. .... 6 ounces.

M.

673. Rheumatic Liniment.

Turpentine .... 1 gallon.
Nitrate potash. .... 4 ounces.
Sulphuric acid. .... 2 ounces.

Make the above in a stone crock and in the open air. Put the nitrate of potash in the turpentine and slowly add the sulphuric acid. Stir well and let stand 24 hours before bottling.

674. Phenacetin in Rheumatism.

The Journal de Medecine de Paris says that useful results are obtained in cases of acute rheumatism by applying phenacetin externally to the painful parts. The following prescription may be used:

Phenacetin. .... 75 grains.
Lanolin. .... 6 drams.
Olive oil. ....

A sufficient quantity.

To be rubbed about the inflamed part.

675. For Sciatica.

Tinct. aconiti rad. ...... 4 grammes.
Tinct. colchici sem. ..... 4 grammes.
Tinct. belladonnae. ...... 4 grammes.
Tinct. cimicifugae. ...... 4 grammes.

M.

Sig: Twelve drops every four to eight hours.

NEURALGIC REMEDIES.

676. Magic Neuralgic Drops.

Tincture gelsem. semp.... 3 drams.
Liq. morph. hydroch. B. P. 3 drams.
Vin. colchic. .... 4 drams.
Aqua chloroformi ad. ..... 3 ounces.

Mix.

Dose: One to two teaspoonfuls every 3 or 4 hours until relieved. Afterwards repeat the dose every six hours until three ounces are taken.

677. Neuralgia Mixture.

Exalgin. .... 1 to 2 grains.
Sp. chloroform. .... 10 minims.
Aquae ad. .... 1 ounce.

M.

Sig.: For one dose. Repeat every four hours.

—Dr. G. G Younger's prescription.

678. Neuralgic Mixture.

Chloral. hydrat. .... 2 scruples.
Potass. brom. .... 160 grains.
Glycerini. .... 3 drams.
Tr. valerian. .... 6 drams.
Aq. chlorof. ad. .... 4 ounces.

M.S.A.

A dessertspoonful to a tablespoonful in water when in pain.

679. Neuralgia Mixture.
Tinct. gelsem. sempervirens 1½ drams.
Tr. quininae. .... 1 ounce.
Tr. quininae ammoniat. ... 1 ounce.
M.
Dose: One teaspoonful in water every second hour until relieved; then a dose twice or thrice daily, between meals, for a few days.

680. For Neuralgia.
Quinine valerianatis. ...... 10 grains.
Tinct. sumbuli. .... 2 drams.
Extracti taraxaci liq ... 6 drams.
Infus. cascarillae ad. ...... 6 ounces.
M.
Sig.: A dessertspoonful three times a day.

681. Neuralgia Mixture.
Ammon. bromide .... 1½ drams.
Tinct. gelsemii. .... 2 drams.
Tinct. gentian co. .... 2 drams.
Aquae chloroformi. q. s. to measure. .... 6 ounces.
Dose: One tablespoonful.
The above mixture gives immense satisfaction.

682. Neuralgia Mixture. (Br. & Col. Dr.)
Quinine sulphate. .... 12 grains.
Potassium bromide. .... 2 drams.
Dilute sulphuric acid. ..... 20 minims.
Tincture gelsemium....... 90 minims.
Spirit chloroform. .... 2 drams.
Distilled water, up to. .... 6 ounces.
A tablespoonful every four hours as long as the pain continues.

683. Neuralgic Powder. (Ch. & Dr.)
Neuralgic powder ("not more than three to be taken in one day"):
Acetanilidi. .... 7 grains.
Pulv. rhei. .... 1 grain.
Soda bicarb. .... 2 grains.
M.

684. Neuralgia Powders.
Antifebrin. .... 5 grains.
Ferri redacti. .... 5 grains.
M. Ft. pulv.
Ter die sd.

685. Neuralgic and Toothache Powders.
Acetanilid .... 5 grains.
Lupulin. .... 5 grains.
Powdered sugar. .... 5 grains.
Make a powder.
Three powders to be taken at intervals of four hours.

686.
Acetanilid .... 5 grains.
Sodium salicylate. .... 5 grains.
Caffeine. .... 1 grain.
Make a powder.
To be taken as above.

The marvelous influence of antipyrin in abating neuralgic headache has led to considerable abuse of the remedy. Some people are peculiarly susceptible to its bad influences. In view of this susceptibility, and of the uncertainty which to an extent exists as to the best moderate dose of antipyrin, we may conclude that 5 grains three times a day is quite sufficient as a beginning dose in the vast majority of cases, and that in a fair proportion of instances even smaller quantities will be equally beneficial.

FOR NERVOUSNESS.

687. Remedy for Neurasthenia.
The following was a favorite prescription of Sir Andrew Clark's for various kinds of neurasthenic debility:
Acid phosphate. .... 1 dram.
Ext. cocae liquid. .... ½ dram.
Ext. damian. liquid. ...... ½ dram.
Tr. nucis vomic. .... 10 minims.
Syrup. zingib. .... 1 dram.
Aq. ad. .... ½ ounce.
Ft. dosis.
Sig: To be taken in water at 11 a. m. and 6 p. m.

688. Nerve Tonic.
Tinct. cinchon. co. .... 2 ounces.
Tinct. lavand. co. .... 2 ounces.
Fl. ext. coca leaves. ...... 2 ounces.
Fl. ext. damiana. .... 2 ounces.
Port wine. .... 8 ounces.
Dose: One tablespoonful three times a day.

689. Nervina.
Coca, ground. .... 16 ounces.
Damiana, ground. .... 16 ounces.
Orange peel, ground. ..... 8 ounces.
Quassia, ground. .... ½ dram.
Bromide of potash. .... 4 ounces.
Alcohol, 188 per cent. .... 32 ounces.
Glycerine. .... 16 ounces.
Water. .... 64 ounces.
Sherry or port wine q. s. to measure .... 1 gallon.

Macerate and percolate the drugs with 32 ounces of alcohol and 32 ounces of water mixed—afterwards run through the other 32 ounces of water; in this dissolve the bromide of potash; mix with the glycerine and add to the percolate and enough wine to make up to 1 gallon.

690.   Nervo-Valeria.
Valerianate of ammonium.. 256 grains.
Aromatic spts. of ammonia. 640 minims.
Fl. ext. valerian. .... 1 ounce.
Simple elixir red q. s. to
  make. .... 1 pint.
Dose: One to two teaspoonfuls.

691.   Nerve Pills.
Phosphorus .... 1-50 grain.
Valerianate zinc. .... ½ grain.
Ext. nux vomica. .... ¼ grain.
Quinine .... ½ grain.
Iron by hydrogen. .... 1 grain.
To make one pill.

692.   Female Tonic for Nervousness.
Black haw, ground........ 30 ounces.
Red clover, ground. ...... 30 ounces.
Yarrow, ground. .... 30 ounces.
Coca, ground. .... 10 ounces.
Eucalyptus, ground. ..... 10 ounces.
Jaborandi. .... 2 ounces.
Ergot. .... 5 ounces.
Cologne spirits, 188 p. c... 2 gallons.
Distilled water. .... 4 gallons.
Simple syrup. .... 1 gallon.
Macerate for seven days—percolate and add the syrup.

HEADACHE REMEDIES.

693.   Migraine Powders.
Caffeine. .... 30 grains.
Phenacetine. .... 30 grains.
Soda bicarb. .... 15 grains.
Fill into 20 capsules, or cachets.
Dose: Two every three hours until relieved.

694.   Headache Capsules.
Caffeine. .... 240 grains.
Phenacetin. .... 7000 grains.
Soda bicarb. .... 1750 grains.
Willow charcoal. .... 480 grains.
Fill into No. 2 capsules.

695.   Headache Powders.   A
Acetanilid. .... 30 grains.
Caffeine. .... 5 grains.
Bicarb. soda. .... 30 grains.
q. s. for ten powders, or cachets.

696.   Headache Powders.   B
Acetanilid. .... 30 grains.
Salicylate of soda. .... 20 grains.
Bicarb. of soda .... 10 grains.
Caffeine. .... 5 grains.
q. s. for ten powders, or cachets.

697.   Headache Powders.   C
Phenacetine .... 30 grains.
Salicine. .... 30 grains.
Rhubarb powdered. .... 5 grains.
Caffeine. .... 5 grains.
q. s. for ten powders, or cachets.

698.   Digestive Pastilles.
Bismuth subnitrate ...... 20 parts.
Calcium phosphate .... 30 parts.
Sodium bicarbonate ...... 10 parts.
Magnesium carbonate .... 200 parts.
Iron carbonate .... 50 parts.
Sugar .... 1,000 parts.
Flavor with peppermint, make in pastilles; three to twelve may be taken daily.

699.   Digestive Pastilles of Borivent.
Bismuth subnitrate ...... 20 parts.
Calcium phosphate .... 30 parts.
Sodium bicarbonate ...... 10 parts.
Magnesium carbonate .... 200 parts.
Iron carbonate .... 50 parts.
Sugar .... 1,000 parts.
Flavor with essence of peppermint, anise, or orange flowers. Make into pastilles of 1 gram each, of which 3 to 12 may be taken daily.

700.   For Chronic Headache.
Arseniate of sodium. ..... ½ grain.
Sulphate of atropine...... ½ grain.
Extract of aconite. .... 7½ grains.
Powdered cinnamon. ..... q. s.
Mix and make into thirty pills.
Sig.: From one to four pills daily.

701. Compound Bismuth Mixture for Indigestion.
Liq. bismuthi. .... 6 drams.
Potassæ bicarb. .... 1½ drams.
Tr. nucis vom. .... 2 drams.
Tr. chlorof. co. .... 2 drams.
Tr. calumba. .... ½ ounce.
Aq. ad. .... 6 ounces.
One-half ounce, 11, 4 and 8.

CREASOTE PREPARATIONS.

702. Creasote Gargle. (Ch. & Dr.)
Creasote. .... 10 minims.
Spirit of chloroform. ...... 1 dram.
Glycerine. .... ½ ounce.
Water to. .... 8 ounces.

Dissolve the creasote in the spirit, and add with brisk shaking to the glycerine and water previously mixed.

If a stronger gargle (5 minims or 10 minims to 1 ounce) is required, the creasote should be mixed with fresh milk (10 minims to 1 dram) and then diluted with water. The emulsion formed is perfect.

703. Ringworm Application. (Ch. & Dr.)
Creasoti. .... 30 minims.
Glycerini. .... 2 drams.
Acid. acetic. glacial. ..... 2½ drams.
Ol. amygdal. ess. .... 10 minims.
Tr. lavand. co. .... 1 dram.

Dissolve creasote and ol. amygdal. in 2 drams of alcohol; add other ingredients, making up to 1 ounce with alcohol.

704. Creasote Pills. (Ch. & Dr.)
I wish to give my experience of creasote pills, which have been discussed in the "Dispensing Notes" for the last two weeks. I have had large quantities to make for a customer at regular periods for three or four years, and I tried all the following excipients with unsatisfactory results: Curd soap, pulv. glycyrrhizae, pulv. althaeae, pulv. acaciae, pulv. tragac. co., ext. malt. All these exude oil, no matter how much powder is used. I then tried flour, with happy results. It leaves the mortar perfectly clean, without the slightest oiliness. Its only fault is a little elasticity; but this is nothing compared to the nasty crumbly oiliness of the other excipients. The form I use is this:

Guaiacol or creasote. ...... ½ ounce.
Flour. .... 1 ounce.

Mass with mucil. acaciae and divide in ten lots of twenty-four pills each.

705. Creasote Pills.
The following formula for "creasote pills" has been sent to us by Mr. A. Fetchner, chemist, of Cairo, who claims the advantages over other excipients in being easy to manipulate, readily soluble in water, and no difficulty in coating:

Creasoti. .... 12 minims.
Glycerini pur. .... 3 minims.
Pulv. succ. glycyrrhizae. .. 12 grains.
Pulv. rad. do. .... 24 grains.

M. Ft. massa. Divide in 12 pills.

Mix the creasote with glycerine in a mortar, then add the pulv. succ. glycyrrh. and rub together for a minute or two (which forms an emulsion with the creasote); lastly add the pulv. rad. glyc. and mass.

A little more powder may be added, if necessary, and by doubling the quantity of glycerine the mass will keep of a pilular consistence any length of time. Roll in finely-powdered cinnamon-bark.

706.
The second is a formula for creasote pills:
Creasote. .... 2 parts.
Pulv. saponis. .... 1 part.
Pulv. benzoin. .... 1 part.

Mix and add—
Pulv. glycyrrh. .... q. s.

These pills are small, of good consistence, do not get hard, and keep their shape.

H. L. Grimes says (Merck's Rep.) that owing to the peculiar and persistently pungent taste of creasote, there is nothing short of the gelatin capsule that will completely mask it. However, as this form of administration is not always eligible, efforts were made to combine the drug with other agents calculated to modify the pungency of the drug to a greater or lesser extent, and make the medicament more acceptable to the palate and to the stomach. In all pharmaceutical preparations of creasote, intended for internal use, none but the purest beech-wood creasote should be used. The three appended formulas have been deduced by experiments and the products have received the approval of many very prominent physicians.

707. Wine of Creasote.
Creasote (Beech-wood) ... 96 minims.
Alcohol. .... 1 fl. ounce.
Oil cinnamon. .... 24 drops.
Oil cloves. .... 12 drops.
Oil anise. .... 12 drops.
Syrup orange-peel. .... 4 fl. ounces.
Sherry wine. .... 8 fl. ounces.
Simple elixir, enough to
make. .... 16 fl. ounces.

Dissolve the creasote and oils in the alcohol, add the wine, syrup and elixir, and filter through purified talcum.

708. Emulsion of Creasote.
Creasote (Beech-wood). .... 768 minims.
Powdered acacia. .... 1080 grains.
Water, enough to make. .. 32 fl. ounces.

Triturate the creasote with the acacia in a dry mortar, and add, all at once, 27 fluid drams of water; stir briskly with the pestle until the nucleus of the emulsion is formed, and add enough water to make 2 pints; finally strain through a cloth.

Perhaps the most admirable combination is:

Creasoted Emulsion of Cod-Liver Oil with
709.   Hypophosphites.

Cod-liver oil.	32 fl. ounces.
Creasote (Beech-wood).	6½ fl. drams.
Powdered acacia.	8 ounces.
Glycerin.	4 fl. ounces.
Syrup orange-peel	2 fl. ounces.
Calcium hypophosphite.	555 grains.
Sodium hypophosphite.	555 grains.
Oil wintergreen.	2 fl. drams.
Oil sassafras.	2 fl. drams.
Oil. cinnamon.	2 fl. drams.
Distilled water, enough to make.	4 pints.

Mix the cod-liver oil, creasote, and essential oils, with the acacia, in a dry mortar; dissolve the hypophosphites in 12 fluid ounces of warm water, pour the solution, all at once, into the mixture of oils, creasote and acacia, and stir briskly in one direction with the pestle until emulsification takes place; then add the glycerine, syrup, and enough water to make 4 pints, and strain through a cloth. Recently-distilled water should preferably be used in these emulsions; but if none is at hand, water that has been freshly boiled and filtered will serve the purpose. In cold weather the water should be slightly warmed, else the emulsion will be very slow in forming. The creasote in the latter emulsion temporarily obtunds the sense of taste to a considerable degree while the preparation is being swallowed, and helps to conceal, in a measure, the unpleasant taste of cod-liver oil.

AGUE PREPARATIONS.

710.   Agueine.

Cherry juice.	¼ gallon.
Proof spirits.	3¼ gallons.
Simple syrup.	¼ gallon.
Water.	1¼ gallons.
Alcohol	¼ gallon.
Tinct. capsicum	10 ounces.
Tinct. ginger.	10 ounces.
Aromatic sulphuric acid.	20 ounces.
Quinine sulphate.	10 ounces.
Fl. ext. mandrake.	8 ounces.
Citrate of iron and ammon.	15 ounces.

711.   Baby Quinine.   A

Tannin.	30 grains.
Quinine sulph.	80 grains.
Soda bicarb.	2 drams.
Peppermint water.	2 ounces.
Simple syrup.	6 ounces.

Dose: One teaspoonful. Shake well label.

712.   Baby Quinine.   B

Cinchonia alkaloid pow'd.	80 grains.
Sugar of milk.	400 grains.
Soda bicarb.	100 grains.
Cinnamon water.	2 ounces.
Simple syrup.	6 ounces.

Rub the cinchonia alkaloid, sugar of milk and soda bicarb. together in a mortar, with a portion of the syrup, until smooth—add the other ingredients and mix well.

Dose: One teaspoonful.

Shake well label.

713.   Tasteless Chill Tonic.

Quinine sulphate.	64 grains.
Cinchonine sulphate.	64 grains.
Soda bicarb.	120 grains.
Saccharin.	15 grains.
Oil of wintergreen.	30 minims.
Fowler's solution.	256 minims.
alcohol.	2 ounces.
Water.	3 ounces.
Cascara arom. formula No. 57, q. s. to make up to	16 fl. ounces.

Dissolve the cinchona salts and oil of wintergreen in the alcohol, using a gentle heat of water bath. Dissolve the saccharin and soda bicarb. in the water.

Mix the solution of cinchona salts with the cascara arom., and then add the solution of saccharin and soda; lastly add the Fowler's solution and mix well.

Dose: One to two teaspoonfuls.

714.   Tasteless Chill Powders.

Cinchonia alkaloid.	25 grains.
Phenacetine.	25 grains.
Sugar of milk.	10 grains.
Soda bicarb.	5 grains.

Mix. Make into ten powders.

Dose: For an adult two powders, follow with a glassful of lemonade half an hour after taking the powders.

Acetanilid, exalgin or antipyrin may be substituted for phenacetine in the above.

KIDNEY AND LIVER MEDICINES.

Whayne's Buchu and Acetate of Potash.
715.

Buchu leaves, ground.	50 pounds.
Juniper berries, ground.	50 pounds.
Oil of wintergreen.	1 pound.
Proof spirits.	q. s.
Caustic potash.	1 pound.
Alcohol.	1 gallon.
Acetic acid.	10 gallons.
Potash bicarb.	q. s.
Water.	9 gallons.
Sugar house syrup.	10 gallons.

Percolate buchu and juniper berries with proof spirits until 30 gallons are obtained. Then run through the percolator the caustic potash dissolved in the 9 gallons of water.

Dissolve the oil of wintergreen in the alcohol and add the sugar house syrup, then neutralize the 10 gallons of acetic acid with potash bicarb. q. s. and mix with the other ingredients; color with caramel, q. s.

716. Diuretic Elixir of Buchu Co.

Buchu leaves, ground.	10 pounds.
Juniper berries, ground.	10 pounds.
Powdered cubebs.	½ pound.
Oil of peppermint.	½ ounce.
Sugar house syrup.	5 gallons.
Water.	q. s.
Proof spirits.	q. s.
Liquor Potassa.	2 pounds.
Caramel.	3 pints.

Mix the oil well with the drugs and macerate with a portion of the proof spirits for seven days, then percolate with proof spirits until the product obtained is 14 gallons; dissolve the liquor potassa in 2 gallons of water and run through the percolator. Add the syrup and caramel and enough water to measure 24 gallons.

717. Liver Invigorator. A

Fl. ext. colombo root.	1 gallon.
Fl. ext. dandelion.	1 gallon.
Fl. ext. virginia snake root.	1 gallon.
Fl. ext. senna.	5 gallons.
Fl. ext. mandrake.	2 gallons.
Proof spirits.	10 gallons.
Tinct. coriander seed (one pound to the gallon).	5 gallons.
Simple syrup.	5 gallons.
Caramel.	½ gallon.
Water.	11½ gallons.

Mix.

718. Liver Invigorator. B

Powdered senna.	2 pounds.
Powdered mandrake.	½ pound.
Powdered rhubarb.	½ pound.
Powdered jalap.	½ pound.
Powdered cloves.	1/8 pound.
Oil of peppermint.	½ ounce.

Mix well, macerate and percolate with 2 gallons of alcohol and one gallon of water; run water through the percolator until the product measures 4 gallons; to this add 1 gallon of simple syrup.

719. Kidney and Liver Cure.

Fl. ext. uva ursi.	1 pound.
Fl. ext. buchu.	1 pound.
Fl. ext. pareira brava.	1 pound.
Fl. ext. dandelion.	1 pound.
Nitrate of potash.	½ pound.
Oil of wintergreen.	½ ounce.
Alcohol.	2 gallons.
Simple syrup.	6 pints.
Caramel.	6 ounces.
Water.	5 gallons.

Mix.

720. Liver Mixture.

Acid nitro. hydrochlor. dil.	½ ounce.
Magnesia sulphate.	1 ounce.
Tinct. capsicum.	1 dram.
Water.	2 ounces.
Cascara arom. formula No. 57, q. s. to make up to 16 fl. ounces.	

721. Hamburg Breast Tea.

Marshmallow root cut.	4 ounces.
Licorice root cut.	1½ ounces.
Orris root cut.	½ ounce.
Coltsfoot leaves bruised.	2 ounces.
Mullein flowers bruised.	1 ounce.
White poppy capsules, bruised.	½ ounce.
Star anise seed, bruised.	1 ounce.

Mix.

722. St. Germain Laxative Tea. (Ger. Ph.)

Senna leaves cut.	16 ounces.
Elder flowers, bruised.	10 ounces.
Fennel seed, bruised.	5 ounces.
Anise seed, bruised.	5 ounces.
Cream of tartar.	4 ounces.

Moisten the senna with a small quantity of water; then sprinkle over it as evenly as possible the cream of tartar; dry thoroughly with a gentle heat; add the other drugs and mix well.

723. Blood and Kidney Tea.

Senna leaves bruised.	16 ounces.
Uva ursi bruised.	2 ounces.
Buchu, bruised.	2 ounces.
Sassafras bark, cut.	10 ounces.
Elder flowers, bruised.	10 ounces.
Fennel seed, bruised.	5 ounces.
Anise seed bruised.	5 ounces.
Coriander seed, bruised.	1 ounce.
Culver's root cut.	1 ounce.

Mix well.

Pack in cartons.

Directions: One teaspoonful to a cup of boiling water, draw for 15 minutes. Sugar may be added if desired. Use twice daily.

724. Kreuzthe—Cross Tea.

The Suddeutsche Apothekar Zeitung gives the following formula for this favorite German domestic remedy:

Species pectoralis.	20 parts.
Herba pulmonariae.	10 parts.
Chamomile flowers.	10 parts.
Elder flowers.	5 parts.
Tilia flowers.	4 parts.
Senna flowers.	4 parts.

Mix.

725. German Herb Tea.

Senna, cut.	17 grammes.
Triticum, cut.	17 grammes.
Fennel seed, bruised.	3 grammes.
Elder flowers.	3 grammes.

LAXATIVES AND APERIENTS

726. Syrup of Figs.

Senna, ground.	48 ounces.
Licorice root, ground.	4 ounces.
Cloves, powdered.	½ ounce.
Granulated sugar.	2 pounds.
Rochelle salts.	1 pound.
Magnesia sulphate.	½ pound.
Oil coriander.	30 drops.
Oil peppermint.	15 drops.
Oil cassia.	60 drops.
Glycerine.	4 pints.
Alcohol.	4 ounces.
Salicylic acid.	2 drams.
Saccharine.	1 dram.
Hot water.	q. s.

Macerate the senna, licorice and cloves with three gallons of hot water for two hours, keeping well covered. Press out by the aid of a tincture press and evaporate down to 1¼ gallons. Dissolve in this the sugar and salts and add the glycerine.

Dissolve the oils, saccharine and salicylic acid in the alcohol, and add.

727. Castroilina.

Senna, ground.	48 ounces.
Wormseed, ground.	4 ounces.
Licorice root, ground.	4 ounces.
Wintergreen leaves, ground	4 ounces.
Fennel seed, ground.	4 ounces.
Anise seed, ground.	4 ounces.
Rochelle salts.	24 ounces.
Glycerine.	4 pints.
Oil of wintergreen.	½ ounce.
Oil of peppermint.	15 drops.
Salicylic acid.	2 drams.
Alcohol.	4 ounces.
Sugar granulated.	2 pounds.
Hot water.	q. s.

Macerate the senna, licorice root, wintergreen leaves, fennel, wormseed and anise with three gallons of hot water for two hours, keeping well covered. Press out by the aid of a tincture press and evaporate down to 1¼ gallons. Dissolve in this the sugar and salts and add the glycerine. Dissolve the oil of wintergreen and salicylic acid in the alcohol and add to the other ingredients.

728. Purgative Tablets.

Jalap, powdered	1 ounce.
Senna, powdered.	1 ounce.
Ginger, powdered.	1 dram.
Sugar, powdered.	1 ounce.
Salicylic acid.	½ dram.
Tamarind pulp., q.s. to make mass.	

Cover with chocolate for laxative fruit pastilles. For compressed tablets, replace the tamarind pulp by mucilage of tragacanth, q. s.

729. Effervescent Purgative Salts. (Ch. & Dr.)

Epsom salts, half dried.	1 ounce.
Soda bicarb.	90 grains.
Tartaric acid.	80 grains.
Saccharin.	3 grains.
Oil of lemon.	2 minims.
Essence of cloves (1 to 10).	5 minims.

Mix thoroughly.

Dose: Two heaped up teaspoonfuls in three-fourths of a tumblerful of cold water.

730. Harrogate Salts.

Pulv. potass. sulph. c. sulph.	1½ ounces.
Pulv. potass. bitart.	5 ounces.
Mag. sulph. dry.	40 ounces.

Put up in 2 ounce packets (first wrapper stearin or parchment paper) and label "The contents of the packet to be put into a wine-bottleful of water, and a wineglassful of the solution taken every morning."

NON-SECRET FORMULAS.

731. Fruit Saline. A
Tartaric acid. .... 13 ounces.
Soda bicarb. .... 14 ounces.
Sugar powdered. .... 40 ounces.

Dry the ingredients separately, then mix well together and sift through fine sieve twice. Preserve in well corked bottles.

732. Fruit Saline. B
Soda bicarb. .... 16 ounces.
Acid tartaric. .... 14 ounces.
Magnesia sulph. dried. .... 2 ounces.
Chlorate of potash. .... 2 drams.
Powdered sugar. .... 16 ounces.

Dry the ingredients separately. Mix well together and sift through fine sieve twice. Preserve in well corked bottles.

733. Fruit Saline. C
Soda bicarb. .... 2 ounces.
Acid. tartaric .... 1½ ounces.
Cream of tartar .... 1½ ounces.
Sulphate of soda, dried .. 1 ounce.
Powdered sugar .... 6 ounces.

Carefully dry before mixing and preserve in a well corked dry bottle.

734. Fruit Saline. D
Rochelle salts .... 1 ounce.
Cream of tartar .... ½ ounce.
Tartaric acid. .... 1 ounce.
Soda bicarb. .... 1 ounce.
White sugar .... 2 ounces.

Carefully dry before mixing and preserve in a well corked dry bottle.

735. Sulpho Saline with Iron.
Sulphate of soda, dried .. 1 ounce.
Soda bicarb. .... 2 ounces.
Acid. tartaric .... 1¾ ounces.
Rochelle salts .... ½ ounce.
Sulphate of iron, dried ... 30 grains.
Powdered sugar .... 4 ounces.
Saccharin .... 10 grains.

Dry the ingredients separately before mixing; sift and mix well.
Preserve in well corked bottles.

EFFERVESCENT POWDERS.

The London Confectioner's Union (Nat. Dr.) gives the following formulae for effervescent powders:

736. Magnesian Lemonade Powders.
Fine white sugar .... 2 pounds.
Magnesium carbonate .... 6 ounces.
Citric acid. .... 4 ounces.
Essence of lemon .... 2 drams.

Rub the essence into the dry ingredients, work well together, sift and bottle.

737. Magnesian Orgeat Powders.
Fine sugar .... 1 pound.
Carbonate of magnesia ... 3 ounces.
Citric acid. .... 1 ounce.
Oil of bitter almonds .... 3 drops.
Vanilla flavoring .... q. s.

Thoroughly amalgamate the dry ingredients. Rub in the oil of almonds and sufficient essence of vanilla to give a slight flavor. Work all well together, sift and bottle.

738. Raspberryade Powder.
Fine sugar .... 2 pounds.
Carbonate of soda .... 2 ounces.
Tartaric acid. .... 2 ounces.
Essence of raspberry .... 4 drams.
Carmine coloring .... q. s.

Rub the essence well into the sugar, and mix this with the soda and acid. Then work in sufficient liquid carmine to make the powder pale red, sift through a fine sieve, and pack in air tight bottles.

739. Ambrosia Powder.
Fine sugar .... 2 pounds.
Carbonate of soda .... 12 drams.
Citric acid. .... 10 drams.
Essence of almonds...... 20 drops.

Amalgamate the whole of the above, and afterwards sift and bottle in the usual manner.

740. Noyeau Powder.
Fine sugar .... 2 pounds.
Carbonate of soda .... 12 drams.
Tartaric acid. .... 10 drams.
Essence of noyeau .... 6 drops.

After the dry ingredients have been mixed and the essence rubbed into them, sift and bottle the powder.

741. Lemon Sherbet (Best).
Fine sugar .... 9 pounds.
Tartaric acid. .... 40 ounces.
Carbonate of soda .... 36 ounces.
Oil of lemon .... 2 drams.

Having thoroughly mixed the dry ingredients, add the lemon, rubbing it well in between the hands; then sift the whole thrice through a fine sieve, and cork down tight.

As oil of lemon is used in this recipe, the blending must be perfect, or when the powder is put in water the oil of lemon will float.

Any other flavoring may be substituted for lemon, and the sherbet named accordingly.

742. Cream Soda Powder.

Fine sugar	30 parts.
Tartaric acid	7 parts.
Carbonate of soda	6 parts.
Finely powd. gum arabic	1 part.
Vanilla flavoring	q s.

Proceed exactly as for best lemon sherbet.

743. Compound Mixture Taraxacum.
(Rocky Mountain Drug.)

Extract taraxacum	8 tr. ounces.
Nitrohydrochloric acid, dilute	4 fl. ounces.
Elixir bismuth	8 fl. ounces.
Syrup ginger	5⅜ fl. ounces.
Tincture nux vomica	260 minims.
Spirits peppermint	15 minims.
Water, enough to make	32 fl. ounces.

744. Aperient Lozenge. (Ch. & Dr.)

Sulphur	5 grains.
Cream tartar	1 grain.
Extract ipecacuanha	1-100.
Capsicine	1-1000.
Calcium bisulphate	¼ grain.
Sugar	8 grains.

Make one lozenge.

This combination is a gentle, efficient aperient remedy for habitual constipation. One, two or three lozenges to be slowly dissolved in the mouth soon after meals, will be sufficient to produce a gentle and pleasant action. The patient, after the lozenge has dissolved, should drink a glass of water to increase the effect.

LINIMENTS.

745. Arnica Liniment.

Gum camphor	2½ ounces.
Laudanum	8 ounces.
Chloroform	2 ounces.
Tinct. arnica flowers	1 gallon.

M. S. A.

746. German Oil Liniment.

Gum camphor	2½ ounces.
Chloroform	4 ounces.
Sulphuric ether	4 ounces.
Chloral hydrate	1 ounce.
Oil origanum	6 ounces.
Oil sassafras	3 ounces.
Turpentine	192 ounces.
Alkanet root q. s. to color red.	

M. S. A.

747. Magic Arnica Liniment.

Refined petroleum	1 pint.
Oil origanum	1 ounce.
Oil terebinth	2 ounces.
Oil cedar	1 ounce.
Oil spruce	1 ounce.
Spirits camphor	1½ ounces.
Oil sassafras	1 ounce.

Color light red with alkanet root.

Giles' Liniment of Iodide of Ammonia.
748.

Iodine	15 grains.
Alcohol	8 ounces.
Camphor	2 drams.
Oil lavender	1 dram.
Oil rosemary	1 dram.
Water of ammon. stronger	1 dram.

Mix.

See also formulas 671, 672, 673.

749. Indian Liniment.

Tincture capsicum	1 ounce.
Oil camphor	½ ounce.
Oil origanum	½ ounce.
Oil pennyroyal	½ ounce.
Oil hemlock	½ ounce.
Alcohol	32 ounces.

Color with red sanders.

750. Liniment for Sprains.

Liquor plumbi acet.	2 ounces.
Ol. origanum	1 ounce.
Acetum	2 ounces.
Aqua	30 ounces.

Make a lotion.

751. British Oil. A

Oil of spike	1 pint.
Oil of juniper wood	1 ounce.
Oil of origanum	½ ounce.

Mix.

752. British Oil. B

Oil of turpentine	8 fl. ounces.
Oil of flaxseed	8 fl. ounces.
Oil of amber	4 fl. ounces.
Oil of juniper	4 fl. drams.
Barbadoes petroleum	3 fl. ounces.
Seneca oil	1 fl. ounce.

Mix.

NON-SECRET FORMULAS.

753. British Oil.
Oil of turpentine .... 8 fl. ounces
Barbadoes petroleum ..... 4 fl. ounces.
Oil rosemary .... 4 fl. drams.
Mix.

754. White Oils Liniment. A
Camphor .... 3 ounces.
Spirit of turpentine ...... 4 pints.
Soft soap .... 1 pound.
Olive oil .... 2 pints.
Solution of ammonia ...... 1 pint.

Dissolve the camphor in the turpentine, and to this add the olive oil. Dissolve the soap in 6 pints of water, add the ammonia, and incorporate this mixture with the oils with the help of an emulsifier. Allow to stand for a day or two, agitating every day; then with water reduce the emulsion to the consistency desired.

755. White Oils Liniment. B
Egg 1
Acetic acid .... 2 ounces.
Distilled water .... 2 ounces.
Oil turpentine .... 4 ounces.

Beat up the egg with the turpentine; then add the acetic acid and water.

756. Red Nose Liniment.
Corrosive sublimate ...... 4 grains.
Muriate of ammonia ...... 8 grains.
Alum .... 8 grains.
Alcohol .... 4 ounces.
Rose water .... 4 ounces.
M. S. A.

757. Liniment for Colic.
Which when warmed and rubbed over the surface of the abdomen very quickly allays the pains of flatulent colic.
Lin. saponis comp. .... 2½ ounces.
Lin. camphorae co. .... 2½ ounces.
Ol. terebinth. rect. ...... 2 ounces.
Sapo. hispan. .... 2 drams.
Ol. cajuput. .... 1 dram.
Ol. limon. .... 1 dram.

Mix, and make a liniment, to be rubbed assiduously or applied warm over the surface of the abdomen.

758. Roberts' Ready Relief.
Alcohol .... 1 gallon.
Cayenne pepper, powdered. 8 ounces.
Ginger, powdered .... 8 ounces.
Spirits of ammonia ...... 8 ounces.
Gum myrrh, powdered .... 1 ounce.
Red saunders .... ½ ounce.

Macerate 7 days and filter.

759. Cream of Camphor Liniment.
Gum camphor .... 1 ounce.
Spirits of turpentine ..... 2 ounces.
Aqua ammonia .... 2 ounces.
Sweet oil .... 2 ounces.

Dissolve the camphor in the turpentine; mix the ammonia and sweet oil, shaking well together.

760. Ringworm Liniment.
Aromatic sulph. acid .... 1 ounce.
Spirits of nitrous ether ... 1 ounce.
Creosote .... 1 ounce.
Mix.

Apply once a day with a feather until well.

761. Stokes' Chest Liniment.
Morphiae acet. .... 6 grains.
Chloroform. puri. .... 1 ounce.
Lin. saponis ad .... 3 ounces.
M. Ft. lin.

To be rubbed into the chest, back and front, every night.

762. Stokes' Rheumatic Liniment.
Ol. terebinthinae .... 1½ ounces.
Acid. acetic. .... 1½ ounces.
Ovi vitelli .... unus
Olei limonis .... 1 scruple.
Aquae rosae ad .... 8 ounces.
M. Ft. lin.

To be rubbed into affected joints.

763. Cyclists' Universal Oil.
Camphorated oil .... 1 ounce.
Sperm oil .... 3 ounces.
Vaseline oil .... 4 ounces.
Mix.

764. Arnica Opodeldoc.
Rad arnica............... aa.
Rad aconite.............. 2 ounces.
Pulvis opii .... 6 drams.
Alcohol .... 15 ounces.
Aqua distil. .... 10 ounces.

Macerate seven days and strain with pressure; then add
White castile soap ...... 3½ ounces.
Gum camphor .... 3 ounces.
Oil lavand. .... 1 ounce.
Oil origanum .... ½ ounce.
Strong ammonia water ... 1¼ ounces.

765. Neuralgic Liniment.
Menthol .... ½ ounce.
S. V. R. .... 1 ounce.
Solve et adde—
Lin. aconiti .... 3 drams.
Ext. opii liq. .... 3 drams.
Aether. ad .... 3 ounces.
M.

Put up in ½-ounce phials, with a brush. Directions: "Paint the liniment over the affected part."

766. White Liniment.
Ol. terebinthinae .... 8 ounces.
Camphorae .... ½ ounce.
Vitell. ovi 2
Ac. acetic. .... 1 ounce.
Tr. arnicae .... 2 ounces.
Aq. ad .... 20 ounces.

Dissolve the camphor in the turpentine contained in a 40-ounce bottle, add the yolk of egg and 10 ounces of water; shake briskly. Then add, 2 ounces at a time, the rest of the water containing the arnica and acetic acid, shaking well the while.

767. Nerve and Bone Liniment. A
Turpentine oil .... 1 gallon.
Linseed oil .... 1 gallon.
Juniper wood oil .... ¾ gallon.
Engine oil, neutral .... 1 gallon.
Origanum oil .... 8 ounces.
Amber oil .... 8 ounces.
Mix.

768. Nerve and Bone Liniment. B
Turpentine oil .... 2 gallons.
Linseed oil .... 2 gallons.
Engine oil .... 2 gallons.
Origanum oil .... 8 ounces.
Camphor oil .... 8 ounces.
Rosemary oil .... 8 ounces.
Mix.

769. Hamlin's Wizard Oil Liniment.
Oil hemlock .... 2 ounces.
Oil cedar .... 2 ounces.
Oil sassafras .... 3 ounces.
Oil origanum .... 3 ounces.
Oil turpentine .... 6 ounces.
Oil linseed, raw .... ½ gallon.
Sulph. ether .... 2 ounces.
Tr. opium .... 2 ounces.
Chloroform .... 2 ounces.
Alcohol .... 1 gallon.
Tr. capsicum .... 3 ounces.
Spts. ammonia .... 2 ounces.
Gum camphor .... 1 ounce.

770. Liniment of Soap and Iod. Potash.
Castile soap, powdered ... 1¼ ounces.
Rose geranium oil .... 5 drops.
Almond oil .... 1¼ ounces.
Iodide of potash .... 4 drams.
Water .... 1¾ ounces.

Rub the castile soap and oils together; dissolve the iodide of potash in the water and mix well.

771 Hydride of Amyl Liniment.
Castor oil .... 1 ounce.
Cocaine hydrochlorate .... 20 grains.
Menthol .... 60 grains.
Chloral hydrate .... 60 grains.
Amyl hydride .... 120 minims.
Alcohol, q. s. to make up to 2 ounces.

Dissolve the cocaine, menthol, chloral hydrate and hydride of amyl in the alcohol, and mix with the castor oil.

Prescribed by Dr. Bennet.

OINTMENTS.

772. Itch Ointment.
White wax .... 2½ pounds.
Petrolatum, yellow .... 5 pounds.
Lac. sulphur .... 1 pound.
Powd. white helebore .... ¼ pound.
Carbolic acid, crystals .... ¼ pound.
Oil rosemary .... ¼ ounce.

773. Ointments for the Itch.
(French Hospital.)
Chloride of lime .... 1 dram.
Rectified spirit .... 2 fl. drams.
Rub together, add of
Sweet oil .... ½ fl. dram.
Soft soap .... 2 ounces.
Oil of lemon .... ½ fl. dram.

Mix perfectly, and then further add of
Common salt .... 1 ounce.
Sulphur .... 1 ounce.

Cheap, very effective, and much less offensive than sulphur ointment.

774.
(Le Gros.)
Iodide of potassium ...... ½ dram.
Lard .... 1 ounce.

Mix. Cleanly, harmless and effective.

775. Kraemer's Pile Ointment.

Beef suet	10 pounds.
Lard	15 pounds.
Solid extract stramon.	1 pound.
Tannic acid.	1 pound.
Calomel	2½ pounds.
Oil rose geranium	2 ounces.
Salicylic acid.	1 ounce.

Melt the fats, and mix in the other ingredients, stirring constantly until cold; run through a paint mill to ensure thorough mixing.

776. Compound Pile Ointment. A

White wax	1 pound.
White petrolatum	2½ pounds.
Powdered opium	1 ounce.
Powdered hydrastia sulph.	1 dram.
Powdered catechu	1 ounce.

Melt the wax and petrolatum and add the other ingredients; stir well and mix thoroughly.

777. Compound Pile Ointment. B

Tannin	2 drams.
Bismuth subnit.	2½ ounces.
Aqueous extract opium.	2 drams.
Petrolatum, yellow	12 ounces.

778. Arnica Salve.

Yellow rosin	2 pounds.
Yellow petrolatum	2 pounds.
Solid extract arnica	2 ounces.

779. Carbolic Ointment.

Lard	12 pounds.
Beef suet	12 pounds.
White wax	2 pounds.
Gum camphor	2 ounces.
Carbolic acid crystals	2½ pounds.
Calomel	2½ pounds.

Melt the lard, suet, wax, and camphor together.

Melt the carbolic acid crystals and add; strain and stir well; when nearly cold add the calomel and mix thoroughly; when cold fill into containers. This is the best carbolic ointment on the market.

780. Boracic Acid Salve.

Boracic acid, powdered	8 ounces.
Yellow rosin	2 pounds.
Yellow petrolatum	2 pounds.
Fl. ext. witch hazel bark	2 ounces.
Solid ext. arnica	½ ounce.
Glycerine	1 pint.
Lanoline	1 pound.

Melt the rosin and petrolatum together and strain.

Mix the witch hazel, boracic acid, extract arnica and glycerine together and heat in a water bath until dissolved. Then add the lanoline and mix thoroughly with the other ingredients.

781. Mercurial Ointment.

Mercury	1 ounce.
Lanoline	1 ounce.
Olive oil	½ ounce.

Kill the mercury by triturating with a few drops of balsam of sulphur, work in the lanoline then the olive oil.

782. Glycerine Ointment.

Starch	3 parts.
Glycerine	10 parts.

The starch, finely pulverized, is digested for about an hour with the glycerine, at the heat of a water bath.

783. Ointment of Iodine.

Ointment of Iodine.—Iodine is very soluble in vaseline, and it is supposed enters partially into combination with the hydrocarbon, giving rise to a considerable effervescence (probable hydrogen being displaced). Iodine dissolves slowly in vaseline if allowed to macerate in it or if rubbed up with it, but for ointment of iodine the following gives the best results:

Iodine	20 grains.
Alcohol	q. s.
Vaseline	1 ounce.

Dissolve the iodine in the alcohol, and mix with the vaseline p'aced on a hot water bath. Very little iodine will be evaporated during the operation.

784. Iodide of Iron Ointment.

Iodide of Iron Ointment.—If iron be added to a solution of iodine in vaseline and repeatedly shaken (the whole kept liquid on a water bath), the almost black color of the iodine disappears, and if an excess of iron be employed the color becomes green, and if it be then filtered the ointment will have a beautiful emerald green color through transmitted light and almost black by reflected light.

    Iodine .... 4 drams.
    Iron filings .... 12 drams.
    Vaseline .... 16 ounces.

This iodide of iron ointment is stable and almost without taste. Prepare from it a jelly by adding an equal quantity of very fine sugar, in which manner it could be easily taken by children. Mr. E. Fougera, of Brooklyn, has also prepared a bromide and chloride in like manner, and suggests its use in keeping the protosalts of iron by enveloping them in it.

785. Ointment for Barber's Itch.
    Creolin .... 1 dram.
    Oleate of mercury .... 4 drams.
    Oxide of zinc .... 4 drams.
    Salicylic acid .... 1 dram.
    Yellow petrolatum .... 1½ ounces.

786. Itch Salve.
    Bismuth subnitrate .... 2 drams.
    Creolin .... 3 drams.
    Sulphur .... 2 drams.
    Yellow petrolatum .... 1 ounce.

787. Oleate of Mercury.
    Red oxide of mercury .... 1 ounce.
    Oleic acid .... 2¾ ounces.
    White petrolatum .... 1¼ ounces.

Add the oxide to the acid at a steam-bath temperature, and, after combination, add the vaseline.

Dilute with acid. oleic or paraffin. molle alb., according as an oleate or an ointment is ordered.

788. Iodide of Potassium Ointment.
    Iodide of potassium ...... 64 grains.
    Hyposulphite of sodium .. 1 grain.
    Glycerine .... 1 dram.
    Benzoated lard .... 1 ounce.
    Water .... 5 minims.

Triturate the iodide with the glycerine, add the benz. lard, and lastly the hyposulphite dissolved in the water, and mix thoroughly.

789. Witch Hazel Ointment.
    Lanolin .... 2 ounces.
    Glycerin .... 2 ounces.
    Fl. ext. witch hazel bark.. 2 ounces.
    Boracic acid .... 2 drams.
    Yellow petrolatum .... 10 ounces.

Dissolve the boracic acid in the glycerine by heat; add the witch hazel and lanoline; and then the petrolatum. Stir well.

790. Ointment for Blistering Horses.
    Croton oil .... 2 drams.
    Euphorbium powd. .... 1 ounce.
    Cantharides powd. .... 1 ounce.
    Turpentine oil .... 3 ounces.
    Petrolatum yellow .... 3 ounces.
Mix.

791. Healing Ointment.
    Petrolatum, white .... 16 ounces.
    Oxide of zinc .... 2 ounces.
    Oleate of mercury .... 1 ounce.
    Boracic acid .... 2 drams.
    Carbolic acid .... 2 drams.

792. Ointment for Chapped Hands.
    Menthol .... 15 grains.
    Salol .... 30 grains.
    Ol. olivae .... ½ dram.
    Lanolini .... 1½ ounces.
M.

Apply night and morning. rubbing in well.

793. Nit Ointment.
The safest preparation on the whole is one made from stavesacre, such as:
    Ol. staphisag. .... 1 ounce.
    Cerae flavae .... 1 ounce.
    Vaselini .... 6 ounces.
    Hyd. sulph. rub. .... 10 grains.
    Ol. bergam. .... 10 minims.
    Ol. cinnam. .... 3 minims.
    Ol. citronell. .... 2 minims.
Ft. ung.

794. Ointment for Boils.   A
Heltzmann is authority for the following:
    Salicylic acid .... 2 drams.
    Soap plaster .... 2 ounces.
    Lead plaster .... 1 ounce.

795. Ointment for Boils.   B
    Ichthyol .... 1 dram.
    Lead plaster .... 2 drams.
    Resin plaster .... 1 dram.

796. Stick Salve.

Rosin	1 pound.
Mutton tallow	1 ounce.
Beeswax	
Burgundy pitch, of each..	½ ounce.
Balsam fir	
Venice turpentine of each	¼ ounce.
Oil spike	
Oil hemlock	
Oil cedar	
Oil origanum	
Oil wormwood	
Laudanum	
Pulverized camphor gum of each	1 dram.

Melt the rosin, tallow, beeswax and pitch together. When a little cool, add the oils, laudanum, etc.; stir in the pulverized camphor, and pour into cold water, then, by greasing the hands, it can be pulled and worked until it becomes intimately mixed, when it can be rolled into suitable sized sticks.

797. Eye Salve. A

White petrolatum	1¼ pounds.
Purified beef suet	1½ pounds.
White precipitate	½ ounce.
Oil of sassafras	1 dram.

798. Eye Salve. B

Yellow oxide of mercury..	96 grains.
Oxide of zinc	60 grains.
Morphine sulphate	30 grains.
White petrolatum	16 ounces.

799. Steer's Opodeldoc.

White castile soap; cut small; 2 pounds; camphor, 5 ounces; oil of rosemary, 1 ounce; oil of origanum, 2 ounces; rectified spirit, 1 gallon; dissolve in a corked bottle by the heat of a water bath, and when quite cool, strain; then add ammonium hydroxide, aqua ammonia, 11 ounces; immediately put it in bottles, cork close, and tie over with bladder. It will be very fine, solid, and transparent when cold. The liquid opodeldoc is prepared by taking 2 ounces castile soap shavings, and dissolving them in one quart alcohol, with gentle heat; then add 1 ounce camphor, ½ ounce oil rosemary, and 2 ounces spirits hartshorn (aqua ammonia).

800. Camphor Ball.

Cerae alb.	5 ounces.
Cetacei.	2 ounces.
Ol. amygdal.	5 ounces.
Ol. coc. nucis	8 ounces.
Flor. camphor.	1 ounce.
Ol. amygd. essent.	10 minims.
Ol. eucalypti	15 minims.

Melt the first four, transfer to the shop-pot, add the camphor and perfumes. Stir, and cover the pot.

Camphor has very little action in healing skin-fissures; it is a mild antiseptic, but the reason that camphor-ball does good is that, being a cerate, it is a protective.

801. Mayer's Ointment.

Prof. J. U. Lloyd, in 1890, contributed an article to the Era on the history of this preparation, for which he gave the following formula from the Eclectic Dispensatory of 1852, with these remarks:

Formula for Mayer's Ointment.—To olive oil, two pounds and a half, add white turpentine, half a pound; beeswax, unsalted butter, of each, four ounces; melt them together and heat to nearly the boiling point. Then add gradually red lead, one pound, and stir constantly until the mixture becomes black or brown; then remove from the fire, and when it has become somewhat cool, add to it a mixture of honey, twelve ounces, powdered camphor, half a pound.

Uses.—"This forms a superior salve, and is useful for all ulcers, cuts, wounds, etc. It has been kept a great secret for a length of time among the foreign population of our country, and is highly prized by those who have used it."

Remarks.—The mixture of olive oil, beeswax and greases (lard will answer instead of butter), should be heated over direct fire until they will effervesce, when a little red lead is added thereto. The vessel containing them should be iron and of four times the capacity of the batch. The red lead should be added cautiously, a tablespoonful at a time for a fifty-pound batch and well stirred after each addition, the red color changing to brown quickly if the temperature is high enough. After the reaction is completed, and the mixture is cool enough to receive the honey without violent effervescence, it should be added and stirred well to evaporate the water. Lastly, when the mixture is cool enough to dissolve the camphor without vaporization, it must be added and dissolved. This point must be determined nicely to prevent the loss of camphor from evaporation, or roughness of the ointment by reason of undissolved particles of camphor.

Mayer's ointment has a dark brown color (not red), and is about the consistence of simple cerate. The prominent odor of camphor overcomes the peculiar odor of the other ingredients, and even the familiar rank odor of olive oil that has been heated in contact with litharge or red lead is scarcely perceptible. Mayer's ointment should be perfectly smooth and free from grit or roughness.

802. Screw Worm Ointment.

Laundry soap, yellow .... 60 pounds.
Yellow rosin .... 5 pounds.
Crude carbolic acid ...... 9½ gallons.

Shave the soap and break up the rosin into small pieces and dissolve by the aid of heat; add the acid. Pour into wide mouth bottles while warm.

803. Neuralgic Ointment.

Menthol .... 45 grains.
Cocaine .... 15 grains.
Chloral .... 10 grains.
Vaseline .... 5 drams.

To be applied to the painful part.

804. Simple Ointment.

Ointment, simple.— Olive oil, 5½ fl. ounces; white wax, 2 ounces; melted together and stirred while cooling.

805.

Prepared lard, 4 pounds; white wax, 1 pound; as the last.

806.

White wax, 2; prepared lard, 3; almond oil, 8; melt together and stir until it becomes solid. The above are mild emollients, useful in healthy ulcers, excoriations, etc., but chiefly as forming the basis of other ointments.

807. Sulphur Ointment.

Sublimed sulphur .... 1 ounce.
Lard .... 4 ounces.

Mix thoroughly, by trituration. These are the proportions of the new Br. and the E. and D. Ph. In the last London Ph. a larger quantity of sulphur is ordered.

808.

The compound sulphur ointment of the London Ph. consists of—

Nitrate of potassa (in fine
  powder) .... 40 grains.
White hellebore (in fine
  powder) .... 10 drams (troy).
Sulphur .... 4 ounces (troy).
Soft soap .... 4 ounces (troy).
Lard .... 1 pound. (troy)

It is said to be more efficacious than the simple ointment; but is apt to irritate a delicate skin.

809. Ointment of White Wax.

1. White wax (pure)...... 2 ounces.
   Prepared lard .... 3 ounces.
   Almond oil .... 3 fl. ounces.

Melt them together, and stir the mixture until it solidifies. This is the unguentum simplex of the new British Pharmacopoeia.

810.

2. White wax .... 2 ounces.
   Olive oil .... 5½ fl. ounces.

As before. A mild emollient, in various applications but chiefly as a basis for other ointments and medicated pommades. On the Continent it is regarded as more healing when made with yellow wax.

811. Spermaceti Ointment.

Spermaceti Ointment.—Simple ointment, emollient dressing, etc.

1. Spermaceti .... 5 ounces.
   White wax (pure)...... 2 ounces.
   Almond oil .... 1 pint.

Melt them together by a gentle heat, and stir constantly until the whole solidifies.

812. Ointment of Creasote.

Creasote .... 1 fl. dram.
Spermaceti ointment .... 1 ounce.

Triturate them together, in a slightly warmed mortar, until perfectly united, and subsequently until nearly cold.

813. Indian Cerate.

For burns, scalds, chapped hands, sore eyes, etc.

Zinci oxidi .... 2 drams.
Cerae japonicae .... 1½ ounces.
Adipis .... 4 ounces.
M. S. A.

814. Pile Ointment. (Era).

(For itching piles.)

Yellow oxide of mercury.. 5 grains.
Petrolatum .... 1 ounce.
Gallic acid .... 20 grains.
Extract of opium .... 10 grains.
Extract of belladonna .. 10 grains.
Simple ointment .... 1 ounce.

Apply night and morning.

815.

Ointment of galls with
  opium .... 20 grains.
Bismuth subnitrate ..... 1 dram.
Powdered opium .... 10 grains.
Soft paraffin .... 1 ounce.

815½. **Bleeding Piles.**
    Tannic acid .... ½ dram.
    Morphine acetate .... 5 grains.
    Liniment subacetate of
        lead .... ½ fl. ounce.
    Simple ointment .... 7 drams.
Triturate the tannic acid with the liniment and then mix all together.

816. **Pile Salve.**
    Tannic acid .... 10 grains.
    Bismuth subnitrate ...... 20 grains.
    Carbolic acid .... 10 minims.
    Morphine sulphate .... 8 grains.
    Petrolatum, enough to
        make .... 1 ounce.
Apply locally night and morning.

817. **Hæmorrhoids.**
    Extract hamamelis .... 3 grains.
    Milk of almonds .... 1¾ drams.
    Cacao butter .... 2½ drams.

818. **Suppositories for Piles.** A
    Ext. ergot. (solid) .... 2 grains.
    Ext. opii .... ¼ grains.
    Ext. nuc. vom. .... ¼ grains.
    Cocain. hydrochlor. .... ¼ grains.
    Ol. theobrom. .... q. s.
    Ft. suppositoria.
    Mitte 12.
(Rub down the extracts and cocaine on a warm slab, and gradually add the ol. theobrom., which should be only just melted, return to the suppository-bath, pouring into the mould as soon as liquefied, using the least possible heat.)

819. **For Painful Piles and Vaginitis.**
    (Journ. Med. and Science.)
    Ext. aconite .... ⅛ grain.
    Ext. belladonna .... ⅛ grain.
    Ext. hydrastis .... 1 grain.
    Ext. lobelia .... 3 grains.
    Cacao butter .... enough.
Make one suppository.

820. **Pile Suppositories.** B
    Iodoform .... 30 grains.
    Extract belladonna .... 3 grains.
    Morphine sulphate .... 1½ grains.
    Cacao butter .... 180 grains.
Mix, and make twelve suppositories.

821 **Pile Suppositories.** C
    Extract witchhazel, powd.. 60 grains.
    Tannin .... 12 grains.
    Opium .... 4 grains.
    Cacao butter .... 180 grains.
Mix, and make twelve suppositories.

ANTIPYRETICS AND ANTISEPTICS.

Kamnafuga—A Substitution Product.
822.
Sir: I send you a formula for publication in The Chemist and Druggist which I think will prove acceptable to the pharmacists of the whole country. Yours respectfully,
R. N. GIRLING.
New Orleans, December 11.
    Acetanilide .... 50 grammes.
    Caffeine .... 2 grammes.
    Tartaric acid .... 3 grammes.
    Sodium bicarbonate ...... 45 grammes.
    Mix thoroughly.
Kamnafuga will be found an excellent antipyretic and analgesic. It should be brought to the notice of the physicians of the whole country, as it is eminently fitted to take the place of a certain high-priced proprietary article which is largely advertised. The low price at which kamnafuga can be sold to the public should bring it into favor with physicians.

823. **Analysis of Ammonol.**
Dr. R. J. Eccles has made an analysis of the proprietary article sold as ammonol, the result of which he publishes in the Druggists' Circular. He concludes his paper by saying that, "The exact determination of the quantities of the various ingredients in a mixture like this is one of great difficulty, and takes much time. The determination with sufficient accuracy to be able to practically duplicate them is not quite so difficult. If the reader who is curious to experiment with such preparations will take 6 parts of acetanilid, 3 parts of sodium bicarbonate and 1½ parts of ammonium carbonate and mix them together he will get a preparation giving all the medicinal results that can be had from ammonol. If he will add 20 centigrams of methyl orange to every 1,000 grams of such a mixture and then incorporate with this enough curcumin to give the whole the same yellow tinge as is possessed by ammonol, he will practically be able to duplicate its various chemical reactions as well as its medicinal. It will be well for druggists to call the attention of medical men who use ammonol to these facts."

824. **Antikamnia.** (Ch. & Dr.)
    Acetanilidi .... 65 grains.
    Sodii bicarb. .... 30 grains.
    Caffeinae cit. .... 5 grains.

825. **Aristol.**
 Iodi .... 98 grains.
 Potas. iodidi .... 120 grains.
 Thymol .... 212 grains.
 Sodae caustic .... 309 grains.
 Sol. calc. chlorinatae ..... q. s.

Dissolve the first two in 8 ounces aq., the next two in 8 ounces more; then mix both solutions in a ½-gallon glass vessel, in which they can be stirred briskly while gradually adding solution chlorinated lime. Be careful towards end so as to leave it only in slight excess. Collect on a filter, and dry in warm place.

826. **Anti Pain Powder.**
 Phenacetin .... 50 grains.
 Caffeine .... 5 grains.
 Sodium bicarb. .... 40 grains.
 Citric acid, powdered .. 5 grains.

827. **Antiseptic Wound-Dressing.**
 (Dr. J. Cornby.)
 Iodoform .... 10.0.
 Cinchona .... 10.0.
 Charcoal .... 10.0.

Soothing Antiseptic Dressing for Contusions.
 (Southern Practitioner.)
828.
 Cocaine hydrochlorate .. 30 grains.
 Camphor .... 40 grains.
 Carbolic acid .... 40 grains.
 Resorcin .... 1 dram.
 Zinc oxide .... 4 drams.
 Lanolin .... 2 ounces.
 Petrolatum .... 2 ounces.

Apply every three hours. Soothing, healing and antiseptic.

829. **Antiseptic Mixture.**
 Alcohol .... 8 ounces.
 Thymol .... 60 grains.
 Menthol .... 10 grains.
 Oil eucalyptus .... 60 drops.
 Oil wintergreen .... 110 drops.
 Glycerine .... 8 ounces.
 Boric acid .... 5 drams.
 Aqua dist. .... 128 ounces.
 Color q. s. ....
 Filter.

CARMINATIVES, ETC.

830. **Diarrhœa Cordial.**
 Laudanum .... 8 ounces.
 Fl. extract catechu aqueous 32 ounces.
 Spirits of camphor .... 8 ounces.
 Essence of peppermint . 5 ounces.
 Tincture of ginger .... 10 ounces.
 Tincture of cloves .... 10 ounces.
 Tincture of cassia .... 10 ounces.
 California port wine .. 96 ounces.
 Proof spirits .... 256 ounces.
 Simple syrup .... 128 ounces.
 Water .... 96 ounces.
 Caramel .... 4 ounces.

831. **Squibb's Diarrhœa Mixture.**
 Tincture of opium ..... 1 fl. ounce.
 Tincture of capsicum .. 1 fl. ounce.
 Spirit of camphor ..... 1 fl. ounce.
 Purified chloroform ... 180 minims.
 Alcohol, enough to make.. 5 fl. ounces.

832. **Thielemann's Diarrhœa Mixture.**
 Wine of opium .... 1 fl. ounce.
 Tincture of valerian .. 1½ fl. ounces.
 Ether .... ½ fl. ounce.
 Oil of peppermint ..... 60 minims.
 Fl. ext. of ipecac. ... 15 minims.
 Alcohol, enough to make.. 4 fl. ounces.

This preparation is practically identical with the "Mixtura Thielemanni" of the Swedish Pharm.

833. **Velpeau's Diarrhœa Mixture.**
 Tincture of opium, compound tincture of catechu (U. S. P.), spirit of camphor, each equal volumes.

834. **Anti-Cholera Mixture.**
 Tr. rhei co. .... 1½ ounces.
 Tr. catechu. .... ½ ounce.
 Tr. zingib. .... 2 drams.
 Ext. glycyrrhiz. liq. . ½ ounce.
 Aq. camphorae ad. ..... 8 ounces.
 M.

835. **For Diarrhœa in Children.**
 Paregoric .... 17 minims.
 Bismuth. subnit. ...... 2 drams.
 Syr. limonis. .... ½ ounce.
 Mist. cretae. .... 1½ ounces.
 M.

Shake well, and give one teaspoonful every three or four hours to a child one year old.

836. Loomis' Diarrhœa Mixture.

Tincture of opium	½ fl. ounce.
Tincture of rhubarb	½ fl. ounce.
Co. tinct. catechu (U. S. P.)	1 fl. ounce.
Oil of sassafras	20 minims.
Compound tincture of lavender, enough to make	4 fl. ounces.

Carminative or Gripe Mixture for Infants.
837.

Sodii bromidi	1 scruple.
Sodii bicarb	½ dram.
Ol. pimentae	1 minim.
Ol. carui	4 minims.
Ol. anisi	2 minims.
Spt. rectificat	½ ounce.
Syrupi	1 ounce.
Aq. ad	8 ounces.

Dissolve the oils in the spirit, and add to 6½ ounces of water containing 1 dram of French chalk. Shake well, and filter. In the filtrate dissolve the salts, and add the syrup.

Dose: One to two teaspoonfuls.

838.

The cramps of cholera are treated by the celebrated Bartholow with the following combination:

Chloral hydrate	3 drams.
Sulphate of morphine	1 grain.
Sulphate of atropine	¼ grain.
Chloroform water	4 fl. drams.
Distilled water	4 fl. drams.

A dose is twenty minims repeated every ten minutes as required.

839. Diarrhœa Mixture.

Tincture capsicum	½ fl. ounce.
Spirit peppermint	1 fl. ounce.
Tincture opium	1½ fl. ounces.
Tincture catechu compound	2 fl. ounces.
Tincture kino	2 fl. ounces.
Tincture rhatany	2 fl. ounces.
Spirit camphor	2 fl. ounces.
Water	2 fl. ounces.

Mix. Dose one teaspoonful.

Diarrhœa Mixture for Children and Adults.
840.

Tr. catechu	½ ounce.
Bismuth. subsalicylat	3 drams.
Pulv. cretae aromat.	3 drams.
Aq. chloroformi ad	8 ounces.

M.

Dose: For an adult, half a wineglassful; from 14 to 18 years, a tablespoonful; from 10 to 14 years, a dessertspoonful, and less for younger children. Repeat twice at intervals of three hours.

841. Thielmann's Cholera Drops.

Oil of peppermint	1 fl. ounce.
Alcohol	8 fl. ounces
Tincture opium and saffron	3 fl. ounces
Tincture ipecac	8 fl. ounces
Tincture valerian	13½ fl. ounces

Mix. Dose: One to two fluid drams.

842. New York "Sun" Cholera Mixture.

Tincture capsicum	1 part.
Tincture opium	1 part.
Tincture rhubarb	1 part.
Spirit peppermint	1 part.
Spirit camphor	1 part.

Mix. Dose, 15 to 30 drops in a wine glass of water.

Sir Andrew Clark's Prescription for Choleraic Diarrhœa.
843.

Acid. sulph aromat	4 drams.
Spiritus aetheris	4 drams.
Tinct. chloroformi co.	1 ounce.
Tinct. camph. comp.	1¼ ounces.
Spiritus menthae pip.	3 drams.
Ext. haematoxyli	4 drams.
Aq. camphorae ad	12 ounces.

Dose: Two tablespoonfuls for the first dose, and one tablespoonful every two, three or four hours afterwards, according to the urgency of the diarrhœa.

This medicine must be preceded by a full teaspoonful of castor oil, and given only if the diarrhœa continues after the action of the oil has ceased.

GONORRHŒA, GLEET, ETC.

844. Mist Gonorrhœa.

Powdered gum tragacanth	30 grains.
Spirits nitrous ether	3 drams.
Liquor potassa	3 drams.
Balsam copaiba	6 drams.
Tincture of cubebs	6 drams.
Oil of cinnamon	6 drops.
Syrup of orange	1 ounce.
Cinnamon, water q. s. to make up to	8 ounces.

Dose: One to two tablespoonsful two to three times a day.

Triturate the gum tragacanth in a mortar with the spirits of nitrous ether, in which the oil of cinnamon has been dissolved; add gradually four ounces of cinnamon water. Mix the liquor potassa with the balsam copaiba in a bottle; add the tincture of cubebs and syrup then add contents of mortar. Make up the product to eight ounces with cinnamon water and shake well.

845. Copaiba Mixture.

Copaibae .... ½ ounce.
Liq. potassae.............. 2 drams.
Aq. ad..................... 3 ounces.
Shake well, and add to the following:
Tinct. cubebae............. 1 ounce.
Tinct. opii................ ½ dram.
Mucil. acaciae............. ½ ounce.
Aq. chloroformi ad......... 5 ounces.
M.
Dose: A tablespoonful thrice daily.

846. Liq. Copaibae Solubilis.

Oil of copaiba............. ½ ounce.
Balsam of copaiba.......... 4 ounces.
Or resin of copaiba........ 2½ ounces.
Freshly slaked lime .... 1½ ounces.
Water to................... 30 ounces.
Carbonate of soda.......... 2 ounces.
Rectified spirit........... 2 ounces.

Rub up the oil and balsam, or the resin, with the lime and 20 ounces of water, then transfer to a glass flask and boil gently for twenty minutes; then dissolve the soda in remainder of the water, and add to first solution. When cold, stand for a week, with occasional shaking; then add the spirit in which a few drops of pimento or cinnamon oil may be dissolved; shake well, and filter through wetted filter-paper.

847. Essence Copaiba, Cubebs and Buchu.

Tinct. cubebs.............. 8 ounces.
Oil of copaiba............. 2 drams.
Fl. extract buchu.......... 4 ounces.
Alcohol .... 8 ounces.
Mix.

Essence of Santal with Buchu and Cubebs
848.

Tincture of cubebs......... 8 ounces.
Fluid extract buchu........ 4 ounces.
Essence of santal.......... 8 ounces.
1 to 15
Spirits of nitre........... 4 ounces.
Mix.

849. Solidified Copaiba.

Calcined magnesia.......... 2 ounces.
Rub well with water, 2 drams, until throughly mixed, then add:
Balsam copaiba............. 2 pounds.

Mix well together and expose in a suitable vessel, to heat of a water bath (212°F) for one half to one hour, stirring frequently. Set aside to solidify. The proportions may be changed to accommodate the heavy balsam

850. Cubeb Paste.

Copaiba balsam............. 10 parts.
Yellow wax................. 10 parts.
Mix by the aid of a gentle heat and add:
Powdered cubebs .... 50 parts.

The mass can be divided into boluses of any suitable size.

851. Injection for Gleet.

Acetate zinc............... 4 grains.
Extract belladonna .... 4 grains.
Colorless hydrastis........ 1 ounce.
Camphor water.............. 1 ounce.
Glycerine .... ½ ounce.
Water, q. s. ad .... 4 ounces.

852. Injection Brou.

Opium powdered............. 30 grains.
Catechu powdered........... 30 grains.
Spanish saffron .... 60 grains.
Glycerine .... 1 ounce.
Water .... 7 ounces.
Macerate seven days and filter.
To this add
Acetate of lead............ 20 grains.
Sulphate of zinc........... 30 grains.

853. Red Wash Injection.

Acetate lead............... 4 ounces.
Sulphate zinc.............. 8 ounces.
Sulphate hydrastia......... 1 ounce.
Fld. ext. spanish saffron.. 4 ounces.
Fld. ext. catechu aqueous . 8 ounces.
Fld. ext. opium aqueous .. 4 ounces.
Glycerine .... 128 ounces.
Aquae dist................. 500 ounces.

854. Gonorrhœa Injection.

Sulphate of hydrastia...... ½ ounce.
Sulphate of zinc........... 128 grains.
Acetate of lead............ 320 grains.
Sulphate of morphia........ 30 grains.
Boracic acid .... 1⅝ ounces.
Dissolved in
Glycerine .... 16 fl. ounces.
Carbolic acid.............. 15 drops.
Water, distilled........... 128 ounces.
Mix.

855. Emulsion of Sandalwood.

Santal wood oil............ 2 ounces.
Cubebs oil................. 2 ounces.
Copaiba oil .... 20 ounces.
Wintergreen oil............ 2 ounces.
Castor oil................. 32 ounces.
Gum tragacanth powd....... 8 ounces.
Gum arabic, powd. .... 32 ounces.
Camphor water.............. 96 ounces.
Glycerine .... 32 ounces.
Salicylic acid............. 1 dram.
Chloride of sodium .... 1 ounce.

EYE WATERS.

856. Rose Eye Water.
  Acetate of zinc............ 480 grains.
  Acetate of lead............ 480 grains.
  Acetate of morphia....... 30 grains.
  Acetic acid dil............ 1 dram.
  Rose water................ 192 ounces.
  Mix.

857. Alum Eye Water.
  Alum .... 8 grains.
  Rose water................ 8 ounces.
Drop night and morning into the eye with a pipette.

858. Witch Hazel Eye Water.
  Distilled ext. of witch hazel 2 ounces.
  Rose water................ 2 ounces.
  Zinc sulphate............. 4 grains.
  Morphia sulphate.......... 1 grain.
See formula 797 and 798 for eye salves.

859. The Care of the Eyes.

At the sanitary convention held at Ann Arbor, Mich., not long ago, Dr. C. J. Lundy, of Detroit, read a paper on "Hygiene in Relation to the Eye," which should have the widest circulation, especially among teachers and school officers. A fruitful source of eye troubles is shown to be the excessive strain upon the muscles and nerves of the eyes due to faulty educational methods, the ill-planned and insufficient lighting of school rooms, poor ink and fine print in school books, and other causes which education might correct. In conclusion, Dr. Lundy laid down the following rules for the better care of the eyes:

1. Avoid reading and study by poor light.
2. Light should come from the side, and not from the back or front.
3. Do not read or study while suffering great bodily fatigue or during recovery from illness.
4. Do not read while lying down.
5. Do not use the eyes too long at a time for near work, but give them occasional periods of rest.
6. Reading and study should be done systematically.
7. During study, avoid the stooping position, or whatever tends to produce congestion of the head and face.
8. Select well printed books.
9. Correct errors of refraction with proper glasses.
10. Avoid bad hygienic conditions and the use of alcohol and tobacco.
11. Take sufficient exercise in the open air.
12. Let the physical keep pace with the mental culture, for asthenopia is most usually observed in those who are lacking in physical development.

Another set of rules which gives additional information on the care of the eyes are drawn up to serve as a guide to students and others working by artificial light:

1. If the work be carried on at a table, the cover should be green.
2. If the light be given from a lamp or candle, it should be so covered with a shade as to prevent the glare from falling on the eye.
3. It will, in addition, be advantageous to have the candle or lamp covered with a globe or chimney of tinted glass; which may be green, blue, or opaline.
4. If gas is used it may be brought down by means of an india-rubber pipe to a lamp placed on the table, which may be arranged as before recommended.
5. If this cannot well be done, the gas globes may be of tinted glass, and the person should wear a shade over the eyes, or should sit with his back to the light.
6. If there is any defect of vision, compensating glasses should be worn, and they may be made of tinted glass.

Reading by firelight is also injurious on account of the glare, the quickly repeated dilatations and contractions of the iris, due to the changes in the intensity of the light, and the frequent alteration of the accommodation of the eye which the latter necessitates. Persons as cooks, compelled to work before a strong fire, should, if they experience any ocular inconvenience from the practice, wear smoked glasses.

CHILBLAINS.

860. Chilblain Liniment. A
  Lin. terebinth co.......... 6 ounces.
  Lin. saponis.............. 6 ounces.
  Tinct. opii............... 2 ounces.
  Lin. camphoras........... 2 ounces.
  M. S. A.

861. Chilblain Liniment. B
  Chloroform .... 1 ounce.
  Camphor .... 1 ounce.
  Liq. ammon. fort......... 1 ounce.
  Lin. opii................. ½ ounce.
  Tr. lavand. co........... ½ ounce.
  Glycerini .... 2 ounces.
  Spt. rectificat. ad........ 10 ounces.
  M. S. A.

To be gently rubbed on the unbroken skin night and morning.

862. Chilblain Liniment. C

Tinct. iodi.	3 drams.
Tinct. cantharidis	1 ounce.
Spt. chloroformi	2 drams.
Spt. aetheris nitrosi	1½ drams.
Aquae ammoniae	2 drams.
Acid. boracici	20 grains.
Zinci acetatis	10 grains.
Plumbi acetatis	6 grains.
Sap. mollis	1 ounce.

M.

One application every night after bathing feet well.

863. Chilblain Liniments (Unbroken). D

a. Potassii iodidi	1½ ounces.
b. Sapo mollis, P. B.	3 ounces.
c. Tr. cantharidis	1 ounce.
d. Glycerini	6 drams.
Aquae	6 ounces.

Dissolve a and b separately in q. s. of water, and add c and d and ol. geranium to perfume and liq. cocci to color.

864. E

Bals. peru	1 dram.
S. V. R.	4 drams.
Acid. hydrochlor	1 dram.
Tr. benz. co.	1 ounce.

865. A Remedy for Chilblains.

Professor Boeck, of Christiana, suggests the following inelegant but most effectual remedy for children's chilblains:

Ichthyoli	1 dram.
Resorcini	1 dram.
Tannini	1 dram.
Aquae	5 drams.

M.

To be painted on each evening.

When thus applied, the fluid in a few minutes forms a varnish on the skin, and causes the chilblain and swelling to disappear. The objection to the remedy is that for a week or a fortnight the parts look black and dirty, and some persons cannot stand the application of resorcin to their skin.

866. Chilblain Liniment. F

Chloroform	½ fl. ounce.
Belladonna liniment	½ fl. ounce.
Water of ammonia strong	½ fl. ounce.
Glycerine	1 ounce.
Soap liniment q. s. to make up to	6 ounces.

Mix.

867. Chilblain Ointment. A

Lanolin	1 ounce.
Vaselin	2 drams.
Ol. cajuput	2 drams.
Ac. boric	2 drams.
Ac. carbolic	20 grains.
Pulv. camphor	40 grains.

Ft. ung.

868. Chilblain Ointment. B

Resin flav.	1 dram.
Cerae flav.	1½ drams.
Ol. olivae	3 drams.
Vaselini	12 drams.
P. zinci oxidi	1½ drams.
Hyd. ox. rub.	45 grains.
Ol. eucalypti	10 minims.

Mix. Ft. ung.

Apply daily to affected parts.

869. Chilblain Ointment. C

Adipis benzoat.	4 ounces.
Ceresinae	1 ounce.
Ol. terebinth	1 ounce.
Camphor	2 drams.
Ol. rosmarinae	15 minims.

Melt the lard and wax, and add the rest of the ingredients, previously mixed together. Stir well.

To be rubbed on the parts affected night and morning.

Chilblain Ointment for Broken Chilblains.
870.

Zinci oxidi	1 dram.
Hydrarg. ox. flav.	2 grains.
Lanolini	½ ounce.
Vaselini	½ ounce.

M.

871. Borosalicylat.

This is the name given to a compound made by bringing together two molecules (676 parts) of sodium salicylate and four molecules (124 parts) of boric acid. They are rubbed together, and the damp mass then dried. It is an antiseptic, and in the following combination is an excellent application for chilblains:

Borosalicylat	5 drams.
Arnica glycerine	1 ounce.
Lanoline or lard	4½ drams.
Vaseline	5½ drams.

Mix.

The arnica glycerine is made by macerating 1 ounce of arnica flowers in 9 ounces (by weight) of glycerine for eight days.

872. **Vance's Chilblain Cream.**
   Ointment of nitrate of mercury. ... 1 ounce.
   Camphor, powdered. ... 1 dram.
   Oil of turpentine. ... 2 drams.
   Olive oil. ... 5 drams.

   Mix, with a gentle heat, in a wedgewood ware mortar and triturate until cold.

873. **Ointments for Chilblains.** A
   Made mustard, (best, very thick). ... 2 drams.
   Glycerine (Price's). ... 1 dram.
   Spermaceti cerate. ... 1½ drams.

   Mix in a slightly warmed mortar, and triturate until cold. For unbroken chilblains, to be applied night and morning.

874. **Ointments for Chilblains.** B
   Gall nuts, (in very fine powder). ... 1 dram.
   Spermaceti cerate. ... 7 drams.
   Glycerine (Price's). ... 2 drams.

   Mix, and rub the whole to a uniform mass. An excellent application to obstinate broken chilblains, particularly when used as a dressing. When the parts are very painful, 1 oz. of compound ointment of galls ("unguentum gallae compositum," L. Ph.) may be advantageously substituted for the galls and cerate ordered above.

875. **Cottereau.**
   Acetate of lead. ... 1 dram.
   Camphor (in powder). ... 1 dram.
   Cherry laurel water. ... 1 dram.
   Tar. ... 1½ drams.
   Lard. ... 1 ounce.

   Mix as before.

876. **Devergie.**
   Creasote. ... 12 drops.
   Goulard's extract. ... 12 drops.
   Extract of opium. ... 2 grains.
   Lard. ... 1 ounce.

   Mix.

877. **Giacomini's.**
   Lead acetate. ... 2 drams.
   Cherry laurel water (distilled). ... 2 fl. drams.
   Lard (hard). ... 1 ounce.

   Mix.

878. **Linnæus.**
   Spermaceti ointment. ... 2½ ounces.
   Balsam of Peru. ... 1 dram.

   Mix, with a gentle heat; when cooled a little, add of hydrochloric acid, 2 fluid drams, and triturate until cold. For unbroken chilblains.

CORN CURES, ETC.

879. **Corn Cure.** A
   Collodion ... 16 ounces.
   Salicylic acid ... 960 grains.
   Ext. cannabis indicus ... 90 grains.
   Sulphuric ether ... 2 fl. ounces.
   Alcohol ... 4 fl. ounces.

   M. S. A.

880. **Corn Cure.** B
   Collodion ... 4 ounces.
   Salicylic acid ... 240 grains.
   Cocaine ... 40 grains.

   M. S. A. Color with chlorophyll.

881. **Corn Solvent.**
   Solution of potassa ... 1 dram.
   Tincture of iodine ... 1 dram.
   Glycerine ... 4 drams.
   Water, enough to complete 1 ounce.

882. **Application for Soft Corns.**
   Acid. salicylic ... 30 grains.
   Sapo. moll ... 1 ounce.

   M. Ft. ungt.

   Apply a small piece on lint each morning.

883. **Corn Salve.**
   Lard ... 2½ pounds.
   Beef suet ... 3¾ pounds.
   Wax ... 1¼ pounds.
   Salicylic acid ... 15 ounces.

   Mix.

884. **Corn and Wart Eradicator.**
   Gum sandarach picked ... 7 drams.
   Gum mastic ... 1 dram.
   Acid salicylic ... 80 grains.
   Extract cannabis indicus ... 40 grains.
   Iodine resublimed ... 6 grains.
   Sulphuric ether ... 2 fl. ounces.

   Dissolve the gums in the ether; strain and add the salicylic acid, iodine and extract of cannabis indicus—shaking well until dissolved.

   Directions: Paint a little on the corn or wart with a camel's hair brush, allow it to dry on, repeat the application three times, let it remain on a week, when the corn or wart may be removed by the finger nails or blunt instrument. It is advisable to soak the feet before using.

885. Dusting Powder for Sweating Feet. A
(Kaposi.)

Sodium salicylate .... 1 dram.
Potassium permanganate.. 2 drams.
Bismuth subnitrate........ 3 ounces.
Talcum, enough to make.. 6 ounces.

Dust freely on feet and into stockings and shoes every morning. Wash feet before retiring, dry well and apply some of the powder.

886. Foot Powder. (Ch. & Dr.) B

Salicylic acid............. 1 dram.
Boric acid................ 2 drams.
French chalk............. 6 drams.

Mix and perfume with a drop of an essential oil.

887. Foot Powder. C

Powdered orris........... ½ ounce.
Powdered boric acid ..... 1 ounce.
Powdered starch.......... 2 ounces.
Powdered Fuller's earth... 2 ounces.
M.

Zinc Cream for Bromidrosis. (Ch. & Dr.) 888.

Zinc oxide................ 1 ounce.
Starch powder............ 4 drams.
Salicylic acid............. 1 dram.
Glycerin .... 4 drams.
Saturated solution boric
   acid in rose water...... 4 ounces.

Useful for painful sweaty feet.

889. For Acne or Pimples.
(Monats. Prakt. Dermat.)

Camphor .... 0.5 grammes.
Salicylic acid............ 0.5 grammes.
Soap (medicinal)......... 1.0 grammes.
Zinc oxide............... 2.0 grammes.
Sulphur, precipitated..... 10.0 grammes.
Whale oil................ 12.0 grammes.

Apply to the affected parts on going to bed and wash off in the morning.

890. For Acne. (Bernard Wolff.)

Mercuric chloride, (gr. 1 to) 2 grains.
Resorcin, (gr. 30 to)...... 1 dram.
Cherry-laurel water....... 2 fl. drams.
Wheat flour.............. 2 drams.
Lanolin, enough to make.. 1 ounce.

891. For Acne of the Face.
(Bull. Gen. Therap.)

Ointment betanaphthol.... 15 grains.
Ointment storax.......... 15 grains.
Lard, benzoinated........ 375 grains.

Application of this mixture should be made with strong friction every night for a week, then interrupted for six days, when it may be repeated if necessary, although it is often useless to do so. If there is an appearance of small acute clusters, which generally show themselves toward the second day, the acne is ordinarily cured or very much ameliorated at the end of a week.

SOOTHING SYRUPS, TEETHING POWDERS, ETC.

892. Soothing Syrup Without Opium.

Simple syrup............. 64 ounces.
Cologne spirits, 188 per
   cent .... 16 ounces.
Oil of anise .... 1 dram.
Oil of caraway .... ½ dram.
Bromide of potash........ 2 ounces.
Water distilled........... 8 ounces.

Dissolve the oils in the spirits. Dissolve the bromide of potash in the water and add all to the syrup.

893. Soothing Syrup With Morphine.

Oil of anise.............. 1 dram.
Oil of caraway .... ½ dram.
Cologne spirits, 188 per
   cent .... 16 ounces.
Morphia sulphate......... 40 grains.
Simple syrup q. s. to measure in all.............. 80 ounces.

Dose: 1 teaspoonful or less according to age; each teaspoonful contains 1/16 grain of morphine.

894. Soothing Syrup (Non-Poisonous).

Sodae bicarb. .... ½ dram.
Sodae brom. .... ½ dram.
Ol. anethi .... 8 minims.
Ol. anisi .... 8 minims.
Spt. rectificat. .... 3 drams.
Aq. chloroformi .... 1½ ounces.
Syr. simplicis ad .... 8 ounces.

Dissolve the oils in the spirit and the soda salts in the water. Mix and filter through magnesia into the syrup. Color slightly with tr. croci.

Dose: Half to a whole teaspoonful alone, or in a little warm water.

895. Soothing Syrup.
Ol. carui .... 10 drops.
Ol. menth. pip. .... 4 drops.
Spt. chloroformi .... 3 drams.
Syrupi rhoeados .... ½ ounce.
Syrupi simplicis .... 19 ounces.

Dissolve the oils in the spirit, and pour upon this hot simple syrup. Shake well and occasionally until cold; then add the syrup of red poppy.

Dose: A teaspoonful.

896. Teething Powder.
G. sent to the C. & D., 1874, p. 148, the subjoined formula, which makes what he has found to be a good teething powder.
Calomel .... 13 drams, 1 scruple.
White sugar ... 26 drams, 2 scruples.
Powdered opium 2 scruples.

Dose: 3 to 6 grains. Each 6-grain powder contains 1-10 g. of opium.

C. contributed the following:
Calomel .... ½ grain.
Pulv. antim. comp. .... 2 grains.
P. ipecac. co. .... 1 grain.

Dose: For a child under six months old half a powder, above that age a whole powder.

Children's Soothing Syrup (Without Poison).
897.
Syr. hyoscyami .... 2 ounces.
Syr. anisi .... 4 ounces.
Potass. bromid. .... 20 grains.
Syrup. ad .... 1 pint.
M.

One teaspoonful for a child a year old.

898. Syr. Hyoscyami.
Ext. hyoscyami .... 30 grains.
Aq. bullientis. .... 4 ounces.

Rub in mortar, filter, make up to 4 fl. ounces, and dissolve therein—
Saccharum .... 8 ounces.

899. Syr. Anisi.
Ol. anisi .... 4 minims.
Simple syrup, hot .... 5 ounces.
Shake well together.

900. Teething Powders.
Chlorate of potash, powdered .... 6 grains.
Bicarbonate of soda .... 6 grains.
Powdered antimony .... 1 grain.
Powdered sugar .... 6 grains.

Mix well, and make into 6 powders.

Dose: One to two powders according to age.

901. Cooling and Teething Powders.
Potass. chlorat. .... 2 grains.
Pulv. glycyrrhiz. .... 2 grains.
Pulv. sacch. alb. .... 4 grains.
M.

The above represents the contents of one packet, and from a quarter to a half of a powder is sufficient for children between two and twelve months old.

902. Children's Soothing Powders.
Calomel .... 60 grains.
Morphine .... 4 grains.
Sugar of milk .... 180 grains.
Mix well and sift twice.

Doses: 2 to 6 months, 2 grains; 6 to 9 months, 3 grains; 9 to 15 months, 4 grains; and ½ grain more for each additional three months.

Children's Soothing Powders (Without Poison).
903.
P. potass. bromid. .... 1 ounce.
P. ipecac. .... 1 dram.
Sacch. lactis. .... 1 ounce.
M.

Two grains for a child a year old.

904. Cooling Powder for Children.
Hydrarg. subchlor. .... 2 drams.
Antim. tart. .... 2½ grains.
Pulv. amyli .... 4 drams.
M.

Doses: 6 months to 1 year, 2 grains; 1 to 2 years, 3 grains; 2 years and upwards, 4 grains.

905. Powder for Children when Relaxed.
Compound aromatic powder of chalk............ 5 grains.
Salicylate of soda .... 1 grain.
M.

906. Whooping Cough Powders.
Powdered senega .... 3 grains.
Lac sulphur .... 12 grains.
Powdered licorice .... 10 grains.
Powdered sugar .... 16 grains.
Mix.
Make into 12 powders.

907. Baby Dusting Powder.
Boric acid. .... 2½ ounces.
Starch .... 5 ounces.
French chalk .... 3 pounds.
Oil of rose-geranium ...... 2 drams.
Mix.

VERMIFUGES.

908.　Oil Vermifuge. (Old Style.)
Olive oil .... 32 ounces.
Castor oil .... 10 ounces.
Oil of wormseed .... 1 ounce.
Oil of peppermint .... 1 dram.

Mix. Fill into 1 ounce long round vials; put two teaspoonfuls of fluid extract of pink root in each bottle before filling with the above.

909.　Worm Syrup.　A
Fl. ext. pink root and
　senna .... 64 ounces.
Essence of peppermint ... 10 ounces.
Distilled water .... 60 ounces.
Simple syrup .... 250 ounces.
Alcohol, 188 per cent...... 32 ounces.
Oil of wormseed .... 5 drams.

Dissolve the oil in the alcohol and add to the other ingredients; mix well.

910.　Worm Syrup.　B
Santonin .... ½ dram.
Liq. potassae .... 2 drams.
Aquae .... 2 ounces.
Sacch. cryst. .... 2 ounces.
Ol. anisi .... 1 minim.
Spt. chloroformi .... ½ dram.

Put the santonin in a flask and pour upon it the liq. potassae, then the water, and boil until dissolved (from five to ten minutes). Then add the sugar, dissolve, and strain. When cold add the oil dissolved in the spirit, and make up to 4 fluid ounces with simple syrup.

911.　Worm Syrup.　C
Santonin .... 4 grains.
Liq. sennae dulc. .... 1½ dram.
Glycerini .... 1 dram.
Syr. anisi ad .... 1 ounce.

Rub the santonin to fine powder, and mix with the glycerine; then add the syrups.

Label: Shake the bottle. Worm-syrup for children. Under one year old, half teaspoonful; one year old, three-quarter teaspoonful; two years old, one teaspoonful; three years old, one and a half teaspoonful; four years old two teaspoonfuls; six years old, two and a half teaspoonfuls; eight years old, three teaspoonfuls. To be given first thing in the morning, fasting.

912.　Worm Syrup.　D
Fluid extract of spigelia.. 5 ounces.
Fluid extract of senna.... 3 ounces.
Oil anise .... 10 minims.
Oil caraway .... 10 minims.
Syrup .... 8 ounces.

Dose: One or more teaspoonfuls at intervals until purging commences.

913.　Remedy for Worms. (J. G. P.)
Santonin .... 10 grains.
Calomel .... 3 grains.
Resin jalap .... 1 grain.

For 3 or 6 powders.

914.　Worm Powders. (C. W. Moister.)　A
Santonin .... 10 grains.
Calomel .... 15 grains.
Scammony, resin, powdered .... 15 grains.
Powdered sugar .... 30 grains.

Mix, and divide into 15 powders. Give one 3 times daily (on an empty stomach) for one day and repeat in 3 days if necessary.

915.　Worm Powders.　B
Santonin .... 10 grains.
Podophyllin .... 4 grains.
Powdered rhubarb .... 15 grains.
Sugar of milk .... 30 grains.

Mix, and divide into 15 powders. Give powders 5 hours apart (on an empty stomach), until 3 have been given.

Omit a day, repeating the dose if necessary.

916.　Tasteless Worm Powder.
Santonin .... 1 ounce.
Pulv. sacch. alb. .... 2 ounces.
M.

Doses: 2 to 5 years, 6 grains; 5 to 10 years, 9 grains.

917.　Worm Lozenges (Plain).
Powdered santonine ...... 4 pounds.
Essence of peppermint.... q. s.
Confectioners' sugar ..... q. s. to

Make into 100 pounds of lozenges; 280 lozenges to the pound; each lozenge contains 1 grain of santonine.

If lozenges containing ½ grain of santonine are desired, have the above amount of santonine put into 200 pounds of lozenges, 280 lozenges to the pound, color with carmine if a pink color is desired.

918. Worm Lozenges (Compound).

Powdered santonine ...... 4 pounds.
Calomel .... 2 pounds.
Podophyllin .... 1400 grains.
Carmine q. s. to color pink.

Make into 100 pounds of lozenges, 280 lozenges to the pound, each lozenge contains 1 grain of santonine, ½ grain of calomel and 1 2/9 grain of podophyllin.

919. Worm Cakes.

White sugar powdered .... 5820 grains.
Powdered scammony ..... 480 grains.
Powdered jalap .... 480 grains.
Calomel .... 960 grains.
Powdered acacia .... 960 grains.
Powdered curcuma ...... 240 grains.
Powdered starch .... 720 grains.
Oil of cinnamon .... 10 drops.
Water q. s. to make a mass cut into 960 cakes.

920. Tapeworm Emulsion.

Emulsion pumpkin seeds .. 4 ounces.
Ethereal ext. male fern.... ½ ounce.
Make an emulsion.

Take half at bedtime after fasting 12 hours. In the morning take a bottle of eff. citrate of magnesia. If the worm is not expelled repeat the dose next evening.

Should any symptoms of vomiting be manifested apply a mustard plaster to the pit of the stomach.

TOOTHACHE REMEDIES.

921. Magic Toothache Drops.

Camphor .... 8 ounces.
Chloral hydrate .... 8 ounces.
Cocaine .... 240 grains.
Alcohol .... 8 ounces.
Mix.

922. Windsor Toothache Drops. A

Oil cloves .... 2 ounces.
Oil peppermint .... ½ ounce.
Creasote .... 1 ounce.
Tinct. aconite .... ½ ounce.
Chloroform .... 2 ounces.
Alcohol .... 2 ounces.
Mix.

923. Windsor Toothache Drops. B

Oil of cajeput .... 4 ounces.
Oil of black pepper ... 6 drams.
Laudanum .... 8 ounces.
Alcohol .... 16 ounces.
Oil of cloves .... 1¼ ounces.

Dissolve the oils in the alcohol and add the laudanum.

924. Toothache Balsam.

Tinct. benzoin co. .... 2¼ ounces.
Chloroform .... 6 fl. drams.
Cocaine hyd. .... 12 grains.
Oil peppermint .... 12 drops.
Oil cloves .... 12 drops.
Oil sassafras .... 12 drops.
Acid. carbolic .... 1 dram.

Dissolve the cocaine, oils and acid in the chloroform and add to the tincture of benzoin co.

925. Toothache Anodyne.

Cocaine hyd. .... 12 grains.
Sulphuric ether .... 1 ounce.
Oil of peppermint .... 1 ounce.

Dissolve the cocaine in the ether and add the oil.

926. Toothache Paint.

Tincture of iodine .... ½ ounce.
Tincture of aconite ...... ½ ounce.
Laudanum .... ¼ ounce.
Carbolic acid .... ½ dram.
Mix.

Paint the gums about the affected teeth every two hours (not oftener) until relieved.

927. Toothache Drops (Nat. Drug.)

A writer in the Journal des Practiciens recommends the following as a quick and excellent remedy for toothache, due to carious teeth:

Crystallized carbolic acid. 1 part.
Cocaine hydrochlorate .... 1 part.
Menthol .... 1 part.
Glycerin .... 20 parts.
Mix and dissolve.

The directions to go with the above are: Remove, if possible, any foreign matter that may be in the cavity, and syringe the latter out with a little warm carbolized water (2 per cent), then saturate a little pledget of cotton with the above solution and place it in the cavity. If necessary, drop on it a little tincture of benzoin, sandarac or collodion to keep it in place.

928. Toothache Tincture. A

Tincture of opium .... 1 ounce.
Tincture of hyosciamus ... 1 ounce.
Tincture of chloroform and morphine .... 1 ounce.

929. Toothache Gum.

Beeswax or hard paraffin wax	2 ounces.
Lard	½ ounce.
Oil of cloves	1 ounce.
Creasote	1 ounce.
Powdered sugar	1 dram.

Melt the beeswax and lard, when cool add the oil of cloves and the creasote; pick absorbent cotton into lint; q. s. to saturate thoroughly with the above mixture and sprinkle with the sugar, then roll into pipes, wrap with waxed paper and place in vials.

930. Painless Tooth Extraction.

H. O. Collier, D. D. S., of Forney, Texas, explains in the Medical World that he uses the following local anesthetic for the painless extraction of teeth.

Cocaine hydrochloride	20 grains.
Chloral hydrate	10 grains.
Carbolic acid	5 grains.
Oil clove	5 minims.
Glycerin	4 fl. drams.
Water	4 fl. drams.

931. Toothache Tincture. B

Camphor	1 dram.
Sang. draconis	1 dram.
Mastic	1½ dram.
Ol. caryoph.	1 dram.
Chloroform	2 ounces.
Spt. rectificat.	2 ounces.

Macerate several days, and filter.

After the toothache is relieved the customer should be recommended to insert a stopping of guttapercha.

932. Toothache Tincture. C

Sp. ammon. co.	3 drams.
Ol. caryoph.	3 drams.
Tannin	½ ounce.
Mastich	½ ounce.
Tr. opii	3 ounces.

933. For Toothache.

Menthol	1 dram.
Chloroform	1 dram.

Dissolve.

Dry out the tooth with absorbent cotton and insert in the hollow a piece of cotton upon which 5 drops of the solution have been placed.

934. Toothache Ball and Stopping.

Resin. flav.	1 ounce, 6 drams.
Gum. juniper.	1 ounce. 6 drams.
S. V. R.	1 ounce.
Spt. aetheris	6 drams.
Acid. carbol.	1 ounce.

935. For Toothache.

Tannin	40 grains.
Creasoti	15 drops.
Aether. sulph.	1 ounce.

M.

936. Odontodol for Toothache.

Hydrochlorate of cocaine.	15 grains.
Elder-flower water	15 minims.
Tincture of arnica	2½ drams.
Mindererus spirit	5 drams.

Mix.

937. Toothache Essence. A

Dr. L. Cyrus Allen states that the following seldom fails to give temporary relief:

Ol. caryophylli	15 minims.
Menthol	2 drams.
Chloroform	1 dram.
Tr. aconiti	3 drams.
Spt. rectificat.	1½ ounces.

M.

Directions: Cleanse out the cavity thoroughly (preferably by syringing) and apply on cotton. Also rub a little on gums.

938. Toothache Essence. B

Menthol	1 ounce.
Methylated chloroform	1 ounce.
Oil of cloves	½ ounce.
Spirits	4 ounces.

Dissolve the menthol in the spirit, add the chloroform and oil of cloves.

This may be rubbed into the face with the fingers, or a few drops may be placed on cotton wool and inserted in the tooth.

939. Roback's Toothache Cordial.

Oil peppermint	15 drops.
Cocaine	6 grains.
Chloroform	1 ounce.
Alcohol	¼ ounce.

M.

BEVERAGES, ETC.

940. Beverage Preservative.
Acid. salicylic .... 1 ounce.
Potass. carb. .... 2 drams.
Aq. bullien. .... 25 ounces.
Glycerin .... 10 ounces.

Dissolve the acid and potass. carb. in the water, and add the glycerine.

941.
Hop-bitter Beer as now sold is a fermented beer containing 2 per cent, or less, of proof spirit. To make it, dissolve 4 pounds of sugar in 10 gallons of hot water, and add the following mixture:

Tincture of lupuline (1 in
20 of S. V. R.).......... 2 ounces.
Oil of cassia .... 6 minims.
Oil of citronella .... 3 minims.
Tincture of capsicum .... 20 minims.

Dissolve, and add
Tincture of chiretta ...... 1 ounce.
Conc. compound infusion
of orange .... ½ ounce.
Caramel to .... 4 ounces.

When the temperature of the syrupy fluid is reduced to 80° F., add ½ ounce of compressed yeast; ferment for twelve hours, skim off the yeast, strain through a felt bag, and bottle.

942. Ginger Wine. (Ch. & Dr.)
Sugar .... 4 pounds.
Water .... 5 pints.

Dissolve by the aid of heat, strain, and add the following mixture:

Soluble essence of ginger. 6 drams.
Tincture of orange .... 2 ounces.
Essence of raspberry ..... 15 drops.
Essence of peppermint.... 3 drops.

943. Curacao Liqueur.
Tincture of fresh orange-
peel .... 1 ounce.
Tincture of tangerine orange 1 ounce.
Oil of orange .... 2 drams.
Rectified spirit .... 12 ounces.
Water .... 10 ounces.
Syrup .... 8 ounces.

Mix, and at the end of a few days filter.

944.
Orange-wine is made by boiling together 23 pounds of sugar and 10 gallons of water. Clarify with the whites of six eggs, and pour upon the peels of 100 Seville oranges. To the syrup add the juice of the oranges, and when the whole is sufficiently cool add 6 ounces of fresh yeast, and ferment for three or four days. Then strain into a barrel, allow to stand for a month, add half a gallon of brandy, and mature for at least three months longer.

945. Beef and Malt Wine.
Extract of beef .... 4 ounces.
Extract of malt .... 8 ounces.
New port wine .... 1 gallon.

Rub down the extracts with sufficient wine to make a thin syrup, add to the bulk, shake, and set aside for a few weeks; then decant the clear portion and filter the sediment.

946. Raspberry Vinegar.
Red raspberries .... ½ gallon.
Malt vinegar .... ¼ gallon.
Water .... 32 ounces.

Macerate 48 hours; press out the juice, and boil with sugar twelve ounces; skim and bottle.

947. Jersey Brandy.
Proof spirits .... 1 gallon.
Sweet spirits of nitre .... 1 ounce.
Orris root crushed .... ½ ounce.
Prunes with pits broken.. 4 ounces.
Sherry wine .... 16 ounces.

Macerate for two weeks and filter.

948. Hop Stout.
To a solution of brown sugar 1 pound and licorice-juice 4 ounces in 2 gallons of water, add the following mixture, and ferment with yeast in the usual way:

Tincture of hops .... ½ ounce.
Oil of cinnamon .... 5 minims.
Ess. of jargonelle pear ... 10 minims.
Tincture of capsicum...... ½ dram.
Conc. infusion of quassia to 1 ounce.

949.
(Non-Alcoholic Hop Stout.)
Hops .... 1 pound.
Boiling water .... 10 gallons.

Infuse for six hours, and strain 8 gallons of the clear liquor. In this dissolve—

Sugar .... 4 pounds.
Caramel .... 4 ounces.
Licorice-juice .... 4 ounces.

Again strain, and when the temperature is at 75° F., add a quart of ext. malt, and 6 ounces of fresh unwashed brewers' yeast. Ferment for thirty hours, strain through twill, and bottle.

950. Raspberry Wine Essence.

Tartaric acid	2 ounces.
Essence of raspberry	1½ ounces.
Tincture of orris	1 ounce.
Cochineal coloring	5 ounces.
Caramel	½ ounce.
Salicylic acid	½ dram.
Water to	20 ounces.

M.

To be put up in 4-ounce bottles, the contents being sufficient to make "wine" with 4 pounds of sugar and three wine-bottlefuls of water. Strawberry and other fruit essences may take the place of the raspberry, but to the extent of 2½ ounces, as the orris must be omitted.

951. Herb Beer Extract.

Extract of licorice	½ ounce.
Gentian-root	½ ounce.
Hoarhound	1 ounce.
Hops	1 ounce.
Ginger	2 ounces.
Water	1 pint.

Boil the first three ingredients in the water, then add the others, and infuse for two hours; strain and wash with warm water to 15 ounces. In this dissolve 4 ounces of glucose, and add the following solution:

Oil of cassia	10 minims.
Oil of wintergreen	6 minims.
Salicylic acid	½ dram.
Rectified spirit	1 ounce.

Mix thoroughly.

For Putting a Foam Upon Aerated Waters.
952.

Quillaia-bark, in coarse powder	4 ounces.
Boiling water	15 ounces.

Simmer gently for fifteen minutes; when almost cool add spt. vini rect. 5 ounces; macerrate for a couple of days, strain and filter.

953. Lemon Squash.

Sugar	32 ounces.
Citric acid	1 ounce.
Water	24 ounces.

Dissolve and add the following, previously mixed and filtered:

Salicylic acid	½ dram.
Oil of lemon	½ dram.
Tincture of lemon-peel	1 ounce.
Tincture of turmeric	½ dram.
Caramel	20 minims.

Shake up the tincture of lemon with the oil now and then during four hours; allow the oil to separate, decant the tincture from it, mix the tincture with the other ingredients, and filter.

954. Aromatic Ginger Ale Essence.

Cort. cinnamom	1 ounce.
Caryophyllae	3 drams.
Sem. cardamom	½ ounce.
Fruct. capsici	1 dram.
Ess. zingib. sol.	2 pints.

Macerate four days and filter. Color with caramel.

955. Ginger Ale Essence.

Ol. ros. geranii	5 minims.
Otto rosae	10 minims.
Ol. caryoph.	10 drops.
Ol. cinnamom.	½ dram.
Tr. capsici	6 drams.
Sacch. ust.	q. s.
Ess. zingib. sol. ad	1 pint.

M.

Use 1½ ounces of essence to the gallon of syrup.

956. Kola Champagne Essence.

Fluid extract of kola	4 ounces.
Tincture of canella	½ ounce.
Tincture of orange	2 ounces.
Essence of cherry	3 drams.
Essence of cloves	2 drams.
Proof spirit to	20 ounces.

Mix.

Two ounces to the gallon of syrup, and color with cochineal.

957. Kola Elixir.

Powdered kola	2 ounces.
Glycerine	14 drams.
Rectified spirit	10 drams.
Cinnamon water	6 ounces.
Essence of vanilla	1 dram.
Tincture of orange	1 ounce.

Macerate for a week, and filter. More essence of vanilla may be added if desired.

958. Punch.

An excellent winter cordial.

Citric acid	2 drams.
Benzoic acid	½ dram.
Brandy	5 ounces.
Rum	1½ ounces.
Sugar	3 ounces.
Boiling water	1 pound.

Mix.

959. Chartreuse.

Oil of melissa	6 minims.
Oil of angelica	½ dram.
Oil of cloves	6 minims.
Oil of peppermint	40 minims.
Oil of hyssop	6 minims.
Oil of nutmeg	6 minims.
Oil of cinnamon	6 minims.
Rectified spirit	1 gallon.
Sugar	8 pounds.
Water to	2½ gallons.

Mix, and color yellow or green as desired.

NON-SECRET FORMULAS.

960. Ginger Beer. A

Jamaica ginger	2½ ounces.
Moist sugar	2 pounds.
Cream tartar	1 ounce.
Lemons, juice and peel	2
Brandy	½ pint.
Good ale yeast	¼ pint.
Water	3½ gallons.

This will produce 4½ dozen bottles of excellent ginger beer, which will keep twelve months. Boil the ginger and sugar for 20 minutes in the water, slice the lemons, and put them and the cream of tartar in a large pan; pour the boiling liquor over them and stir well; when milk warm, add the yeast; cover and let it remain 2 or 3 days, skimming frequently; strain through a cloth into a cask, and add the brandy. Bung down very close; at the end of two weeks draw off and bottle; cork very tightly. If it does not work well, add a very little more yeast.

961. Ginger Beer. B

Brown sugar	2 pounds.
Boiling water	2 gallons.
Cream tartar	1 ounce.
Bruised ginger root	2 ounces.

Infuse the ginger in the boiling water, add the sugar and cream of tartar; when lukewarm strain; then add ½ pint good yeast. Let it stand all night, then bottle; if you desire you can add one lemon and the white of an egg to fine it.

962. English Ginger Beer.

Water	3 gallons.
Pulverized ginger	6 ounces.
Sugar	4 pounds.
Cream tartar	4 ounces.

Boil, and when cold add 2 tablespoonfuls of yeast. Allow it to stand over night, then filter and bottle.

963. Ginger Beer Powder.

Jamaica ginger, powdered	1 ounce.
Sodium bicarbonate	7 ounces.
Sugar	1¾ pounds.
Oil of lemon	1 fl. dram.

Make into powders.

964. Ginger Beer Powder.

The London Chemist and Druggist says that a powder may be prepared thus:

Ginger, bruised	¼ ounce.
Cream of tartar	¾ ounce.
Essence of lemon	4 drops.

Mix.

Some sugar may be added if it be thought desirable to make the packet look bigger. For use this powder is to be added to a gallon of boiling water, in which dissolve 1 pound of lump sugar, and when the mixture is nearly cool two or three tablespoonfuls of yeast are to be added. The mixture should be set aside to work for four days, when it may be strained and bottled.

965. Hop Beer.

Water	5 quarts.
Hops	6 ounces.

Boil three hours, strain the liquor, add:

Water	5 quarts.
Bruised ginger	4 ounces.

Boil a little longer, strain, and add:

Sugar	4 pounds.

When milk warm,

Yeast	1 pint.

Let it ferment; in 24 hours it is ready for bottling.

966. Lemon Beer. A

Boiling water	1 gallon.
Lemon, sliced	1
Bruised ginger	1 ounce.
Yeast	1 teacupful.
Sugar	1 pound.

Let it stand 12 to 20 hours, and it is ready to be bottled.

967. Lemon Beer. B

Put in a keg.

Water	1 gallon.
Sliced lemon	1
Ginger	1 tablespoonful.
Syrup	1 pint.
Yeast	½ pint.

Ready for use in 24 hours. If bottled, tie down the corks.

968. Maple. A

Boiling water	4 gallons.
Maple syrup	1 quart.
Essence of vanilla	½ ounce.

Add

Yeast	1 pint.

Proceed as with ginger pop.

969. Maple. B

Boiling water	4 gallons.
Maple syrup	1 quart.
Essence of spruce	½ ounce.

Add

Yeast	1 pint.

Let it ferment for 24 hours, and then strain and bottle it. In a week or more it will be ready for use.

NON-SECRET FORMULAS.

970. Maple. C
Boiling water .... 6 gallons.
Maple syrup .... 1½ quarts.
Essence of spruce .... ¾ ounce.
Add
Yeast .... 1½ pints.

971. Molasses Beer.
Molasses .... 14 pounds.
Hops .... 1½ pounds.
Water .... 36 gallons.
Yeast .... 1 pound.
Boil the hops in the water, add the molasses and ferment.

972. Ottawa Beer.
Sassafras .... 1 ounce.
Allspice .... 1 ounce.
Yellow dock .... 1 ounce.
Wintergreen .... 1 ounce.
Wild cherry bark .... ½ ounce.
Coriander .... ½ ounce.
Hops .... ¼ ounce.
Molasses .... 3 quarts.
Put boiling water on the ingredients, and let them stand 24 hours. Filter, and add
Brewer's yeast .... ½ pint.
Leave again 24 hours, then put it in an ice cooler, and it is ready for use. It is a wholesome drink, if it is used in moderation.

973. Peruvian Beer, Carbonated.
Syrup .... ½ gallon.
Add
Extract of cinchona or
Peruvian bark .... 1 ounce.
This may be flavored with 1 ounce of essence sarsaparilla or root beer.

974. Root Beer. A
Boiling water .... 5 gallons.
Add
Molasses .... 1½ gallons.
Allow it to stand for 3 hours, then add:
Bruised sassafras bark.... ¼ pound.
Wintergreen bark .... ¼ pound.
Sarsaparilla root .... ¼ pound.
Fresh yeast .... ½ pint.
Water, enough to make 15 to 17 gallons.
After this has fermented for 12 hours it can be drawn off and bottled.

975. Root Beer. B
Pour boiling water on
Sassafras .... 2½ ounces.
Wild cherry bark .... 1½ ounce.
Allspice .... 2½ ounces.
Wintergreen bark .... 2½ ounces.
Hops .... ½ ounce.
Coriander seed .... ½ ounce.
Molasses .... 2 gallons.
Let the mixture stand 1 day. Strain, add—
Yeast .... 1 pint.
Enough water to make... 15 gallons.
This beer may be bottled the following day.

976. Root Beer. C
Sarsaparilla .... 1 pound.
Spice wood .... ¼ pound.
Guaiacum chips .... ½ pound.
Birch bark .... ½ pound.
Ginger .... ¼ ounce.
Sassafras .... 2 ounces.
Prickly ash bark .... ¼ ounce.
Hops .... ½ ounce.
Boil for 12 hours over a moderate fire with sufficient water, so that the remainder shall measure 3 gallons, to which add—
Tincture of ginger .... 4 ounces.
Oil of wintergreen .... ½ ounce.
Alcohol .... 1 pint.
This prevents fermentation.

977. Root Beer. D
To make root beer, take of this decoction 1 quart.
Molasses .... 8 ounces.
Water .... 2½ gallons.
Yeast .... 4 ounces.
This will soon ferment and produce a good, drinkable beverage. The root beer should be mixed, in warm weather, the evening before it is used, and can be kept for use either bottled or drawn by a common beer pump. Most people prefer a small addition of wild cherry bitters or hot drops to the above beer.

978. Spruce Beer. A
Hops .... 2 ounces.
Chip sassafras .... 2 ounces.
Water .... 10 gallons.
Boil half an hour, strain, add—
Brown sugar .... 7 pounds.
Essence of spruce .... 1 ounce.
Essence of vanilla........ 1 ounce.
Ground pimento .... ½ ounce.
Put in a cask and cool, add—
Yeast .... 1½ pints.
Let it stand 24 hours, fine, draw it off to bottle.

979. Spruce Beer. B
Hops .... 8 ounces.
Chip sassafras .... 2 ounces.
Water .... 10 gallons.
Boil half an hour, strain, and add—
Brown sugar .... 7 pounds.

Essence of spruce .... 1 ounce.
Essence of ginger .... 1 ounce.
Ground pimento .... ½ ounce.
Put into a cask, and cool, add—
Yeast .... 1½ pints.

Let it stand 24 hours, fine, draw it off to bottle.

980. Spruce Beer. C
Water .... 6 gallons.
Essence of spruce .... 1 pint.
Pimento .... 10 ounces.
Ginger .... 10 ounces.
Hops .... 1 pound.
After boiling about 10 minutes, add—
Moist sugar .... 24 pounds
Warm Water .... 22 gallons.

When the ingredients are well mixed, and luke-warm, add—
Yeast .... 1 quart.

Let it ferment 24 hours. Strain, and bottle.

981. Spruce Beer. D
Sugar .... 1 pound.
Essence of spruce .... ½ ounce.
Boiling water .... 1 gallon.

Mix well and when nearly cold add ½ a wineglass of yeast, and the next day bottle.

982. Spruce Beer. E
Essence of spruce .... ½ pint.
Pimento .... 5 ounces.
Ginger, bruised .... 5 ounces.
Hops .... ½ pound.
Water .... 3 gallons.
Boil the whole for 10 minutes, then add—
Moist sugar .... 12 pounds.
Warm water .... 11 gallons.

Mix well and when luke-warm add 1 pint of yeast. After the liquor has fermented for about 24 hours, bottle it.

983. Spruce Beer. F
Water, 16 gallons; boil half, put the water thus boiled to the reserved cold half, which should be previously put into a barrel or other vessel; then add 16 pounds molasses, with a few spoonfuls of the essence of spruce, stirring the whole together; add half pint of yeast, and keep it in a temperate situation with the bung hole open for two days, or till fermentation subsides; then close it up or bottle it off, and it will be fit to drink in a few days.

984. White Spruce Beer.
5 pounds loaf sugar are dissolved in 5 gallons of boiling water, then 2 fl. ounces of spruce are added. When almost cold add a gill of yeast. Place in warm place and after 24 hours strain through a piece of flannel and bottle.

985. Table Beer.
"Table beer of a superior quality may be brewed in the following manner, a process well worth the attention of the gentleman, the mechanic, and the farmer, whereby the beer is altogether prevented from working out of the cask, and the fermentation conducted without any apparent admission of the external air. I have made the scale for one barrel in order to make it more generally useful to the community at large; however, the same proportions will answer for a greater or less quantity, only proportioning the materials and utensils. Take one peck of good malt, ground, 1 pound of hops, put them in twenty-gallons of water, and boil them for half an hour; then run them into a hair cloth bag or sieve, so as to keep back the hops and malt from the wort, which, when cooled down to 60° by Fahrenheit's thermometer, add to it 2 gallons of molasses, with 1 pint, or a little less, of good yeast. Mix these with your wort, and put the whole into a clean barrel, and fill it up with cold water to within six inches of the bung hole (this space is requisite to leave room for fermentation), bung down tight. If brewed for family use, would recommend putting in the cock at the same time, as it will prevent the necessity of disturbing the cask afterward. In one fortnight this beer may be drawn and will be found to improve."—Eng. Mech.

986. Beer Tonic.
Syrup of Baume, 22° .... 5 gallons.
Oil of wintergreen .... 2 drams.
Oil of sassafras .... 2 drams.
Oil of allspice .... ½ dram.
Oil of sweet orange ...... 2 drams.

Mix the oil with 12 ounces of alcohol and add to the plain syrup. Then add 35 gallons of water at blood heat, and ferment with sufficient yeast. To this add
Salicylic acid .... 1 dram.

Dissolved in conjunction with 1 dram of baking soda in a small glass of water. After it has ceased effervescing, add to the fermenting beer. The object of using this minute quantity is to prevent putrefactive fermentation. The natural vinous ferments will not be obstructed by it.—American Bottler.

987. Root Beer Extract.

Tincture of ginger.	12 ounces.
Extract of vanilla.	12 ounces.
Oil of sassafras.	4 ounces.
Oil of wintergreen.	2 ounces.
Oil of anise.	1 ounce.
Oil of orange.	¼ ounce.
Oil of cloves.	¼ ounce.
Alcohol.	½ gallon.
Simple syrup.	3½ gallons.
Tinct. soap bark.	4 ounces.
Salicylic acid.	1 dram.
Caramel.	1¼ gallons.
Water q. s. to make up to.	6 gallons.

Dissolve the oils and salicylic acid in the alcohol; mix the syrup, water and caramel and add the other ingredients.

988. Acid Solution of Phosphates.

Potassium phosphate	1 part.
Magnesium phosphate	2 parts.
Sodium phosphate.	1 part.
Calcium phosphate.	3 parts.
Ortho-phosphoric acid.	48 parts.

Water sufficient to make 768 parts. Mix and dissolve.

Acid phosphate fruit syrup contains 8 ounces of this solution to the finished gallon, the latter consisting of from 6½ to 7 pints (usually the latter) of simple syrup, the remainder being the material which go to make up the fruit flavor.

LIQUEURS, ETC.

The following formulas for bitters, cordials, German and French liqueurs, are taken from Finchett's Cordial and Liqueur Makers' Guide. Where spirits of wine is prescribed, use cologne spirits 188 per cent.

989. Ten Gallons of Peppermint.

Mix half an ounce of best oil of peppermint with a pint of strong spirits of wine, shaking it about well; put this into your cask. Next put in three gallons of clean rectified spirit proof. Dissolve thirty pounds of good lump sugar in three gallons of hot water; put this to your other ingredients, and fill the cask up to within an inch of the top with water. Fine it with one ounce of alum, dissolved in boiling water; put it into the cask hot, and stir it about well; then put in half an ounce of salts of tartar, and rouse it up again; in a day or two it should be perfectly bright.

990. Ten Gallons of Cloves.

Mix one ounce of oil of cloves with a pint of strong spirits of wine, put it in your cask; then add three gallons of clean rectified spirit proof, and stir the whole well together. Dissolve twenty-eight pounds of lump sugar in three gallons of boiling water; put this to the other ingredients, and fill the cask to within an inch of the top with water. Fine it down with one ounce of alum, dissolved in boiling water, and put into the cask hot; afterwards put in half an ounce of salts of tartar, and rouse it up well; in a day or two it will be perfectly bright. This cordial is usually colored pink; sometimes red, brown, etc.

991. Ten Gallons of Rum Shrub.

Procure one gallon and three quarters of bitter seville orange juice (or, what is preferable, buy the oranges, cut them in half, and squeeze them yourself); put it into your cask, and add three gallons of proof rum. Dissolve thirty pounds of lump sugar in three gallons of boiling water, and put it to the other ingredients, and fill the cask to within an inch of the top with water. Fine it down as follows: Pound fine one ounce of chalk, and lay it in front of a fire until perfectly dry, stir this into the cask; and lastly, add half a pint of ale finings, stirring it up again. It will very likely be upwards of a week before it is fit for use.

992. Ten Gallons of Aniseed.

Mix one ounce and a dram of oil of aniseed with a pint of strong spirits of wine, shaking it up well; put it in your cask, and add three gallons of clean rectified spirit proof. Dissolve thirty-two pounds of lump sugar with three gallons of boiling water, and mix it with the other ingredients. Fill your cask to within an inch of the top with water, and fine with two ounces of alum dissolved in boiling water, and put into the cask hot, afterwards adding one ounce of salts of tartar, and rouse well up.

993. Ten Gallons of Carraway.

Mix one ounce of oil of Carraway with a pint of strong spirits of wine, shaking it well in a bottle; put it in your cask, and add two gallons more of spirits of wine. Dissolve thirty-four pounds of lump sugar in four gallons of boiling water, and put it to the other articles. Fill the cask up with water, and fine down with two ounces of alum dissolved in boiling water, and put into the cask hot. Afterwards add one ounce of salts of tartar, and rouse the whole well together.

994. Ten Gallons of Noyeau.

Mix half an ounce of essential oil of bitter almonds with a quart of strong spirits of wine, and shake it well; put it into your cask, and add a quarter of an ounce of oil of cassia, dissolved in another pint of spirits of wine.

Next put in three gallons of clean rectified spirit proof, and rouse them up well. Dissolve thirty-two pounds of good lump sugar in three gallons of boiling water, and mix all together. Fill up the cask with water, and fine with two ounces of alum dissolved in boiling water, put into the cask hot; and lastly, one ounce of salts of tartar. Stir the whole well together.

995. Ten Gallons of Raspberry.

Buy the fruit fresh gathered, and squeeze it through a bag made of cheese cloth. When you have got five gallons of juice, put it in your cask, with thirty pounds of common lump sugar dissolved in two gallons of boiling water. Add two gallons of strong spirits of wine, and rouse the whole well together. Now draw off about half a gallon of the mixture, and stir into it a quarter of a pint of brandy coloring; return this to the cask, and rouse well up again. Fine it down with half a pint of ale finings.

996. Ten Gallons of Gingeretta.

Bruise two pounds of good ginger with a hammer, and steep it in five quarts of spirits of wine for a fortnight in a close stoppered bottle, shaking it up frequently; pour off the spirit, and put into the cask. Continue to put a quart of water into the bottle with the ginger every day, pouring it off each time, until by tasting it you find all the spirit has been washed out; put this likewise into the cask. Add two gallons of white sherry wine, a quarter of a pint of brandy coloring, thirty pounds of lump sugar, and a quarter of an ounce of citric acid, dissolved in three gallons of boiling water. Fill the cask up with water, and fine it down with half a pint of ale finings.

997. Ten Gallons of Orange Bitters.

Take five pounds of dry Seville orange peel cut into small pieces, one ounce of carraway seeds, and six ounces of coriander seeds, bruised. Steep all in three gallons of proof spirit for a month; pour off the spirit through a hair sieve, and return all the seed into the bottle; wash out all the remaining spirit in the ingredients, by putting a quart of water daily, and pouring off each time, until by tasting you find there is none left. Add twenty pounds of lump sugar dissolved in two gallons of boiling water, and half a pint of brandy coloring; fill up the cask with water. Fine it down with two ounces of alum dissolved in boiling water, and put into the cask hot; afterwards stir in one ounce of salts of tartar.

998. Three Gallons of Wormwood Bitters.

Take two drams of oil of orange, one dram of oil of carraway, one dram of oil of wormwood, a quarter-ounce of almond cake, half-ounce of coriander seeds, half-ounce of Virginia snake root. Mix the oils with a quart of spirits of wine; also the other ingredients, well bruised, with another quart of spirits of wine. Let them stand a fortnight, and shake frequently; then strain, and add five pounds of sugar dissolved in hot water. Fine it with half an ounce of alum boiled in half a pint of water.

999. Ten Gallons of Lemonade.

Dissolve one pound of citric, and half a pound of tartaric acid in three gallons of boiling water, add seven gallons of capillaire; and if wanted to keep any time, also add a quart of spirits of wine. Mix well together.

1000. Ten Gallons of Capillaire.

Break eighty pounds of finest lump sugar into a copper, and add five gallons of water; keep stirring it until it boils; then add a tablespoonful of pyroligneous acid, and stir it well in; keep boiling a quarter of an hour, and leave it in the copper until cold; draw off clear from the sediment.

1001. Ten Gallons of Cherry Brandy.

Buy the largest black cherries you can get, —mash them first in a tub, and squeeze them through a bag made of sampler cloth, until you have five gallons of juice, which put into your cask, with two gallons of strong spirits of wine. Dissolve twenty-six pounds of lump sugar in two gallons of boiling water; add a quarter of a pint of brandy coloring; also a dram of oil of cloves, mixed with half a pint of spirits of wine. Fine it down with two ounces of alum, dissolved in boiling water, and put into the cask hot; afterwards add one ounce of salts of tartar, and stir the whole well together.

1002. Ten Gallons of Cinnamon.

Mix one ounce of oil of cinnamon with a quart of strong spirits of wine, shaking it up well in a bottle; next put in three gallons of clean rectified spirit proof. Dissolve twenty-six pounds of lump sugar in three gallons of boiling water; put this into the cask with the spirit, and fill up to within an inch of the top with water. Fine it down with two ounces of alum dissolved in boiling water, and put into the cask hot; afterwards add one ounce of salts of tartar, and rouse the whole well up.

1003. Ten Gallons of Lovage.

Mix five drams of oil of nutmegs, five drams of oil of cassia, and three drams of oil of carraway, in a quart of strong spirits of wine; shake it up well in a bottle; put it into the cask, with two gallons more of spirits of wine. Dissolve twenty pounds of lump sugar in hot water; add this to the spirit, with a quarter of a pint of coloring, and fill the cask up with water. Fine it down with two ounces of alum, dissolved in boiling water, and put into the goods hot; afterwards add one ounce of salts of tartar, and stir the whole well together.

1004. Ten Gallons of Usquebaugh.

Take two drams each of oil of juniper aniseed, nutmeg, and cloves, and one dram of oil of cassia; mix the whole of them, one after the other, with two gallons of strong spirits of wine. Add twenty pounds of lump sugar dissolved in boiling water, and a quarter of a pint of coloring. Fill up the cask with water, and fine with one ounce of alum dissolved in boiling water, and put into the cask hot; and lastly, half an ounce of salts of tartar. Stir the whole well together.

1005. Coloring Materials for Liqueurs.

Red.—Steep four ounces of raspings of red sanders wood in a pint of strong spirits of wine for a fortnight; strain and filter.

1006.

Red.—Steep three ounces of cochineal, finely powdered, in a pint of strong spirits of wine for a fortnight; add two drams of powdered alum and filter through blotting paper.

1007.

Blue.—Steep four drams of indigo in a bottle, with two ounces of sulphuric acid, for several days, frequently putting the bottle into hot water; add half a pint of distilled water and filter.

1008.

Yellow.—Steep one ounce of saffron in half a pint of spirits of wine for a week, and filter.

1009.

Green.—Mix equal parts of blue and yellow coloring as above, and it will make a good green.

1010.

Violet.—Mix one part of blue with two of red liquor as above,—the product will be a fine violet.

1011.

Pink.—Steep four ounces of Cudbear in a quart of strong spirit for a fortnight, and filter.

1012. Brandy Coloring.

Put twenty-eight pounds of lump sugar into a brass or iron pan with one gallon of water, and boil it until quite black on the top. Add one gallon and a half of boiling water, and boil it ten minutes longer.

1013. Yellow Coloring.

Two ounces of turmeric or saffron root bruised, put into a pint of spirits of wine for a month, shaking it frequently; filter through blotting paper.

1014. British Brandy.

To ten gallons of cleanest rectified spirit put two ounces of bitter almond meal, half an ounce of mace pounded, half an ounce of orris root sliced, and one ounce of cassia buds ground; shake it frequently for a fortnight, and then add one ounce of terra japonica finely pulverized, two ounces of sweet spirits of nitre, and half a pound of prunes. Let it be well roused up; and after it has stood another fortnight, it will be fit for use. Color with brandy coloring, if you need it darker.

1015. Spirit Beading.

To put a fine bead on fifty gallons of weak spirits.—Take one dram of oil of vitriol, and one dram of oil of sweet almonds; rub them together in a marble mortar, and when well incorporated, add by degrees half a pint of spirits of wine; mix with the spirits, and rouse up well.

1016. Gin Flavoring.

Take one ounce of oil of juniper, one dram of oil of sweet fennel, four ounces of essence of angelica, and an ounce of tincture of capsicums; mix altogether in a quart of strong spirits of wine; add to it one gallon of capillaire. If gin is reduced to a very low strength, add as much as will fetch up the flavor.

Finings for a Butt of Sherry Wine.
1017. (120 Gallons.)

Put two ounces of isinglass into a jar with one quart of sherry, near the fire; when soft, beat and whisk it up to a froth with the whites of six eggs; thoroughly mix the whole with a gallon of the wine, and return it to the cask; rouse the whole well up. This will answer equally well for marsala, madeira, etc.

Finings for a Pipe of Port Wine.
1018. (120 Gallons.)

Take the whites and shells of sixteen eggs, and beat them up to a froth in a tub; add half a gallon of the wine, and whisk it well up again; put the mixture into the cask, and rouse the whole well up. The same for red cape.

Finings for a Pipe of White Cape.
1019. (120 Gallons.)

The same as for a butt of sherry, with the addition of a quart of milk with the cream taken off.

1020. Ale and Porter Finings.

Take any quantity of isinglass, and put it into a tub or pan with sufficient hard ale or porter to cover it; as the glass swells, keep adding more liquid, until the whole is formed into a stiff jelly; rub it through a hair sieve, and add hard ale or porter until the whole is of the consistency of thick cream. A pint of this is sufficient for a barrel of ale or porter.

1021. Finings for Gin, Whisky, etc.

For 100 gallons, take two ounces of roach alum, and boil it in a quart of water for a few minutes; put it into the liquor hot, and add one ounce of salts of tartar; rouse well up.

1022. To Make 100 Gallons of Gin.

To eighty-two gallons of clean rectified spirit proof add the following:

Oil of juniper (English)	1½ ounces.
Essence of angelica	1½ ounces.
Oil of sweet fennel	¼ ounce.
Oil of bitter almonds	½ ounce.
Oil of coriander	1 ounce.
Oil of carraway	½ ounce.

Mix the whole of the oils with a gallon of spirits of wine 60 o. p., having first taken the precaution of rubbing them down in a mortar with a little lump sugar; add this to the spirit, and after having well mixed the whole, add seventeen gallons of water. Fine it down with

Alum	4 ounces.
Salt of tartar	4 ounces.

1023. To Make Up Gin for Sale.
(For 100 Gallons.)

Oil of juniper	1 ounce.
Oil of bitter almonds	½ ounce.
Oil of carraway	½ ounce.
Oil of cassia	¼ ounce.
Oil of vitriol	¼ ounce.

Rub the whole of these down in a mortar with a little sugar and a quart of spirits of wine 60 o. p. Boil 1 ounce of chillies in a quart of water gently, until it has reduced to a pint, and strain. Put the whole into the gin, with forty-five pounds of lump sugar, and twenty-five gallons of water. This gin, which is in reality about 35 u. p., will taste as full of flavor and as strong as 17 u. p.

1024. To Improve a Puncheon of Rum.

After the rum has been racked into the vat and reduced to the selling strength, add six gallons of good old sound porter, four pounds of honey well mixed with a gallon of the rum, and a pound of green tea. The addition of a couple of pounds of prunes is, I think, an improvement; they should be struck with a hammer, to break the stones. After all is in the vat, rouse it well up, night and morning, for three days. If the honey prevents its going bright in the usual time, add half a pint of ale finings, which will have the desired effect.

FOREIGN LIQUEURS.

1025. Directions for Mixing and Managing, etc.

As the following recipes contain merely the names and quantities of the several ingredients, the instructions for the method of proceeding with them must be particularly attended to,—viz.:

All dry substances, such as cloves, cinnamon, etc., should be ground. Leaves and flowers, orange peel, figs, etc., and all fresh and soft substances, must be cut up into the smallest possible pieces, and always used fresh, if they can be procured; if not, use them dry; but double the quantity will in many instances be required. Almonds and fruit kernels must be beaten to a paste in a marble mortar, with a small quantity of spirit, to prevent them oiling.

When the several ingredients have been prepared as above, put them into a jar, well corked up, with the quantity of spirit ordered, and allow it to remain a month, shaking it frequently every day, and if possible, kept in a very warm situation; at the expiration of this time, pour off the spirit, and add the quantity of water ordered in the recipe; let this stand a few days, shaking it up as before; then pour off, press out all the liquid, and mix with the spirit; add the sugar and coloring matter, and filter through a flannel bag. If essential oils are ordered, a small quantity of the pure spirit should be kept back to mix with them, and added to the other materials previous to filtering.

In a few instances, gold and silver leaf is ordered, which is prepared in the following manner:—get a few leaves, such as are used by gilders, and spread them on a plate which has a little thin sirop on it; cover the leaf also with the sirop, and with two forks tear it into small pieces about the size of a canary seed. These precautions are necessary, as, if you attempt to break them in a dry state, one-half will go into dust, and spoil the appearance of the liquor; it should not be added until the liqueur is in the bottles.

GERMAN LIQUEURS.

1026.　　Eau de Sultane Zoraide.
Lemon peel .... 8 ounces.
Orange peel .... 8 ounces.
Figs .... 8 ounces.
Dates ... . 4 ounces.
Jessamine flowers .... 4 ounces.
Cinnamon .... 3 ounces.
Spirits of wine, 60 o. p... 19 quarts.
Orange flower water ..... 2 quarts.
Pure water .... 12 quarts.
Capillaire .... 8 quarts.
Color rose.

1027.　　Eau des Princesses.
Lavender flowers .... 4 ounces.
Figs .... 4 ounces.
Orange peel .... 4 ounces.
Balm .... 4 ounces.
Cinnamon .... 3 ounces.
Camomile .... 1 ounce.
Rosemary leaves .... 1 ounce.
Bitter almonds .... 1 ounce.
Cloves .... 6 drams.
Spirits of wine, 62 o. p... 19 quarts.
Essence of amber .... 50 drops.
Water .... 14 quarts.
Capillaire .... 8 quarts.
A little gold leaf.

1028.　　Eau de Rebecca.
Veronica .... 5 ounces.
Pimento .... 5 ounces.
Junipers .... 5 ounces.
Grains of Paradise .... 2 ounces.
Cumin .... 1½ ounce.
Ginger .... 1½ ounce.
Cinnamon .... 1½ ounce.
Cloves .... 1 ounce.
Spirits of wine, 60 o. p... 19 quarts.
Water .... 14 quarts.
Capillaire .... 8 quarts.

1029.　　Eau des Nobles.
Petals of roses .... 1 pound.
Orange peel .... 12 ounces.
Cinnamon .... 6 ounces.
Cloves .... 1 ounce.
Nutmegs .... ½ ounce.
Spirits of wine, 60 o. p.... 19 quarts.
Essence of vanilla .... 50 drops.
Water .... 14 quarts.
Capillaire .... 8 quarts.
Color red.

1030.　　Elixir Vital de Tanchon.
Lemon peel .... 10 ounces.
Orange flowers .... 10 ounces.
Jessamine flowers .... 4 ounces.
Cinnamon .... 4 ounces.
Coriander .... 2 ounces.
Cumin .... 2 ounces.
Cloves ... . 2½ ounces.
Nutmegs .... 2½ ounces.
Spirits of wine, 60 o. p... 19 quarts.
Essence of ambergris..... 3 drams.
Orange flower water .... 8 quarts.
Pure water .... 6 quarts.
Capillaire .... 8 quarts.
Color green.

1031.　　Eau de Legitimité.
Flowers of jessamine ..... 12 ounces.
Marjoram .... 6 ounces.
Coriander .... 4 ounces.
Thyme .... 3 ounces.
Anniseed .... 2 ounces.
Cinnamon .... 2 ounces.
Cardamom .... 1 ounce.
Spirits of wine, 60 o. p.... 19 quarts.
Essence of vanilla ...... 1 dram.
Rose water .... 2 quarts.
Pure water .... 12 quarts.
Capillaire .... 8 quarts.
Color red.

1032.　　Eau des Templiers.
Orange peel .... 8 ounces.
Lemon peel .... 8 ounces.
Laurel berries .... 4 ounces.
Jujubes .... 2 ounces.
Cinnamon .... 2 ounces.
Anniseed .... 2 ounces.
Rosemary leaves .... 4 ounces.
Spirits of wine .... 19 quarts.
Water .... 6 quarts.
Essence of vanilla ...... 2 drams.
Essence of amber .... 1 dram.
Orange flower water ..... 4 quarts.
Rose water .... 4 quarts.
Capillaire .... 8 quarts.
Color sky blue.

1033. Eau de Fantasie.

Lemon peel	1 pound.
Cinnamon	3 ounces.
Pine apple	3 ounces.
Cardamom	2 ounces.
Cloves	½ ounce.
Spirits of wine, 60 o. p.	19 quarts.
Water	14 quarts.
Capillaire	8 quarts.

1034. Eau de Jacques.

Petals of roses	8 ounces.
Orange peel	4 ounces.
Lemon peel	4 ounces.
Veronica	3 ounces.
Fennel	3 ounces.
Cinnamon	1 ounce.
Cloves	1 ounce.
Cassia	½ ounce.
Spirits of wine, 60 o. p.	19 quarts.
Essence of amber	1 dram.
Rose water	8 quarts.
Pure water	8 quarts.
Capillaire	8 quarts.

Color green.

1035. Eau de Côte.

Cinnamon	1 pound.
Peel of 12 lemons	
Oil of peppermint	1 dram.
Spirits of wine	19 quarts.
Water	15 quarts.
Capillaire	8 quarts.

Color yellow.

1036. Eau de Chypre.

Orris root	6 ounces.
Lemon peel	6 ounces.
Cinnamon	2 ounces.
Spirits of wine, 60 o. p.	19 quarts.
Oil of bergamot	60 drops.
Oil of amber	½ dram.
Orange flower water	6 quarts.
Pure water	8 quarts.
Capillaire	8 quarts.

Color red.

1037. Eau Batave.

Juniper berries	12 ounces.
Lemon peel	8 ounces.
Cinnamon	3 ounces.
Nutmeg	1 ounce.
Cloves	½ ounce.
Spirits of wine, 60 o. p.	19 quarts.
Water	14 quarts.
Capillaire	8 quarts.

1038. Eau d'Absinthe.

Wormwood	4 pounds.
Peel of 26 lemons	
Spirits of wine, 60 o. p.	19 quarts.
Water	4 quarts.
Capillaire	8 quarts.

Color green.

1039. Alkermés Italien.

Laurel leaves	2 pounds.
Cloves	2 pounds.
Cinnamon	2 ounces.
Nutmeg	3 ounces.
Spirits of wine, 60 o. p.	19 quarts.
Water	7 quarts.
Capillaire	7 quarts.

Color deep scarlet.

1040. Eau des Barbades.

Lemon peel	1½ pounds.
Cloves	2 ounces.
Cinnamon	8 ounces.
Spirits of wine	19 quarts.
Oil of citron	2 drams.
Oil of bergamot	2 drams.
Water	7 quarts.
Capillaire	1 quart.

1041. Eau Nuptiale.

Parsley seed	6 ounces.
Carrot seed	5 ounces.
Aniseed	2 ounces.
Orris root	2 ounces.
Mace	1½ ounces.
Spirits of wine, 60 o. p.	19 quarts.
Rose water	7 pints.
Pure water	11 quarts.
Capillaire	9 quarts.

Color yellow.

1042. Eau d'Amour.

Bitter almonds	12 ounces.
Lemon peel	12 ounces.
Cinnamon	6 ounces.
Mace	1 ounce.
Cloves	1½ ounces.
Lavender flowers	8 ounces.
Spirits of wine, 60 o. p.	19 quarts.
Muscat wine	8 quarts.
Oil of amber	36 drops.
Water	7 quarts.
Capillaire	7 quarts.

Color rose.

1043. Eau de Vertu.

Junipers	6 ounces.
Orange peel	4 ounces.
Lemon peel	4 ounces.
Rosemary leaves	3 ounces.
Angelica seeds	2 ounces.
Cloves	2 ounces.
Ginger	2 ounces.
Mastic	2 drams.
Storax	2 drams.
Spirits of wine, 60 o. p.	19 quarts.
Water	14 quarts.
Capillaire	8 quarts.

Color violet.

1044. Eau de Sorcier-Comte.

Orange flowers	1 pound.
Rose flowers	1 pound.
Lemon peel	8 ounces.
Orange peel	8 ounces.
Cloves	2 ounces.
Cinnamon	2 ounces.
Spirits of wine, 60 o. p.	19 quarts.
Water	6 quarts.
Essence of vanilla	1 dram.
Essence of amber	1 dram.
Rose water	4 quarts.
Orange flower water	4 quarts.
Capillaire	8 quarts.

A little gold leaf.

1045. Creme Romantique.

Lemon peel	4 ounces.
Mace	4 ounces.
Lavender flowers	4 ounces.
Marjoram	4 ounces.
Cinnamon	2 ounces.
Cloves	1 ounce.
Spirits of wine, 60 o. p.	19 quarts.
Essence of vanilla	1 ounce.
Rose water	5 quarts.
Capillaire	8 quarts.
Water	9 quarts.

Color rose.

1046. Eau de Tubinge.

Lemon peel	6 ounces.
Angelica root	3 ounces.
Aniseed	3 ounces.
Orange peel	3 ounces.
Cinnamon	2 ounces.
Nutmegs	1 ounce.
Junipers	1 ounce.
Cloves	½ ounce.
Grains of paradise	½ ounce.
Gentian	½ ounce.
Spirits of wine, 60 o. p.	19 quarts.
Essence of citron	36 grains.
Essence of amber	36 drops.
Water	14 quarts.
Capillaire	8 quarts.

Color rose.

1047. Eau de Florence.

Lemon peel	1½ pounds.
Cinnamon	3 ounces.
Mace	1½ ounce.
Cloves	½ ounce.
Spirits of wine, 60 o. p.	19 quarts.
Oil of lemon	2 ounces.
Balm water	2 quarts.
Pure water	12 quarts.
Capillaire	8 quarts.

Color nearly black.

1048. Rosolis de Turin.

Orange flowers	2 pounds.
Rose buds	2 pounds.
Flowers of jessamine	1½ pounds.
Cloves	2 ounces.
Cinnamon	3 ounces.
Spirits of wine, 60 o. p.	19 quarts.
Water	16 quarts.
Capillaire	8 quarts.

Color deep scarlet.

1049. Eau d'Ardelle.

Mace	4 ounces.
Cloves	4 ounces.
Spirits of wine, 60 o. p.	19 quarts.
Water	13 quarts.
Capillaire	10 quarts.

Color violet.

1050. Eau Cordiale de Caladon.

Lemon peel	2 pounds.
Cloves	6 drams.
Fennel seed	2 ounces.
Cardamom	1 ounce.
Aniseed	½ ounce.
Spirits of wine, 60 o. p.	19 quarts.
Water	15 quarts.
Capillaire	7 quarts.

1051. Eau d'Or.

Lemon peel	2 pounds.
Cinnamon	3 ounces.
Coriander	2 ounces.
Mace	1½ ounces.
Spirits of wine, 60 o. p.	19 quarts.
Capillaire	2 gallons.
Water	14 quarts.

Color yellow, and add a little gold leaf.

1052. Eau de Montpellier.

Oil of bergamot	4 drams.
Oil of lemon	2 drams.
Cloves	2 ounces.
Cinnamon	2 ounces.
Spirits of wine, 60 o. p.	19 quarts.
Capillaire	8 quarts.
Water	14 quarts.

Color blue.

1053. Citronat.
- Lemon peel .... 2 pounds.
- Spirits of wine, 60 o. p.... 19 quarts.
- Oil of orange .... 50 drops.
- Oil of bergamot .... 36 drops.
- Oil of amber .... 50 drops.
- Orange flower water .... 2 quarts.
- Pure water .... 10 quarts.
- Capillaire .... 10 quarts.

Color yellow.

1054. Eau d'Argent.
- Lemon peel .... 1 pound.
- Cloves .... 2 ounces.
- Angelica seed .... 1½ ounces.
- Aniseed .... 1½ ounces.
- Orris root .... 1½ ounces.
- Cinnamon .... 2 ounces.
- Spirits of wine, 60 o. p.... 19 quarts.
- Balm water .... 2 quarts.
- Pure water .... 12 quarts.
- Capillaire .... 8 quarts.

Color pink, and add a little silver leaf.

1055. Eau de Mille Fleurs.
- Orange flowers .... 12 ounces.
- Quince pepins .... 9 ounces.
- Lavender flowers .... 6 ounces.
- Orris root .... 5 ounces.
- Mint .... 5 ounces.
- Balm .... 4 ounces.
- Cinnamon .... 4 ounces.
- Thyme .... 2 ounces.
- Cloves .... 1½ ounces.
- Spirits of wine, 60 o. p.... 19 quarts.
- Water .... 13 quarts.
- Capillaire .... 10 quarts.

Color green.

1056. Elixir de J. Saint Aure.
- Lavender flowers .... 8 ounces.
- Rose flowers .... 8 ounces.
- Orange flowers .... 8 ounces.
- Lemon peel .... 5 ounces.
- Cinnamon .... 1 ounce.
- Cloves .... 1 ounce.
- Nutmeg .... 1 ounce.
- Spirits of wine, 60 o. p.... 19 quarts.
- Rose water .... 3 quarts.
- Orange flower water .... 3 quarts.
- Peppermint water .... 3 quarts.
- Balm water .... 3 quarts.
- Cinnamon water .... 3 quarts.
- Capillaire .... 9 quarts.

Color rose.

1057. Eau de Yalpa.
- Marjoram .... 3 ounces.
- Cinnamon .... 3 ounces.
- Fennel seed .... 2 ounces.
- Thyme .... 2 ounces.
- Sweet basil .... 2 ounces.
- Bitter almonds .... 2 ounces.
- Figs .... 2 ounces.
- Balm .... 2 ounces.
- Carrot seed .... 1 ounce.
- Sage .... 1 ounce.
- Cardamom .... ½ ounce.
- Cloves .... ½ ounce.
- Spirits of wine, 60 o. p.... 19 quarts.
- Essence of vanilla .... 50 drops.
- Essence of amber .... 50 drams.
- Water .... 14 quarts.
- Capillaire .... 8 quarts.

Color scarlet.

1058. Eau Divine.
- Lemon peel .... 1½ pounds.
- Coriander .... 4 ounces.
- Mace .... 1 ounce.
- Cardamom .... 1 ounce.
- Spirits of wine, 60 o. p.... 19 quarts.
- Oil of bergamot .... 1½ drams.
- Oil of neroly .... 2 drams.
- Water .... 14 quarts.
- Capillaire .... 8 quarts.

1059. Eau de Pucelle.
- Juniper berries .... 1½ pounds.
- Fennel seed .... 4 ounces.
- Angelica seed .... 3 ounces.
- Cinnamon .... 3 ounces.
- Cloves .... 1 ounce.
- Spirits of wine, 60 o. p.... 19 quarts.
- Water .... 13 quarts.
- Capillaire .... 10 quarts.

Color yellow.

1060. Eau de Paix.
- Orange peel .... 6 ounces.
- Lemon peel .... 6 ounces.
- Rosemary flowers .... 4 ounces.
- Angelica root .... 4 ounces.
- Sweet almonds .... 4 ounces.
- Cardamom .... 1 ounce.
- Aniseed .... 1 ounce.
- Nutmeg .... 1 ounce.
- Cinnamon .... 1 ounce.
- Cloves .... 1 ounce.
- Spirits of wine, 60 o. p.... 19 quarts.
- Water .... 7 quarts.
- Capillaire .... 8 quarts.

Color violet.

1061. Eau Royale.

Orange peel	10 ounces.
Lemon peel	10 ounces.
Jessamine flowers	8 ounces.
Mace	4 ounces.
Cinnamon	4 ounces.
Cloves	2 ounces.
Nutmegs	1 ounce.
Spirits of wine, 60 o. p.	19 quarts.
Oil of amber	20 drops.
Oil of vanilla	2 ounces.
Orange flower water	2 ounces.
Pure water	12 quarts.
Capillaire	8 quarts.

Color red.

1062. Eau de Santé.

Lemon peel	6 ounces.
Lavender flowers	4 ounces.
Rosemary leaves	4 ounces.
Jessamine flowers	4 ounces.
Mint	4 ounces.
Angelica root	3 ounces.
Marjoram	3 ounces.
Grains of paradise	2 ounces.
Spirits of wine, 60 o. p.	19 quarts.
Water	14 quarts.
Capillaire	8 quarts.

Color green.

1063. Eau Américaine.

Orange peel	1 pound.
Rosemary leaves	4 ounces.
Lavender flowers	4 ounces.
Cinnamon	3 ounces.
Cloves	2 ounces.
Nutmegs	1 ounce.
Spirits of wine, 60 o. p.	19 quarts.
Water	14 quarts.
Capillaire	8 quarts.

Color green.

1064. Eau du Dauphin.

Orange peel	8 ounces.
Junipers	4 ounces.
Veronica	6 ounces.
Coriander	2 ounces.
Angelica root	2 ounces.
Ginger	2 ounces.
Rosemary leaves	1 ounce.
Cinnamon	1 ounce.
Myrrh	1 ounce.
Aniseed	1 ounce.
Spirits of wine, 60 o. p.	19 quarts.
Water	14 quarts.
Capillaire	8 quarts.

1065. Eau de Didon.

Orange peel	8 ounces.
Lemon peel	8 ounces.
Figs	8 ounces.
Balm	4 ounces.
Grains of paradise	2 ounces.
Chamomile	2 ounces.
Cinnamon	1 ounce.
Aniseed	1 ounce.
Nutmeg	½ ounce.
Spirits of wine, 60 o. p.	19 quarts.
Water	14 quarts.
Capillaire	8 quarts.

Color blue.

1066. Eau des Epicuriens.

Orange peel	9 ounces.
Lemon peel	9 ounces.
Figs	9 ounces.
Cinnamon	4 ounces.
Marjoram	3 ounces.
Cloves	2 ounces.
Nutmegs	1 ounce.
Spirits of wine, 60 o. p.	19 quarts.
Water	14 quarts.
Capillaire	8 quarts.

Color red.

1067. Eau de Napoleon.

Lemon peel	10 ounces.
Cloves	3 ounces.
Cinnamon	3 ounces.
Jessamine flowers	6 ounces.
Nutmegs	2 ounces.
Spirits of wine	19 quarts.
Essence of vanilla	2 drams.
Rose water	4 quarts.
Orange flower water	4 quarts.
Peppermint water	2 quarts.
Pure water	4 quarts.
Capillaire	8 quarts.

Color blue.

1068. Crême Voizot.

Lemon peel	4 ounces.
Orange peel	2 ounces.
Rosemary leaves	1 ounce.
Balm	1 ounce.
Peppermint	½ ounce.
Cinnamon	1 ounce.
Mastic	4 drams.
Storax	4 drams.
Cloves	4 drams.
Nutmegs	4 drams.
Spirits of wine, 60 o. p.	19 quarts.
Rose water	4 quarts.
Orange flower water	4 quarts.
Peppermint water	4 quarts.
Balm water	4 quarts.
Essence of vanilla	1 dram.
Capillaire	8 quarts.

Color green.

1069. Crême Mojon.
Cinnamon	2 ounces.
Mace	2 ounces.
Cloves	2 ounces.
Nutmeg	4 drams.
Rosemary leaves	3 ounces.
Spirits of wine, 60 o. p.	19 quarts.
Orange flower water	4 quarts.
Rose water	4 quarts.
Essence of amber	1 dram.
Essence of vanilla	2 drams.
Essence of bergamot	2 drams.
Pure water	7 quarts.
Capillaire	8 quarts.

Color rose.

1070. Aqua Bianca.
Oil of bergamot	1 dram.
Oil of citron	1 dram.
Oil of lemon	1 dram.
Oil of amber	1 dram.
Oil of peppermint	1 dram.
Spirits of wine, 60 o. p.	19 quarts.
Rose water	6 quarts.
Pure water	8 quarts.
Capillaire	9 quarts.

1071. Elixir Moupon.
Essence of cinnamon	1 dram.
Essence of aniseed	1 dram.
Essence of peppermint	1 dram.
Essence of cloves	1 dram.
Essence of vanilla	1 dram.
Spirits of wine, 60 o. p.	19 quarts.
Rose water	6 quarts.
Orange flower water	4 quarts.
Pure water	6 quarts.
Capillaire	9 quarts.

Color rose.

1072. Eau d'Orient.
Fennel	1 pound.
Dates	12 ounces.
Lemon peel	12 ounces.
Orange peel	12 ounces.
Pine apple	4 ounces.
Grains of paradise	2 ounces.
Pimento	2 ounces.
Spirits of wine, 60 o. p.	19 quarts.
Water	14 quarts.
Capillaire	8 quarts.

Color blue.

1073. Eau de Selia.
Lemon peel	2 ounces.
Rosemary leaves	1 ounce.
Lavender flowers	1 ounce.
Cinnamon	1 ounce.
Cloves	½ ounce.
Mace	½ ounce.
Aniseed	½ ounce.
Bark	½ ounce.
Spirits of wine, 60 o. p.	19 quarts.
Essence of vanilla	50 drops.
Rose water	2 quarts.
Orange flower water	2 quarts.
Balm water	2 quarts.
Pure water	8 quarts.
Capillaire	8 quarts.

Color red.

DANZICK LIQUEURS.

1074. Eau Miraculeuse.
Orange peel	1 pound.
Lemon peel	1 pound.
Cinnamon	6 ounces.
Ginger	6 ounces.
Rosemary leaves	2 ounces.
Galanga	1 ounce.
Mace	1 ounce.
Cloves	1 ounce.
Orris root	1½ ounces.
Spirits of wine, 60 o. p.	19 quarts.
Capillaire	8 quarts.
Water	14 quarts.

Color red.

1075. Eau Cordiale.
Lemon peel	2½ pounds.
Balm	5 ounces.
Aniseed	4 ounces.
Coriander	4 ounces.
Cinnamon	8 ounces.
Mace	2 ounces.
Nutmegs	1 ounce.
Spirits of wine, 60 o. p.	19 quarts.
Capillaire	8 quarts.
Water	14 quarts.

Color sky blue.

1076. Krambambuli.
Aniseed	3 ounces.
Camomile flowers	3 ounces.
Cinnamon	2 ounces.
Sage	1½ ounce.
Lavender flowers	1½ ounce.
Marjoram	1½ ounce.
Galanga	1½ ounce.
Nutmeg	1½ ounce.
Cardamom	1½ ounce.
Spirits of wine, 60 o. p.	19 quarts.
Capillaire	8 quarts.
Water	15 quarts.

Color yellow.

1077. Eau de Baal.

Sage	5 ounces.
Orange peel	5 ounces.
Cinnamon	5 ounces.
Cloves	1 ounce.
Rosemary leaves	2 ounces.
Fennel seed	2 ounces.
Aniseed	2 ounces.
Camomile	3 ounces.
Galanga	1½ ounce.
Vanilla	1½ ounce.
Spirits of wine, 60 o. p.	19 quarts.
Capillaire	8 quarts.
Water	14 quarts.

Color red.

1078. Eau Aérienne "Luft Wasser."

Figs	12 ounces.
Cumin	5 ounces.
Leaves of rosemary	4 ounces.
Fennel seed	4 ounces.
Cinnamon	5 ounces.
Sage	2 ounces.
Sassafras	2 ounces.
Lavender flowers	4 ounces.
Camomile flowers	4 ounces.
Orris root	4 ounces.
Spirits of wine, 60 o. p.	19 quarts.
Capillaire	8 quarts.
Water	14 quarts.

1079. Rosolis.

Fresh lemon peel	10 ounces.
Cinnamon	3 ounces.
Cloves	1 ounce.
Aniseed	1 ounce.
Cardamom	1 ounce.
Angelica root	1 ounce.
Spirits of wine, 60 o. p.	19 quarts.
Capillaire	8 quarts.
Water	7 quarts.

Color pale rose.

1080. Eau des Prelats.

Orange peel	1 pound.
Lemon peel	12 ounces.
Cinnamon	3 ounces.
Marjoram	3 ounces.
Lavender flowers	2 ounces.
Rosemary flowers	2 ounces.
Vanilla	½ ounce.
Spirits of wine, 60 o. p.	19 quarts.
Essence vanilla	4 ounces.
Medoc wine	3 quarts.
Orange flower water	4 quarts.
Distilled water	4 quarts.
Capillaire	8 quarts.

1081. Eau des Favorites.

Aniseed	8 ounces.
Cinnamon	8 ounces.
Orange flowers	6 ounces.
Juniper berries	6 ounces.
Orange peel	3 ounces.
Rosemary leaves	3 ounces.
Thyme	1 ounce.
Penny royal	2 ounces.
Mint	2 ounces.
Sage	2 ounces.
Spirits of wine, 60 o. p.	19 quarts.
Orange flower water	4 quarts.
Water	10 quarts.
Capillaire	8 quarts.

1082. Amer d'Angleterre.

Lemon peel	10 ounces.
Cumin	6 ounces.
Cinnamon	4 ounces.
Thyme	2 ounces.
Sage	2 ounces.
Galanga	2 ounces.
Cloves	1½ ounce.
Nutmegs	1 ounce.
Orange flower water	4 quarts.
Spirits of wine, 60 o. p.	19 quarts.
Water	18 quarts.
Capillaire	8 quarts.

Color brown.

1083. Persicot.

Bitter almonds	3 pounds.
Lemon peel	6 ounces.
Cinnamon	2 ounces.
Cloves	½ ounce.
Nutmegs	½ ounce.
Spirits of wine, 60 o. p.	19 quarts.
Capillaire	8 quarts.
Water	14 quarts.

Color pale yellow.

1084. Liqueur des Évêques.

Orange peel	3½ pounds.
Cinnamon	10 ounces.
Medoc wine	10 quarts.
Spirits of wine, 60 o. p.	19 quarts.
Capillaire	8 quarts.
Water	6 quarts.

1085. Liqueur Limonade.

Lemon peel	2 pounds.
Cinnamon	4 ounces.
Nutmeg	½ ounce.
Spirits of wine, 60 o. p.	19 quarts.
Oil of lemon	30 drops.
Capillaire	8 quarts.
Water	14 quarts.

Color pale yellow.

1086. Liqueur de Girofle.
- Cloves .... 12 ounces.
- Orris root .... 3 ounces.
- Cinnamon .... 2 ounces.
- Cardamom .... ½ ounce.
- Spirits of wine, 60 o. p. .. 19 quarts.
- Capillaire .... 8 quarts.
- Water .... 14 quarts.

Color pink.

1087. Eau de Lisette.
- Lemon peel .... 2 pounds.
- Cinnamon .... 3 ounces.
- Dates .... 1 pound.
- Raisins .... 8 ounces.
- Figs .... 8 ounces.
- Mace .... 1 ounce.
- Spirits of wine, 60 o. p. .. 10 quarts.
- Capillaire .... 10 quarts.
- Water .... 14½ quarts.

A little gold leaf. Color red.

1088. Eau des Princesses.
- Lavender flowers .... 1 pound.
- Lemon peel .... 5 ounces.
- Aniseed .... 4 ounces.
- Cinnamon .... 4 ounces.
- Camomile .... 2 ounces.
- Oil of lemon .... 30 drops.
- Oil of amber .... 30 drops.
- Spirits of wine, 60 o. p. .. 19 quarts.
- Capillaire .... 10 quarts.
- Water .... 13½ quarts.

A little gold leaf. Color red.

1089. Eau d'Amour.
- Lemon peel .... 20 ounces.
- Bitter almonds .... 4 ounces.
- Figs .... 16 ounces.
- Cinnamon .... 5 ounces.
- Lavender .... 4 ounces.
- Mace .... 4 ounces.
- Spirits of wine, 60 o. p. .. 19 quarts.
- Capillaire .... 8 quarts.
- Muscat wine .... 4 quarts.
- Water .... 13½ quarts.

Color rose, and add a little gold leaf.

1090. Liqueur de Punch.
Two pounds lemon peel infused in a close vessel with 19 quarts boiling water several hours; when cold filter and add—
- Rum .... 10 quarts.
- Brandy .... 8 quarts.
- Lemon juice .... 1 quart.
- Sugar .... 29 pounds.

1091. Liqueur de Cumin.
- Cumin .... 2 pounds.
- Aniseed .... 2 ounces.
- Cinnamon .... 1 ounce.
- Orris root .... 1 ounce.
- Angelica root .... ½ ounce.
- Cloves .... ½ ounce.
- Spirits of wine, 60 o. p. .. 19 quarts.
- Capillaire .... 7 quarts.
- Water .... 15 quarts.

1092. Eau de Musetier.
- Lemon peel, dry .... 6 ounces.
- Cinnamon .... 4 ounces.
- Rosemary leaves .... 2 ounces.
- Sage .... 2 ounces.
- Lavender flowers .... 2 ounces.
- Cloves .... 12 ounces.
- Spirits of wine, 60 o. p. .. 19 quarts.
- Capillaire .... 8 quarts.
- Water .... 5 quarts.
- Rose water .... 15 quarts.

Color green.

1093. Christophelet
- Figs .... 10 ounces.
- Orris root .... 4 ounces.
- Aniseed .... 4 ounces.
- Cinnamon .... 2 ounces.
- Sage .... 2 ounces.
- Coriander .... 2 ounces.
- Cardamom .... 1 ounce.
- Galanga .... 1 ounce.
- Saffron .... 4 ounces.
- Wine (Medoc) .... 8 quarts.
- Spirits of wine, 60 o. p. .. 19 quarts.
- Capillaire .... 8 quarts.
- Water .... 7 quarts.

1094. Eau Carminative.
- Lemon peel .... 6 ounces.
- Orange peel .... 6 ounces.
- Cumin .... 4 ounces.
- Juniper berries .... 3 ounces.
- Aniseed .... 3 ounces.
- Chamomile .... 3 ounces.
- Mint .... 2 ounces.
- Nutmeg .... 1 ounce.
- Spirits of wine, 60 o. p. .. 19 quarts.
- Capillaire .... 8 quarts.
- Water .... 14 quarts.

1095. Usquebaugh.
- Cinnamon .... 12 ounces.
- Lavender .... 3 ounces.
- Cloves .... 2 ounces.
- Aniseed .... 2 ounces.
- Nutmegs .... 2 ounces.
- Cardamom .... 1 ounce.
- Spirits of wine, 60 o. p. .. 19 quarts.
- Capillaire .... 8 quarts.
- Water .... 13 quarts.

Color yellow.

1096. Eau d'Or.

Fresh lemon peel	1½ pounds.
Fresh orange peel	10 ounces.
Cinnamon	2 ounces.
Aniseed	2 ounces.
Juniper berries	1½ ounces.
Nutmegs	1 ounce.
Orris root	1 ounce.
Flowers of rosemary	1 ounce.
Cardamom	½ ounce.
Cloves	½ ounce.
Spirits of wine, 60 o.p.	19 quarts.
Capillaire	8 quarts.
Water	14 quarts.

A small quantity of gold leaf.

1097. Eau d'Argent.

Flowers of the lily	12 ounces.
Bitter almonds	8 ounces.
Peppermint	2 ounces.
Nutmegs	2 ounces.
Cinnamon	4 ounces.
Aniseed	2 ounces.
Angelica root	1 ounce.
Cloves	½ ounce.
Spirits of wine, 60 o.p.	19 quarts.
Capillaire	8 quarts.
Water	14 quarts.

A small quantity of silver leaf.

1098. Liqueur d'Oranges.

Orange peel	4 pounds.
Coriander seed	½ pound.
Spirits of wine, 60 o.p.	19 quarts.
Capillaire	8 quarts.
Water	19 quarts.

Color deep yellow.

1099. Eau des Abbés.

Lemon peel	1½ pounds.
Orange peel	¾ pound.
Aniseed	½ pound.
Juniper berries	¼ pound.
Sage	2 ounces.
Peppermint	2 ounces.
Spirits of wine, 60 o.p.	19 quarts.
Capillaire	8 quarts.
Water	15 quarts.

Color deep red.

1100. Annisette.

Aniseed	2½ pounds.
Lemon peel	12 ounces.
Cumin	4 ounces.
Orris root	3 ounces.
Spirits of wine, 60 o.p.	19 quarts.
Capillaire	8 quarts.
Water	18 quarts.

1101. Parfait Amour.

Lemon peel	2 pounds.
Cinnamon	6 ounces.
Orange flowers	4 ounces.
Rosemary leaves	2 ounces.
Mace	1 ounce.
Cloves	1½ ounces.
Saffron	1½ ounces.
Cardamom	1½ ounces.
Spirits of wine, 60 o.p.	19 quarts.
Water	14 quarts.
Capillaire	8 quarts.

Color rose.

1102. Eau Forcifère.

Chamomile	8 ounces.
Juniper berries	6 ounces.
Orange peel	6 ounces.
Rosemary leaves	4 ounces.
Cinnamon	2 ounces.
Cloves	1 ounce.
Cardamom	½ ounce.
Spirits of wine, 60 o.p.	19 quarts.
Capillaire	8 quarts.
Water	14 quarts.

1103. Eau de Vie de Dansick.

Petals of roses	2 pounds.
Orange flowers	8 ounces.
Lemon peel	8 ounces.
Bitter almonds	8 ounces.
Mastic	2 ounces.
Spirits of wine, 60 o.p.	19 quarts.
Water	14 quarts.
Capillaire	8 quarts.

FRENCH LIQUEURS.

1104. Ratafia de Violette.

Orris root	4 ounces.
Spirits of wine	12 quarts.
Water	9 quarts.
Capillaire	3 quarts.

Color violet.

1105. Vespetro.

Angelica seed	3 ounces.
Coriander seed	2 ounces.
Fennel seed	½ ounce.
Aniseed	½ ounce.
Lemons sliced	6 ounces.
Orange sliced	6 ounces.
Spirits of wine, 60 o.p.	12 quarts.
Water	9½ quarts.
Capillaire	3 pints.

NON-SECRET FORMULAS.

1106. Ratafia de Benjoin.
Benjoin in powder.	4	ounces.
Boiling water.	7	quarts.
Spirits of wine.	4	quarts.
Sugar.	1½	pounds.

1107. Liqueur des Muscades.
Mace.	3	ounces.
Nutmegs.	3	ounces.
Orris root.	3	ounces.
Cinnamon.	3	ounces.
Orange peel.	2	ounces.
Lemon peel.	2	ounces.
Rosemary leaves.	2	ounces.
Marjoram	1	ounce.
Aniseed	1	ounce.
Fennel seed.	1	ounce.
Cardamom.	4	ounces.
Camomile.	4	ounces.
Spirits of wine, 60 o.p.	19	quarts.
Capillaire.	7	quarts.
Water.	15	quarts.

1108. Liqueur de Romarin.
Rosemary leaves.	1½	pounds.
Cinnamon.	5	ounces.
Lavender flowers.	2	ounces.
Spirits of wine, 60 o.p.	19	quarts.
Capillaire.	7	quarts.
Water.	15	quarts.

Color green.

1109. Liqueur de Cumin.
Cumin.	2	pounds.
Aniseed	3	ounces.
Oil of cumin.	1	dram.
Spirits of wine, 60 o.p.	19	quarts.
Capillaire.	8	quarts.
Water.	14	quarts.

1110. Liqueur de Cannelle.
Cinnamon.	2	pounds.
Spirits of wine, 60 o.p.	19	quarts.
Capillaire.	7	quarts.
Water.	15	quarts.

Color red.

1111. Persicot.
Bitter almonds.	2	pounds.
Spirits of wine, 60 o.p.	19	quarts.
Capillaire.	7	quarts.
Water.	14	quarts.

1112. Eau de Manheim.
Aniseed	12	ounces.
Fennel seed.	10	ounces.
Lemon peel.	8	ounces.
Cinnamon.	4	ounces.
Cloves.	2	ounces.
Spirits of wine, 60 o.p.	19	quarts.
Capillaire.	5	quarts.
Water.	16	quarts.

1113. Eau de Feichmeier.
Juniper berries.	2	ounces.
Chamomile	1½	ounces.
Lemon peel.	1½	ounces.
Orange peel.	1½	ounces.
Aniseed	1½	ounces.
Fennel seed.	1½	ounces.
Cumin.	1½	ounces.
Pimento.	1½	ounces.
Cinnamon.	1½	ounces.
Peppermint.	1½	ounces.
Marjoram	1½	ounces.
Spirits of wine, 60 o.p.	19	quarts.
Cherry juice.	12	pounds.
Water.	5	pounds.
Capillaire.	15	pounds.

1114. Eau de Capucins.
Celery.	10	ounces.
Orange peel.	8	ounces.
Lemon peel.	8	ounces.
Cinnamon.	6	ounces.
Cumin.	2	ounces.
Nutmeg.	2	ounces.
Fennel.	2	ounces.
Spirits of wine, 60 o.p.	19	quarts.
Capillaire.	7	quarts.
Water.	15	quarts.

1115. Eau Céleste.
Oil of cloves.	50	drops.
Oil of fennel.	36	drops.
Oil of cumin.	36	drops.
Oil of aniseed	15	drops.
Oil of lemon.	½	ounce.
Spirits of wine.	19	quarts.
Cinnamon water.	3	quarts.
Pure water.	12	quarts.
Capillaire.	7	quarts.

Color sky blue.

1116. Elixir Stomachique.
Orange peel.	12	ounces.
Coriander.	4	ounces.
Cinnamon.	1	ounce.
Cloves.	1	ounce.
Nutmegs.	½	ounce.
Saffron.	½	ounce.
Spirits of wine, 60 o.p.	10	quarts.
Peppermint water.	12	quarts.
Capillaire.	3	quarts.

1117. Elixir Vital.

Lemon peel.	4	ounces.
Orange peel.	2	ounces.
Cinnamon.	2	ounces.
Orris root.	2½	ounces.
Cardamom.	1	ounce.
Mace.	1	ounce.
Cloves.	½	ounce.
Musk.	10	grains.
Rose water.	2	quarts.
Water.	10	quarts.
Capillaire.	3	quarts.
Spirits of wine, 60 o.p.	10	quarts.

1118. Huile de Venus.

Carrot seed.	8	ounces.
Cumin.	6	ounces.
Cinnamon.	4	ounces.
Mace.	1	ounce.
Spirits of wine, 60 o.p.	10	quarts.
Water.	8	quarts.
Capillaire.	1	quart.

Color green.

1119. Eau de Scubac.

Lemon peel.	6	ounces.
Coriander.	4	ounces.
Aniseed	2	ounces.
Juniper berries.	2	ounces.
Cinnamon.	2	ounces.
Angelica root.	1½	ounces.
Saffron.	1	ounce.
Spirits of wine, 60 o.p.	10	quarts.
Orange flower water.	2	quarts.
Pure water.	8	quarts.
Capillaire.	4	quarts.

1120. Elixir Stomachique.

Orange peel.	2	ounces.
Lemon peel.	2	ounces.
Galanga.	1½	ounces.
Cardamom.	1½	ounces.
Marjoram	1	ounce.
Nutmeg.	1	ounce.
Cinnamon.	1	ounce.
Rosemary leaves.	6	drams.
Angelica root.	6	drams.
Cloves.	4	drams.
Lavender flowers.	4	drams.
Spirits of wine, 60 o.p.	10	quarts.
Water.	12	quarts.
Capillaire.	3	quarts.

1121. Crème des Barbades.

Lemon peels.	6	
Orange peels.	6	
Cinnamon.	6	drams.
Cloves.	6	drams.
Mace.	2	drams.
Spirits of wine, 60 o.p.	10	quarts.
Water.	8	quarts.
Capillaire.	5	quarts.

1122. Marasquin de Zara.

Raspberries, red.	6	pounds.
Cherries, with the kernels.	4	pounds.
Orange flowers.	2	pounds.
Spirits of wine, 60 o.p.	10	quarts.
Water.	8	quarts.
Capillaire.	5	quarts.

1123. Marasquin.

Prunes with the kernels.	6	pounds.
Raspberries.	3½	pounds.
Cherry tree leaves.	1	pound.
Bitter almonds.	10	
Orris root.	1	ounce.
Spirits of wine, 60 o.p.	10	quarts.
Water.	8	quarts.
Capillaire.	5	quarts.

1124. Elixir des Anges.

Cinnamon.	4	ounces.
Galanga.	2	ounces.
Cloves.	1½	ounces.
Nutmeg.	1	ounce.
Orange peel.	1	ounce.
Lemon peel.	1	ounce.
Ginger.	6	drams.
Orris root.	4	drams.
Cardamom.	4	drams.
Rose water.	12	quarts.
Spirits of wine, 60 o.p.	12	quarts.
Capillaire.	4	quarts.

1125. Eau de Pologne.

Raisins	6	ounces.
Aniseed	1	ounce.
Cinnamon.	1	ounce.
Cloves.	1	ounce.
Fennel.	1	ounce.
Mint.	1	ounce.
Rosemary.	1	ounce.
Marjoram	1	ounce.
Galanga.	1	ounce.
Spirits of wine.	18	quarts.
Rose water.	14	quarts.
Capillaire.	7	quarts.

1126. Liqueur d'Orange.

Orange peel.	2	pounds.
Spirits of wine.	19	quarts.
Orange flower water.	4	quarts.
Pure water.	10	quarts.
Capillaire.	7	quarts.

Color green.

1127. Liqueur de Menthe.
Peppermint leaves.	3 pounds.
Aniseed	3 ounces.
Spirits of wine, 60 o. p.	19 quarts.
Capillaire.	7 quarts.
Peppermint water.	6 quarts.
Pure water.	8 quarts.

1128. Liqueur d'Angelique.
Lemon peel.	16 ounces.
Angelica.	5 ounces.
Orange peel.	4 ounces.
Cinnamon.	4 ounces.
Mace.	2 ounces.
Lavender flowers.	2 ounces.
Cloves.	1 ounce.
Marjoram.	1 ounce.
Rosemary leaves.	1 ounce.
Orris root.	1 ounce.
Spirits of wine, 60 o.p.	19 quarts.
Rose water.	16 quarts.
Orange flower water.	2 quarts.
Pure water.	2 quarts.
Capillaire.	8 quarts.

1129. Crême de Chocolat.
Cocoa berries, ground.	4 pounds.
Cinnamon.	6 ounces.
Cloves.	2 drams.
Vanilla.	2 drams.
Spirits of wine, 60 o.p.	10 quarts.
Water.	8 quarts.
Capillaire.	5 quarts.

1130. Crême de Roses.
Rose leaves, dry.	8 pounds.
Spirits of wine, 60 o.p.	12 quarts.
Oil of roses.	20 drops.
Water.	8 quarts.
Capillaire.	5 quarts.

1131. Crême de Macaron.
Bitter almonds.	11 ounces.
Cinnamon.	6 drams.
Cloves.	6 drams.
Cardamom.	6 drams.
Spirits of wine, 60 o.p.	10 quarts.
Rose water.	2 quarts.
Orange flower water.	2 quarts.
Pure water.	4 quarts.
Capillaire.	5 quarts.

1132. Liqueur Stomachique.
Orange peel.	6 ounces.
Lemon peel.	4 ounces.
Aniseed	2 ounces.
Galanga.	1½ ounces.
Cinnamon.	1½ ounces.
Orris root.	1½ ounces.
Sweet basil.	1½ ounces.
Chamomile	1½ ounces.
Lavender flowers.	1 ounce.
Rosemary leaves.	1 ounce.
Vanilla.	1½ ounces.
Nutmeg.	1½ ounces.
Mace.	1½ ounces.
Cardamom.	1½ ounces.
Spirits of wine, 60 o.p.	19 quarts.
Capillaire.	7 quarts.
Water.	15 quarts.

1133. Liqueur de Girofle.
Cloves.	2 pounds.
Spirits of wine, 60 o.p.	19 quarts.
Capillaire.	7 quarts.
Water.	15 quarts.

Color pink.

1134. Liqueur de Roses.
Petals of roses.	5 pounds.
Cinnamon.	3 ounces.
Fennel seed.	1 ounce.
Spirits of wine, 60 o.p.	19 quarts.
Capillaire.	7 quarts.
Water.	15 quarts.

Color rose.

1135. Rosolis.
Cinnamon.	8 ounces.
Cardamom.	4 ounces.
Nutmeg.	4 ounces.
Orris root.	4 ounces.
Spirits of wine, 60 o.p.	19 quarts.
Capillaire.	7 quarts.
Rose water.	15 quarts.

Color rose.

1136. Liqueur de Citron.
Lemon peel.	3 pounds.
Spirits of wine, 60 o.p.	19 quarts.
Capillaire.	7 quarts.
Water.	15 quarts.

Color yellow.

1137. Eau Vert Stomachique.
Spirits of wine, proof.	25 quarts.
Coriander.	2 ounces.
Aniseed	1 ounce.
Angelica seed.	2 ounces.
Cloves.	1 ounce.
Saffron.	2 drams.
Mace.	2 drams.
Cinnamon	1 ounce.
Carrot seed.	½ ounce.
Essence of bergamot.	1 dram.
Peel of oranges	8
Sugar, 13 pounds dissolved in 4 quarts of water.	

Color green.

1138. Eau des Amis.
Oil of citron .... 20 drops.
Oil of bergamot .... 10 drops.
Spirits of wine, proof. .... 12 quarts.
Sugar. .... 12 pounds.
Water. .... 6 quarts.
Figs. .... 8 ounces.
Raisins. .... 8 ounces.
Color pale yellow.

1139. Eau de Vie d'Andaye.
Orleans brandy. .... 24 quarts.
Aniseed .... 4 ounces.
Coriander. .... 4 ounces.
Orris root. .... 8 ounces.
Sugar. .... 12 pounds.
Water. .... 4 quarts.
Color pale yellow.

1140. Eau de la Cote.
Spirits of wine, proof .... 6 quarts.
Cinnamon. .... 4 ounces.
Dates. .... 4 ounces.
Figs. .... 4 ounces.
Bitter almonds. .... 2 ounces.
Nutmeg. .... ½ ounce.
Peel of oranges 2
Sugar. .... 5 pounds.
Water. .... 2 quarts.

1141. Creme de Framboises.
Raspberries. .... 2 pounds.
Spirits of wine, proof. .... 4 quarts.
Water. .... 2 quarts.
Sugar. .... 5 pounds.

1142. Huile d'Anis.
Oil of aniseed .... 10 drops.
Spirits of wine, proof .... 2 quarts.
Capillaire. .... 5 quarts.

1143. Huile de Roses.
Spirits of wine, proof. .... 10 quarts.
Sugar. .... 20 pounds.
Rose water. .... 5 quarts.
Color rose.

1144. Eau des Chevaliers de la Legion d'Honneur.
Spirits of wine, proof. .... 6 quarts.
Orange peel. .... 10 ounces.
Lemon peel. .... 6 ounces.
Distilled water. .... 2 quarts.
Sugar. .... 4 pounds.
Oil of citron. .... 8 drops.
Color red.

1145. Huile de Vanille.
Spirits of wine, proof. .... 10 quarts.
Sugar. .... 20 pounds.
Tincture of vanilla. ...... 2 drams.
Water. .... 5 pounds.

1146. Cremes des Barbades.
Peels of oranges 6
Cinnamon. .... 4 ounces.
Mace. .... 2 drams.
Cloves. .... 1 dram.
Coriander. .... 1 ounce.
Bitter almonds. .... 1 ounce.
Nutmeg. .... 1 dram.
Spirits of wine, proof. .... 15 quarts.
Sugar. .... 15 pounds.
Water. .... 10 quarts.

1147. Nectar des Dieux.
Spirits of wine, proof. .... 6 quarts.
Honey. .... 4 ounces.
Coriander. .... 2 ounces.
Orange peel. .... 1 ounce.
Tincture of vanilla. ...... ½ dram.
Cloves. .... 2 drams.
Benjoin. .... 4 drams.
Spirit of orange flowers... 3 ounces.
Sugar. .... 6 pounds.
Water. .... 1 quart.
Color deep red.

1148. Nectar de la Beauté.
Peels of oranges 9
Cinnamon. .... 2 ounces.
Mace. .... 2 drams.
Aniseed .... 4 ounces.
Coriander. .... 4 ounces.
Juniper berries. .... 2 ounces.
Angelica seed. .... 1 ounce.
Saffron. .... 1 dram.
Spirits of wine, proof. .... 16 quarts.
Sugar. .... 9 pounds.
Water. .... 2 quarts.
Rose water. .... 1 quart.
Color rose.

1149. Elixir de Garus.
Myrrh. .... 2 drams.
Aloes .... 2 drams.
Cloves. .... 3 drams.
Nutmegs. .... 3 drams.
Saffron. .... 1 ounce.
Cinnamon. .... 5 drams.
Spirits of wine, proof. .... 5 quarts.
Sugar. .... 6 pounds.

1150. Nectar du General Foy.
Spirits of wine, proof. .... 1 quart.
Rose water. .... 2 quarts.
Tincture of vanilla. .... ½ dram.
Color rose.

1151. Nectar des Grecs.
Spirits of wine, proof. .... 10 parts.
Peels of oranges 4
Coffee, ground. .... 2 ounces.
Cinnamon. .... 1 ounce.
Tincture of vanilla. .... 1 dram.
Sugar. .... 10 pounds.
Water. .... 2 quarts.
Color red.

1152. Parfait Amour.
Spirits of wine, proof. .... 12 quarts.
Orange peel. .... 6 ounces.
Cloves. .... 2 drams.
Water. .... 6 quarts.
Sugar. .... 10 pounds.
Color rose.

1153. Rosolis.
Red roses. .... 8 ounces.
Orange flowers. .... 4 ounces.
Cinnamon. .... 2 drams.
Cloves. .... 1 dram.
Spirits of wine, proof. .... 10 quarts.
Water. .... 8 quarts.
Sugar. .... 6 pounds.
Extract of jessamine ..... 2 ounces.
Color red.

1154. Larmes de Missolonghy.
Bitter almonds. .... 1 pound.
Angelica seed. .... 2 ounces.
Mace. .... 1 dram.
Spirits of wine, proof. .... 10 quarts.
Sugar. .... 5½ pounds.
Water. .... 1 quart.
Orange flower water. ..... 1 quart.
Essence of cinnamon ..... 1 dram.
Essence of bergamot ..... 1 dram.
Color rose.

1155. Alkermès.
Cinnamon. .... 2 drams.
Cloves. .... 2 drams.
Nutmeg. .... 4 drams.
Spirits of wine, proof. .... 4 quarts.
Sugar. .... 5 pounds.
Rose Water. .... 1 pint.
Color red.

1156. Missilimakinac.
Spirits of wine, proof. .... 8 quarts.
Cloves. .... 2 drams.
Mace. .... 1 dram.
Water. .... 3 quarts.
Orange flower water. ..... 1 pint.
Rose water. .... 1 pint.
Essence of jessamine. ..... ½ ounce.
Tincture of amber. .... 10 drops.
Sugar. .... 7 pounds.

1157. Amiable Vainqueur.
Spirits of wine, proof. .... 25 quarts.
Essential oil of citron. .... 1 ounce.
Essential oil of neroli .... ½ ounce.
Essential oil of angelica.. ½ ounce.
Tincture of vanilla. .... 1 dram.
Sugar. .... 12 pounds.
Water. .... 4 quarts.

1158. Elixir Columbat.
Spirits of wine, proof. .... 8 quarts.
Oil of citron. .... 20 drops.
Peels of oranges 12
Cinnamon. .... 2 ounces.
Mace. .... 2 drams.
Saffron. .... 1 dram.
Angelica root. .... 1 dram.
Juniper berries. .... 2 drams.
Sugar. .... 12 pounds.
Water. .... 2 quarts.
Orange flower water. ..... 1 quart.
Color rose.

1159. Citronelle.
Spirits of wine, proof. .... 8 quarts.
Peels of oranges 68
Cloves. .... 1 dram.
Nutmeg. .... 1 dram.
Sugar. .... 5 pounds.
Water. .... 2 quarts.
Color yellow.

1160. La Félicité.
Spirits of wine, proof. .... 8 quarts.
Cardamoms. .... ½ ounce.
Angelica root, dry .... ¼ ounce.
Orris root. .... 1 ounce.
Mace. .... 1 dram.
Tops of sweet basil. ...... 2 drams.
Peels of lemons 8
Sugar. .... 5 pounds.
Water. .... 1 quart.
Color rose.

1161. **Plaisir des Dames.**
  Spirits of wine, proof.... 5 quarts.
  Bitter almonds............ 8 ounces.
  Angelica seed............. 2 ounces.
  Cinnamon.................. ½ ounce.
  Coriander................. ½ ounce.
  Sugar..................... 6 pounds.
  Water..................... 2 quarts.
  Color violet.

1162. **Gaîté Française.**
  Spirits of wine, proof.... 8 quarts.
  Cloves.................... ½ ounce.
  Cinnamon.................. ½ ounce.
  Cardamom.................. 1 pound.
  Peels of oranges.......... 6
  Sugar..................... 5 pounds.
  Water..................... 1 quart.
  Color rose.

1163. **Amour Sans Fin.**
  Two lemons, minced fine.
  Two oranges, minced fine.
  Spirits of wine, proof.... 3 quarts.
  Sugar..................... 5 pounds.
  Water..................... 3 quarts.
  Rose water................ ½ pint.
  Color yellow or rose.

1164. **Ratafia de Cerises.**
  Cherries with their stones
    well mashed............. 8 pounds.
  Spirits of wine, proof.... 3 quarts.
  After macerating 15 days, press out all the juice, and for every pint of the liquor add 3 ounces sugar; by the same manner it may be made with gooseberries and strawberries.

1165. **Ratafia de Noyeau.**
  Apricot kernels........... 4 ounces.
  Spirits of wine, proof.... 2 quarts.
  Sugar..................... 2 pounds.
  Water..................... 1 pint.

1166. **Ratafia des Quatre Graines.**
  Spirits of wine, proof.... 12 quarts.
  Celery seed............... 2 ounces.
  Angelica seed............. 4 ounces.
  Coriander seed............ 4 ounces.
  Fennel seed............... 2 ounces.
  Sugar..................... 8 pounds.
  Water..................... 5 quarts.

1167. **Ratafia d'Anis et de Carvi.**
  Aniseed................... 1 ounce.
  Carraway seed............. 1 ounce.
  Coriander seed............ 1 ounce.
  Fennel seed............... 1 ounce.
  Spirits of wine, proof.... 2 quarts.
  Sugar..................... 1 pound.
  Water..................... 1 pint.

1168. **Ratafia des Cassis.**
  Currant leaves............ 4 ounces.
  Ripe currants............. 6 pounds.
  Cloves.................... ½ dram.
  Cinnamon.................. 1 dram.
  Spirits of wine, proof.... 6 quarts.
  Sugar..................... 4 pounds.
  Water..................... 1 quart.

1169. **Ratafia d'Absinthe.**
  Wormwood.................. 4 pounds.
  Juniper berries........... 8 ounces.
  Cinnamon.................. 2 ounces.
  Angelica root............. 4 drams.
  Spirits of wine, proof.... 17 quarts.
  Water..................... 1 quart.
  Orange flower water....... 6 ounces.
  Sugar..................... 2½ pounds.

1170. **Ratafia d'Angelique.**
  Angelica seeds............ 2 ounces.
  Bitter almonds............ 2 ounces.
  Spirits of wine, proof.... 6 quarts.
  Sugar..................... 3 pounds.
  Water..................... 1 quart.

1171. **Ratafia d'Anis.**
  Aniseed................... 1 ounce.
  Spirits of wine, proof.... 2 quarts.
  Sugar..................... 1 pound.
  Water..................... 1 pint.

1172. **Ratafia de Celery.**
  Spirits of wine, proof.... 5 quarts.
  Celery seed............... 8 ounces.
  Coriander seed............ 1 ounce.
  Cloves.................... 1 dram.
  Sugar..................... 3 pounds.
  Water..................... 2 quarts.

1173. **Ratafia dit Escubac.**
  Saffron................... 2 ounces.
  Jujubes................... 4 ounces.
  Dates..................... 3 ounces.
  Raisins................... 3 ounces.
  Aniseed................... 1 dram.
  Coriander seed............ 1 dram.
  Cinnamon.................. 1 dram.
  Sugar..................... 4 pounds.
  Spirits of wine, proof.... 8 quarts.
  Water..................... 2 quarts.

1174. Guignolet d'Anges.
Spirits of wine, proof	12 quarts.
Cherries, with the stones	1 pound.
Raspberries	1 pound.
Gooseberries	1 pound.
Red currants	1 pound.
Oil of cinnamon	10 drops.
Oil of cloves	10 drops.
Sugar	7 pounds.
Water	2 quarts.

1175. China-China.
Bitter almonds	1 pound.
Angelica seed	2 ounces.
Mace	1 dram.
Spirits of wine, proof	9 quarts.
Sugar	5 pounds.
Distilled water	2 quarts.
Orange flower water	8 ounces.
Oil of cinnamon	10 drops.

Color pale yellow.

1176. La Valeureuse.
Spirits of wine, proof	6 quarts.
Water	4 quarts.
Essence of roses	2 ounces.
Essence of orange flowers	8 ounces.
Essence of jessamine	3 ounces.
Sugar	6 pounds.

Color rose.

1177. Coquette Flatteuse.
Spirits of wine, proof	10 quarts.
Peels of lemons	9
Peels of oranges	5
Tops of hyssop., dry	5 ounces.
Musk roses	1 ounce.
Sugar	8 pounds.
Water	2 quarts.

Color red.

1178. Persicot.
Bitter almonds	12 ounces.
Cinnamon	½ dram.
Spirits of wine, proof	12 quarts.
Sugar	6 pounds.
Water	2 quarts.

Color red.

1179. Vespetro.
Angelica seeds	4 drams.
Carraway seeds	4 drams.
Coriander seeds	4 drams.
Fennel seeds	4 drams.
Peels of oranges	2
Spirits of wine, proof	5 quarts.
Sugar	4 pounds.
Water	3 pints.

Color red.

1180. Goutte Nationale.
Spirits of wine, proof	4 quarts.
Peels of oranges	6
Coriander seed	1 ounce.
Sassafras peas	1 ounce.
Cinnamon	1 dram.
Sugar	3 pounds.
Water	1 quart.

Color rose.

1181. Suvenir d'un Brave.
Spirits of wine, proof	15 quarts.
Cloves	½ ounce.
Cinnamon	¼ ounce.
Bitter almonds	4 pounds.
Peels of oranges	4
Sugar	8 pounds.
Water	2 quarts.

Color rose.

1182. Espoir des Grecs.
Spirits of orange flowers	4 ounces.
Spirit of roses	5 ounces.
Spirit of tuberose	2 ounces.
Tincture vanilla	1 dram.
Spirits of wine, proof	5 quarts.
Sugar	8 pounds.
Water	5 quarts.

Color crimson.

1183. Escubac.
Saffron	1 ounce.
Juniper berries	4 ounces.
Dates	2 ounces.
Raisins	2 ounces.
Jujubes	4 drams.
Aniseed	1 dram.
Coriander	1 dram.
Cinnamon	2 drams.
Mace	1 dram.
Cloves	1 dram.
Spirits of wine, proof	5 quarts.
Capillaire	4 quarts.

1184. Curacao.
Spirits of wine, proof	10 quarts.
Peels of oranges	40
Cinnamon	2 drams.
Mace	1 dram.
Sugar	7 pounds.
Water	3 quarts.

Color pale yellow.

1185. Elixir de Genievre.
Juniper berries	2 ounces.
Spirits of wine, proof	2 quarts.
Sugar	3 pounds.
Water	1 quart.

1186. Rosolio de Turin.
Raisins.	8 ounces.
Orange flowers.	8 ounces.
Jessamine flowers.	8 ounces.
Cinnamon.	1 ounce.
Cloves.	1 ounce.
Spirits of wine, proof.	6 quarts.
Sugar.	6 pounds.
Water.	2 quarts.

Color red.

1187. Elixir Stomachique de Violette.
Syrup of violets.	8 ounces.
Raspberry juice.	6 ounces.
Spirits of wine, proof.	2 quarts.
Sugar.	4 pounds.
Water.	1 quart.

1188. Elixir Barathier.
Myrrh.	1 ounce.
Aloes.	2 ounces.
Saffron.	1 ounce.
Cloves.	1 ounce.
Cinnamon.	1 ounce.
Nutmeg.	1 ounce.
Spirits of wine, proof.	6 quarts.
Orange peels.	2 ounces.
Sugar.	6 pounds.
Water.	3 quarts.

Color pale yellow.

1189. Baume Consolateur.
Spirits of wine, proof.	12 quarts.
Mace.	2 drams.
Distilled water.	4 quarts.
Spirit of jessamine.	1½ ounces.
Spirit of orange flowers.	1 ounce.
Spirit of roses.	1 ounce.
Tincture vanilla.	½ ounce.
Sugar.	10 pounds.

Color violet.

1190. Baume des Grecs.
Angelica seed.	2 ounces.
Coriander seed.	1 ounce.
Fennel seed.	2 drams.
Aniseed	2 drams.
Lemons, minced small	2
Spirits of wine, proof.	5 quarts.
Sugar.	2½ pounds.
Water.	1 quart.

Color rose.

1191. Eau des Pacificateurs de la Grèce.
Spirits of wine, proof.	6 quarts.
Orange flower water.	1 pint.
Water.	1 quart.
Sugar.	3 pounds.
Peels of oranges	6

Color red.

1192. Eau des Chevaliers de Saint Louis.
Apricot kernels.	1 pound.
Bitter almonds.	8 ounces.
Cherry stone kernels.	8 ounces.
Spirits of wine, proof.	10 quarts.
Rose water.	12 ounces.
Distilled water.	5 quarts.
Sugar.	6 pounds.

Color red.

1193. Huile de Jasmin.
Spirits of wine, proof.	10 quarts.
Sugar.	20 pounds.
Oil of jessamine.	1 dram.
Water.	5 quarts.

1194. Huile des Jeunes Mariés.
Aniseed	2 ounces.
Fennel seed.	2 ounces.
Angelica seed.	1 ounce.
Cumin seed.	1 ounce.
Carraway seed.	1 ounce.
Coriander.	3 ounces.
Spirits of wine, proof.	6 quarts.
Distilled water.	3 quarts.
Sugar.	10 pounds.

Color yellow.

1195. Huile de Rhum.
Jamaica rum, proof.	10 quarts.
Water.	6 quarts.
Sugar.	20 pounds.

1196. Eau de Noyeau de Phalsbourg.
Spirits of wine, proof.	15 quarts.
Apricot kernels.	20 ounces.
Peach kernels	8 ounces.
Prune kernels.	8 ounces.
Sugar.	7½ pounds.
Distilled water.	4 quarts.
Orange flower water.	1 quart.

1197. Eau de Vie de Danzick.
Spirits of wine, proof.	18 quarts.
Carraway seed.	3 ounces.
Celery seeds.	3 ounces.
Aniseed	4 ounces.
Peels of oranges	2
Sugar.	12 pounds.
Water.	4 quarts.

Add a small quantity of gold leaf, and color pale yellow.

1198. Eau des Financiers.
Spirits of wine, proof.	2 quarts.
Mace.	1 dram.
Peels of oranges	6
Sugar.	6 pounds.
Water.	3 pints.
Orange flower water.	¼ pint.

Color pale yellow.

1199. **Eau Archiepiscopale.**
Orange peels. 2
Fresh balm. .... 1 ounce.
Mace. .... 1 dram.
Spirits of wine, proof. .... 2 quarts.
Water. .... 2 quarts.
Spirit of jessamine .... 4 drams.
Orange flower water. ..... 1 pint.
Sugar. .... 1½ pounds.
Color violet.

FORMULÆ OF THE NEW YORK HOSPITAL.

FOR EXTERNAL USE.

1200. **Antiseptic Solutions.**
Sol. acid carbolic. .... 1-20 water.
Sol. acid carbolic. .... 1-30 water.
Sol. acid carbolic. .... 1-40 water.
Sol. acid boracic. .... 1-30 water.
Sol. thymol. .... 1-1000.
Distilled water is preferred; it will make a clearer solution than ordinary water.

1201. **Carbolic Spray.**
Sodii bicarb. ....
Sodii biborat.......aa. 1 dram.
Acidi carbolici. .... 40 grains.
Glycerinae. .... 7 drams.
Aquae ....ad 8 ounces.
M.

1202. **White Wash.**
Potassii sulphuret.,
Zinci sulphat......aa. 1 dram.
Aquae. .... 4 ounces.
Dissolve each in two ounces water and mix.

1203. **Red Wash.**
Zinci sulphat. .... 2 scruples.
Spts. lavand. co. ...... 1 fl. dram.
Aquae. .... 1 pint.
Cochineal coloring. ... q. s.
M.

1204. **Ward Gargle.**
Tannin. .... ½ dram.
Sol. potass. chlorat. sat. 8 ounces.
M.

1205. **Muriate of Ammonia Wash.**
Ammonii chloridi. .... ½ ounce.
Tinct. opii. .... 1 ounce.
Aquae. ....ad 2 pints.
M.

1206. **Lead and Opium Wash.**
Liquor plumbi subacet. 3 drams.
Aquae. .... 1 pint.
Tr. opii. .... 4 drams.
M.

1207. **Alkaline Tar Water.**
Picis liquidae. .... 2 ounces.
Potassae causticae. ... 1 ounce.
Aquae. .... 5 ounces.
M.

1208. **Compound Tincture of Green Soap.**
Oil of cade,
Green soap,
Alcohol, equal parts.
M.

1209. **Churchill's Tincture of Iodine.**
Iodinii. .... 1 dram.
Potassii iodidi. .... 2 dram.
Aquae destill. ....
Alcohol. ....aa 2 fl. ounces.

1210. **Iodoform Cylinders.**
Iodoform. .... 2½ drams.
Tragacanth. .... 15 grains.
Mucilag. acaciae. ..... q. s.
Divide into 10 cylinders, 1½ in. long.

1211. **Epilating Stick.**
Wax. .... 3 ounces.
Shellac. .... 4 ounces.
Rosin. .... 6 ounces.
Burgundy pitch. ...... 10 ounces.
Damar. .... 12 ounces.
Melt together and roll into sticks of different diameters.

1212. **Parasiticide.**
Acidi carbol. .... 10 grains.
Ungt. hydrarg. nitrat. .
Sulphur. precip. ....aa. 1 dram.
Ungt. simplicis. ...... 1 ounce.

1213. **Colorless Evaporating Lotion.**
Ammon. hydrochlor. .. 12 grains.
Spts. vini rect. .... 34 minims.
Aquae. .... 1 ounce.

1214. **Lotion of Calamine and Zinc Oxide.**
Pulv. calamin. prep.,
Zinci oxidi. ....aa 1 dram.
Glycerinae. .... 2 drams.
Aquae. .... 4 ounces.

1215. **Stimulating Lotion.**
Arnicae tinct. .... 20 minims.
Spts. rosmarin. .... 15 minims.
Aq. dest. .... 1 ounce.

OINTMENTS.

1216. Carbolized Vaseline (Saturated).
Vaselinae. .... 20 ounces.
Acid. carbolic, crystal. 1 ounce.
Melt each separately and mix.

1217. Ointment of Chrysophanic Acid; Concentrated.
Acid. chrysophanic. .. 1 ounce.
Ung. simplicis. .... 4 ounces.
Melt the ointment, and while hot add the acid, stirring till dissolved.

1218. Brown Ointment.
Pulv. acid. salicylic. .. 40 grains.
Bals. peruvian. .... 1 dram.
Vaselinae. .... 1 ounce.

1219. Ointment of Salicylic Acid.
Pulv. acid. salicylic... 1 dram.
Vaselinae. .... 1 ounce.

1220. Ointment of Iodoform.
Iodoform. .... 1 dram.
Vaselinae. .... 1 ounce.
Reduce the iodoform to powder and add to the vaseline; heat by water bath till dissolved.

1221. Ointment of Peruvian Balsam.
Bals. peru. .... 2 drams.
Cerat. simpl. .... 1 ounce.
M.

1222. Dusting Powder.
Camphor .... 1 dram.
Talc.
Zinc oxide, each. ..... 6 drams.
M.

1223. Compound Oil of Cade Ointment.
Ol. cadini. .... f. 1 dram.
Ungt. zinci oxidi. ..... 1 ounce.

1224. Compound Iodoform Ointment.
Pulv. iodoform,
Acidi tannici .... aa. 1 dram.
Vaselinae. .... 1 ounce.

1225. Ointment of Tar and Oxide of Zinc.
Ungt. picis. .... 4 drams.
Zinci oxidi. .... 1 dram.
Cerat. simpl. .... 1½ ounce.

1226. Lead and Zinc Ointment.
Plumbi acetat. .... 10 grains.
Zinci oxidi.
Hydrarg. chlor. mitis. .
Ungt. hydr. nitratis..aa. 20 grains.
Adipis recentis,
Olei palmae purific ..aa. ½ ounce.

1227. Ointment of Mercury and Iodide of Potassium.
Ungt. hydrarg.,
Ungt. iodin. co. .....aa. 1 ounce.

1228. Tannic Acid Ointment (Stronger).
Acidi tannici. .... 1 dram.
Ungt. simplic. .... 1 ounce.

1229. Eczema Drying Salve.
Plumbi glycerat. ..... 1 dram.
Ungt. zinci oxid. ...... 1 ounce.

MIXTURES.

1230. Emulsion of Cod Liver Oil with Solution of Saccharated Lime.
(75 per cent. emulsion.)
Ol. morrhuae. .... 6 ounces.
Ol. anisi. .... ½ dram.
Ol. sassafras .... 10 drops.
Liquor. calc. sacchar... 2 ounces.
M.
Not compatible with acids.

1231. Chlorate of Potassa Mixture.
Ammon. muriat.,
Potass. chlorat. .....aa. 1 dram.
Ext. glycyrrh. .... ½ dram.
Aquae cinnam. .....ad 4 ounces.
Dose, a tablespoonful.

1232. Mixture of Iodide of Potassium and Hoffman's Anodyne.
Potass. iodid. .... 3 drams.
Spts. ether. co. .... 1 ounce.
Syr. pruni virg. .... 3 ounces.
M. Dose, a teaspoonful.

1233. Cough Mixture.
Ether. sulph. .... 3 drams.
Tinct. hyoscyam.,
Syr. pruni virg.,
Syr. tolutan. ....aa 1 ounce.
Aquae. ....ad 4 ounces.
Dose, two to four drams.

1234. **Chloroform Cough Mixture.**
Morphiae acet. .... 3 grains.
Tr. belladonnae. ...... 4 drams.
Spts. chloroformi. ..... 6 drams.
Syr. senegae. .... 1 ounce.
Syr. pruni virg. ... .ad 4 ounces.

1235. **Hydrocyanic Mixture.**
Potassii cyanidi. ..... 2 grains.
Syrupi tolut.,
Liq. morph. sulph. U.
S. P. ....aa 1 ounce.
Dose, a teaspoonful.

1236. **Ward Cough Mixture.**
Fld. ext. pruni virg... 3 ounces.
Sol. potassii cyanidi. .. 8 grains.
Sol. morph. magendie.. ½ ounce.
Syr. simplicis. .... 10 ounces.
Aquae. .... 18 ounces.
Dose, a teaspoonful p. r. n.

Mixture of Sulphate of Magnesia
1237. **and Iron.** A
Magnes. sulph. .... 1 ounce.
Ferri sulph. .... 16 grains.
Acidi sulph. dil. ...... 2 f. drams.
Syr. zingib. .... 1 f. ounce.
Aquae. .... 7 ounces.
M.

Mixture of Sulphate of Magnesia
1238. **and Iron.** B
Magnes. sulph. .... 1 ounce.
Ferri sulph. .... 1 dram.
Acidi sulph. aromat. .. 2 drams.
Tinct. gentian. .... 1 ounce.
Aquae. .... 3 ounces.
M. Teaspoonful after eating.

Mixture of Sulphate of Magnesia
1239. **and Iron.** C
Ferri sulph. .... 16 grains.
Magnes. sulph. .... 1 ounce.
Ac. sulph. arom. ...... ½ f. ounce.
Aq. menthae pip. .. .ad 1 pint.
M.

1240. **Mixture of Iron and Cinchona.**
Ferri et ammon. citratis. .... 1 dram.
Tinct. nucis vom. ..... 2 drams.
Tinct. cinchon. co. .... 4 ounces.
M. Dose, a teaspoonful.

1241. **Alkaline Mixture.** A
Potass. acetat. .... 2 drams.
Potass. et sodii tartrat. 1 ounce.
Syr. zingiberis. .... 1 f. ounce.
Aquae. .... 3 ounces.
M.

1242. **Alkaline Mixture.** B
(Dr. Hawley.)
Potass. citrat. .... 1½ ounces.
Syr. limonis,
Aquae. ....aa 3 ounces.

1243. **Nitrous Acid Mixture.**
(Dr. Kelly.)
Tr. opii deod. .... 2 f. dram.
Acidi nitrosi. .... ½ f. dram.
Aq. camphorae......... ad 4 ounces.

Mixture of Hydrargyrum and Iodide
1244. **of Potassium.** A
Hydrarg. bichlor. ..... 1 grain.
Potass. iodid. .... 2 drams.
Tr. cardam. co. ......
Tr. gentian. ....aa 1 ounce.
M. Dose, one dram.

Mixture of Hydrargyrum and Iodide
1245. **of Potassium.** B
Hydrarg. bichlor. ..... 1¼ grains.
Potass. iodid. .... 3 drams.
Tr. cardamom. co. .... 2 ounces.
M. Dose, one dram.

Mixture of Hydrargyrum and Iodide
1246. **of Potassium.** C
Hydrarg. biniod. ..... ½ grain.
Potass. iodidi. .... 1 dram.
Syr. sarsap. co. ...... 1 ounce.
M. Dose, one dram three times a day.

1247. **Townsend's Mixture.**
Hydrarg. biniod. ...... 1 grain.
Potass. iodidi. .... 5 dram.
Syr. aurant. cort. ..... 2 f. ounces.
Tr. card. comp. .... 2 f. drams.
Aquae q. s. ....ad 4 f. ounces.

1248. **Mendelson's Tonic.**
Acidi arseniosi. .... 1/5 grain.
Ferri et quin. cit. ..... 80 grains.
Tr. cinch. comp...... .ad 2 f. ounces.

1249. Kelly's Tonic.
Tr. nucis vomicae. .... 2 f. drams.
Acid. nitromuriat. dil.. 3 f. drams.
Tr. cinch. co. .... 1½ f. ounces.
Tr. gent. co. .... ad 3 f. ounces.
Dose, two drams in water, three times a day.

1250. Knapp's Tonic.
Pulv. cubeb. .... 3 drams.
Tr. cinch. co. .... 4 f. ounces.

1251. Hamilton's Tonic.
Strychniae sulph. ..... 8 grains.
Cinchonidiae sulph..... 1 ounce.
Tr. ferri chlor. .... 6 ounces.
Syr. zingiberis,
Acid. phosphoric dil..aa. 16 ounces.
Dose, one teaspoonful three times a day.

1252. Effervescing Mixture.
(Dr. Draper.)
R. Acidi citrici,
Ferri et quiniae cit. ..aa. 4 drams.
Aquae,
Syr. limonis ....aa. 2 f. ounces.
M.

1253.
R. Potass. bicarb. .... 4 drams.
Aquae. ....ad 4 ounces.
M. One fluid dram of each in two drams of water, to be mixed at the time of taking.

1254. Mixture of Rhubarb and Soda.
R. Pulv. rhei. .... 14 grains.
Sodii bicarb. .... 1½ drams.
Aq. menth. pip. ....ad 2 f. ounces.

1255. Rochelle Salt Mixture.
Sodii et potass. tart. .. 960 grains.
Ferri et potass. tart. . 320 grains.
Aquae menth. pip. ... 4 fl. ounces.
Aquae q. s. ...... ad 1 pint.
M.

1256. Mixture of Squill, Compound.
(Dr. Kelly.)
Ammon. chlor. .... 2 drams.
Potass. chlorat. ...... 1 dram.
Syr. scillae co. .... ½ fl. ounce.
Syr. tolut. .... 6 fl. drams.
Liq. ammon. acet. ad 8 fl. ounces.

1257. Mixture of Quinia, Compound.
Quiniae sulph. .... 2 drams.
Acid. sulph. ar. .... 4 fl. drams.
Tinct. cinch. co. ad 3 fl. ounces.

1258. Carminative Mixture.
(Dr. Kelly.)
Tr. opii .... 20 drops.
Ol. anisi, ...
Ol. caryophyl.. ......
Ol. gaulth. .... aa 2 drops.
Tr. asafoetidae .... 1 fl. dram.
Magnes. carbon. ...... 1 dram.
Aquae menthae pip. ad 3 fl. ounces.

1259. Anti-Rheumatic Mixture.
(Mistura Antiarthritica.)
Potassii iodidi .... 5 drams.
Vini colchici. sem. .. 1 ounce.
Tr. cimicifugae rac. .. 2 ounces.
Tr. stramon. .... ½ ounce.
Tr. opii camp. .... 1½ ounces.
M.
Dose: One dram three times a day.

1260. La Fayette Mixture.
Bals. copaivae ....
Spts. ether. nit. ......
Spts. lavand. co. .. aa 4 ounces.
Liquor potassae ...... 4 drams.
Mucilag. acac. ......ad 2 pints.

MISCELLANEOUS.

1261. Syrup of Hypophosphites, Compound.
Calcii hypophos., ...
Sodii hypophos. ...... aa 2 grains.
Potassii hypophos., ...
Ferri hypophos. ...... aa 1 grain.
Acidi hypophos. solut. q. s.
Glycerinae ....
Aquae .... aa q. s. ad 1 dram.
M.

1262. Bitter Wine of Iron.
Ferri et quiniae cit. .. 64 grains.
Tr. aurant. amar. .... 2 fl. drams.
Elix. simplicis .... 1 fl. ounce.
Vini xerici .... 2 fl ounces.
Aquae .... q. s. ad 4 fl. ounces.
M.

1263. **Errhine Powder.**
(Dr. B. Robinson.)
Pulv. cubebae .... ½ ounce.
Sodae bicarb. .... 2 drams.
Acidi salicylic .... 10 grains.
Sacch. albi. .... 2 drams.
Misce. fiat pulvis.

1264. **Fasciculus Sennæ Comp.**
Fol. sennae ....
Quassiae .... aa 2 drams.
Potass. bitart. .... 1 ounce.
Semin. anisi .... ½ ounce.
M.

1265. **Suppositories of Ergot.**
Ext. ergot. aquos. (Squibb) 2 scruples.
Ol. theobromae .... 1 dram.
M.
Div. in supposit. No. 12.

Concentrated Solution of Acetate of
1266. **Ammonia.**
Acid. acetic. .... 2 ounces.
Aquae fervent. .... 2 ounces.
Ammonii carbonat. ... q. s.
Ft. sol. neutral. Evaporate to two ounces. This keeps well.

1267. **Solution of Acetate of Ammonia.**
Liq. ammon. acet. conc. 1 ounce.
Aquae acidi carbonici . 15 ounces.
M.

HYPODERMIC SOLUTIONS.

1268. **Carbolized Distilled Water.**
Acidi carbolici .... 1 part.
Aquae destillatae ..... 909 parts.

1269. **Ext. Ergot Solution.**
Ext. ergot (Squibb's) . 1 part.
Aquae destil. carbol. . 5 parts.

1270. **Magendie's Sol. Morphia.**
Morphiae sulph. ...... 80 grains.
Aquae destil. carbol. . 5 fl. ounces.
M. and filter .

1271. **Lente's Solution of Quinia.**
Sulph. quiniae .... 80 grains.
Acid. sulph. dil. ...... q. s.
Aquae ...... ad 1 fl. ounce.
Heat to boiling and add
Acid. carbolic .... 5 grains.

1272. **Sol. Pilocarpia Muriate.**
Pilocarpiae mur. ..... 1 grains.
Aquae dest. carbol. ... 50 minims.
Dose: Ten minims.

1273. **Sol. Apomorphia Muriate.**
Apomorphiae muriat. cryst. 1 grain.
Aquae dest......... ... 80 minims.
Dose: Ten minims for emetic.
To be prepared only at the time it is wanted.

POWDERS.

The following powders are sent to the wards and dispensed in bulk, and measured out to the patient in a small measure equal to about 20 grains.

1274. **Pulvis S. I. C.**
Sodii bicarb. .... 600 parts.
Ipecac. .... 1 part.
Cubebae .... 300 parts.
M.
Dose: One measure.

1275. **Pulvis P. B. S.**
Pepsinae ....
Bismuth. subnitr. ....
Sodii bicarb. .... aa 100 parts.
Dose: One measure.

1276. **Pulvis B. I. C. S.**
Bismuth. subnitr. ..... 200 parts.
Ipecac. .... 3¼ parts.
Cubebae .... 200 parts.
Sodii bicarb. .... 400 parts.
M.
Dose: One measure.

PILLS.

1277. **Triplex Pills.**
Hydrarg. mass. ....
Pulv. aloes ....aa 2 grains.
Pulv. scammon. res. .. 1 grain.
M.
Ft. pil. No. 1.

1278. **Laxative Pills.**
Podophyll. res. .... 1/3 grain.
Ext. bellad. .... ¼ grain.
Ext. nuc. vom. .... 1/3 grain.
M.
Ft. pil. No. 1.

1279. **Compound Podophyllin Pills.**
Res. podophyll. ...... ½ grain.
Ext. nuc. vom. .... 1/3 grain.
Aloes purif. .... 1 grain.
Ol. anisi .... 1/6 drop.
M.
Ft. pil. No. 1.

1280. **Rhubarb and Soda Pills.**
Rhei. pulv. ....
Sodii bicarb. ...... aa 1½ grains.
Ipecac. .... 1/10 grain.
M.
Ft. pil. No. 1.

1281. **Carmalt's Pills.**
Res. podophylli. ...... ¼ grain.
Ext. nuc. vom. ....
Aloes purif. .... aa 1/6 grain.
Ext. hyoscyami .... ½ grain.
M.
Ft. pil. No. 1.

1282. **Fothergill's Pills.**
Morph. mur. .... 1/6 grain.
Atropiae sulph. .... 1/60 grain.
Pulv. capsici .... ½ grain.
Pil. aloes et myrrhae . 1½ grains.
M.
Ft. pil. No. 1.

1283. **Clark's Pills.**
Quiniae sulph. .... 3 1/3 grains.
Pulv. capsici .... 1 grain.
Pulv. opii .... 1/3 grain.
M.
Ft. pil. No. 1.

1284. **Pills of Lead and Opium.**
Plumbi acet. .... 2 grains.
Pulv. opii .... 1 grain.
M.
Ft. pil. No. 1.

1285. **Diuretic Pills.**
Pulv. scillae ....
Pulv. digitalis. ....
Massae hydrarg. ..... aa 2 grains.
M.
Ft. pil. No. 1.

1286. **Blaud's Pills.**
Ferri sulph. ....
Potass. carb. .... aa 2½ grains.
M.
Ft. pil. No. 1.

1287. **Pills of Aloes and Iron.**
Ferri sulph. exsic. .... ½ dram.
Pulv. aloes purif. .... 1 scruple.
Pulv. aromat. .... 1 dram.
Conf. rosae .... 1 scruple.
M.
Fiant pil. No. 40.

1288. **Antiperiodic Pills.**
Quin. sulph. .... 1 dram.
Pulv. capsici .... 15 grains.
Pulv. zingib. .... 30 grains.
M.
Div. in pil. No. 30.

Pills of Hydrarg., Colocynth, and
1289. **Ipecac.**
Ext. colocynth. co.....
Mass. hydrarg. ..... aa 10 grains.
Pulv. ipecac. .... 2 grains.
M.
Div. in pil. No. 4.

1290. **Pills of Nux Vomica, Compound.**
Ext. nucis vomicae .. 24 grains.
Pulv. rhei ....
Pulv. aloes .... aa 36 grains.
Podophylli resinae ... 8 grains.
M.
Ft. massa div. in pil. No. 48.

On the Preparation of Hydrobromic and
1291. **Hydriodic Acids.***

By J. H. Kastle and J. H. Bullock.

It is doubtful if any of the methods proposed for the preparation of these two acids have ever come into general use. That such is the case is shown by the fact that the whole treatment of the chemistry of these two acids is quite brief in even the better text-books and treatises on chemistry. And yet it is just by the aid of these compounds that the greatest knowledge can be gained concerning the chemistry of the halogen family, and it is through the study of these hydrogen compounds that we can make the most satisfactory comparison of chlorine, bromine and iodine. If, for example, it can actually be shown the student, in the case of hydrochloric and hydriodic acids, that both of these substances are heavy, colorless gases, which fume in the air, have powerful acid odors and dissolve in water with great readiness, forming strongly acid solutions, one of which remains unaltered under ordinary conditions—the other changing; and, further, that one of these compounds cannot

*Reprinted from Amer. Chem. Journ.

be decomposed by heat alone, whereas the other can with the greatest ease; that one is readily attacked by oxidizing agents, the other not—if these phenomena can actually be brought before the student, it is more than likely that he will have some clear conceptions as to the real resemblances and differences existing between chlorine and iodine. On the other hand, if he is shown a great deal about hydrochloric acid and little or nothing about the corresponding iodine compound, as is usually the case, he will probably quit the subject with no clear conceptions as to the nature of the latter compound, and in some instances he may even be troubled with doubts as to its existence. And, further, if attractive and brilliant experiments are possible at all they are possible with just such unstable compounds as these.

Realizing the importance of having the unstable halogen acids at their disposal, chemists have made quite a number of attempts to devise satisfactory methods for their preparation. Of the many methods which have been proposed for the preparation of hydrobromic acid two are certainly worthy of notice as yielding good results. One of these, described by Erdmann, consists in bringing bromine slowly into benzene containing a little ferrous bromide, and purifying the resulting hydrobromic acid gas by passing it through a tube containing ferric bromide and finally through one containing anthracene. The other method, that of Champion and Pellet, consists in leading bromine into paraffin heated to 185° C.

It is believed, however, that the method herein proposed for making hydrobromic acid is simpler and better than either of the above, for these reasons: First, the materials used are easy to obtain; second, no brominating agent is necessary, and third, the formation of the hydrobromic acid gas proceeds regularly, smoothly and rapidly without the aid of heat, and with little or no attention after the flow of bromine has once been regulated.

Of the methods proposed for the preparation of hydriodic acid, that involving the use of red phosphorus, iodine and water seems to have come into most general use. The objection to this method is that, unless great precautions are taken in the beginning, explosions are liable to occur. Hence, it is believed that the method here recommended for the preparation of this acid has advantages over the old method involving the use of red phosphorus, for the reason that no precautions whatever need be taken in preparing the acid rapidly by the process here described.

1292. Preparation of Hydrobromic Acid.

The method here proposed for the preparation of this acid takes advantage of the reaction between bromine and naphthalene. Any one who has ever had occasion to bring these two substances together has doubtless remarked the great ease with which they react upon each other. When brought together even at ordinary temperatures torrents of hydrobromic acid are evolved. Therefore it occurred to one of us (Kastle) that this reaction might be employed in the preparation of hydrobromic acid. Such, indeed, has proven to be the case, the mode of procedure being as follows: About 15 to 20 grams of naphthalene are dissolved in a small quantity of orthoxylene and the solution placed in a Florence flask of one-half to one liter capacity. The flask is connected, by means of a bent glass tube, with a double-neck Woulff's bottle, which is partially filled with a solution of concentrated hydrobromic acid,* holding a small quantity of red phosphorus in suspension, and in turn is connected with a U-tube containing red phosphorus and one or more drying tubes partly filled with phosphorus pentoxide. Attached to the farther end of the drying tubes is a tube for the delivery of the dry hydrobromic acid gas. The bromine is introduced into the solution of naphthalene in the flask by means of a tap-funnel, the end of which dips beneath the surface of the liquid. On allowing the bromine to flow slowly into the solution of the naphthalene action takes place at once and hydrobromic acid is rapidly evolved. By passing the gas through the concentrated aqueous hydrobromic acid containing red phosphorus in suspension it is deprived of any free bromine that may pass over along with it (which, by the way, is never present in any considerable quantity), so that, after passing through the U-tube containing dry red phosphorus and the drying tubes, it is obtained as a perfectly colorless gas. With this simple apparatus, and working with the quantities given in the above, the acid can be prepared quite as rapidly as hydrochloric acid can be prepared from sulphuric acid and salt, and with no more trouble or attention for the reason that, if the flow of bromine into the solution of the naphthalene be once properly regulated, the formation of the acid proceeds regularly and automatically. In order to obviate the use of xylene, which is

---

*The object in using a concentrated solution of hydrobromic acid is that this solution allows all of the hydrobromic acid gas to pass through, and, at the same time, dissolves and retains any free bromine better than water, thereby giving the red phosphorus a chance to combine with it.

not always easily obtained, some experiments were tried in which kerosene boiling above 150° C. was used as a solvent for the naphthalene. It was found to work just as satisfactorily as the purest orthoxylene. And, lastly, to put the method entirely within the reach of all lecturers upon chemistry, some experiments were tried with moth balls,* which were found to consist almost, if not entirely, of naphthalene, in the place of the pure naphthalene. This preparation, viz., the moth balls, was found to serve the purpose quite as well as the purest naphthalene, as will be seen from the following results:†

I.—50 grams of bromine, with 15 grams of naphthalene, dissolved in 50 cc. of orthoxylene, gave 21 grams of hydrobromic acid. Theory=26 grams of HBr.

II.—90 grams of bromine, with 15 grams of naphthalene, dissolved in 50 cc. xylene, gave 33 grams of hydrobromic acid. Theory=46 grams.

III.—105 grams of bromine, with 12.8 grams of naphthalene, dissolved in 20 grams of xylene, gave 40.5 grams of hydrobromic acid. Theory=53.5 grams HBr.

IV.—95 grams of bromine, with 12 grams of naphthalene (in form of moth balls) dissolved in a small quantity of kerosene, gave 47.5 grams of hydrobromic acid. Theory=48.5 grams HBr.

V.‡—95 grams of bromine, with 12 grams of naphthalene (in form of moth balls) dissolved in a small quantity of kerosene, gave 60.5 grams of hydrobromic acid. Theory = 48.5 grams of HBr.

In all there was obtained 202.5 grams of hydrobromic acid, the theory being 222.5 grams for the quantity of bromine used, a loss of only 9.1 per cent.

In addition to these experiments, which were conducted with the view of finding out the quantity of hydrobromic acid set free, the method has been tried upon the lecture table with entire success. The gas was collected, handled and experimented with with the greatest ease. The method is certainly to be recommended for lecture work and for the preparation of large quantities of the acid.

1293. Preparation of Hydriodic Acid.

The method here proposed for the preparation of this acid depends upon a reaction first observed by Etard and Moissan, viz., that when iodine and common resin (colophony) are heated together hydriodic acid is evolved. Not having access to the original papers of Etard and Moissan upon this subject, we are unable to judge from the abstract whether it was ever proposed to utilize the reaction in the preparation of the acid, or whether it was simply their object to call attention to it as being one of the reactions of which iodine is capable. Be this as it may, it is certain that this simple mode of preparation of hydriodic acid has escaped the notice of American chemists; at least it has never come into general use; and hence it cannot be amiss to call attention to it with such modifications as have been found advantageous.

When a mixture of iodine and common resin, in about equal parts by bulk, is heated, hydriodic acid, together with small quantities of iodine, are evolved. The mixture foams considerably, however, and a black, disagreeable liquid distills over. To obviate this and to render the hydriodic acid as pure as possible the following method was tried successfully:

Ten grams of finely divided iodine are mixed with an equal bulk of finely powdered resin and this mixture is then intimately mixed with a little more than an equal bulk of white sand. The mixture of iodine, resin and sand is then placed in a small glass retort, the neck of which, accurately fitted with a cork, is connected with one of the necks of a double-neck Woulff's bottle, and extends for some distance into the Woulff's bottle. The other neck of the Woulff's bottle is connected with a U-tube containing red phosphorus. This U-tube in turn is connected with a calcium chloride cylinder, which is filled with alternate layers of glass-wool and phosphorus pentoxide, the calcium chloride cylinder being connected with a tube for the delivery of the gas.

On gently heating the retort containing the mixture of iodine, resin and sand hydriodic acid gas is freely evolved, together with small quantities of iodine and the brownish liquid to which reference has already been made.

---

*As the name indicates, these moth balls are used for protecting clothing against moth. The preparations sold under that name in this part of the country has been found to consist almost, if not entirely, of naphthalene, and may be obtained at any drug store for 5 or 10 cents a pound.

†In the quantitative experiments the mixture of naphthalene and bromine was gently warmed toward the end of the reaction, in order to drive off any small quantities of hydrobromic acid which might remain dissolved in the bromnaphthalene.

‡That more than the theoretical quantity of hydrobromic acid was obtained in this experiment is accounted for by the fact that, during the operation, the wash bottle containing the concentrated hydrobromic acid got quite hot, so that hydrobromic acid distilled over into the vessel in which the acid was finally collected.

Both of the latter are condensed in the Wouiff's bottle, and if any iodine escapes condensation at this point it is held back by the red phosphorus in the U-tube through which the gases next pass. On passing through the cylinder containing the phosphorus pentoxide the hydriodic acid is dried completely, so that it may be collected in cylinders by displacement of air as a perfectly colorless gas. Without special precaution 5.4 grams of hydriodic acid were made from 10 grams of iodine by this method.

It should be said, further, that the method is a rapid one and in every way adapted to work on the lecture table. The apparatus once set up and the mixture put in the retort, one can easily collect, in a few minutes, a sufficient quantity of the dry gas to illustrate its remarkable and beautiful properties. For example, the apparatus having been set up, the gas was prepared and collected in quantities sufficient for the following experiments, and the experiments themselves performed all in about a quarter of an hour:

1.—Introduction of lighted taper into the gas.

2.—Action of dry chlorine on gaseous hydriodic acid to show formation, first of iodine and then of iodine trichloride.

3.—Decomposition of the gas into its elements by passing it through a heated tube.

4.—Oxidation of the gas by fumes of nitric acid.

5.—Absorption of the gas by water, and preparations of aqueous hydriodic acid.

In view of these results there can be no doubt as to the efficiency of this method of preparing hydriodic acid.

In conclusion it may be said that both of the methods above described for these two acids are highly satisfactory. The materials used are such as are easily accessible to all. There are no explosions attending the formation of these acids, nor is there any troublesome phosphonium bromide or iodide produced to clog up the apparatus, as is the case with the methods involving the use of phosphorus. The methods are rapid and practically free from the objections which may be urged against the other methods which have previously been proposed for the preparation of these two acids.

1294. How to Calculate Equivalent Weights.

(From the Druggists Circular.)

The atom of hydrogen is the unit of the atomic system of weights; when we say that the atomic weight of oxygen is 16, we mean that its atom or smallest conceivable particle weighs sixteen times as much as the equal sized atom of hydrogen. But as we cannot fix a precise size for the atoms, we cannot state their absolute weight; we cannot reckon them in grains or fractions of grains. But this causes no difficulty in arriving at practical results. The proportions of all the atoms which go to form a given molecule remaining constant, the theoretical unit of weight may be translated into any practical unit desired. If we consider the hydrogen atom to weigh 1 grain, the oxygen atom will weigh 16 grains, and consequently the molecule of water containing two hydrogen atoms and one oxygen will weigh 18 grains. Grams may, of course, be substituted for grains with the same results, and so may any other unit from ounce to ton. The officinal phosphate of sodium, the proportion of phosphorus in which forms the subject of one of our correspondent's questions, consists of a molecule weighing 358; that is, its weight is 358 times that of an atom of hydrogen. This molecule contains one atom of phosphorus, the weight of which is 31. Now, if we translate our weights into grams, we can make the definite statement that 358 grams of sodium phosphate contain 31 grams of phosphorus. This being established, we can easily calculate by simple proportion (or "rule of three") the amount of phosphorus in any given quantity of the phosphate. If, for instance, we wish to know the amount of phosphorus in 800 grams we would state it thus: As 358 (the weight of the molecule) is to 31 (the weight of the phosphorus atom), so is 800 to the figures sought:

$$358 : 31 :: 800 : 69.273.$$

The gram being taken as the unit the answer is, of course, in grams.

Our correspondent's second question, although apparently different, amounts to exactly the same thing. To ascertain the quantity of a given element or compound required to form a certain weight of a new compound into which it is to enter, the problem must be stated in the same way, only being careful to note whether in the case of complex reactions any portion of the original atoms escape as gases or otherwise.

1295. Granular Effervescing Preparations. (Ch. & Dr.)

The demand for granular effervescent preparations by prescription is largely on the increase. We may have a demand for 2 grains to dram hydrobromate of caffeine one hour, and later 5 grains, or possibly a combination with bromide of sodium. Consequently, we must be prepared at short notice to dispense, if possible, variously medicated effervescent granules. In making them citric acid is a necessary constituent, the water of crystallization being required to give a coherent mass that can be granulated by pressing through a sieve. As the medication varies so must the relative amount of citric and tartaric acids to suit the medicament; thus a hydrous or deliquescent substance requires less of the former and more of the latter. The U. S. P. uses alcohol for damping the ingredients of a caffeine preparation and omits citric acid. The heat applied should not exceed 100° C., otherwise the granules are colored and carbonic acid is driven off. But a strong heat obviates the use of the B. P. proportion of citric acid, and examination of trade-samples shows that this fact is known and acted upon by manufacturers.

As to neutrality, theoretically and practically the granules are generally slightly acid. In some cases it is necessary to make an exactly neutral granule if the therapeutic action is to be maintained. For example, piperazine only acts in alkaline solution, and it requires care to compound, as it must not be allowed to combine with the acid; so the proper way of making it is to thoroughly mix the piperazine with the bicarbonate, and any pre-decomposition in the granule takes place between the acids and the soda, for which they have greater affinity. Pharmaceutically, the order of mixing has also a great deal to do with the product. Piperazine is invariably granulated without heat at all, the formula being adjusted to yield a coherent mass when simply mixed in the proper order.

The effervescent citro-tartrate of sodium affords a basis suitable generally for medication where the quantity of medicament is small—such as citrate of caffeine 2 grains to 1 dram; antipyrin 5 grains; iron carbonate 5 grains; iron and arsenic, iron and quinine, and so on. Another type is the sulphate and phosphate of sodium, and the sulphate of magnesium granules where the medicament forms 50 per cent, although ultimately, when dried, actually about 25 per cent of the two former and 40 per cent of latter. These are naturally much less effervescent than the former type, although the sugar is entirely left out of sodium salt preparations for this and physiological reasons. In the magnesium preparation the granule is overburdened with medicament and sugar, leaving only 50 per cent of available effervescing material.

There is a demand for granules medicated with insoluble substances, such as euonymin, phenacetin, sulphonal, salicin, quinine salicylate, and bismuth salts. These are neither elegant nor palatable, and in all cases should be pointed out to prescribers as unsuitable modes of exhibition, excepting, perhaps, the bismuth salts, where the nascent carbonic acid would increase the effect. Liquids, the active principles of which are not dissipated on heating, may be mixed with the sugar or the bicarbonate, and dried before incorporation with the acids. Such potent remedies as strychnine and arsenic can only be diffused evenly by adding them in solution to the sugar or bicarbonate, and drying at a low temperature before mixing with acids. In addition to two pharmacopoeial granules without sugar, there are others of that nature in frequent demand, sugar being contra-indicated. Such prepartions are not so uniform unless sifted and made with a fine sieve, because the binding power of the sugar is absent, but they give a brisker effervescence.

As to the size of granules, the author uses No. 12 and No. 6 sieves, and finds the former most suitable for granules with a large percentage of medicament or sugar. The small granules produced by it are more quickly decomposed in water, but more prone to caking in the bottle unless dried until pulverulent. It is a mistake to sacrifice to uniformity or size either the effervescence or color of the granules. Consequently, for all practical purposes, and so that they may keep under varied conditions, a No. 6 or No. 9 is the most suitable sieve.

1296.   **Granular Effervescents.**

Referring to the B. P. method, as exhibited in sodii phos. eff., the author said that the heat of a water-bath is best. The granulation may be done admirably with a fork having three or four prongs so bent as to be from 3/16 inch to ¼ inch apart. In effervescent salts there are two essentials—base and active principle. After many experiments the author had found the following the best base:

Bicarbonate of soda............ 17 parts.
Citric acid. .... 6 parts.
Tartaric acid. .... 6 parts.
White sugar .... 9 parts.

The finished preparation is slightly acid, which is an advantage. The active ingredient is mixed with the base in the proportion required. The method of granulation which Mr. Clarke favored is as follows:

Place an enamelled basin with an oval bottom over a water-bath, and when quite hot and dry add, say, ½ pound of the ready-mixed powder. Allow to remain about a quarter of a minute (longer or shorter, according to temperature), when the powder begins to "cake." Now take the fork, and so manipulate it as to make the whole of the salt pass through its prongs. Remove from the source of heat and continue trituration, gradually diminishing the pressure until the granules become cold and brittle. The size of the granules depends greatly upon the rate of trituration, therefore too much energy is to be avoided.

The drying, he explained, is best done by the sun. The mixture loses 1/19 of its weight by granulation.

1297. Caffeine Citrate Effervescens.
Citrated caffeine .... 4 parts.
Bicarbonate of sodium .... 46 parts.
Tartaric acid .... 24 parts.
Citric acid .... 16 parts.
Refined sugar .... 10 parts.
                         100 parts.
All in powder.

This preparation contains rather over 4 per cent of citrated caffeine. The dose is 1 dram.

1298.
Mag. cit. gran. the quantity of magnesium sulphate should not exceed ½ ounce to the pound. The following is a good formula:
Bicarbonate of soda .... 17 ounces.
Tartaric acid. .... 13 ounces.
Citric acid .... 2 ounces.
Sulph. of magnesium (dried) 1 ounce.
Sugar .... 1½ pounds.

1299.
Granular citrate of magnesia is prepared on the large scale by heating the ingredients in shallow steam-pans, and passing the pasty mass through sieves with large meshes. Citric and tartaric acids must be used.

1300. Lemon Kali.
Pulv. sacch. alb. .... 2 pounds.
Pulv. acid. tart. .... 1 pound.
Sodae bicarb. .... 1 pound.
Ol. limonis. .... 2 drams.
Mix and sift twice.

1301. Summer Saline.
Sodae bicarb. .... 2 ounces.
Ac. tartarici .... 1½ ounces.
Pot. acid. tart. .... 1½ ounces.
Sodae sulph. exsic. .... 1 ounce.
Sacch. alb. .... 6 ounces.
Mix, and pass through a fine sieve.

1302. Cheltenham Salts.
Glauber salts, Epsom salts, common salt, equal parts, powder.
Mix.
Dose: One-half ounce.

1303. Saline.
(The popular form for Eno substitute.)
Pulv. acid. tartaric. .... 2 ounces.
Sodae bicarb. .... 2 ounces.
Mag. sulph. .... 1 ounce.
Pulv. pot. bitart. .... 2 ounces.
Mag. cit. efferves. .... 2 ounces.
Pulv. sacch. alb. .... 4 ounces.
M.

1304. Effervescing Cheltenham Salts.
Tartaric acid, dried .... 25 parts.
Tartrate of iron .... 1 part.
Seidlitz salt .... 120 parts.
Mix.
Dose: A teaspoonful in a glass of water.

1305. Hydrobromate of Caffeine Granular.
Soda bicarbonate. .... 16 ounces.
Tartaric acid. .... 15 ounces.
Bromide of potash, powdered. .... 4 ounces.
Caffeine. .... 4 drams.
Sugar, powdered. .... 6 ounces.

Mix well and sift through a fine sieve; dampen a portion of the mixture at a time with strong alcohol. Make into a compact ball and force through a sieve of proper mesh to make granules of the size desired, dropping them on trays lined with paper; dry very carefully by the heat of the sun or moderate artificial heat, and fill into wide mouth bottles, taking care that the bottles are absolutely dry. Cork tightly to exclude the air. Other granular effervescent preparations may be made in the same manner by substituting in the formula in proper proportions any other active ingredient desired.

Should granulation by means of heat of the water bath be preferred (see foregoing remarks) replace one-third of the tartaric acid, with powdered citric acid.

1306. Pyro Caffeine Compound.
Soda bicarbonate. .... 16 ounces.
Tartaric acid. .... 15 ounces.
Bromide of potash, powdered. .... 4 ounces.
Caffeine. .... 4 drams.
Acetanilid, powdered. ..... 1 ounce.
Celery seed, powdered. ... 2 ounces.
Alcohol. .... 6 ounces.

Macerate the celery seed for three days in the alcohol, and percolate.

Mix the other powders thoroughly and sift well; dampen with the percolate and granulate. See remarks on granulation after the formula for hydrobromate of caffeine.

1307. On the Preparation of Compressed Tablets.*

There is one form in which medicine is very frequently used at the present time, that gives the retail druggist ample opportunity to show his individual skill and meet the many demands of his customers without resorting to the products of others; I mean compressed tablets.

The enterprising manufacturers not only will furnish them direct to the physician, but will solicit orders also from the druggist. No pent-up Utica is theirs, the whole boundless domain of physics is embraced in their all-absorbing love. Nor will the doctor, prone to the easy paths in the practice of medicine, stop his ears to the seductive arguments of the traveling salesman. The manufacturer sees the opening for trade, the retail druggist tries to ignore it. But it is useless; the doctors want compressed goods, and if they cannot get them from the retail druggist first-handed they will get them where they can. It is useless to say that they are not used, or that they cannot be made by the retail druggist. They are used and the retail druggist can furnish them in a better condition for administration than is often done by the manufacturer. The druggist can fill a doctor's own prescription, leaving the doctor no excuse for using that of others. He can make them hard or pliable, to suit the wants of the physician. By this means, the patient, the doctor and the druggist are brought nearer together, between whom there should be mutual confidence. It is urged by many druggists that they can buy tablets at a lower price than they can make them. This is not so for goods of the best quality; further, there are some compressed goods which are popular as domestic remedies, which change in appearance by keeping long, if made properly. For instance, soda mint tablets, such as usually put on the market, if they have the full amount of oil in them and ammonia they will turn yellow; if they have not they are of but little use, and the buyer is disappointed or cheated. A druggist could make up a small quantity at a time and have them fresh; customers always want things fresh.

Soda mint is very easily made. Mix 1 pound of soda, gum arabic 1 ounce, oil of peppermint 3 drams; and carbonate of ammonia 1 dram; dampen with alcohol and water, run through a No. XX sieve and dry. Make into 5-grain tablets, and sell them to your customers as the best in the market; for they are of your own make. These will be what they profess to be, and your patrons will soon find it out.

If you understand the principles of pharmacy, you can soon learn how to make compressed tablets, and, learning how, you will become better druggists. Of course, as graduates, you know the chemical relation of drugs, how and when chemical reactions take place; this will serve a good purpose here. For some time past there have been used many tablets of calomel and bicarbonate of soda. Your chemistry will tell you if these salts be mixed wet, and granulated, decomposition will take place, and the question would be, how to avoid it? You might do so in several ways; but I will mention only one. Take bicarbonate of soda 10½ drams, gum arabic ½ dram, mix and dampen with water, run through a No. 40 sieve, dry and put into a bottle; add calomel 1½ drams, and shake this until every granule is coated. The calomel will adhere to the small particles of soda hardened with the gum; this will obviate any necessity of talc. The object is to prevent the soda and calomel coming together in a damp condition. Make up into 1-grain tablets, each of which will contain 1-12 of a grain of calomel. This illustrates pretty well how chemical incompatibles may be put together in a compressed form and still retain their individuality, and, still better, how in some cases a dangerous result may be avoided from mixing together articles innocent in themselves; but deleterious as factors in a product. The soda hardened with the gum is scarcely in the least hygroscopic, and the tablets made with it, in the manner stated, will keep without change fully as long as a druggist who has them for sale desires. The calomel being put in last answers the purpose of its indications as a medicine, and at the same time as a protection against adhesion to the dies and punches. In all these combinations a certain amount of brains is a sine qua non, and may be written on the formula Quantum sufficit. Here as elsewhere the dictum of the teacher cannot give individual skill, nor can the dreams of theory take the place of applied knowledge.

At the start remember, and never let it be forgotten, that facts established cannot be changed, and it is with facts you have to deal. The metal of which the dies and punches are made is a fixed unalterable fact. You may change the form, the peculiar construction of the punches or die, but so long as the face of them presents a smooth surface to the material to be compressed, it is always the same. Remembering this, you will not ascribe the fault to the die or punch if your material adheres to them. The punch should be perfectly smooth and have sharp edges,

---

*Read by J. A. McFerran, M. D., at a pharmaceutical meeting Philadelphia College of Pharmacy. From Am. Jr. Ph.

and move freely in the dies. They should be made of tool steel and tempered just hard enough to prevent bending under pressure—beyond this you should expect nothing, and if the material adheres to them, you must look to the material as the thing at fault. As a rule you should cause the cohesive property of the material to be greater than the adhesive, and when, by experiment, you find where the fault is, all that you have to do is to apply your knowledge of the nature of the different excipients to correct it. There are some materials that are neither cohesive nor adhesive: for instance, if an ounce of pulverized charcoal were ordered to be made into 40 lozenges, you would have no trouble in their sticking to the dies and punches, but you would have a great deal in getting any cohesion between the different particles of the material. The question here would be to add something that would cause a cohesion greater than adhesion, and, at the same time, not destroy the effect of the charcoal as a remedy. Here dextrin, wax, gelatin, gum arabic and tragacanth, mastich, etc., present themselves, as the different particles of the charcoal must actually be glued together.

If you were ordered to make 480 grains of salicylate of soda into 96 tablets, you might add some pulverized acacia, dampen with alcohol and water, run through a No. 30 sieve and dry. Just before using stir in some talc to prevent sticking. There are other ways without the use of talc, but it is better to learn this way first.

The coal oil products will claim your attention very often. Most of them are not soluble in water, and when pressed alone may prove useless on account of their insolubility. A small quantity of starch added to the mixture may often become of great service. Say you take salol, phenacetin, starch; dampen with alcohol, run through a No. 20 sieve, shake over a gas jet to slightly warm to granulate and dry; a moderate heat assists in granulating. There is no need of anything to prevent sticking.

There is a point that it is well to remember; any liquid that is not a solvent to any of the ingredients in the compound will act as a protection against adhesion to the dies. In the manufacture of refined naphthalin into tablets, the material will stick to the dies if something is not used to prevent. As naphthalin is not soluble in water, water should be used to dampen, and this is effectual against adhesion.

In making tablet triturates you will find sugar of milk alone makes the tablets too brittle: to correct this add about one part in 8 of cane sugar as the base, dampen with alcohol, and make up damp, unless they contain extracts; in that case you would have to make up dry and use the talc to prevent sticking. The talc should always be stirred in after the material has been granulated and dried. When talc is objectionable, white cosmoline or albolin can be used pretty freely, if you have a machine that will feed a damp and sluggish material. By putting the tablets into some absorbent powder after they are made and apply heat, most of it will disappear.

Learn the nature of each article that you wish to compress and take advantage of your knowledge of the solubility in different menstrua, and when the contrary nature of the different articles in a combination precludes the use of this knowledge, fall upon such correctives as experience and your own thoughts suggest to meet the particular case. In making up compounds, reduce all to a fine powder as far as practicable; in this way you will make more regular granulations and finer looking tablets. Take the familiar brown mixture; gum and licorice, each 2 pounds.; opium, 219 grains.; benzoic acid, 219 grains; camphor, 140 grains; oil of anise, 219 grains; tartar emetic, 110 grains; nitrate of potash, 1,750 grains; sugar sufficient for 10 pounds. If these be thoroughly mixed and ground to a fine powder, put into a wide receiver, and hang a wet sponge to the under side of the lid; the material will absorb enough moisture to dampen during one night; next morning run through a No. 30 sieve and dry; on account of the extracts and the sugar you cannot do without talc or lycopodium to prevent sticking. If you prefer, you can use diluted alcohol and dampen with a hand atomizer.

In filling prescriptions of small quantities there is often no need of elaborate work in granulating; sometimes when not incompatible powdered soap rubbed up with the articles ordered prepares them to be run through a sieve; simply dampening with ether puts a powder into a granular condition. And when running out a pound might require something to prevent sticking, 10 to 20 tablets would require nothing. Wetting with alcohol and drying will almost always leave the mass grainy. It does not matter how fine your material is, all you want is that it will tumble and not hold together on account of the moisture in it. I might talk for a week about material; but I wish to say something about how to make the tablets.

In the first place do not get the fidgets, see that everything is in place and that your machine is clean. Choose the set of dies required; and in this machine designed especially for druggists you will find by lifting a small shaft and removing a pin you can take off the feeder. Turning a few turns on this thumb screw you can pull out the die holder; while this is out you can see if the internal part of the machine is clean. The die holder being out, put in a top punch the size you wish, put the die into the die holder, insert the bottom punch, put in the die holder with its containing die and punch, fasten into place by turning thumb-screw slip on the feeder, drop the small vertical shaft into place and you are ready for work. Weigh out the quantity for one tablet, pour it into the die and screw up the bottom punch until the material comes even with the plate. Turn on the pressure and when the top punch is at its lowest depth, turn the knob at the top of the eccentric strap until you feel the pressure. Make two or three tablets to see whether the weight is all right, then put on more pressure if necessary and finish your work. The first tablets should not be pressed much; when you are sure of your weight you can powder the trial ones between your fingers and return to the feeder. The small cup should be used in making up small quantities. Put it in by taking off the top of the feeder and simply putting the cup into its place; the motion of the feeder in going backward and forward will cause the material to drop into the die; the remnant of one or two tablets can be brushed into the die and there is no need of wasting any material at all. The feeder is so constructed that there can be no leakage from beneath the feed. The lower punch is so constructed that there is the least amount of friction possible. One great fault in making tablets is in using too much pressure, running at the rate of 60 per minute, the pressure should scarcely be felt on small tablets; but by taking a tablet between the fingers a little experience will tell you whether to put on or take off pressure which is easily done by simply turning the knob to the right or left. In making tablets whenever you hear a rubbing sound when the tablet is ejected you may know that the material needs correcting. As the feeder is so easily taken off you can remove it with its contents without wasting a particle, correct the material by adding talc, or what else is needed; put it back and proceed. Do not undertake to make tablets too fast; a regular easy motion is the best, and you will accomplish more than by trying to do a great deal in a short time. I am sure this machine will do all that is required by a retail druggist, as well as it is possible for a machine to do it. It is strong, it takes up but little room, is easily kept clean and is so simple that any one can understand it and run it. You can make quinine tablets, hypodermic tablets and such things as you wish to avoid excipients in; besides, by the construction of the feeder you can make up the flat friable triturates faster and more regular than on plates, and that too without the use of talc or other insoluble excipients. The how to make those things does not properly belong to my short talk on tablets; any one wishing to learn can do so on a proper occasion.

Here are quinine tablets made without gum, oil, starch, or talc and other tablets of different sizes and shapes, made on a machine similar to this, which should be evidence conclusive that a retail druggist can make his own tablets and furnish physicians who desire to think for themselves, any tablet that they wish.

1308. Preparation of Compressed Tablets.* B

The tablet machine should be kept scrupulously clean, and the surface of the dies and punches smooth and polished. Before commencing operations two or three tablets should be made from weighed quantities of material, to enable the operator to adjust the pressure and size for the work in hand. Excessive pressure should be carefully guarded against,† and a regular, easy motion of the machine aimed at. The soluble substances therefore should be compressed as lightly as possible. Unduly light pressure, on the other hand, is accompanied by a greater tendency for the material to stick to the face of the punches. Coblentz states that the pressure should be regulated so that the tablets may readily be broken in half by the fingers, but should not break to pieces when dropped upon the floor. "Capping," i. e., the splitting off of the surface of the tablet, may be remedied by slightly dampening the granulated material with water, reducing the pressure, or by changing the weight of the tablet.

The three main points in tablet making are, (a) to regulate carefully the pressure, (b) to insure proper cohesion of the particles of substance under compression, and (c) to prevent adhesion of those particles to any part of the machine. The skillful dispenser, with his knowledge of what is best to use in any given case as a pill excipient, will not experience any difficulty in deciding whether gum

*Reprinted from Pharmaceutical Journal.

†A case recently occurred in a Northern town which forcibly illustrated the mischief that may result from compressing insoluble substances too much. The patient, acting under medical instructions, had been taking compressed tables of salol for some length of time; prepared by a wholesale firm. Later, an operation for intestinal obstruction became necessary, and the surgeon was astonished to find the whole of the tablets unaltered in the intestine.

arabic or tragacanth, syrup, dextrin, wax, mastic, or other adhesive agents should be employed. And he will also be fully aware that to prevent adhesion to the dies, etc., some liquid must be used which is not a solvent of the substance undergoing compression. The rapid disintegration and solution of tablets is facilitated by adding finely powdered starch, from 1/20th to 1/10th the weight of material, to the granulated substance ready to be compressed. On the other hand, glucose, which should be diluted with 25 per cent. of water before use, renders tablets hard and tough, so that they will not readily disintegrate. This is frequently an advantage when it is desired that the tablets should dissolve slowly in the mouth. To prevent adhesion to the die a little powdered French chalk may be sifted into the material just before compression. White paraffinum molle (2 per cent. dissolved in sufficient ether) often facilitates the compression of a dry powder, and improves the appearance of the finished tablets, if diffused through the granulated material, the latter being subsequently sifted and dried before compression.

1309. Preparation of the Material.

Experience proves that it is not desirable to have the substances to be compressed in a very fine state of subdivision, as a fine powder cannot be satisfactorily compressed into uniform and well-finished tablets. The granular product obtained by grinding hard crystals represents the condition that should be aimed at, powdered ammonium chloride and potassium chlorate, as supplied in commerce, being good examples of what is required. In many cases, however, it will be found necessary to reduce the substance to fine powder first, and granulate afterward. In dispensing small quantities the material may be obtained in the desired condition by simply damping with ether or alcohol by means of an atomizer, or by rubbing up with a little powdered soap, and afterward passing through a sieve.

With larger quantities of material, cane sugar and powdered gum are chiefly used, the former being preferable, as tablets prepared with it disintegrate more rapidly. Coblentz (Handbook of Pharmacy) recommends the addition to the substance to be granulated of 1/10th of its weight of cane sugar and 1/20th of its weight of gum. On the large scale white dextrin may often replace the gum. After thoroughly mixing, sufficient water should be added to render the powder of such consistence that it can readily be shaken through a No. 12 sieve without sticking to it or clogging the openings. Care should be taken to add the water in small quantities at a time, and to mix thoroughly after each addition. The powder is next passed through a No. 20 sieve and dried, after which a lubricant is added to enable the particles of powder to move freely over each other and prevent them sticking to the die and punches.

Finely powdered French chalk, lycopodium, powdered boric acid or an odorless hydrocarbon oil may be employed for this purpose. The better the granulated material has been dried the smaller the quantity of lubricant required. Coblentz says 10 to 12 drops of hydrocarbon oil, added by means of a spray, is usually sufficient for each pound, with French chalk, not exceeding one-fourth the weight of material, added after the oil. If, however, the tablets are to be dissolved boric acid should be used as the lubricant, clear solutions being thus obtainable. In many cases, of course, this latter addition would be undesirable, as in the case of mercuric chloride, in which chemical action would take place. When the lubricant added is a powder, it should be scattered over the material spread out on paper, and the whole slightly shaken up in a bottle. By this means the granules are not broken down, and they become coated very thinly with the lubricating powder. It is above all things necessary that the operator should be familiar with the nature of the substance or mixture to be compressed, as this must to a great extent guide him in selecting a suitable granulating medium and lubricant. As McFerran pertinently observes (see Phar. Jour. (3), XXIII., 974), "learn the nature of each article that you wish to compress, and take advantage of your knowledge of the solubility in different menstrua, and when the contrary nature of the different articles in a combination precludes the use of this knowledge, fall back upon such correctives as experience and your own thoughts suggest to meet the particular case." Tablet making is an art which requires not only carefully detailed instructions, but considerable experience and knowledge of the capabilities of the particular machine used.

Manipulation in Special Cases.[*]
1310.

AMMONIUM CHLORIDE, in a slightly moist and finely granulated condition, can be compressed into tablets without any preparation.

---

[*] For convenience of reference details are here given of a number of special cases considered by Coblentz (Handbook of Pharmacy), McFerran (Pharm. Jour. (3), xxiii., 972) and Remington (Practice of Pharmacy), whose writings may be consulted for further particulars. Though sieves with meshes of various sizes are mentioned, a No. 30 sieve will usually prove fine enough in almost every case.

1311.

CALOMEL WITH SODIUM BICARBONATE requires special treatment. Sodium bicarbonate, 630 grains, and gum arabic, 30 grains, are mixed and damped with water, then passed through a No. 40 sieve, dried and bottled. Calomel, 90 grains, is added in the bottle, and the latter shaken until all the granules are coated. Finally compress into tablets (McFerran).

1312.

CHARCOAL and similar spongy bodies must be in impalpable powder, and should be granulated by the addition of at least 25 per cent. of cane sugar. They require no lubricant, as a rule, and should be fed to the machine in very fine granular form. The granules should be passed through a No. 12 sieve, dried and then reduced until they will pass through a No. 60 to 80 sieve. A solution of gelatin may be employed instead of sugar, in which case a little French chalk should be added afterwards.

1313.

EFFERVESCING MIXTURES should have their constituents granulated separately and mixed in a perfectly dry granular condition just before being compressed.

1314.

EXTRACTS require varying treatment, according to their condition. Powdered extracts should be mixed with starch powder before treating by the foregoing general process of Coblentz. Solid extracts should be rubbed to a syrupy consistence by the aid of a little water; the excess of water is then absorbed by the addition of about 25 per cent. of starch powder, the mixture being left sufficiently moist to form a proper consistence or granulation. Fluid extracts should be evaporated to a syrupy consistence and then treated in the same manner as solid extracts.

1315.

HYGROSCOPIC OR DELIQUESCENT BODIES will need the addition of gum in the proportion of one-tenth the weight of substance, water being used for moistening.

1316.

HYPODERMIC TABLETS may be made with sugar of milk as a basis, but dried neutral sodium sulphate and purified sodium chloride or ammonium chloride are frequently preferable.

1317.

INSOLUBLE SUBSTANCES, such as acetanilid, phenacetin, sulphonal, etc., are best granulated with one-tenth their weight of cane sugar, water being used for moistening.

1318.

PEPSIN in powder should be prepared by adding to it one-tenth its weight of cane sugar, then spraying with diluted alcohol (50 per cent.) and mixing to insure moistening of all the particles. The powder should then be capable of passing through a No. 80 sieve, and, after drying, is ready for compression. Scale pepsin requires only to be reduced to No. 80 or 40 powder and then lubricated.

1319.

POTASSIUM BROMIDE AND IODIDE simply require crushing, and should then be treated in the same way as ammonium chloride.

1320.

POTASSIUM CHLORATE should be used in the same condition as ammonium chloride, and is very readily compressed.

1321.

QUININE SULPHATE requires similar treatment to charcoal, but if, instead of French chalk, a little finely powdered arrow-root or ethereal solution of white pariffinum molle be added, the tablets will disintegrate more readily.

1322.

RHUBARB AND SODA, in combination, require one-tenth their weight of cane sugar, and should be granulated by means of a mixture of liquid glucose, 1 volume; water and alcohol, 3 volumes.

1323.

SALICYLIC ACID should be treated like charcoal, quinine sulphate and substances of similar nature.

1324.

SALOL AND PHENACETIN can be made into tablets by adding starch, moistening the mixture with alcohol, passing through a No. 20 sieve, then slightly warming, granulating and drying prior to compression.

1325.

SALTS containing water of crystallization should be reduced to fine powder, then mixed with one-twentieth their weight of powdered gum arabic, moistened and passed through a No. 12 sieve. The granules must then be dried and again powdered, mixed with one-tenth their weight of cane sugar, and moistened with just enough water to pass again through a No. 12 sieve. After drying, first spontaneously but finally by the aid of heat, pass the mixture through a No. 20 sieve, lubricate and compress.

1326.

SCALE PREPARATIONS generally require the same treatment as scale pepsin, which see.

1327.

SODA-MINT tablets are prepared by mixing sodium bicarbonate, 1 pound; gum arabic, 1 ounce; oil of peppermint, 180 grains; ammonium carbonate, 60 grains; damp with alcohol and water, pass through a No. 20 sieve and dry (McFerran).

1328.

SODIUM BICARBONATE requires the addition of 5 per cent. of acacia, then moisten with water, sift and dry.

1329.

SODIUM SALICYLATE should be mixed with powdered gum, moistened with alcohol and water, passed through a No. 20 sieve and dried.

1330.

SUGAR OF MILK, when used as a vehicle for powders to be compressed into tablets, should be moistened with a mixture of 1 part of syrup and 2 parts of water.

1331. The Manufacture of Compressed Tablets.

(Western Druggist.)

BY F. R. LEDER.

Notwithstanding the howl that is being raised in certain quarters against tablet-triturates and compressed tablets these goods seem to be daily increasing in popularity. Although these goods are ever increasing in demand, it is a fact that but few pharmacists prepare their own tablets but depend entirely upon the manufacturers or wholesalers for their supplies. Why is this so? Is the manufacture of these goods so difficult as to deter the pharmacist from making them? This seems to be the idea entertained by many, but it is far from being correct.

With the proper appliances and a little practice and experience there is no reason why any intelligent pharmacist should not be able to produce either tablet-triturates or compressed tablets the equals of those of the large manufacturers. Edward Squibb has been quoted as saying that in preparing large quantities of compressed tablets, the heavier particles settle to the bottom and that often an assay of the finished tablets will show that the different ingredients are not equally distributed throughout the tablets. If this is the case, is it not a strong argument in favor of the pharmacist preparing his own compressed tablets? If he do so, he is not compelled to crowd his shelves with compressed goods of the large manufacturers, but can prepare them as wanted in quantities to suit the demand, thus dispensing freshly-made goods and being absolutely sure as to their composition.

It is not my purpose to consider tablet-triturates in this paper, but to confine myself entirely to the consideration of compressed tablets, and to enter into the detail of their manufacture as fully as is possible in a paper of this kind.

Some drugs compress readily without any special treatment, while others, being unadhesive, must be especially treated before they can be successfully compressed. It has been found that fine powders do not work satisfactorily in making compressed tablets, as a fine powder does not feed evenly and does not compress regularly. The powder is granulated by adding the proper adhesive and moistener, then passing through a sieve and drying. In the selection of the proper adhesive the pharmacist must use his judgment and strive to leave the finished tablet as soluble as possible. Among the articles used as adhesives, sugar, starch and acacia are most prominent, but glucose and dextrin also are sometimes used. Sugar, if it gives the necessary adhesiveness, is to be preferred to acacia, because the tablets made with it are more soluble. Sometimes it is necessary to use both sugar and acacia in order to make a powder sufficiently adhesive. In this case five per cent. of acacia and ten per cent. of sugar is the proportion generally recommended. Acacia should be used in all combinations of a hygroscopic nature. Glucose is used only where it is desired to make a hard tablet for slow solution in the mouth. Starch is recommended in tablets containing considerable quantities of fluid extracts or tinctures. As remarked above, it should be the aim to make tablets as soluble as possible, and this is best accomplished by granulating the powder with a considerable quantity of some soluble substance, such as starch or sugar.

It only stands to reason that substances which are considered insoluble in powder form, are much more so when compressed, unless mixed with some soluble substance which, dissolving out, brings about the disintegration of the tablet.

1332. Materials.

Every part of the material that is desired to be compressed should be reduced to a very fine powder, then mixed thoroughly and the proper amount of adhesive added and mixed with the powder, the whole then moistened and passed through a sieve and dried. The moistening must be carefully done and must not be carried far enough to make the mixture stick to the sieve in passing through. Water, if carefully used, is the most generally useful moistener, although in some cases 70 per cent alcohol is recommended. I have in my own experience found a No. 20 tinned iron sieve to answer nicely. The granulated powder should be thoroughly dry before attempting to compress, for if not so, it sticks to the dies, and even when thoroughly dried, this is often a source of much annoyance. In order to overcome this tendency to adhere to the dies, it is customary to add some substance, such as talcum or white petrolatum, or, in case of hypodermic tablets, powdered C. P. boric acid, in small proportions. The more carefully the powder is prepared the less lubrication it will need, and only as much should be used as is absolutely necessary. White petrolatum is best used as a two per cent. ethereal solution with an atomizer. The use of liquid petrolatum is not to be recommended, except in case the ether might have some solvent action that would be undesirable for the reason that a slight excess, which it is difficult to guard against, makes the tablets adhere. The petrolatum, however, solidifies as soon as the ether evaporates and is much to be preferred. The dry granulated powder is sprayed with this solution and stirred with a spatula, or mixed on paper, then allowed to become dry, and then passed through the sieve. Both petrolatum and talcum are sometimes necessary. The talcum should be added to the powder after the petrolatum, and not until the powder has become dry. It is generally stirred in with a spatula or mixed in a wide-mouth bottle by gentle agitation. Not to exceed three per cent. of the weight of the powder to be compressed should be used. Boric acid is used, but not to exceed one and one-half or two per cent.

In making tablets as much pressure only should be used as is absolutely necessary. The molds should be kept absolutely clean and highly polished. It is impossible to make a smooth tablet with a rough die. Use no hard substance in removing adhering portions of tablets, for fear of scratching the dies. Some substances already in granular form compress readily without any preparation. Among these are granulated bromide of potash, iodide of potash, muriate of ammonia, chlorate of potash, and bisulphate of quinine compresses nicely without any treatment, but as it sticks to the dies, it must have some lubricant added. Three per cent. of powdered talcum added in the manner directed above will overcome this. As the bisulphate of quinine is more soluble than the sulphate, it is generally preferred on this account, and the fact that it needs no adhesive makes it popular for use in tablets. The formula given below will fully illustrate the mode of preparing powders for compression:

1333.

    Phenacetin. .... 1000 grains.
    Powdered sugar. .... 100 grains.

Mix carefully, then moisten with water, pass through a sieve and dry. When dry, spray with ethereal solution of petrolatum and mix on paper. Allow the ether to evaporate and pass through the sieve again. Make 200 tablets. In this same manner tablets can be made of phenacetin and salol, antikamnia, antipyrin, chlorate acid, trional, sulphonal, bismuth subnitrate, bismuth subgallate, quinine salicylate, quinine sulphate, and many others. Petrolatum will generally be preferable as a lubricant, or it can be used in connection with talcum, or talcum alone can be used. Another illustration are tablets of benzoate of soda:

1334.

    Benzoate of soda. .... 1000 grains.
    Powdered acacia. .... 60 grains.

Mix thoroughly and moisten with water, then proceed exactly as in making tablets of phenacetin. In this way, using powdered acacia as an adhesive, tablets are generally made of such chemicals as benzoate of lithium salicylate of soda, etc.

As tablets containing acacia are not as soluble as those containing sugar, it is a good rule, where the substance is not readily soluble and where acacia is necessary as an adhesive, to use both sugar and acacia. Such substances as charcoal require either the addition of considerable quantities of sugar or of acacia before they can be successfully compressed. Some authorities direct the addition of 25 per cent. of powdered sugar, others direct acacia, my own experience, however, leads me to favor a combination of 15 per cent. of powdered sugar and 8 per cent. of acacia. Sulphur and its combinations are also granulated in a similar manner.

1335.

Hypodermic tablets are usually made as tablet-triturates, and these are to be preferred to the compressed form; but where it is desired to make them by compression, pure cane sugar should be used as a vehicle. Cane sugar is much to be preferred to either the dried sulphate of soda, or chloride of sodium, or sugar of milk, as recommended in the standard works on pharmacy. Let a person take a tablet made with dried sulphate of soda as the vehicle and drop it into water; he will find that it dissolves with difficulty. Some years ago it was used by some manufacturers, but they are all using powdered cane-sugar to-day.

1336.

Powdered boric acid should be used to prevent the material adhering to dies; 2 per cent. will usually be found efficient. The powder should be granulated and dried, and then the proper amount of boric acid added as directed above.

There is a large class of tablets that contain active alkaloids and very potent remedies which constitute only a small portion of the body of the tablet, the balance usually being sugar of milk. The writer prefers to add 10 per cent. of powdered cane-sugar before granulating. They can be lubricated with either powdered talcum or white petrolatum. As an example, the following formula is offered:

1337.

Strychnine sulphate.	3 grains.
Powdered sugar.	30 grains.
Powdered sugar of milk.	267 grains.

Mix thoroughly, moisten with water, granulate and dry. Lubricate with talcum or petrolatum, and make 300 tablets.

Tablets containing extracts are best made from the powdered extracts, as they are more easily mixed with sugar than the ordinary solid extract. If it is desired to use solid extracts, not in powdered form, they should be rubbed to a smooth paste with some suitable solvent, and then rubbed with a small quantity of starch and the solvent evaporated, the whole then to be mixed with a suitable quantity of milk sugar and granulated. Tablets made from tinctures are made in this manner, and many times these furnish all the moisture that is needed to granulate. Salts containing much water of crystallization should be reduced to a fine powder and then dried and mixed with 5 per cent. of acacia and 8 per cent. of sugar, and moistened with water and granulated by passing through the sieve and then drying very thoroughly and then lubricating. To this class belong such tablets as alum, sulphate of zinc, etc. Tablets containing pepsin and pancreatin in a pure state should be mixed with sugar of milk, to which 5 or 10 per cent. of powdered cane-sugar has been added and carefully moistened with water, granulated in the usual way and dried.

To make effervescent tablets the acid should be granulated with a part of the powdered sugar and dried. The rest of the ingredients containing the soda, etc., should be granulated with the rest of the sugar and dried, and then the two thoroughly mixed by agitation in some closed vessel. These can be lubricated with petrolatum if desired, or the whole of the ingredients may be dried separately and mixed, then moistened with alcohol and granulated and dried as directed in the U. S. Pharmacopoeia, for making effervescent salts. The first is generally preferred, although it is simply a question of choice.

1338.

Tablets of calomel and bicarbonate of soda call for special treatment, in order to prevent chemical action between the soda and calomel. McFerran recommends that the soda bicarbonate be mixed with 5 per cent. of powdered acacia, dampened with water and granulated, and then the calomel mixed with the same by agitating them together in a wide-mouth bottle until thoroughly mixed. The writer prefers, however, to proceed differently, using the following process:

Calomel.	200 grains.
Soda bicarbonate.	200 grains.
Sugar, powdered.	30 grains.
Acacia, powdered.	16 grains.

Mix the calomel and 20 grains of sugar, moisten and granulate; then mix the soda with 10 grains of sugar and the acacia and moisten and granulate. When both are dry mix in a mortar, reducing to fine powder, and moisten with alcohol and granulate and dry. Then make 200 tablets. In a similar manner other tablets containing chemicals likely to react on each other when moist are made.

Tablets containing extract of licorice are best moistened carefully with water and need no adhesive added.

1339.   Tablets of Soda Mint.

Bicarbonate of soda.	400 grains.
Powdered acacia.	60 grains.
Carbonate of ammonia.	25 grains.
Oil of peppermint.	16 grains.

Mix thoroughly and moisten with water, granulate and dry. Lubricate with petrolatum. Make 100 tablets.

Tablets containing resins are sometimes moistened with 70 or 80 per cent alcohol; this, dissolving a portion of the resin, gives them the necessary adhesiveness in many cases. In some cases, however, water is to be preferred in such combination, for the reason that alcohol often tends to make hard granules that compress with difficulty and make a very hard tablet.

It is not to be expected that the pharmacist will succeed in perfectly preparing every combination on first trial, but there is no reason why any competent pharmacist should depend on the manufacturer entirely for his supplies.

If in doubt what adhesives to use with any combination, it is well to use 5 per cent. of powdered acacia and 10 per cent. of sugar. There are few powders that cannot be nicely granulated in this manner.

Many fail in trying to compress tablets before they are dry, and as a consequence have the powder stick to the dies. Some think that the harder you can compress a tablet the better. Nothing can be further from the truth, for only as much pressure should be used as is absolutely necessary. In selecting an adhesive, do so with a view of leaving the resulting tablet as soluble as possible. It is a general practice to compress tablets with as little adhesive as possible. This is done mainly to keep the size of the tablet as small as possible. The writer believes that in making tablets of such insoluble substances as salol, sulphonal, etc., that the presence of even as much as 25 per cent. of powdered sugar would not be objectionable in any way and would add materially to the solubility of the tablet.

I have thought best not to speak of the different machines on the market for making compressed tablets; my observation is that care is necessary to do nice work with any one of them, and, with care, they all will do nice work. Each one possibly has its peculiar merits; but the one essential to success in making tablets is the careful preparation of the ingredients for compression, for it is impossible for any machine to do nice work with a powder not properly prepared.

1340. Manufacture of Tablet Triturates.
(Ph. Era.)

Tablet triturates consist of medicine, which, if a dry solid, has been triturated with sugar of milk until a thorough and complete division and distribution of it has been made. In the case of pasty or fluid bodies, these are mixed in a wet state with sugar of milk, the whole dried, and then finely subdivided by trituration. The powder in either case is then formed into a pasty mass with varying proportions of alcohol and water, or other suitable menstruum, and afterward molded into tablets of uniform size and weight.

The formula for each separate combination is arrived at in the following way:

The mold is filled with finely powdered sugar of milk, which has been wetted to a pasty mass with dilute alcohol. The tablets are then pressed from the mold, thoroughly dried, and weighed. This weight is generally 65 grains for 50 tablets for the rubber molds now usually supplied, making a tablet weighing slightly less than 1 1-3 grains when filled with plain milk sugar. The weight of the plain sugar of milk tablet is slightly increased with the increased solvent action of the menstruum, as more sugar enters the solution, making the tablet more compact. The next step is to ascertain how much milk sugar must be omitted from the previously ascertained amount in order to make room for medicinal constituents. For this purpose 130 grains of milk sugar are weighed off, which is equivalent to 100 finished tablets of plain sugar of milk. From these 130 grains a bulk is taken, equivalent, as nearly as possible, to that of the substance to be incorporated, and the weight noted. The active ingredient, if a dry solid, is now mixed with the remaining portion of sugar of milk by thorough trituration. In the case of solid extracts, tinctures and other fluids, these are mixed with the remaining portions of sugar of milk, if necessary, by the aid of water or some other menstruum which dissolves them perfectly, then the mass is dried and powdered.

After the mixture has been made, dried and thoroughly triturated, it is wetted with a suitable menstruum, and molded, care being taken to scrape the mortar as clean as possible in order not to waste any of the material. The tablets are then carefully dried. If there be any mass in excess of that required for the 100 tablets, it shows that not enough milk sugar has been taken from the original 130 grains. The weight of this excess is generally equal to that of an equal bulk of milk sugar. Hence it will only be necessary, at the next trial, to remove as much more milk sugar as the bulk of this excess amounts to.

If there should be less than 100 tablets, the weight of the number deficient is ascertained by determining the average weight of the finished tablets, and deducting the calculated weight of the missing tablets from the weight of the bulk of sugar of milk originally separated. At the next trial the amount of milk removed from the original 130 grains should be as much less as the weight of the missing tablets amounted to. In each case the formula finally found, by actual experiment, to yield a correct result, should be noted in a special book for the purpose of future reference.

It is important that all the ingredients and the mixture of powders ready for molding should be in the finest possible state of subdivision. If they are coarse, the tablets will not show a smooth, finished appearance. In tablets composed nearly all of milk sugar, if the latter be in a coarse powder, it necessitates the addition of more water to the alcohol than it required when the sugar of milk is in a very fine powder. The menstruum selected should possess a slight solvent action upon one or more of the ingredients, but the latter, should not be too freely soluble, since the mass is then molded with difficulty, and the tablets prepared therefrom will be uneven, sometimes being cracked on the surface and very hard. It should possess sufficient solvent action to make a firm yet not too hard a tablet, one that will hold firmly together when shaken in a vial, and which should readily disintegrate upon the addition of water. It is, however, impossible to prepare all the various combinations in such a form that they readily dissolve or diffuse upon the addition of water, the rapidity of disintegration depending upon the proportion and soluble character of the constituents.

The menstrua generally used are alcohol, absolute alcohol, alcohol and water, and chloroform. For tablets composed nearly entirely of sugar of milk, a menstruum composed of nearly three volumes of alcohol and one volume of water is preferable. For bodies insoluble in alcohol the proportion of water is raised in proportion to the increase of active ingredient. The menstruum must, therefore, be so adjusted that it will dissolve enough of either the milk sugar or of the active ingredient, to make a sufficiently firm tablet.

In preparing the powder for molding, it should be wetted to a pasty consistence, the mold placed upon a smooth surface, a pill tile answering admirably, and the wetted powder pressed into the spaces with a horn or ivory spatula, which is drawn over the mold. Sometimes the mass adheres to the spatula and is drawn from the holes. This is remedied by dipping the spatula in the menstruum used for wetting the mixture before drawing it over the surface. The mold is then reversed by sliding it toward and off the edge of the tile without raising it, the spatula is drawn over the other side of the mold, and the latter then again drawn toward and off the edge. The tablets are now pressed out by the punch-pin plate and allowed to dry a few minutes upon the punch pins, then shaken off by striking the pin plate forcibly upon the counter covered with a sheet of paper to receive the tablets.

Practical Suggestions About Lozenges.*
1341.

In the manufacture of lozenges the paste is formed the same way as a biscuit maker mixes flour with water to make the dough, except that a thick solution of East India or Turkey gum is used for the mixing, instead of water, and finely powdered loaf sugar instead of flour. The paste, when made, is rolled out in the same manner as the baker treats the dough, and during this process sufficient starch powder to prevent it sticking to the slab is used. The thickness of the sheet of paste may be regulated either by the gauge at each end of the rolling-pin, or judged by the sight, and must be, according to the lozenges to be made, from an eighth to a quarter inch thick. To make lozenges on the smallest scale, there must be employed a smooth marble slab, four feet long by two feet wide, to cut the lozenges upon, also a smooth stone slab of a lesser size to mix the paste on; a good palette knife, 15 or 18 inches long; a hand-brush, made with long, soft hairs; and small pieces of linen cloth to run through cutters when clogged with the paste; lozenge trays, made with smoothly planed seasoned deal, four feet long by two feet wide, with edges one inch deep; a hot closet or drying-room, with racks fitted round it to place the trays of lozenges upon, and heated, free from dust and smoke; small gallipots with some clean water must be kept near the cutting slab to place the cutters in to free them from the paste which clings to the edges, and must be wiped dry with the cloth named above.

In rolling the paste out to the required thickness, it must be lifted up with the palette knife two or three times to see that it does not stick to the slab, then to be taken up by rolling it round the pin, and after dusting the slab with more powder replace the sheet of paste, the upper side downwards, smoothing the surface of the same by dusting it with powder and using the brush over it. In cutting out the lozenges, commence with a straight line as close to the left edge as possible, and however slowly you may progress at first, keep parallel with that all through the sheet. In emptying the cutters, place the lozenges evenly and closely together on the trays, which must first be thoroughly dried and covered with the starch powder.

Recipes and mixings for some of the most familiar kinds of lozenges are here given for beginners.

1342. The Ordinary Peppermint Lozenges.

For twenty-eight pounds of finely powdered loaf or icing sugar, after making a bay in the center of the sugar placed on the slab, pour

*Brit. Baker, Confect. and Purv.

into it 2 quarts of thick gum mucilage; on that pour 1 ounce of either Mitcham or the best American oil of peppermint; work these two well together. When sufficiently mixed, stir in the sugar from all around the sides of the bay, and add to the mixture an eggspoon of smalts; work this in, and make the whole into a good stiff paste with as much of the sugar as can be used, and keep it ready on the mixing slab, with a damp, clean cloth covered over it for use. Take from the bulk about 2 pounds in weight, and work it with the hands into a compact square piece, keeping it free from sticking on the slab with the powdered starch; then proceed to roll, and cut it out in the shapes desired, and follow the preliminary instructions given above. The cuttings left on the slab from each sheet of paste must be mixed with each portion taken from the mixture to continue the process until the whole is used up. This is an example for all peppermint lozenges, the only difference in the quality or high-priced article being in the quantity and quality of the oil of mint used in making them, consisting of from ¼ ounce to 1½ ounces of the essential oil extra to that here given for the same quantity of sugar, and which are sold at a higher price and stamped "extra."

1343. Ginger Lozenges.

Work into the same quantity as given above of sugar and gum, 1 pound of finely powdered best Jamaica ginger, ¼ ounce of extract of ginger, ½ ounce of essence of lemon, and enough vegetable yellow to make the mixture a primrose color, and proceed to finish as directed previously.

1344. Cough-No-More Lozenges.

All the cough lozenges sold differ either in color, shape or taste. A good and effectual lozenge may be made as follows: Work into the paste of gum and sugar given some thick dissolved solazzi licorice to make it of a brown color, with 2 ounces of powdered ipecacuanha, 1 ounce of anise seed, 1 dram of acetate of morphine, and 1 ounce of powdered tartaric acid. The drugs to be carefully and thoroughly incorporated with the gum mucilage before mixing that with the sugar.

1345. Bath, or Coltsfoot Lozenges.

The same mixture of gum and sugar as for coughs, leaving out the anise seed, but putting more dissolved licorice, 1 ounce tartaric acid and 1 ounce of oil of lemon previously stirred well in with the gum.

1346. Black Currant Lozenges for the Voice, Sore Throats, Etc.

To 4 pounds of the black-currant extract, the consistence of thick honey, work in 10 or 12 pounds of finely powdered sugar, 1 pound of powdered Turkey gum, with 2 ounces of tartaric acid.

This recipe makes a better lozenge for the purpose mostly required if half a dram of capsicum is added.

1347. Otto of Rose Lozenges.

To the same amount of gum and sugar as given in the first recipe, work into the gum 1 dram of otto of rose with 1 ounce of the French oil of geranium, 2 ounces of powdered tartaric acid, and color the whole mass with liquid carmine to a nice delicate pink.

1348. Bronchial Lozenges, Brown. A

Ext. of licorice, powd.	10 pounds.
Oleo resin of cubebs	1 pound.
Powdered sugar q. s. to make	150 pounds.

1349. Bronchial Lozenges. B

Cubeb-powder	½ ounce.
Stockholm tar	½ ounce.
Oil of wintergreen	20 minims.
Solution of potash	6 drams.
Orange-flower water to	4 ounces.

Macerate for twenty-four hours in a warm place, shaking occasionally; then filter through kaolin.

Marshmallow	2 ounces.
Hoarhound	2 ounces.
Licorice	2 ounces.
Aniseed	2 ounces.
Lobelia-seeds	½ ounce.
Hops	½ ounce.
Ipecacuanha	2 drams.
Cayenne	2 drams.

Roughly bruise, and add to 1 gallon of water; boil, and allow to simmer for some hours; press and strain, then evaporate to about 30 ounces; add the infusion of cubebs, diluted with 4 ounces of rectified spirit, and filter.

Use this as stock solution, to be added to any of the usual sugar-pastes, about 2 ounces to every 14 pounds of finished lozenges. A good plan is to arrange with some lozenge-maker to make and stamp the lozenges, using your medicated solution.

MEDICINAL LOZENGES
OF THE UNITED STATES AND BRITISH PHARMACOPŒIAS, LONDON HOSPITAL AND OTHER POPULAR FORMULÆ.

OFFICINAL LOZENGES OF THE U. S. P.

1350. Ammonium Chloride.
Ammonium chloride ...... 2 grains.

1351. Catechu.
Catechu .... 1 grain.

1352. Chalk.
Prepared chalk .... 4 grains.

1353. Cubeb.
Oleo resin cubeb .... ½ grain.

1354. Ginger.
Tinct. ginger .... 2 minims.

1355. Iron.
Hydrated oxide iron ...... 5 grains.

1356. Licorice and Opium.
Ext. licorice .... 2 grains.
Ext. opium ....1/20 grain.

1357. Magnesia.
Calc. magnesia .... 3 grains.

1358. Morphine and Ipecac.
Morphine sulph. .... 1/40 grain.
Ipecac. .... 1/12 grain.

1359. Peppermint.
Oil peppermint .... 1/6 minim.

1360. Rhatany.
Ext. rhatany .... 1 grain.

1361. Soda Bicarbonate.
Soda bicarbonate .... 3 grains.

1362. Santonin (U. S. P. 1870).
Santonin .... ½ grain.

1363. Santoninate Soda.
Santoninate soda .... 1 grain.

1364. Tannic Acid.
Tannic acid .... 1 grain.

OFFICINAL LOZENGES OF THE B. P.

1365. Bismuth.
Bismuth subnitrate .... 2 grains.
Magnesia carbonate ...... 2½ grains.
Precipitated chalk .... 3 2/3 grains.

1366. Catechu.
Catechu .... 1 grain.

1367. Iron.
Reduced iron .... 1 grain.

1368. Ipecac.
Ipecac. .... ¼ grain.

1369. Morphine.
Morphine mur. .... 1/36 grain.

1370. Morphine and Ipecac.
Morphine mur. .... 1/36 grain.
Ipecac. .... 1/12 grain.

1371. Soda Bicarbonate.
Soda bicarbonate .... 5 grains.

1372. Tannic Acid.
Tannic acid .... ½ grain.

LOZENGES OF THE LONDON HOSPITAL FOR DISEASES OF THE THROAT.

FORMULÆ SUGGESTED BY DR. MORRELL MACKENZIE.

(Made with Black and Red Currant Paste.)

1373. Aconite.
Tinct. aconite, B. P. ..... ½ minim.

1374. Ammonium Chloride.
Ammonium chloride ...... 2 grains.

1375. Benzoic Acid.
Benzoic acid .... ½ grain.

LOZENGES OF THE LONDON HOSPITAL.

1376. Borax.
Borax .... 3 grains.

1377. Carbolic Acid.
Carbolic acid .... 1 grain.

1378. Catechu.
Pale catechu .... 2 grains.

1379. Cubeb.
Cubeb .... ½ grain.

NON-SECRET FORMULAS.

1380. Guaiac.
Resin guaiac .... 2 grains.

1381. Kino.
Kino. .... 2 grains.

1382. Logwood.
Ext. logwood .... 2 grains.

1383. Lettuce.
Ext. lettuce .... 1 grain.

1384. Potassium Chlorate.
Potassium chlorate .... 3 grains.

1385. Potassium Citrate.
Potassium citrate .... 8 grains.

1386. Potassium Bitartarate.
Potassium bitartarate .... 3 grains.

1387. Pellitory Root.
Pellitory root .... 1 grain.

1388. Rhatany.
Ext. rhatany .... 3 grains.

1389. Sedative.
Ext. opium .... 1/10 grain.

1390. Tannic Acid.
Tannic acid .... 1½ grains.

UNOFFICINAL LOZENGES.

1391. Ammonium Chloride and Licorice.
Ammon. mur. .... 2 grains.
Ext. licorice .... 8 grains.

1392. Ammonium Chloride and Cubebs.
Ammon. mur. .... 2 grains.
Cubebs .... 1 grain.

1393. Bismuth and Charcoal.
Bismuth subnit. .... 2 grains.
Charcoal .... 5 grains.

1394. Bronchial.
Oleoresin cubeb .... 1/5 grain.
Tolu .... 1/5 grain.
Oil sassafras .... 1/10 grain.
Ext. licorice .... 7 grains.

1395. Brown Mixture.
Ext. licorice .... 3 grains.
Opium .... 1/20 grain.
Acid benzoic .... 1/20 grain.
Camphor .... 1/20 grain.
Tartar emetic .... 1/40 grain.
Oil anise .... 1/20 grain.

1396. Brown Mixture and Muriate Ammonia.
Mist. glyc. comp., U. S. P. 85 minims.
Ammon. mur. .... 3 grains.

1397. Chlorodyne.
Each lozenge represents 2 drops chlorodyne.

1398. Cocaine and Cubeb Compound.
Cocaine mur. .... 1/12 grain.
Cubebs .... 1 grain.
Ext. licorice .... 3 grains.
Benzoic acid .... ½ grain.
Chlorate potass. .... 2 grains.

1399. Coryza.
Oleoresin cubeb .... 1/5 grain.
Tolu .... 1/5 grain.
Oil sassafras .... 1/10 grain.
Ext. licorice .... 7 grains.

1400. Ginger and Soda Bicarbonate.
Tinct. ginger. .... 10 minims.
Soda bicarb. .... 2 grains.

1401. Guaiac.
Res. guaiac .... 2 grains.

1402. Ipecac and Squill.
Ipecac. .... ¼ grain.
Squill .... ½ grain.

1403. Jackson's Ammonia.
Ammon. mur. .... 1 grain.
Morph. mur. .... 1/24 grain.
Hyoscyamus .... ½ grain.
Slippery elm bark .... 3 grains.
Ext. licorice .... 3 grains.
Tolu .... 1/5 grain.

1404. Jackson's Pectoral.
Ipecac. .... 1/15 grain.
Kermes mineral .... 1/15 grain.
Morph. mur. .... 1/20 grain.
Tolu .... 1/5 grain.
Oil checkerberry .... 1/20 minim.
Ext. licorice .... 2 grains.

1405. Kermes Mineral.
Kermes mineral .... ½ grain.

1406. Kino.
Kino. .... 2 grains.

1407. Pepsin, Bismuth and Ginger
Pepsin sacch. .... 2 grains.
Bismuth subnit. .... 3 grains.
Ginger .... 1 grain.

1408. **Pepsin, Bismuth and Charcoal.**
  Pepsin sacch. .... 5 grains.
  Bismuth subnit. .... 2 grains.
  Charcoal .... 5 grains.

1409. **Pepsin and Charcoal with Magnesia and Ginger.**
  Pepsin sacch. .... 2 grains.
  Charcoal .... 3 grains.
  Magnesia .... 2 grains.
  Ginger .... 1 grain.

1410. **Pepsin and Lactophosphate Lime.**
  Pepsin sacch. .... 3 grains.
  Lactophosphate lime ...... 2 grains.

1411. **Potassium Chlorate and Cubeb.**
  Potass. chlorate .... 2 grains.
  Cubeb .... 2 grains.
  Ext. licorice .... 1 grain.
  Oil sassafras .... 1/5 minim.

1412. **Potassium Chlorate and Guaiac.**
  Potass. chlorate .... 1 grain.
  Res. guaiac .... 2 grains.
  Ipecac .... ⅛ grain.

1413. **Rose Leaf and Alum.**
  Red rose leaf .... 1 grain.
  Alum .... 1 grain.

1414. **Rhatany Compound.**
  Ext. rhatany .... 1 grain.
  Cubeb .... ¼ grain.
  Potass. chlorate .... 2 grains.

1415. **Rhubarb and Magnesia.**
  Rhubarb .... 2 grains.
  Magnesia .... 2 grains.

1416. **Rhubarb and Ginger.**
  Rhubarb .... 2 grains.
  Ginger .... 1 grain.

1417. **Rhubarb, Ginger and Soda.**
  Rhubarb .... 2 grains.
  Ginger .... 1 grain.
  Soda bicarb. .... 2 grains.

1418. **Squill Compound.**
  Squill .... 1½ grains.
  Senega .... 1½ grains.
  Tartar emetic .... 1/25 grain.

1419. **Sulphur Compound.**
  Sulphur .... 5 grains.
  Cream tartar .... 2 grains.
  Ext. ipecac .... 1/100 grain.
  Ext. capsicum .... 1/500 grain.
  Arsenious acid .... 1/1000 grain.
  Calcium sulphide .... 1/10 grain.

1420. **Wild Cherry.**
  Morphine sulph. .... 1/50 grain.
  Ipecac .... 1/50 grain.
  Kermes mineral .... ¼ grain.
  Oil bitter almond .... 1/100 minim.
  Fluid extract wild cherry. 1/10 minim.
  Tinct. verat. virid. ..... 3/10 minim.

1421. **Wistar's.**
  Opium .... 1/10 grain.
  Ext. licorice .... 2 grains.
  Oil anise .... 1/30 minim.

COMPRESSED TABLETS.

1422. **Absorbent Dyspeptic.**
  Pepsin .... 1 grain.
  Charcoal .... 2 grains.
  Soda bicarb. .... 2½ grains.

1423. **Acetanilid Aromatic.**
  Acetanilid .... 5 grains.
  Oil gaultheria .... q. s.

1424. **Acetanilid Compound (Bower's).**
  Acetanilid .... 3 grains.
  Monobromated camphor ..... 2 grains.
  Citrate caffeine .... ½ grain.

1425. **Acetanilid Compound (Hoag).**
  Cit. caffeine .... ½ grain.
  Sodium bromide .... 5 grains.
  Acetanilid .... 2 grains.

1426. **Acetanilid Compound (Pitcher).**
  Acetanilid .... 2 grains.
  Fl. ext. gelsemium .... 1 minim.

1427. **Acetanilid Compound.**
  Acetanilid .... 4 grains.
  Fl. ext. gelsemium .... 2 minims.

1428. **Acetanilid Compound.**
  Acetanilid .... 3 grains.
  Tullys powder .... 3 grains.

1429. Acetanilid Compound.
Acetanilid .... 2½ grains.
Caffeine citrate .... 1 grain.
Gelsemin (Eclectic) ...... 1/10 grain.

1430. Acetanilid and Caffeine.
Acetanilid .... 3 grains.
Caffeine .... 1 grain.

1431. Acetanilid and Quinine.
Acetanilid .... 3 grains.
Quinine sulph. .... 2 grains.

1432. Acetanilid and Salol.
Acetanilid .... 2½ grains.
Salol. .... 2½ grains.

1433. Acetanilid and Soda.
Acetanilid .... 4½ grains.
Bicarb. soda .... ¼ grain.
Salicylate soda .... ¼ grain.

1434. Ammonium Chloride and Licorice.
Ammonium chloride ...... 2 grains.
Ext. licorice .... 3 grains.

1435. Anti-Constipation.
Ext. cascara sagrada ..... 1 grain.
Ext. nux vom. .... ⅛ grain.
Ext. bellad. .... ⅛ grain.
Powd. ipecac. .... ⅛ grain.
Podophyllin .... ⅛ grain.

1436. Anti-Dyspeptic (Bradley's).
Powd. cubeb .... 5/8 grain.
Powd. rhubarb .... ½ grain.
Bismuth subnitrate .... 2 grains.
Sugar .... 2½ grains.
Oil peppermint .... ¼ minim.

1437. Antacid.
Carbonate lime .... 3½ grains.
Carbonate magnesia ...... 2½ grains.
Chloride sodium .... 1 grain.

1438. Antifermentive No. 1.
Salicylate soda .... 2 grains.
Powd. ginger .... 2 grains.
Powd. capsicum .... 1/10 grain.
Powd. cardamom comp. .. ¼ grain.

1439. Antifermentive No. 2.
Salicylate soda .... 2 grains.
Gingerine .... 1/12 grain.
Powd. capsicum .... 1/20 grain.
Powd. cardamom comp. ... ¼ grain.

1440. Anti-Malarial.
Powd. nux vomica .... ¼ grain.
Powd. capsicum .... ½ grain.
Ext. hyoscyamus .... ½ grain.
Quinine sulphate .... 3 grains.

1441. Antiseptic Tablets.
Corrosive sublimate .... 7.30 grain.
Ammonium muriate .... 7.70 grain.
The strength of these tablets is so adjusted that one dissolved in a pint of water gives a 1 to 1000 solution.

1442. Bismuth (Hunt).
Bismuth subnitrate .... 5 grains.
Sugar milk .... 2 grains.

1443. Bismuth and Charcoal.
Bismuth subnitrate .... 2 grains.
Charcoal .... 5 grains.

1444. Borax Compound.
Borax. .... 1 grain.
Powd. sugar .... 4 grains.
Oil checkerberry .... ½ minims.

1445. Brown Mixture and Ammonium Muriate.
Brown mixture ....1 teaspoonful.
Ammonium mur. ....1 grain.

1446. Calomel and Capsicum.
Calomel .... 2 grains.
Capsicum .... ½ grain.

1447. Calomel and Ipecac Comp. (Dr. Stimson).
Calomel .... 1 grain.
Powd. ipecac. .... 1 grain.
Powd. opium .... ¼ grain.

1448. Calomel and Rhubarb Compound.
Calomel .... 2½ grains.
Powd. rhubarb .... 2½ grains.
Cinnamon .... 1 grain.

1449. Calomel and Soda.
Calomel .... ½ grain.
Soda bicarbonate .... 3 grains.

1450. Camphor and Acetanilid.
Camphor monobromated .. 1 grain.
Acetanilid .... 2 grains.

1451. Camphor, Opium and Hyoscyamus.
Camphor .... 1 grain.
Powd. opium .... ½ grain.
Ext. hyoscyamus .... 1 grain.

NON-SECRET FORMULAS.

1452. Cascara Compound.
Ext. cascara sagrada ...... 2 grains.
Podophyllin .... ⅛ grain.
Ext. belladonna .... 1-16 grain.

1453. Cocaine Throat.
Cocaine mur. .... 1-12 grain.
Powd. cubebs .... 1 grain.
Benzoic acid .... ½ grain.
Chlorate potass. .... 2 grains.
Licorice .... q. s.

1454. Coryza (Richard's).
Quinine sulph. .... ½ grain.
Ammon mur. .... ½ grain.
Camphor .... ½ grain.
Powd. opium .... 1-10 grain.
Ext. belladonna .... 1-10 grain.
Ext. aconite .... 1-10 grain.

1455. Cystitis (For Acid Urine).
Boracic acid .... 2 grains.
Bicarb. potass. .... 2 grains.
Ext. buchu .... 1 grain.
Ext. dog grass .... 1 grain.
Ext. corn silk .... ½ grain.
Ext. hydrangea .... ½ grain.
Atropia sulph. .... 1-500 grain.

1456. Cystitis (For Alkaline Urine).
Benzoic acid .... 3 grains.
Biborate soda .... 2 grains.
Ext. buchu .... 1 grain.
Ext. dog-grass .... 1 grain.
Ext. corn silk .... ½ grain.
Ext. hydrangea .... ½ grain.
Atropia sulph. .... 1-500 grain.

1457. Damiana Compound.
Ext. damiana .... 2 grains.
Phosphorus .... 1-30 grain.
Ext. nux vomica .... ¼ grain.

1458. Diarrhœa Tablets.
Bismuth subnitrate .... 3 grains.
Pepsin sacch. .... 2 grains.
Aromatic chalk powd. .... 2 grains.

1459. Diffusive Malarial.
Corrosive sublimate ...... 1-50 grain.
Ammon. mur. .... 2 grains.
Cinchona sulph. .... 1-10 grain.
Cinchonidia sulph. .... 1-10 grain.
Quinine sulph. .... 1-10 grain.

1460. Diuretic.
Powd. digitalis .... 1 grain.
Ext. buchu .... 1 grain.
Nitrate potass. .... 1 grain.
Powd. squills .... 1 grain.

1461. Emmenagogue (Biguad's).
Powd. soc. aloes .... 1½ grains.
Powd. rue .... ¾ grain.
Powd. saffron .... ¾ grain.
Powd. licorice .... ¾ grain.

1462. Gonorrhœa.
Powd. cubebs .... 1 grain.
Solidifiable copaiba ..... 1 grain.
Iron sulphate .... ¼ grain.
Oil sandalwood .... ¼ grain.
Oil wintergreen .... 1-10 minim.
Venice turpentine .... ¼ grain.

1463. Guaiac Compound.
Powd. guaiac .... 1 2-3 grains.
Ammonia muriate .... 1 2-3 grains.
Ext. licorice .... ½ grain.

1464. Headache and Neuralgia.
Bromide soda .... 5 grains.
Cit. caffeine .... ½ grain.
Acetanilid .... 1 grain.
Ext. hyoscy. .... ½ grain.
Morphine sulph. .... 1-50 grain.

1465. Hypophosphites and Quinine.
Hypophos. quinine .... 1 grain.
Hypophos. iron .... ½ grain.
Hypophos. lime .... ½ grain.
Hypophos. soda .... ¼ grain.
Hypophos. potass. .... ¼ grain.
Hypophos. manganese ...... ¼ grain.
Hypophos. strychnine ..... 1-64 grain.

1466. Hypophosphites, Quinine and Creasote.
Hypophos. quinine .... 1 grain.
Hypophos. iron .... ½ grain.
Hypophos. lime .... ½ grain.
Hypophos. soda .... ¼ grain.
Hypophos. potass. .... ¼ grain.
Hypophos. manganese ...... ¼ grain.
Hypophos. strychnine ..... 1-64 grain.
Creasote .... ½ minim.

1467. Iron, Arsenic and Strychnine.
Powd. iron .... 2 grains.
Arsenious acid .... 1-80 grain.
Strychnine sulph. .... 1-60 grain.

1468. Iron, Quinine and Aloes Compound (Duncan).
Powd. iron .... 2 grains.
Quinine sulph. .... 2 grains.
Strychnine sulph. .... 1-40 grain.
Arsenious acid .... 1-40 grain.
Powd. aloes .... ⅛ grain.

1469. Iron, Quinine and Strychnine Phosphates.
Iron phosphate .... 1 grain.
Quinine phosphate .... 1 grain.
Strychnine phosphate ..... 1-60 grain.

1470. Laryngitis.
Bromide potass. .... 1¼ grains.
Chlorate potass. .... ⅝ grain.
Powd. ipecac. .... 1-12 grain.
Ext. licorice .... 1¼ grains.
Powd. squill .... 1 grain.

1471. Lead and Bismuth Compound.
Lead acetate .... 1 grain.
Bismuth subnit. .... 2 grains.
Powd. camphor. .... ⅛ grain.
Powd. opium .... ¼ grain.

1472. Mercury Compound. A
Calomel .... 1-24 grain.
Tartar emetic .... 1-120 grain.
Nit. potass. .... 2½ grains.
Ext. licorice ....
Oil sassafras ....
Oil wintergreen .... q. s.

1473. Mercury Compound. B
Calomel .... 1-12 grain.
Tartar emetic .... 1-30 grain.
Nit. potass. .... 5 grains.
Ext. licorice ....
Oil sassafras ....
Oil wintergreen .... q. s.

1474. Mercury Compound. C
Calomel .... 1-6 grain.
Tartar emetic .... 1-30 grain.
Nit. potass. .... 1-10 grain.
Ext. licorice ....
Oil sassafras ....
Oil wintergreen .... q. s.

1475. Mercury and Rhubarb.
Blue mass. .... 2 grains.
Co. rhubarb pil. .... 1 grain.

1476. Migrane. A
Acetanilid .... 2 grains.
Monobromated camphor ...... ½ grain.
Citrate caffeine .... ½ grain.

1477. Migrane. B
Acetanilid .... 3 grains.
Monobromated camphor ...... 2 grains.
Citrated caffeine .... 1 grain.

1478. Nerve Tonic. A
Zinc phosphide .... 1-10 grain.
Ext. nux vomica .... ¼ grain.
Powd. iron .... 2 grains.

1479. Nerve Tonic. B
Zinc phosphide .... 1-10 grain.
Ext. nux vomica .... ¼ grain.
Powd. iron .... 2 grains.
Arsenious acid .... 1-20 grain.

1480. Pepsin, Pancreatin and Lactophosphate Lime.
Pure pepsin .... 1 grain.
Pure pancreatin .... 1 grain.
Lactophosphate lime .... ¼ grain.
Celery seed .... ¼ grain.

1481. Pepsin, Bismuth and Charcoal.
Pepsin concentrated .... 2 grains.
Bismuth subnitrate .... 2 grains.
Charcoal .... 2 grains.

1482. Pepsin, Bismuth and Ginger.
Pepsin sacch. .... 2 grains.
Bismuth subnitrate .... 3 grains.
Powd. ginger .... 1 grain.

1483. Podophyllin and Colocynth Compound.
Podophyllin .... 1-5 grain.
Ext. colocynth comp. ...... 1½ grains.
Ext. jalap .... 1 grain.
Ext. hyoscyamus .... 1-5 grain.

1484. Quinine Compound.
Quinine sulph. .... 1 grain.
Arsenious acid .... 1-40 grain.
Powd. iron .... 1 grain.
Strychnine sul. .... 1-40 grain.
Oleoresin black pep. ...... 1-3 grain.

1485. Quinine Tannate Compound.
Quinine tannate .... 1 grain.
Bismuth subnitrate .... 1 grain.
Powd. opium .... ¼ grain.

1486. Rhubarb and Bismuth Compound.
Powd. rhubarb .... 2 grains.
Powd. ginger .... ½ grain.
Soda bicarb. .... 1 grain.
Bismuth subnitrate .... 2 grains.

1487. Rhubarb, Bismuth, Ginger and Soda.
Powd. rhubarb .... 2 grains.
Bismuth subnitrate .... 3 grains.
Powd. ginger .... ½ grain.
Bicarbonate soda .... ½ grain.

1488. Rhubarb and Ginger Compound.
Powd. ginger .... 2½ grains.
Bicarbonate soda .... 1¼ grains.
Powd. rhubarb .... 1¼ grains.
Powd. cardamom .... ⅝ grain.
Oil peppermint .... 1-20 drop.

1489. Rhubarb and Ipecac Compound. A
Powd. rhubarb .... 1 grain.
Bicarb. soda .... 5 grains.
Powd. ipecac. .... ⅛ grain.
Oil peppermint. .... 1-20 drop.

1490. Rhubarb and Ipecac Compound. B
Powd. rhubarb .... 2 grains.
Powd. ipecac. .... ⅛ grain.
Soda bicarb. .... 5 grains.
Oil peppermint. .... 1-20 drop.

1491. Rhubarb and Ipecac Compound. C
Powd. rhubarb .... 2 grains.
Soda bicarb. .... 5 grains.
Powd. ipecac. .... ¼ grain.
Tr. nux vom. .... 5 minims.
Oil peppermint. .... 1-20 drop.

1492. Rhubarb and Soda.
Powd. rhubarb .... 1½ grains.
Soda bicarb. .... 1½ grains.
Oil peppermint. .... 1-7 drop.

1493. Saccharated Carbonate Iron. A
Carbonate iron .... 2 grains.
Sugar .... 1 grain.

1494. Saccharated Carbonate Iron. B
Carbonate iron .... 5 grains.
Sugar .... 2½ grains.

1495. Saccharated Calomel.
Calomel .... 1 grain.
Soda bicarb. .... 2 grains.
Sugar .... 3 grains.

1496. Salol Compound.
Salol .... 3 grains.
Acetanilid .... 2 grains.

1497. Salol and Phenacetine.
Salol .... 2½ grains.
Phenacetine .... 2½ grains.

1498. Salol and Phenacetine (Half Strength).
Salol .... 1¼ grains.
Phenacetine .... 1¼ grains.

1499. Sodium Salicylate Compound.
Sodium salicylate .... 2 grains.
Cerium oxalate .... 1 grain.

1500. Sulphur Compound. A
Sulphur .... 5 grains.
Bitartarate potass .... 1 grain.

1501. Sulphur Compound. B
Sulphur .... 2½ grains.
Cream tartar .... 2½ grains.

1502. Throat.
Benzoic acid .... 1-5 grain.
Paregoric .... 10 minims.
Tinct. belladonna .... 1 minim.
Ext. licorice .... 3 grains.

1503. Tonic Gout.
Quinine sulph. .... 2 grains.
Ext. digitalis .... ¼ grain.
Ext. colchicum seed .... 1 grain.

1504. Triple Bromides, No. 1.
Bromide of ammonium ....
Bromide of potassium ....
Bromide of sodium .....aa. 2½ grains.

1505. Urethritis.
Acetate of zinc .... 2 grains.
Corrosive sublimate .... 1-5 grain.

One of these tablets dissolved in two ounces of water makes a solution the strength of which is about 1 to 5000 of corrosive sublimate.

1506. Viburnum Compound.
Ext. viburnum prunifolium 1 grain.
Ext. viburnum opulus ..... 1 grain.
Ext. aletris ferinosa ..... ½ grain.
Ext. helonias dioca .... ½ grain.
Ext. squaw vine .... ¼ grain.
Caulophylin .... ¼ grain.

1507. Zinc Sulphate Comp. (for Injection).
Sulphate zinc .... 1 grain.
Bichloride mercury .... 1-40 grain.
Boracic acid .... 1 grain.

TABLET TRITURATES.

1508. Aconite and Belladonna. A
Aconite .... 1-100 grain.
Belladonna .... 1-100 grain.

1509 Aconite and Belladonna. B
Tinct. aconite .... 1 minim.
Tinct. belladonna .... 1 minim.

1510. Aconite and Belladonna. C
Tinct. aconite .... ½ minim.
Tinct. belladonna .... ½ minim.

1511. Aconite and Bryonia. A
Aconite .... 1-100 grain.
Bryonia .... 1-100 grain.

1512. Aconite and Bryonia. B
Tinct. aconite .... 1 minim.
Tinct. bryonia .... 1 minim.

1513. Aconite Compound.
Morphine sulph. .... 1-50 grain.
Tartar emetic .... 1-100 grain.
Ext. aconite .... 1-100 grain.

1514. Aconite and Gelsemium.
Tinct. aconite .... 2 minim.
Tinct. gelsemium .... 1 minim.
Tinct. belladonna .... 2 minim.

1515. Aconite and Ipecac.
Tinct. aconite .... ½ minim.
Wine ipecac. .... 1 minim.

1516. Aconite and Tartar Emetic.
Aconite .... 1-50 grain.
Tartar emetic .... 1-50 grain.

1517. Aloin, Belladonna and Hyoscyamus.
Aloin (Merck's) .... ¼ grain.
Ext. belladonna .... ¼ grain.
Ex. hyoscyamus .... ¼ grain.

1518. Aloin, Belladonna and Podophyllin.
Aloin (Merck's) .... ⅛ grain.
Ext. belladonna .... ⅛ grain.
Podophyllin .... ⅛ grain.

1519. Aloin, Belladonna and Nux.
Aloin (Merck's) .... 1-5 grain.
Ext. belladonna .... ⅛ grain.
Ext. nux vomica .... 1-6 grain.

1520. Aloin, Belladonna, Podophyllin and Nux.
Aloin (Merck's) .... 1-10 grain.
Ext. bellad. .... 1-10 grain.
Podophyl. .... 1-10 grain.
Ext. nux vomica .... 1-10 grain.

1521. Aloin and Belladonna Compound, No. 1.
Aloin (Merck's) .... 1-5 grain.
Ext. belladonna .... ⅛ grain.
Strychnine .... 1-60 grain.

1522. Aloin and Belladonna Compound, No. 2.
Aloin (Merck's) .... 1-5 grain.
Ext. belladonna .... ⅛ grain.
Strychnine sulph. .... 1-120 grain.

1523. Aloin Compound, No. 1.
Aloin (Merck's) .... ⅛ grain.
Podophyllin .... ⅛ grain.

1524. Aloin Compound, No. 2.
Aloin (Merck's) .... ¼ grain.
Podophyllin .... ¼ grain.

1525. Aloin and Cascarin Compound, No. 1.
Aloin, (Merck's) .... 1-5 grain.
Ext. bellad. .... ⅛ grain.
Cascarin .... ¼ grain.
Strychnine sulph. .... 1-60 grain.

1526. Aloin and Cascarin Compound, No. 2.
Aloin (Merck's) .... ¼ grain.
Podophyllin .... ¼ grain.
Cascarin .... ¼ grain.
Ext. belladonna .... ⅛ grain.

1527. Aloin, Iron and Strychnine.
Aloin (Merck's) .... 1-10 grain.
Powd. iron .... 1 grain.
Strychnine sulph. .... 1-60 grain.

1528. Aloin and Strychnine Compound.
Aloin (Merck's) .... 1-5 grains.
Ext. bellad. .... ⅛ grain.
Strychnine sulph. .... 1-60 grain.
Powd. ipecac. .... 1-16 grain.

1529. Aloin, Strychnine, Belladonna and Cascara Segrada.
Aloin (Merck's) .... 1-5 grain.
Strychnine .... 1-120 grain.
Ext. bellad. .... ⅛ grain.
Ext. cascara sagrada ..... ½ grain.

NON-SECRET FORMULAS.

1530. Aloin, Strychnine, Belladonna and Ipecac.
Aloin (Merck's) .... 1-5 grain.
Strychnine .... 1-60 grain.
Ext. belladonna .... ⅛ grain.
Ipecac. .... 1-16 grain.

1531. Ammonium Chloride Compound.
Ammonium chloride ...... ¼ grain.
Ext. licorice .... 1-10 grain.
Powd. cubebs. .... ⅛ grain.

1532. Ammonium Chloride Compound and Codeine.
Ammonium chloride ...... ¼ grain.
Ext. licorice .... 1-10 grain.
Powd. cubebs. .... ⅛ grain.
Codeine .... 1-25 grain.

1533. Ammonium Chloride Compound and Ipecac.
Ammonium chloride ...... ¼ grain.
Ext. licorice .... 1-10 grain.
Powd. cubebs. .... ⅛ grain.
Powd. ipecac. .... 1-15 grain.

1534. Ammonium Chloride Compound with Morphine.
Ammonium chloride ...... ¼ grain.
Ext. licorice .... 1-10 grain.
Cubebs. .... ⅛ grain.
Morphine sulph. .... 1-50 grain.

1535. Ammonium Chloride Compound and Tartar Emetic.
Ammonium chloride ...... ¼ grain.
Ext. licorice .... 1-10 grain.
Powd. cubebs. .... ⅛ grain.
Tartar emetic .... 1-60 grain.

1536. Ammonium, Chloride and Hyoscyamus Compound.
Ammonium chloride ...... 1 grain.
Tartar emetic .... 1-24 grain.
Ext. hyoscyamus .... 1-6 grain.

1537. Anæsthetic.
Camphor .... ¼ grain.
Hydrochlorate morphine .. 1-24 grain.
Oil cajuput .... 1-24 grain.

1538. Anodyne.
Camphor .... ¼ grain
Ext. hyoscyamus .... ⅛ grain.
Morphine sulph. .... 1-60 grain.
Oil capsicum .... 1-60 grain.

1539. Anti-Dyspeptic.
Strychnine sulph. .... 1-120 grain.
Powd. ipecac. .... 1-3 grain.
Black pepper .... ⅛ grain.
Oil gaultheria .... 1-10 grain.

1540. Antimony and Ipecac.
Tartar emetic .... 1-100 grain.
Ipecac. .... 1-100 grain.

1541. Antimony Comp. (Plummer's).
Antimony comp. (Plummer's).. 1-10 grain.
Sulphurated antimony .... 1-40 grain.
Powd. guaiac. .... 1-20 grain.
Calomel .... 1-40 grain.

1542. Arsenic Compound.
Arsenious acid .... 1-30 grain.
Piperine .... 1-5 grain.

1543. Arsenic and Iron. A
Arsenious acid .... 1-30 grain.
Powd. iron .... 1 grain.

1544. Arsenic and Iron. B
Arsenious acid .... 1-60 grain.
Powd. iron .... 1-5 grain.

1545. Arsenic and Iron. C
Arsenious acid .... 1-100 grain.
Powd. iron .... 1 grain.

1546. Arsenic and Iron. D
Arsenious acid .... 1-60 grain.
Powd. iron .... 1 grain.

1547. Arsenic and Strychnine.
Arsenious acid .... 1-100 grain.
Strychnine sulph. .... 1-60 grain.

1548. Atropia Compound.
Atropia sulph. .... 1-400 grain.
Tartar emetic .... 1-100 grain.

1549. Belladonna Compound.
Corrosive sublimate ..... 1-100 grain.
Tinct. belladonna .... 1 minim.
Powd. ipecac. .... 1-10 grain.

1550. Bismuth Compound.
Bismuth subnitrate ...... ½ grain.
Cerium oxalate .... ½ grain.

1551. Bismuth and Calomel Compound.
Bismuth .... 1 grain.
Calomel .... 1-40 grain.
Powd. ipecac. .... 1-60 grain.

Bismuth and Ipecac Compound,
1552.   No. 1.
    Bismuth subnitrate .... 1 grain.
    Calomel .... 1-10 grain.
    Powd. ipecac. .... 1-20 grain.
    Opium .... 1-40 grain.

Bismuth and Ipecac Compound,
1553.   No. 2.
    Bismuth subnitrate .... ½ grain.
    Cerium oxalate .... ½ grain.
    Powd. ipecac. .... 1-20 grain.

1554. **Bismuth and Nux Vomica.**
    Bismuth subnitrate .... 1 grain.
    Ext. nux vomica .... ⅛ grain.

1555.   **Bronchitis.**
    Ext. belladonna .... 1-40 grain.
    Dover's powder .... 1-10 grain.
    Powd. ipecac. .... 1-20 grain.
    Quinine sulph. .... ¼ grain.

1556. **Bronchitis Without Quinine.**
    Ext. belladonna .... 1-40 grain.
    Dover's powder .... 1-10 grain.
    Powd. ipecac. .... 1-20 grain.

1557.   **Brown Mixture.**
    Ext. licorice .... 1-10 grain.
    Camphor .... 1-25 grain.
    Benzoic acid .... 1-25 grain.
    Oil anise .... 1-25 grain.
    Powd. opium .... 1-25 grain.
    Tartar emetic .... 1-60 grain.

1558. **Brown Mixture (Half Strength).**
    Ext. licorice .... 1-10 grain.
    Camphor .... 1-50 grain.
    Benzoic acid .... 1-50 grain.
    Oil anise .... 1-50 grain.
    Powd. opium .... 1-50 grain.
    Tartar emetic .... 1-120 grain.

1559.   **Cactus Compound.**
    Fluid ext. cactus......... 1 minim.
    Tinct. strophanthus ...... 3 minims.

1560.   **Caffeine Compound.**
    Caffeine citrate .... 1 grain.
    Nitroglycerin .... 1-200 grain.

1561. **Calomel, Aloin and Podophyllin.**
    Calomel .... 1-10 grain.
    Aloin .... 1-10 grain.
    Podophyllin .... 1-20 grain.

1562.   **Calomel Compound.**   A
    Calomel .... ½ grain.
    Opium .... ⅙ grain.
    Ipecac. .... ⅛ grain.

1563.   **Calomel Compound.**   B
    Calomel .... 1-50 grain.
    Morphine sulph. .... 1-100 grain.
    Tartar emetic .... 1-100 grain.

1564.   **Calomel Compound.**   C
    Calomel .... ¼ grain.
    Podophyllin .... 1-12 grain.
    Soda bicarb. .... ½ grain.

1565.   **Calomel Compound.**   D
    Calomel .... 1-10 grain.
    Soda bicarb. .... 1 grain.

1566.   **Calomel Compound.**   E
    Calomel .... 1 grain.
    Soda bicarb. .... 1 grain.

1567.   **Calomel and Codeine.**
    Calomel .... 1-12 grain.
    Codeine .... ⅛ grain.

1568.   **Calomel and Ipecac.**   A
    Calomel .... ¼ grain.
    Powd. ipecac. .... ¼ grain.

1569.   **Calomel and Ipecac.**   B
    Calomel .... ⅛ grain.
    Powd. ipecac. .... ⅛ grain.

1570.   **Calomel and Ipecac.**   C
    Calomel .... 1-6 grain.
    Powd. ipecac. .... 1-6 grain.
    Powd. opium .... 1-6 grain.

1571. **Calomel, Ipecac and Opium.**
    Calomel .... ¼ grain.
    Dover's powder .... 1 grain.

1572. **Calomel, Ipecac and Soda, No. 1.**
    Calomel .... 1-5 grain.
    Ipecac. .... 1-10 grain.
    Soda bicarb. .... 1 grain.

1573. **Calomel, Ipecac and Soda, No. 2.**
    Calomel .... ⅛ grain.
    Ipecac. .... 1-12 grain.
    Soda bicarb. .... ½ grain.

1574. **Calomel, Ipecac and Soda, No. 3.**
    Calomel .... ⅛ grain.
    Ipecac. .... ¼ grain.
    Soda bicarb. .... 1 grain.

NON-SECRET FORMULAS. 149

1575. Calomel and Morphine Compound.
Calomel .... ½ grain.
Morph. sul. .... ¼ grain.
Tartar emetic .... 1-16 grain.

1576. Calomel and Opium. A
Calomel .... ¼ grain.
Opium .... ¼ grain.

1577. Calomel and Opium. B
Calomel .... ⅛ grain.
Opium .... ⅛ grain.

1578. Calomel and Opium Compound. A
Calomel .... ½ grain.
Opium .... ⅛ grain.
Ipecac. .... ¼ grain.

1579. Calomel and Opium Compound. B
Calomel .... ¼ grain.
Opium .... 1-16 grain.
Ipecac. .... ⅛ grain.

1580. Calomel and Podophyllin.
Calomel .... ⅛ grain.
Podophyllin .... ⅛ grain.

1581. Calomel, Podophyllin and Ipecac.
Calomel .... 1-10 grain.
Podophyllin .... 1-30 grain.
Powd. ipecac. .... ⅛ grain.

1582. Calomel and Soda Compound.
Calomel .... ½ grain.
Soda bicarb. .... ½ grain.
Podophyllin .... 1-12 grain.

1583. Cannabis Indica and Codeine.
Tinct. cannabis indica .... 1 minim.
Codeine .... 1-25 grain.

1584. Capsicum Compound. A
Capsicum .... 1-10 grain.
Nux vomica .... ¼ grain.

1585. Capsicum Compound. B
Ext. nux vomica .... ¼ grain.
Powd. capsicum .... 1-10 grain.
Powd. ipecac. .... 1-12 grain.

1586. Capsicum Compound. C
Powd. capsicum .... 1-5 grain.
Ext. nux vomica .... ½ grain.

1587. Cardiac.
Sulphate sparteine .... 1-10 grain.
Tinct. stropanthus .... 3 minims.
Caffeine citrate .... ¼ grain.
Codeine .... 1-20 grain.

1588. Cardiane.
Tinct. stropanthus .... 2 minims.
Tinct. cactus .... 1 minim.
Sparteine sulph. .... 1-20 grain.
Digitalin .... 1-120 grain.

1589. Cascarin Compound.
Aloin .... ¼ grain.
Podophyllin .... ¼ grain.
Cascarin .... ¼ grain.

1590. Cathartic. A
Leptandrin .... 1-32 grain.
Podophyllin .... 1-6 grain.
Aloin .... 1-16 grain.
Ext. hyoscyamus .... 1-16 grain.
Gamboge .... 1-64 grain.
Oleoresin capsicum .... 1-128 drop.
Oil peppermint .... 1-128 drop.

1591. Cathartic. B
Aloin .... 1-10 grain.
Ext. nux vomica .... 1-10 grain.
Ext. coloc. comp. .... 1-10 grain.
Podophyllin .... 1-5 grain.
Oleoresin capsicum .... 1-128 drop.
Oil croton .... 1-15 drop.

1592. Cerium Oxalate Compound.
Cerium oxalate .... 1 grain.
Powd. ipecac. .... 1-120 grain.

1593. Chlorosis.
Protochlo-. iron .... ¼ grain.
Bichloride mercury .... 1-120 grain.
Chloride quinine .... ⅛ grain.

1594. Cocaine Compound.
Potass. chlorate .... 1 grain.
Cocaine muriate .... 1-50 grain.

1595. Cold. A
Morphine sulph. .... 1-32 grain.
Tartar emetic .... 1-32 grain.
Ext. licorice .... 1-10 grain.
Oil checkerberry .... q. s.

1596. Cold. B
Antimony sul. .... 1-12 grain.
Ext. conium .... 1-12 grain.
Powd. ipecac. .... 1-6 grain.
Potass. nitrate .... 1-6 grain.
Ammonia muriate .... 1-6 grain.

1597. Cold. C
Aconite .... 1-10 grain.
Camphor .... 1-10 grain.
Powd. opium .... 1-10 grain.
Nitrate potass. .... 1-10 grain.

1598. Conium Compound.
Ext. conium .... 1-30 grain.
Cubebs .... 1-10 grain.
Ext. licorice .... 1-10 grain.

1599. Conium Compound with Codeine.
Ext. conium .... 1-30 grain.
Cubebs .... 1-10 grain.
Ext. licorice .... 1-10 grain.
Codeine .... 1-25 grain.

1600. Copper and Opium.
Sulph. copper .... 1-30 grain.
Tinct. opium, deodorized.. ¼ minim.

1601. Corrosive Sublimate Compound
Corrosive sublimate ...... 1-32 grain.
Powd. ipecac. .... ⅛ grain.

1602. Cough Mixture.
Ammonia muriate .... ¼ grain.
Paregoric .... 5 minims.
Corrosive sublimate ...... 1-96 grain.

1603. Diaphoretic. A
Morphine sulph. .... 1-32 grain.
Strychnine sulph. .... 1-95 grain.
Atropine sulph. .... 1-150 grain.
Arsenious acid .... 1-100 grain.
Aconitia .... 1-1000 grain.

1604. Diaphoretic. B
Morphine sulph. .... 1-24 grain.
Tinct. aconite .... ½ minim.
Tartar emetic .... 1-60 grain.
Powd. ipecac. .... ⅛ grain.

1605. Diarrhœa. A
Calomel .... ⅛ grain.
Morphine sulph. .... 1-16 grain.
Capsicum .... 1-16 grain.
Powd. ipecac. .... 1-32 grain.
Camphor .... 1-16 grain.

1606. Diarrhœa. B
Powd. opium .... ¼ grain.
Camphor .... ¼ grain
Powd. ipecac. .... ⅛ grain.
Acetate lead .... 1-6 grain.

1607. Digitalis Compound. A
Tinct. digitalis .... 2 minims.
Brucia .... 1-100 grain.

1608. Digitalis Compound. B
Tinct. digitalis .... 2 minims.
Strychnine sulph. .... 1-100 grain.

1609. Digitalis and Iron Compound.
Ext. digitalis .... 1-10 grain.
Iron phosphate .... ¼ grain.
Strychnine sulph. .... 1-60 grain.

1610. Digitalis and Strophanthus.
Tinct. digitalis .... 3 minims.
Tinct. stropanthus .... 2 minims.

1611. Dipsomania.
Nitrate strychnine .... 1-60 grain.
Chloride gold .... 1-40 grain.

1612. Diuretic.
Caffein .... ¼ grain.
Nitrate potassium .... ½ grain.
Carbonate lithia .... ¼ grain.

1613. Dover's Powder Compound. A
Quinine sulph. .... ½ grain.
Dover's powder .... ½ grain.

1614. Dover's Powder Compound. B
Dover's powd. .... 2½ grains.
Calomel .... ¼ grain.

1615. Dyspeptic.
Strychnine sulph. .... 1-40 grain.
Powd. ipecac. .... ⅛ grain.
Powd. rhubarb .... ¼ grain.
Capsicum .... ⅛ grain.

1616. Euonymin Compound.
Euonymin .... ¼ grain.
Podophyllin .... ⅛ grain.
Aloin .... ⅛ grain.

1617. Expectorant.
Fld. ext. belladonna ...... ⅛ minim.
Powd. ipecac. .... 1-10 grain.
Ext. licorice .... ⅛ grain.
Codeine .... 1-16 grain.
Ext. senega .... 1-10 grain.

1618. Fever.
Dr. H. J. Kenyon.
Tinct. aconite .... 1 minim.
Morphine sulph. .... 1-20 grain.
Tartar emetic .... 1-50 grain.
Ipecac. .... ⅛ grain.

1619. Fever.
Dr. T. G. Davis.
Tinct. aconite .... 1-5 minim.
Tinct. bryonia .... 1-10 minim.
Tinct. belladonna .... 1-10 minim.

1620. Fever and Ague.

Sulphate copper .... 1-10 grain.
Powd. opium .... ⅛ grain.
Sulphate quinine .... ½ grain.
Podophyllin .... 1-12 grain.

1621. Hæmatic.

Arsenious acid .... 1-120 grain.
Powd. iron .... 1-10 grain.
Corrosive sublimate ...... 1-200 grain.
Nux vomica .... 1-20 grain.

1622. Headache.

Acetanilid .... 1 grain.
Ext. belladonna .... ⅛ grain.
Ext. gelsemium .... ¼ minim.

1623. Heart Tonic.
Gardiner's.

Nitroglycerin .... 1-100 grain.
Tinct. stropanthus .... 1 minim.
Fluid ext. digitalis .... 1 minim.
Strycnnine .... 1-60 grain.
Powd. iron .... 1 grain.

1624. Heart Tonic and Stimulant. A

Nitroglycerin .... 1-100 grain.
Tinct. digitalis .... 2 minim.
Tinct. stropanthus .... 2 minim.
Tinct. belladonna .... ¼ minim.

1625. Heart Tonic and Stimulant. B

Tinct. digitalis .... 2 minim.
Tinct. stropanthus .... 2 minim.
Tinct. belladonna .... ¼ minim.
Nitroglycerin .... 1-200 grain.

1626. Hepatica.

Pil. hydrarg. .... ½ grain.
Ext. coloc. comp. .... ½ grain.
Ext. hyoscyamus .... ⅛ grain.

1627. Hepatica.
Dr. H. J. Kenyon.

Euonymin .... ⅛ grain.
Podophyllin .... 1-20 grain.
Ipecac. .... ⅛ grain.
Calomel .... ⅛ grain.
Aloin .... 1-12 grain.

1628. Hydrarg and Ipecac Compound.

Blue mass .... 1 grain.
Powd. ipecac .... ⅛ grain.
Powd. opium .... ¼ grain.

1629. Hydrarg and Podophyllin.

Blue mass .... 1 grain.
Podophyllin .... ¼ grain.

1630. Hydrastin Compound.

Hydrastin .... 1-10 grain.
Podophyllin .... 1-20 grain.

1631. Hyoscyamus and Codeine.

Ext. hyoscyamus .... ⅛ grain.
Codeine .... 1-16 grain.

1632 Ignatia Compound.

Powd. ignatia .... 1-100 grain.
Powd. ipecac .... 1-10 grain.

1633. Indigestion. A

Saccharated pepsin .... 1-40 grain.
Carbo veg. .... 1-40 grain.
Subnitrate bismuth .... 1-40 grain.

1634. Indigestion. B

Carbo veg. .... 1-40 grain.
Powd. rhubarb .... 1-40 grain.
Pepsin .... 1-40 grain.
Subnitrate bismuth .... 1-40 grain.

1635. Iron and Aloes Compound.

Strychnine sulph. .... 1-60 grain.
Arsenious acid .... 1-30 grain.
Ext. aloes .... 1-12 grain.
Powd. iron .... 1 grain.

1636. Iron, Arsenic and Brucia. A

Powd. iron .... 1-10 grain.
Arsen. acid .... 1-100 grain.
Brucia .... 1-33 grain.

1637. Iron, Arsenic and Brucia. B

Powd. iron .... 1-10 grain.
Arsen. acid .... 1-100 grain.
Brucia .... 1-100 grain.

1638. Iron, Arsenic and Brucia. C

Powd. iron .... 1 grain.
Arsen. acid .... 1-100 grain.
Brucia .... 1-100 grain.

1639. Iron, Arsenic and Nux.

Powd. iron .... 1 grain.
Arsenious acid .... 1-100 grain.
Ext. nux vomica .... ⅛ grain.

1640. Iron and Arsenic.

Powd. iron .... 1 grain.
Arsenious acid .... 1-30 grain.

1641. Iron and Arsenic Compound. A

Powd. iron .... 1 grain.
Arsen. acid .... 1-100 grain.
Ignatia .... 1-40 grain.

NON-SECRET FORMULAS.

1642. Iron and Arsenic Compound.   B
  Powd. iron .... 1 grain.
  Arsen. acid .... 1-50 grain.
  Ignatia .... 1-40 grain.

1643. Iron, Arsenic and Strychnine.   A
  Powd. iron .... 1 grain.
  Arsen. acid .... 1-100 grain.
  Strychnine .... 1-60 grain.

1644. Iron, Arsenic and Strychnine.   B
  Powd. iron .... 1 grain.
  Arsen. acid .... 1-50 grain.
  Strychnine .... 1-60 grain.

1645. Iron, Arsenic and Strychnine.   C
  Powd. iron .... 1 grain.
  Arsenious acid .... 1-50 grain.
  Strychnine sulph. .... 1-100 grain.

1646. Iron, Arsenic and Strychnine.   D
  Powd. iron .... 1 grain.
  Arsenious acid .... 1-20 grain.
  Strychnine sulph. .... 1-30 grain.

1647. Iron and Mercury Compound.   A
  Reduced iron .... 1 grain.
  Corrosive sublimate ..... 1-60 grain.
  Strychnine sulph. .... 1-60 grain.
  Arsenious acid .... 1-60 grain.

1648. Iron and Mercury Compound.   B
  Reduced iron .... 1 grain.
  Corrosive sublimate ..... 1-50 grain.
  Arsenious acid .... 1-100 grain.

1649. Iron and Mercury Compound.   C
  Powd. iron .... 1 grain.
  Strychnine sulph. .... 1-60 grain.
  Corrosive sublimate ..... 1-60 grain

1650. Iron and Phosphorus Compound.
  Powd. iron .... 1 grain.
  Arsenious acid .... 1-40 grain.
  Strychnine sulph. .... 1-60 grain.
  Phosphorus .... 1-100 grain.

1651. Iron, Quinine and Arsenic.
  Powd. iron .... ½ grain
  Quin. sul. .... ½ grain.
  Arsenious acid .... 1-100 grain.

1652. Iron, Quinine, Arsenic and Strychnine.
  Powd. iron .... ½ grain.
  Quinine sulph. .... ½ grain.
  Arsenious acid .... 1-100 grain.
  Strychnine .... 1-120 grain.

1653. Iron and Quinine Sulphate.
  Powd. iron .... ½ grain.
  Quinine sulph. .... ½ grain.

1654. Iron, Quinine and Strychnine.
  Powd. iron .... ½ grain.
  Quinine sul. .... ½ grain.
  Strych. .... 1-120 grain.

1655. Iron and Strychnine.
  Powd. iron .... 1 grain.
  Strychnine sulph. .... 1-60 grain.

1656. Laxative Compound.
  Ext. cascara sagrada .... ½ grain.
  Aloin .... ⅛ grain.
  Podophyllin .... 1-10 grain.
  Oil peppermint .... 1-10 grain.

1657. Lithia Carbonate and Soda Arseniate.
  Lithia carbonate .... 1 grain.
  Soda arsen. .... 1-30 grain.

1658. Mercury Compound.
  Blue mass .... ½ grain.
  Opium .... ⅛ grain.
  Ipecac .... ¼ grain.

1659. Mercury Iodide Compound.   A
  Mercury iodide red ...... 1-32 grain.
  Powd. ipecac. .... ⅛ grain.

1660. Mercury Iodide Compound.   B
  Mercury iodide red ...... 1-16 grain.
  Powd. ipecac. .... ⅛ grain.

1661. Mercury Iodide Compound.   C
  Mercury iodide red ...... 1-100 grain.
  Powd. belladonna .... 1-100 grain.
  Bichromate potass. ...... 1-100 grain.

1662. Mercury and Belladonna Compound.
  Mercury iodide red ...... 1-200 grain.
  Powd. ipecac. .... 1-20 grain.
  Belladonna .... 1-100 grain.

1663. Mercury and Charcoal.   A
  Mercury protiodide ...... ¼ grain.
  Carbo veg. .... 1-10 grain.

1664. Mercury and Charcoal.   B
  Mercury protiodide ...... 1-6 grain
  Carbo veg. .... 1-10 grain.

1665. Mercury and Hyoscyamus.
Mercury protiodide .... ¼ grain.
Ex. hyoscyamus .... ¼ grain.

1666. Mercury and Ipecac.
Mercury protiodide .... 1-3 grain.
Powd. ipecac. .... ⅛ grain.

1667. Mercury and Ipecac Compound.
Blue mass .... ½ grain.
Ex. hyoscyamus .... ½ grain.
Powd. ipecac. .... ¼ grain.

1668. Mercury and Iron.
Mercury protiodide .... ¼ grain.
Powd. iron .... 1 grain.

1669. Mercury and Opium.
Mercury protiodide .... 1-5 grain.
Powd. opium .... 1-12 grain.

1670. Mercurial Tonic.
Mercury protiodide .... ⅛ grain.
Iron citrate .... ½ grain.

1671. Morphine Compound. A
Morphine sulph. .... ⅛ grain.
Atropia sulph. .... 1-150 grain.

1672. Morphine Compound. B
Morphine sulph. .... ¼ grain.
Atropia sulph. .... 1-150 grain.

1673. Morphine Compound. C
Morphine sulph. .... ⅛ grain.
Atropia sulph. .... 1-200 grain.

1674. Morphine Compound. D
Morphine sulph. .... ¼ grain.
Atropia sulph. .... 1-150 grain.

1675. Morphine and Aconite. A
Morphine sulph. .... 1-32 grain.
Ext. aconite .... 1-100 grain.

1676. Morphine and Aconite. B
Morphine sulph. .... ⅛ grain.
Ext. aconite .... 1-25 grain.

1677. Morphine and Aconite. C
Morphine sulph. .... 1-32 grain.
Tinct. aconite .... 1 minim.

1678. Morphine and Belladonna. A
Morphine sulph. .... ⅛ grain.
Ext. belladonna .... ¼ grain.

1679. Morphine and Belladonna. B
Morphine sulph. .... ⅛ grain.
Ext. belladonna .... ⅛ grain.

1680. Nerve Tonic. A
Zinc phos. .... 1-10 grain.
Ext. nux vom. .... ¼ grain.
Powd. iron .... 1 grain.

1681. Nerve Tonic. B
Zinc phosphide .... 1-10 grain.
Ext. nux vomica .... ¼ grain.
Arsenious acid .... 1-20 grain.

1682. Nerve Tonic. C
Zinc phosphide .... ⅛ grain.
Ext. nux vomica .... ¼ grain.
Ext. cannabis indica ...... ⅛ grain.

1683. Nerve Tonic. D
Ext. cannabis indica ..... ⅛ grain.
Hyoscyamia .... 1-400 grain.
Zinc phosphide .... 1-10 grain.

1684. Neuralgic.
Quinine sul. .... ½ grain.
Morphine sul. .... 1-80 grain.
Strych. sul. .... 1-120 grain.
Arsen. acid .... 1-80 grain.
Ext. aconite .... ⅛ grain.

1685. Neuralgic.
Dr. H. J. Kenyon.
Zinc phosphide .... 1-16 grain.
Strych. .... 1-60 grain.
Ext. cannab. ind. .... ⅛ grain.
Soda arsen. .... 1-20 grain.
Aconitia, duq. .... 1-400 grain.

1686 Nitroglycerin Compound. A
Nitroglycerin .... 1-100 grain.
Tinct. digitalis .... 2 minims.

1687. Nitroglycerin Compound. B
Nitroglycerin .... 1-100 grain.
Tinct. stropanthus .... 2 minims.

1688. Nux Vomica Compound. A
Ext. nux vom. .... 1-64 grain.
Ext. belladonna .... 1-32 grain.
Ipecac. .... 1-16 grain.
Aloin .... ⅛ grain.
Podophyllin .... ¼ grain.

1689. Nux Vomica Compound. B
Ext. nux vomica .... 1-16 grain.
Arsenious acid .... 1-80 grain.
Pepsin .... 1-32 grain.
Aromatics .... q. s.

NON-SECRET FORMULAS.

1690. **Nux Vomica Compound.** C
Ext. nux vomica .... 1-20 grain.
Arsenious acid .... 1-100 grain.
Sulphur .... 1-20 grain.

1691. **Nux and Arsenic.**
Nux vomica .... 1-10 grain.
Arsenious acid .... 1-50 grain.

1692. **Nux and Bryonia.** A
Nux vomica .... 1-100 grain.
Bryonia .... 1-100 grain.

1693. **Nux and Bryonia.** B
Tinct. nux vomica .... 1 minim.
Tinct. bryonia .... 1 minim.

1694. **Nux and Cantharides.**
Nux vomica .... 1-100 grain.
Cantharides .... 1-100 grain.

1695. **Nux and Carbo Veg.** A
Nux vomica .... 1-100 grain.
Carbo veg. .... 1-10 grain.

1696. **Nux and Carbo Veg.** B
Nux vomica .... ½ grain.
Carbo veg. .... ¼ grain.

1697. **Nux and Pepsin.** A
Nux vomica .... 1-100 grain.
Pepsin .... 1-10 grain.

1698. **Nux and Pepsin.** B
Nux vomica .... 1-10 grain.
Pepsin .... 1 grain.

1699. **Nux and Pepsin.** C
Nux vomica .... 1-10 grain.
Pepsin .... ½ grain.

1700. **Nux and Pepsin Compound.**
Nux vomica .... 1-100 grain.
Pepsin .... ¼ grain.
Bimuth subnit. .... 1 grain.
Calomel .... ¼ grain.

1701. **Nux and Phosphorus.**
Ext. nux vomica .... ¼ grain.
Phosphorus .... 1-50 grain.

1702. **Nux and Sulphur.**
Nux vomica .... 1-100 grain.
Sulphur .... 1-100 grain.

1703. **Nux and Sulphur Compound.**
Nux vom. .... 1-20 grain.
Sulphur .... 1-10 grain.
Arsen. acid .... 1-100 grain.

1704. **Opium and Camphor.**
Powd. opium .... ¼ grain.
Camphor .... ¼ grain.

1705. **Opium and Lead.** A
Powd. opium .... 1-16 grain.
Lead acetate .... ¼ grain.

1706. **Opium and Lead.** B
Powd. opium .... ⅛ grain.
Lead acetate .... ¼ grain.

1707. **Pepsin Compound.**
Powd. pepsin .... ¼ grain.
Ext. nux vomica .... 1-32 grain.
Powd. ipecac. .... 1-16 grain.

1708. **Pepsin and Bismuth.**
Pepsin .... ¼ grain.
Bismuth subnitrate .... 1 grain.

1709. **Pepsin and Calomel.**
Pepsin .... ¼ grain.
Bismuth subnitrate .... 1 grain.
Nux vomica .... 1-100 grain.
Calomel .... 1-40 grain.

1710. **Pepsin and Charcoal.**
Pepsin .... ¼ grain.
Carbo veg. .... ¼ grain.

1711. **Pepsin and Pancreatin.**
Pepsin .... ¼ grain.
Pancreatin .... ¼ grain.

1712. **Podophyllin and Leptandrin.**
Podophyllin .... ¼ grain.
Leptandrin .... ½ grain.

1713. **Podophyllin, Nux and Hyoscyamus.**
Podophyllin .... ½ grain.
Ext. nux vomica .... 1-16 grain.
Ext. hyoscyamus .... ⅛ grain.

1714. **Quinine, Iron and Arsenic.**
Quin. sul. .... ½ grain.
Powd. Iron .... ½ grain.
Arsen. acid .... 1-120 grain.

1715. **Quinine and Licorice.**
Quinine sulph. .... 1-10 grain.
Ext. licorice .... 1-10 grain.

1716. **Rhubarb and Ipecac.**
Powd. rhubarb .... ¼ grain.
Powd. ipecac. .... 1-10 grain.

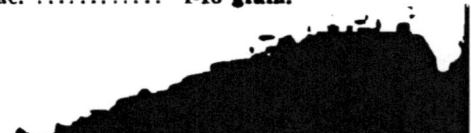

NON-SECRET FORMULAS.

1717. **Rhubarb and Soda.**
Powd. rhubarb .... ½ grain.
Soda bicarb. .... ½ grain.

1718. **Santonin and Calomel.** A
Santonin .... ¼ grain.
Calomel .... ⅛ grain.

1719. **Santonin and Calomel.** B
Santonin .... ½ grain.
Calomel .... ½ grain.

1720. **Santonin and Podophyllin.** A
Santonin .... ¼ grain.
Podophyllin .... 1-20 grain.

1721. **Santonin and Podophyllin.** B
Santonin .... ½ grain.
Podophyllin .... 1-20 grain.

1722. **Sciatica.**
Tinct. aconite .... 3-4 minim.
Tinct. belladonna .... 3-4 minim.
Tinct. colchicum .... 3-4 minim.
Tinct. cimicifuga .... 3-4 minim.

1723. **Senega Compound.**
Tinct. squills .... 1 minim.
Tinct. senega .... 1 minim.
Tinct. ipecac. .... 1 minim.

1724. **Sick Headache.**
Irisin .... 1-10 grain.
Podophyllin .... 1-20 grain.
Sanguinarin .... 1-20 grain.
Nux vomica .... 1-20 grain.
Euonymin .... ¼ grain

1725. **Stomachic.**
Pepsin .... ¼ grain.
Ext. nux vomica .... ¼ grain.
Carbo veg. .... ¼ grain.
Powd. capsicum .... ¼ grain.

1726. **Strychnine Muriate Compound.**
Corrosive sublimate ...... 1-20 grain.
Ext. belladonna .... 1-10 grain.
Strychnine mur. .... 1-40 grain.

1727. **Sulphur and Ipecac.**
Sulphur .... 1-10 grain.
Powd. ipecac. .... 1-10 grain.

1728. **Tartar Emetic Compound.**
Powd. opium .... ⅛ grain.
Tartar emetic .... 1-16 grain.
Calomel .... ½ grain.

1729. **Tartar Emetic and Morphine.** A
Tartar emetic .... 1-100 grain.
Morphine sulph. .... 1-30 grain.

1730. **Tartar Emetic and Morphine.** B
Tartar emetic .... 1-100 grain.
Morphine sulph. .... 1-100 grain.

1731. **Tartar Emetic and Opium.**
Tartar emetic .... 1-100 grain.
Powd. opium .... 1-50 grain.

1732. **Tartar Emetic, Opium and Camphor.**
Tartar emetic .... 1-100 grain.
Powd. opium .... 1-20 grain.
Camphor .... 1-10 grain.

1733. **Throat.**
Potass. iodide .... 1-10 grain.
Salt .... 1-10 grain.
Sugar .... ½ grain.

1734. **Tincture Aconite and Belladonna.**
Tinct. aconite .... 1 minim.
Tinct. belladonna .... 1 minim.

1735. **Tincture Aconite and Gelsemium.**
Tinct. aconite .... 2 minims.
Tinct. gelsemium .... 1 minim.
Tinct. belladonna .... 2 minims.

1736. **Tincture Strophanthus Compound.** A
Tinct. stropanthus .... 2 minims.
Tinct. digitalis .... 3 minims.

1737. **Tincture Strophanthus Compound.** B
Tinct. stropanthus .... 2 minims.
Tinct. digitalis .... 3 minims.
Nitroglycerin .... 1-100 grain.

1738. **Tincture Strophanthus Compound.** C
Dr. O. O. Pike.
Tinct. stropanthus .... 2 minims.
Tinct. digitalis .... 3 minims.
Tinct. nux vomica .... 2 minims.

1739. **Tonic.**
Dr. Hammond.
Iron pyrophos. .... ½ grain.
Quinine sulph. .... ½ grain.
Strychnine sulph. .... 1-120 grain.

1740. **Tonic Alterative.** A
Corrosive sublimate ...... 1-50 grain.
Strychnine sulph. .... 1-100 grain.
Powd. ipecac. .... 1-20 grain.

1741. Tonic Alterative.
Corrosive sublimate .... 1-30 grain.
Strychnine sulph. .... 1-60 grain.
Powd. iron .... 1 grain.

1742. Tonic. Hawkin's.
Strychnine sulph. .... 1-200 grain.
Ext. cannab. indica ...... 1-16 grain.
Phosphorus .... 1-400 grain.
Atropia sulph. .... 1-600 grain.

1743. Tonsilitis.
Tinct. aconite .... 1-5 minim.
Tinct. bryonia .... 1-10 minim.
Tinct. belladonna .... 1-10 minim.
Red iodide mercury ...... 1-100 grain.

1744. Tully's Powder Compound. A
Tully's powder .... 2½ grains.
Calomel .... ¼ grain.

1745. Tully's Powder Compound. B
Tully's powder .... 2½ grains.
Podophyllin .... 1-10 grain.

1746. Zinc Phosphide and Nux Vomica.
Zinc phosphide .... 1-10 grain.
Ext. nux vomica .... ¼ grain.

UNOFFICINAL PILLS.

1747. Roback's Pills.
Gum gamboge .... 100 pounds.
Socotrine aloes .... 100 pounds.
Powdered may apple ..... 16½ pounds.
Powdered cayenne .... 4 pounds.
Mix and mass.
Make into 3 grain pills.

1748. Sir Andrew Clark's Pills.
Ferri sulph .... ½ grain.
Aloin .... ½ grain.
Ext. nuc. vom. .... 1-3 grain.
Ext. belladon. .... ¼ grain.
Myrrhae pulv. .... 1½ grains.
M. Ft. pil. sec. art.

1749. Antibilious and Liver Pills.
Pulv. antim. tart. .... 48 grains.
Pil. hydrarg. ....
 1 ounce, 1 dram, 36 grains.
Pulv. gambogiae ....
 1 ounce, 1 dram, 36 grains.
Pulv. capsici. ....
 2 drams, 1 scruple, 24 grains.
M. Ft. mass. Divide in 4-gr. pills.
One at bedtime.

1750. Pills for Chronic Constipation.
Aloes .... 4 grains.
Strychniae sulphat. ...... ¼ grain.
Extract belladonnae ...... 1¼ grains.
Ipecac. pulv. .... 5½ grains.
M. Divid. in pil. 12.
Sig.: One every evening.

1751. Arsenical Pills for the Complexion.
These contain very little arsenic. The following is a safe prescription:
Ferri arseniatis .... 2 grains.
Ferri redact. .... 1½ drams.
Pil. rhei co. .... 2 scruples.
Ext. nucis vom. .... 10 grains.
Glycer. tragac. .... q. s.
Ft. mass. et div. in pil. 60.
One thrice daily with food.
For lozenges and tablets use arseniate of soda, 1-30 grain in each.

1752. Gravel and Lumbago Pills.
Potass. nitrat. .... 2 grains.
Pulv. ipecac. .... ½ grain.
Pulv. scillae .... ½ grain.
Ext. belladonnae .... ¼ grain.
Ext. gentianae .... q. s.
Ft. pil.
A pill to be taken thrice daily with half a tumblerful of B. P. potash-water.

1753. Digestive Pills.
Pulv. ext. coloc. co. ..... 1 dram.
Bismuth. trisnit. .... 1 dram.
Ext. hyoscyam. .... ½ dram.
Cayenne. .... 1 scruple.
Sp. vin. ten. .... q. s. ut ft. mass.
4-grain pills.
One an hour before dinner.

1754. Neuralgic Pills.
Quininae sulph. .... 1 grain.
Ext. aloes aq. .... ½ grain.
Ferri sulph. ex. .... 1½ grains.
Ext. bellad. .... ⅛ grain.
Ext. gentian. .... 1½ grains.
Pulv. capsici .... 1 grain.
Pulv. camph. .... 1 grain.
M. Ft. pil. 2.

1755. Pills for Spermatorrhœa.
Zinci valer. .... 3 grains.
Ext. bellad. .... 1-6 grain.
Quininae sulph. .... 1 grain.
Conf. rosae .... q. s. ut ft. pil. 1.
Mitte 24.
Sig.: One t. d. s.

1756. Toothache Pills.

Pulv. rhei	12 grains.
Quininae sulph.	24 grains.
Camphor.	12 grains.
Ext. hyoscyam.	36 grains.

M. Ft. pil. 24.

One every four hours until relieved.

1757. Menthol.

Gelatine	1 ounce.
Glycerine (by weight)	2½ ounces.
Orange-flower water	2½ ounces.
Menthol	5 grains.
Rectified spirit	1 dram.

Soak the gelatine in the water for two hours, then heat on a water-bath until dissolved and add 1½ ounces of the glycerine. Dissolve the menthol in the spirit, mix with the remainder of the glycerine, add to the glyco-gelatine mass, and pour into an oiled tin tray (such as the lid of a biscuit-box). When the mass is cold divide it into ten dozen pastilles.

Menthol pastilles are an excellent remedy for tickling cough as well as laryngitis. They should be freshly prepared, and cut oblong, so that the patient may take half of one, or less, as he finds them suit.

1758. Tonic Female Pills.
(Ch. and Dr.)

This is not at all a desirable trade to cultivate, as in some cases it is really abortives that are wanted. The following pill has been in use for twenty years in legitimate practice, and it has never been abused:

Ergotini	1 dram.
Quininae sulph.	½ dram.
Pulv. glycyrrhiz.	½ dram.
Pulv. tragacanth.	8 grains.

Ft. massa, et div. in pil. 30.

One thrice a day immediately before food when the period is delayed or prolonged.

1759. Pruritus Ani.

Regulate the bowels with the late Sir Andrew Clark's pill taken once, twice, or thrice a day, namely:

Aloin	½ grain.
Ferri sulph.	½ grain.
Ext. nucis vomicae	½ grain.
Pulv. myrrhae	½ grain.
Saponis	½ grain.

If no relief is obtained add—

Acidi arseniosi	1-20 grain.

1760.

Also use the following lotion, suggested by Dr. A. Cooper Key in the British Medical Journal:

Pulv. sodae bibor.	20 grains.
Glycerini	2 drams.
Naphthae rectificat.	½ ounce.
Aq. flor. sambuci ad	6 ounces.

M. Ft. lotio.

Or—

1761.

Calaminae levig.	1½ drams.
Acid. hydrocy. (Scheele's).	½ dram.
Glycerini	2 drams.
Liq. calcis ad	8 ounces.

M. Ft. lotio.

1762.

The following cooling-lotion for pruritus is recommended by the Practitioner:

Liq. ammonii acetatis	2 ounces.
Acidi hydrocyanici diluti	1 dram.
Spiritus rectificati	3 drams.
Aquae rosae ad	8 ounces.

To be applied locally.

1763. Little Liver Pills. A

Aloin	1-10 grain.
Jalap resin	1-16 grain.
Podophyllin	1-5 grain.
Ext. nux vomica	1-20 grain.
Extract hyoscyamus	1-20 grain.
Oleoresin capsicum	1-20 grain.

1764. Little Liver Pills. B

Jalap resin.	1-16 grain.
Leptandrin	1-16 grain.
Aloin	⅛ grain.
Podophyllin	¼ grain.
Powdered gamboge	1-32 grain.
Powdered capsicum	1-64 grain.
Extract hyoscyamus	⅛ grain.
Oil peppermint	1-128 grain.

1765. Chill Pills.

Quinine	40 grains.
Ext. cinchona	30 grains.
Oil of black pepper	12 drops.

Make into 24 pills in capsules or sugar coated.

Directions: After a chill take at bedtime a dose of Co-Cathartic pills, early next morning take two of the chill pills; and the same number every two hours until 14 are taken.

The following day take one pill every two hours, until 5 are taken.

1766. Martindale's Phosphorus Pills.
(Ch. and Dr.)

Phosphorus	10 grains.
Oil of theobroma	490 grains.
Bisulphide of carbon	200 grains.
Or q. s. to	750 grains.
Take of above sol.	54 grains.
Acacia	18 grains.
Syrup	18 grains.

Divide into 24 pills.

3 grains = 1-33 grain phosphorus.

Ten grains of phosphorus is dissolved in 200 fl. grains of purified carbon bisulphide, and 490 grains of shredded cocoa-butter added and dissolved by shaking; then the solution is made up to 750 fl. grains with bisulphide.

The solution keeps indefinitely, but it is apt to become solid in cold weather; the heat of the hand, however, suffices to liquefy it. The desired quantity of it is mixed with powdered acacia, stirred for a little and the syrup added, when a mass suitable for rolling is soon produced. The pills may be varnished with sandarac, but should be thoroughly dried after varnishing, otherwise they may stick together in the bottle. They keep well if the coating is perfect. They also take the pearl coating well. The pills are more easily made, more quickly assimilated, and do not cause so much disturbance as others. Mr. Martindale has put them to a number of tests, and he referred to the objections which may be urged against the mass, particularly its comparative softness. This, he said, can be obviated by using glucose instead of syrup, and as to the permanence of the pill in warm climates, he could only say that he had carried one in the pocket without affecting it, and when put in water at 90° F., a pill did not fail.

1767. Phosphorus Pills.

Phosphorus	1 grain.
Chloroform	10 minims.
Dissolve and mix with	
Powdered ficorice	1 dram.
Water	20 minims.
Then mass with	
Ext. nux vomica	10 grains.
Powd. tragacanth.	q. s.

Divide into 50 pills.

1768. Antimalarial Pills.

Phosphorus	1-100 grain.
Strychnia	1-64 grain.
Arsenious acid	1-20 grain.
Iron by hydrogen	1½ grains.
Quinine sulph.	1½ grains.
Purified aloes	¼ grain.

1769. Neuralgic Pills.
Brown Sequard's.

Ext. henbane	2-3 grain.
Ext. conium	2-3 grain.
Ext. ignatia bean	½ grain.
Ext. opium	½ grain.
Ext. aconite	⅛ grain.
Ext. cannabis indica	¼ grain.
Ext. stramon	1-5 grain.
Ext. belladonna	1-6 grain.

METHODS AND TABLES FOR PERCENTAGE SOLUTIONS.

Western Druggist.
1770.

In view of the ever-recurring question concerning the method of calculating percentage solutions we find ourselves compelled to refer to this frequently discussed subject once more, devoting more space to it than ordinarily, so as to cover the question.

Percentum means, for each hundred. Percentage by weight means that all ingredients shall be weighed; percentage by volume means that all ingredients shall be measured. A 1-per-cent cocaine solution, hence, contains 1 grain of cocaine and 99 grains of water; a 2-per-cent. cocaine solution necessarily contains 2 grains of cocaine hydrochlorate and 98 grains of water, and so on. A fluid ounce (480 minims) of distilled water at normal temperature weighs approximately 455.5 grains, so that 1 per cent of 1 fluid ounce is as the proportion, 100:1::455.5:4.555. Subtracting 4.5 grains from 455.5 grains gives us 451 grains of water in which to dissolve 4.5 grains of cocaine, the resulting solution weighing 455.5 grains. In this calculation we have assumed 1 grain of cocaine to occupy the same space as one minim of water. But this is not the case and our 1-per-cent. cocaine solution measures probably two or three minims less than 1 fluid ounce.

If it be desirable to dispense exactly 1 fluid ounce of the solution in question, the only practical way to proceed, on a small scale and extemporaneously, is to prepare a little more than wanted and throw away the surplus. To insure the full volume of 480 minims, take 455.5 grains as a starting point; to this add the percentage required in grains, say 4. We then have 459.5 grains as the weight of the finished product, 4 per cent of which is 100:4::459.5:18.38. The 18.38 subtracted from the whole 459.5, gives us 441.12 grains of water and 18.38 grains of cocaine in a total of 459.5 grains of finished solution. This will measure more than 480 and less than 494.88

minims, depending on the bulk the cocaine assumes in liquefied form.

The calculations, it must be borne in mind, are based on water as a solvent and on a low percentage. The principle, but not the figures, holds good with respect to fluids specifically lighter or heavier than water, while in high percentages, exceeding, say, 10 percent, the increase in bulk is, especially for expensive material and large quantities, sufficiently serious to require preliminary experimental determinations.

An exceedingly practical method for preparing a fluid ounce of a solution of a given percentage has been suggested by an esteemed correspondent, H. M. Wilder, of Philadelphia. His method is in effect the same as explained above, excepting that it does not require careful calculations. Its only possible drawback could be that the excess obtained being about one-tenth of an ounce (difference between 456 and 500 grains) would make the waste (when 4 p. c. or over) when operating with costly material quite appreciable; especially when more than one fluid ounce of solution be dispensed. Mr. Wilder's method, which he has employed for many years, is as follows:

In order to make one fluid ounce of 4-per cent solution, he takes the nearest round number, which is 500. He dissolves 5 times 4 grains of the salt in 500 less 20 grains of the menstruum (water or other solvent of similar specific gravity) and concludes that he now has a 4-per-cent solution. If he now measures off one fluid ounce, he must necessarily have a fluid ounce of a 4-per-cent solution. As to the surplus of solution, that is thrown away; what little loss that may amount to is more than compensated for by the ease of calculation, without bothering oneself about fractions.

In 1891 C. C. Sherrard, of Detroit, Mich., published in the New Idea tables for preparing solutions, which, on account of their practicality deserve reproduction. We quote Mr. Sherrard's article in full:

"With a view of economizing time, the following tables for preparing percentage solutions have been carefully figured out. Many pharmacists closely engaged in the practice of their art will find that these tables will save them much valuable time and also remove the possibility of error incidental to rapid calculation and figuring. That there is a need for such a table is shown by the frequent requests for information of this sort. The table is simple and requires but little explanation. There are two tables, the first giving percentage solutions, as, for instance, 4 per-cent. cocaine muriate solution; the second gives parts in 1,000 or 5,000, as, for instance, corrosive sublimate 1 in 1,000. The use of the first is as follows: Run down column 1 until the correct percentage wanted is found, then move to the right along the line until the column is found giving the amount of fluid measure to be made up; at the intersection will be found the weight of salt required. For example, suppose it is desired to make 4 fluid ounces of 4 per-cent. cocaine muriate solution, run down the left hand column to 4, then along to the right till we reach the column headed 4 fluid ounces. At the intersection of the two will be found 72.91, and this is the number of grains needed. It must be remembered that this is the amount of water to take, and not q. s. water to make the volume. Also that these tables are true only for water, and not for alcohol or other fluid. The second table is similarly employed:

FOR MAKING ANY QUANTITY OF PERCENTAGE SOLUTIONS.

To Make	For each 1 fl. oz. of water take of the drug or salt. Grains.	For each 2 fl. oz. of water take of the drug or salt. Grains.	For each 8 fl. ozs. of water take of the drug or salt. Grains.	For each 4 fl. ozs. of water take of the drug or salt. Grains.	For each 5 fl. ozs. of water take of the drug or salt. Grains.	For each 10 fl. ozs. of water take of the drug or salt. Grains.	For each 16 fl. ozs. of water take of the drug or salt. Grains.
1 per ct..	4.557	9.114	13.671	18.228	22.785	45.57	72.912
2 per ct..	9.114	18.228	27.342	36.456	45.570	91.14	145.824
8 per ct..	13.671	27.352	41.013	54.684	68.355	136.71	218.416
4 per ct..	18.228	36.456	54.684	72.912	91.14	182.28	291.648
5 per ct..	22.785	45.57	68.355	91.14	113.925	227.85	346.56
10 per ct..	45.57	91.14	136.71	182.28	227.85	455.7	729.12
15 per ct..	68.355	136.71	205.065	273.42	341.775	683.55	1093.68
20 per ct..	91.14	182.28	273.42	364.56	455.70	911.4	1458.24
25 per ct..	113.925	227.85	341.775	455.70	569.625	1139.25	1822.80
40 per ct..	182.28	364.56	546.84	729.12	911.4	1822.8	2916.48

FOR MAKING ANY QUANTITY OF SOLUTION WHEN STATED IN PARTS PER THOUSAND HUNDRED, ETC.

To make a solution of	For each 1 fl. oz. of water take of the drug or salt. Grains.	For each 2 fl. ozs. of water take of the drug or salt. Grains.	For each 3 fl. ozs. of water take of the drug or salt. Grains.	For each 4 fl. ozs. of water take of the drug or salt. Grains.	For each 5 fl. ozs. of water take of the drug or salt. Grains.	For each 10 fl. ozs. of water take of the drug or salt. Grains.	For each 16 fl. ozs. of water take of the drug or salt. Grains.
1 in 1,000	.4557	.9114	1.3671	1.8228	2.278	4.557	7.291
1 in 500	.9114	1.8228	2.7342	3.6456	4.557	9.114	14.582
1 in 400	1.139	2.278	3.4177	4.557	5.695	11.392	18.228
1 in 300	1.519	3.035	4.557	6.076	7.59	15.19	24.304
1 in 200	2.2785	4.557	6.8355	9.114	11.39	22.785	36.456
1 in 100	4.557	9.114	13.671	18.228	22.785	45.57	72.912
1 in 50	9.114	18.228	27.342	36.456	45.57	91.14	145.824
1 in 25	18.228	36.456	54.684	72.912	91.14	182.28	291.648
1 in 10	45.570	91.140	136.710	182.280	227.85	455.70	729.120
1 in 5	91.14	182.28	273.42	364.56	455.7	911.4	1458.24

Providing other amounts of a solution than those given in the tables are required, it will be a very simple mathematical calculation to determine the amount of drug or salt required for a specified amount of solution. For example, if 4 fluid ounces of a 4-per-cent solution is required, follow down the 4 fluid ounce column until opposite 4 per cent; the number of grains required are 72.912 grains. Now, to make 8 fluid ounces, just twice as much (145.824 grains) is required. In a similar manner, any solution of any percentage strength may readily be found by consulting the proper column and per-cent.

For all dispensing and administering purposes in any prescribed doses the figures herewith given are correct, and for such purpose this article is especially designed.

In further explanation, we may say that, in giving the above figures, the resulting solution is absolutely correct as regards percentage composition, though it may measure slightly more than the water taken, owing to the increase in volume, which always takes place in some degree when a solid passes into solution in a given amount of liquid. This expansion is not appreciable for small amounts of the solid, say up to 5 per cent, but at 25 per cent or more it may be noticeable. However, as before stated, this expansion has been considered, and the resulting solution, notwithstanding the increase in volume, is correct for the percentage given. From the foregoing explanation it is quite clear that, if a dram of 1-2 per-cent. solution be prescribed, exactly 2 per-cent. of that dram is the salt in the solution, the other 98 per cent. being the water."

The following simple rule was communicated a few years ago to a pharmaceutical journal by John P. Judge, of Philadelphia:

Rule: Multiply the weight (in grains) of a dram of water by the number of drams desired, multiply this product by the percentage desired. Dividing all this by 100 gives the percentage. The result will be the number of grains to be added to the quantity of solution desired. For easy memorizing, the rule may be run off thus: Multiply the weight of a dram by the number of drams and this by the percentage. Divide by 100 for percentage.

Everyone who uses this rule is struck by its simplicity, facility, compactness and exactness.

SOLUTIONS, ETC.

1771. Clemen's Arsenical Solution.

The following is the mode of preparation of the liquor arsenici bromatus, used in the treatment of diabetes mellitus:

Carbonate potassium...... 1 dram.
Arsenious acid............ 1 dram.
Distilled water........... 10 ounces.

Boil until a clear solution is formed, and when cold add

Bromine .... 2 drams.
Water .... 12 ounces.

This is allowed to stand until the color disappears when it is ready for use.

Dose: One to 5 drops once or twice a day.

NON-SECRET FORMULAS.

1772. Colorless Hydrastis.
Hydrastis white alkaloid.. 20 grains.
Water .... 8 ounces.
Glycerine .... 8 ounces.
Dissolve alkaloid in 1 or 2 drops of muriatic acid; add water; filter, and add glycerine.

1773.
Homoeopathic diluted tinctures are made from the mother-tinctures, as follows: The mother-tincture is regarded as tincture 1x when it is made of 1-to-10 strength. One part of this mother-tincture vigorously shaken with 9 parts of alcohol yields tincture 2x; 1 part of 2x with 9 parts of alcohol yields tincture 3x. The centesimal scale is similarly worked. One part of mother-tincture with 9 parts of alcohol yields a tincture 1c.; 1 part of this with 99 parts of alcohol yields a tincture 2c, and so on. For full instructions as to all homoeopathic preparations, see Keene & Ashwell's "Companion to the British Homoeopathic Pharmacopoeia."

1774. Liquor Eastoni.
Iron wire.................. 2½ drams.
Phosphoric acid (s.g. 1.5)..
    2 ounces. 6 drams.
Water .... 3 ounces.
Mix in a flask and heat gently until action ceases, then add—
Powdered strychnine...... 10 grains.
Phosphate of quinine...... 4 drams.
Hypophosphorous acid..... ½ dram.
Water to.................. 10 ounces.
Dissolve and filter.
One part of this solution is to be mixed with 3 parts of thick syrup.

1775. Solution of Saccharin, N. F.
Saccharin .... 512 grains.
Soda bicarb............... 240 grains.
Alcohol .... 4 fl. ounces.
Water, q. s., to make..... 16 fl. ounces.
Dissolve the saccharin and the soda bicarb in 10 fluid ounces of water; filter the solution; add the alcohol to the filtrate, and pass enough water through the filter to make 16 fluid ounces. Each fluid dram represents four grains of saccharin.

1776. Saccharin.
British Unofficial Formulary.
Saccharin .... 480 grains.
Bicarbonate of sodium.... 240 grains.
Alcohol .... 2½ fl. ounces.
Distilled water, q. s.
Rub the saccharin and bicarbonate of sodium in a mortar, with ½ pint of distilled water gradually added. When dissolved add the spirit; filter, and wash the filter with sufficient distilled water to produce 1 pint of elixir.
Each fluid dram contains 3 grains of saccharin.

1777. Cochineal Coloring.
Cochineal .... 1 ounce.
Potassium carbonate...... 1 ounce.
Potassium bitartrate...... 1 ounce.
Alum .... 1 ounce.
Water .... 14 ounces.
Boil till effervescence ceases; filter, and add water to make 16 fluid ounces, in which dissolve 16 ounces of sugar.

ELIXIRS OF CHLORIDES.

The Indiana Pharmacist comments upon the fad for the combining of chlorides or iodides into certain preparations, as elixirs, and offers a few formulas for those most called for (with a little modification and substitution of the iodide for the chloride the elixirs of the iodides can be made in the same manner)..

1778. Elixir One Chloride.
Corrosive sublimate....... 2 grains.
Water .... 8 ounces.
Syrup orange............. 8 ounces.
Dose: Teaspoonful after each meal.

1779. Elixir Two Chlorides.
Tincture chloride of iron.. 1 ounce.
Solution chloride of arsenic 2 drams.
Simple syrup, to make.... 16 ounces.
Dose: Teaspoonful after each meal.

1780. Elixir Three Chlorides.
Corrosive sublimate....... 3 grains.
Chloride of ammonia...... 2 ounces.
Solution chloride of arsenic 3 drams.
Simple syrup, to make.... 16 ounces.
Dose: Teaspoonful after each meal.

1781. Elixir Four Chlorides.
Corrosive sublimate....... 4 grains.
Solution chloride of arsenic 3 drams.
Hydrochloric acid, dilute.. 4 drams.
Tincture chloride of iron.. 8 drams.
Simple syrup, to make.... 16 ounces.

1782. Elixir Five Chlorides.
Corrosive sublimate....... 3 grains.
Solution chloride of arsenic 3 drams.
Hydrochloric acid, dilute.. 3 ounces.
Tincture iron chloride..... 3 ounces.
Ammonia chloride......... 3 ounces.
Simple syrup, to make.... 16 ounces.
Dose: Teaspoonful after each meal.

1783. Hoffman's Red Drops.

Gum camphor	¼ ounce.
Powd. capsicum	1 ounce.
Oil peppermint	¼ ounce.
Oil cassia	¼ ounce.
Alcohol	1 gallon.
Aniline red	5 grains.
Caramel	1 ounce.
Laudanum	1 pint.
Water	4 pints.

1784. Sedative Liquor.

Powd. black haw	2 ounces.
Water	8 ounces.
Alcohol	8 ounces.
Sulph. hydrastis	1 dram.
Water	2 ounces.
Sugar, color	⅛ ounce.
Fl. ext. Jam. dogwood	2 ounces.
Fl. ex. valerian (Eng.)	1 ounce.
Simple syrup	2 ounces.
Simple elixir, or elix. lact. pepsin, q. s., to make	1 quart.

Percolate the black haw with the 8 ounces of water and 8 ounces of alcohol; dissolve the hydrastis in the 2 ounces of water and mix all the ingredients, adding enough simple elixir or elixir of lactated pepsin to make up to 32 ounces.

1785. Solution of Ferric Salicylate.

A permanent solution of ferric salicylate may be made as follows:

Potassium citrate	2 drams.
Glycerine	1 ounce.
Ferric salicylate	80 grains.
Water, enough to make	4 ounces.

Dissolve the citrate in the glycerine with the aid of heat; add the salicylate of iron in small portions, stirring after each addition until dissolved, and lastly the water, also added gradually. Heat to boiling and filter while hot. The glycerine may be omitted, but if so, the solution will gradually precipitate. A solution thus prepared is of a deep brown color in bulk, lighter and transparent in thin layers, odorless and having a sweetish ferruginous taste. It contains 2½ grains of ferric salicylate to the teaspoonful, but the amount may be increased or decreased as desired.

1786. Improved Styptic Colloid.
Dr. Circular.

Collodion	100 parts.
Carbolic acid	10 parts.
Tannin	5 parts.
Benzoic acid (from the gum)	5 parts.

Mix the ingredients in the order above written until perfect solution is effected. This preparation has a brown color, and leaves, on evaporation, a strongly adherent pellicle. It instantly coagulates blood, forming a consistent clot, and a wound rapidly cicatrizes under its protection.

1787. Ioduretted Glycerin.

Iodine	48 grains.
Pot. Iodid	96 grains.
Aqua	2 drams.
Glycerin	4 ounces.

1788. Hall's Solution of Strychnine.

Pure crystals strychnine	16 grains.
Water	7½ fl. ounces.
Alcohol	7½ fl. ounces.
Acetic acid	½ fl. ounce.
Comp. tinct. cardamom	½ fl. ounce.
Mix for solution.	

Dose: Twenty to 30 drops once or twice a day.

1789. Solution for Storm Glass.

Ammon. chlor	30 grains.
Potass. nit	30 grains.
Camphor	30 grains.
Spt. vin. rect	1 ounce.
Aquae	1 ounce. 1 dram.

Weigh S. V. R. into bottle; add camphor and dissolve; then add other solids, lastly the water (warm); shake, and when dissolved, filter into the glass.

The above quantities are all by weight.

SOLUTIONS.

1790. Malate of Iron.
Am. Journ. Pharm.

Cranberry juice	14 fl. ounces.
Iron, in the form of fine wire and perfectly clean,	1 ounce.
Alcohol	2 fl. ounces.

The iron is added to the cranberry juice contained in a suitable vessel and set aside in a warm place, being occasionally agitated, for several days. It is then boiled for a half to one hour, adding water from time to time to replace the amount evaporated. Filter and wash the filter with sufficient water to yield 14 fluid ounces of filtrate, add the alcohol and again filter if necessary. This yields a reddish liquid of a slightly acid and not unpleasant ferruginous taste.

Solution of Bromides Compound, to Replace Bromidia.

1791.

Bromide of potash	40 ounces.
Chloral hydrate crystals	40 ounces.
Fl. ext. cannabis ind	1 ounce.
Fl. ext. hyoscyamus	1 ounce.
Simple elixir	2 pints.
Hot water	7 pints.
Chloroform water, q. s., to make	10 pints.

Dissolve the bromide of potash and chloral hydrate in the hot water; mix the fluid extracts with the simple elixir, and add; make up to 10 pints with chloroform water. The latter is made by agitating 60 minims of chloroform with 25 ounces of distilled water in a gallon bottle. Shake vigorously until the chloroform is dissolved in the water. The water contains ½ per cent of chloroform.

1792. Hydrangea, Lithiated.

Fluid ext. of Hydrangea	2½ fl. ounces.
Tinct. valerianate ammonia	½ fl. ounce.
Benzoate of lithia	256 grains.
Carbonate of lithia	128 grains.
Alcohol, 188 per-cent	2 ounces.
Caramel	1 dram.
Distilled water, q. s. to make up to	16 ounces.

1793. Solution of Cocaine, Four Per Cent.

Cocaine	73 grains.
Glycerine	½ fl. ounce.
Water, distilled	3½ fl. ounces.

For methods and tables for percentage solutions, see number 1771.

1794. Solution of Magnesia Cit., Improved Era.

Citric acid (crystals)	1 dram.
Sulphate of magnesia	1 ounce.
Simple syrup	8 fl. ounces.
Ext. of lemon	10 drops.
Bicarb of potash (crystals)	2 scruples.
Water, q. s., to make	12 fl. ounces.

Place the acid and epsom salts together in a 12-ounce citrate of magnesia bottle, and add simple syrup and extract of lemon; agitate for a moment and add the water, and lastly the bicarb of potash, and cork immediately.

1795. Household Ammonia.

Hot water	1 gallon.
Sal. soda	2 pounds.
Aqua ammonia, 16°	2 pints.

When the sal. soda is dissolved and the solution is cold, add the aqua ammonia.

1796. Liquor Potassa.

Carbonate of potash	1 pound.
Slaked lime	12 ounces.
Distilled water	1 gallon.

Dissolve the carbonate of potash in the water, and having heated the solution to the boiling point, in a clean iron vessel, gradually mix with it the slaked lime and continue the boiling for ten minutes with constant stirring; then remove the vessel from the fire; when cool, put into a large bottle and when settled down decant off into 1 pound glass stoppered bottles.

1797. Liquor Ferro-Mangani-Peptonati.

Iron peptonate (25 p. c. iron)	24.0 grams.
Liquid manganese glucosate (2 p. c. manganese)	50.0 grams.
Sol. soda, s. g. 1.170	10.0 grams.
Syrup	200.0 grams.
Alcohol, 90 p. c.	100.0 grams.
Tinct. orange	3.0 grams.
Aromatic tincture	1.5 grams.
Tinct. vanilla	1.5 grams.
Acetic ether	5 drops.
Water, distilled, enough.	

Dissolve the iron peptonate in 200 grams of hot water; allow to cool, then add first the syrup, next the soda solution, and then 90 grams of distilled water, whereby the precipitate, previously formed, is redissolved. To the manganese glucosate add a few drops of soda solution, to render faintly but distinctly alkaline, and add this to the preceding solution. Finally add 320 grams of distilled water, then the alcohol, and lastly the flavors.

This preparation contains 0.6 per-cent of metallic iron and 0.1 per cent of manganese. Its reaction is alkaline.

1798. Liquor Ferri Peptonati.

Iron peptonate in scales, containing 25 p. c. of iron	24.0 grams.
Water, boiling	200.0 grams.
Syrup	200.0 grams.
Solution soda (G. P.) dilute (1 + 9)	100.0 grams.
Water distilled	370.0 grams.
Alcohol, 90 p. c.	100.0 grams.
Tinct. orange peel	3.0 grams.
Tinct. aromatic (G. P.)	1.5 grams.
Tinct. vanilla (G. P.)	1.5 grams.
Acetic ether	5 drops.

Dissolve the iron peptonate in the boiling water; allow to cool; add the syrup; then gradually add the soda solution, when a precipitate forms, but which will be redissolved. To the clear solution add the remainder of the ingredients. The finished preparation is of alkaline reaction and contains 0.6 per-cent of metallic iron.

It is obvious that the percentage of iron peptonate may be changed as well as the flavoring ingredients, to suit requirements, and in this connection attention is called to the stock solutions of the National Formulary for preparing aromatic elixirs.

1799. Dieterich's Solution Peptonated Iron.

Dried egg albumen	1 part.
Pepsin, pure	0.05 part.
Solution of oxychloride of iron (Germ. Pharm.)	12 parts.
Syrup	3 parts.
Brandy	10 parts.
Distilled water	100 parts.

Dissolve the egg albumen in 19 parts of distilled water, add the pepsin and digest during four hours at 40° C. (104° F.). On the other hand, mix the iron solution with the syrup and 55 parts of distilled water. Mix this liquid with the solution of the peptonized albumen, and heat the whole in a steam-bath to 90-96° C. Then allow it to cool; add the brandy; finally, enough water to make 100 parts. Let the mixture stand during eight days, then pour off the clear solution from the insignificant sediment.

1800. Fowler's Solution, New Method.

Carb. of potash	37 grains.
Arsenious acid, powdered	37 grains.
Dilute alcohol	1 ounce.
Co. tincture of lavender	2 drams.
Water, distilled, q. s., to make	8 ounces.

Dissolve the carbonate of potash in two drams of the distilled water; add the arsenious acid in powder and dissolve. Mix the co. tincture of lavender with the dilute alcohol and five ounces of distilled water, and then add the solution of arsenic and potash; filter. Make up to 8 fluid ounces with distilled water.

1801. Donovan's Solution. U. S.

Iodide of arsenic	37 grains.
Iodide of mercury, red	37 grains.
Distilled water, q. s., to measure	8 ounces.

Triturate the iodides with a half ounce of water until dissolved; filter, and pass enough water through the filter to make the solution measure 8 fluid ounces.

COD LIVER OIL PREPARATIONS, ETC.

Cod Liver Oil Emulsion (50 Per Cent) with Hypophosphites.
1802.

Soap bark, rough ground	1½ ounces.
Irish moss, white, picked	1½ ounces.

Boil the soap bark in a quart of water; boil down to 15 ounces; filter and set aside.
Boil the Irish moss in a quart of water down to 15 ounces; strain.

Hypophosphite of calcium	1024 grains.
Hypophosphite of sodium	1024 grains.
Hypophosphite of potass	512 grains.
Salicylic acid	½ dram.
Glycerine	2 ounces.
Solution of saccharin	1 dram.
Oil of wintergreen	1 dram.
Oil of bitter almonds	½ dram.
Cod liver oil	31 ounces.

Dissolve the hypophosphites in the decoction of soap bark and mix with the mucilage of Irish moss; place in an emulsifying machine with the saccharine solution.

Mix the essential oils with the cod liver oil and add slowly to the above, working the emulsifier rapidly. Dissolve the salicylic acid in the glycerine and add to the other ingredients.

Work the emulsion well for 10 minutes. This emulsion contains 5 grains of hypophosphites to the teaspoonful.

1803. Cod Liver Oil Emulsion (33 Per Cent).

Soap bark, rough ground	3 ounces.
Irish moss, white picked	3 ounces.

Boil the soap bark in a half gallon of water; boil down to 30 ounces; filter and set aside.
Boil the Irish moss in a half gallon of water down to 30 ounces, strain.

Cod liver oil	32 ounces.
Oil of wintergreen	2 drams.
Oil of bitter almonds	1 dram.
Glycerine	4 ounces.
Salicylic acid	1 dram.
Solution of saccharin	1 dram.

Add the solution of saccharin to the decoction of soap bark and mix with the mucilage of Irish moss; place in an emulsifying machine.

Mix the essential oils with the cod liver oil and add slowly to the above; working the emulsifier rapidly.

Dissolve the salicylic acid in the glycerine and add to the other ingredients.

Work the emulsion well for 10 minutes. Extract of malt, extract of beef; hypophosphites, celery, coca, kola, jamaica rum, or other tonics and invigorators may be added to the above as required.

NON-SECRET FORMULAS.

1804. Cod Liver Oil Emulsion (with Gums).
Gum arabic .... 12 ounces.
Gum tragacanth. .... 4 ounces.
Cod liver, oil Norwegian.. 50 ounces.
Oil of wintergreen .... 2 drams.
Oil of bitter almonds...... 1 dram.
Solution of saccharine..... 2 drams.
Distilled water .... 96 ounces.
Hypophosphite of lime..... 2 ounces.
Hypophosphite of soda ... 2 ounces.
Chloride of sodium........ 1 ounce.
Salicylic acid .... 2 drams.
Glycerine .... 4 ounces.

Mix the esential oils with the cod liver oil.

Make a mucilage of the gums with a portion of the water; place in an emulsifying machine and slowly add the oils; stirring rapidly.

Dissolve the hypophosphites and chloride of sodium in another portion of the water and add; dissolve the salicylic acid in the glycerine; add the solution of saccharine and mix well for at least ten minutes.

1805. Cremor Morrhuæ.
Cod liver oil .... 6 ounces.
The yolk of 1 egg.
Tragacanth (in powder)... 10 grains.
Elixir of saccharin .... 30 minims.
Simple tincture of benzoin. 45 minims.
Spirit of chloroform ...... 3 drams.
Flavoring oils .... 12 minims.
Distilled water to .... 12 ounces.

Measure 4 ounces of the water, triturate the tragacanth with a little of the oil, then add the yolk of egg, and stir briskly, adding water as the mixture thickens. When of a suitable consistence, add the remainder of the oil and water alternately, with constant stirring, avoiding frothing. Transfer to a pint bottle, add the other ingredients, previously mixed, shake well and add distilled water, if necessary, to make the product measure 12 ounces.

1806. Extract of Malt and Cod Liver Oil.
(Ch. & Dr.)
Cod liver oil ..... 8 ounces by measure.
Extract of malt .. 8 ounces by weight.
Yolks of 2 eggs
Pulv. tragac. ver. .... 16 grains.
Aqua fervens. .... 1 ounce.
Ess. limonis opt. .... 10 minims.
Ess. amygd. amarae ...... 10 minims.

Weigh the extract of malt in a half-pint graduate, and add the aqua ferv. to thin it, stirring quickly; beat up the two yolks in a large mortar with the pulv. tragac., and add the oil and extract alternately, lastly the ess. lemon and almonds.

1807. Aromatic Cod Liver Oil. A
Cod liver oil .... 1,000 parts.
Lemon oil .... 5 parts.
Oil of neroli .... 2 parts.
English peppermint oil..... 1 part.
Vanillin .... 0.1 part.
Coumarin .... 0.01 part.

Dissolve the last two ingredients in the essential oils by the aid of a gentle heat, and mix the solution with the cod liver oil.

1808. Iodo-Ferrated Cod Liver Oil. A
Iron, in fine powder....... 2 parts.
Iodine .... 4 parts.
Ether .... 10 parts.
Cod liver oil to make...... 1,000 parts.

Rub the iron, iodine, ether, and 40 parts of cod liver oil together until a black mixture results, then add sufficient cod liver oil to make 1,000 parts by weight.—Dieterich's Manual.

1809. Aromatic Cod Liver Oil. B
Chloroform .... 6 minims.
Ol. cinnamom .... 8 minims.
Ol. morrhuae .... 20 ounces.
M.

1810. Cod Liver Oil Emulsion.
Ol. morrhuae .... 10 ounces.
Ol. cinnam. .... 5 minims.
Pulv. acaciae .... 2 ounces.
Liq. calc. sacch. .... ½ dram.
Aq. .... 5 ounces.

Mix the oils with the powdered gum in a large mortar, and add all at once the liquor and water previously mixed. Stir briskly until a crackling emulsion is obtained, then add the following solution gradually, and with constant stirring:

Elixir. saccharin .... 1½ drams.
Ess. vanillae .... 10 minims.
Spt. chloroformi .... 2 drams.
Sodii hyphosphit. .... 2 scruples.
Calcii hypophos.......... 1 scruple.
Aq. flor. aurant. .... 1 ounce.
Aq. ad .... 4 ounces.

The whole should measure 20 ounces. Oil of wintergreen 3 minims may replace the essence of vanilla if desired.

1811. Iodized Cod Liver Oil. B
Cod liver oil .... 8 ounces.
Oil of bitter almonds ..... 5 drops.
Oil of wintergreen .... 5 drops.
Powdered iodide of iron .. 2 drams.

Finely powder the iodide and mix with the oil; warm on a water bath and strain.

NON-SECRET FORMULAS.

1812. Cod Liver Oil with Rock and Rye.
Gaduol (Merck's)	32 grains.
Alcohol	1 ounce.
Rye whisky	11 ounces.
Rock candy syrup	4 ounces.

Dissolve the gaduol in the alcohol and add to the rye whisky; then add the rock candy syrup.

1813. Wine of Cod Liver Oil.
Gaduol (Merck's)	32 grains.
Alcohol, 188 per cent	1 ounce.
Port wine	13 ounces.
Simple elixir, red, q. s. to make	16 ounces.
Magnesia carbonate	¼ ounce.

Dissolve the gaduol in the alcohol and add to the carbonate of magnesia in a mortar; triturate well, slowly adding the wine; filter; and add simple elixir q. s. to measure 16 ounces.

1814. Cod Liver Oil Mixture.
It makes a really delicious emulsion:
Yolks of 2 eggs	
Powdered sugar	4 ounces.
Essence oil almonds	2 drops.
Orange flower water	2 ounces.

Mix carefully, and add an equal bulk of cod liver oil.—Heder.

1815. Petroleum Emulsion.
Oil of sweet almonds	3 ounces.
Pure white petrolatum or vaseline	5 ounces.
Mucilage of dextrin (1 in 3)	5 ounces.
Syrup of tolu	2 ounces.
Lemon, rose, or almond essence	q. s.
Water to	16 ounces.

Mix.

Place the mucilage in a warm mortar; melt together the oil and petrolatum, and, while still warm, add gradually to the mucilage, ensuring that each portion is thoroughly incorporated before adding the next; lastly, add flavoring, syrup, and water q. s.

1816. Phosphorus Butter.
Fresh butter	17½ ounces.
Potassium iodide	4 grains.
Potassium bromide	15 grains.
Sodium chloride	2 drams.
Phosphorus	1-7 grain.

About one-third of an ounce is to be taken daily, spread on bread.

This is proposed as a substitute for cod liver oil in hot weather.—Bulletin of Pharmacy.

1817. Emulsion of Petroleum with Hypophosphites. A
(McDonnell.)
Paraffin oil (liquid petrolatum)	16 ounces.
Acacia	8 ounces.
Glycerin	4 ounces.
Calcium hypophosphite..(?)	256 grains.
Sodium hypophosphite...(?)	256 grains.
Water enough to make	48 fl. ounces.

Add the acacia to the oil and mix thoroughly (in a large mortar), then add one pint of water (all at once) and rub briskly until the emulsion is formed. Dissolve the hypophosphites in a half pint of water, to which add the glycerin; then add all the emulsion and rub well together—and any water necessary to make up the measure of three pints of finished product.

1818. Emulsion of Petroleum with Hypophosphites. B
Liquid petrolatum	4 ounces.
Oil of sweet almonds	2 ounces.
Powdered acacia	1½ ounces.
Glycerin	1½ ounces.
Hypophosphite of sodium	128 grains.
Hypophosphite of calcium	128 grains.
Lime water enough to make	1 pint.

This is made up in a way similar to the preceding.

The addition of suitable flavoring material might improve these preparations somewhat.

1819. Tasteless Cod Liver Oil.
Western Druggist.
Fl. ext. wild cherry	2 fl. ounces.
Fl. ext. licorice	3 fl. ounces.
Glycerin	1 fl. ounce.
Syrup	1 fl. ounce.
Liquid ext. malt	6 fl. ounces.
Syrup hypophosphites	3 fl. ounces
Gaduol	64 grains.
Fuller's earth	4 drams.
Caramel as desired.	

Mix the gaduol with the glycerin, and triturate with the fuller's earth; add the fluid extracts, syrup and malt, shake well and let stand one day, ocasionally shaking, filter, and to the filtrate add the syrup hypophosphites, and mix well.

1820. Castor Oil Emulsion. A
Era.
Castor oil	4 troy ounces.
Powdered gum arabic	1 troy ounce.
Distilled water	1½ troy ounces.
Cinnamon water	3 fl. ounces.

Syrup .... 3 fl. ounces.
Spirit of cinnamon ..... 12 minims.
Emulsify the oil with the gum and distilled water, then add the other ingredients with constant trituration. This emulsion contains 83 per cent of castor oil.

1821. Castor Oil Emulsion. B
Castor oil .... 1 fl. ounce.
Powdered acacia .... 3 drams.
Oil bitter almonds ..... 2 minims.
Oil cloves .... 1 minim.
Saccharin .... 1 grain.
Water to make .... 4 fl. ounces.

Mix the oil with the gum in a dry mortar, add one-half fl. ounce of water at once, stirring until emulsion is formed. Then add the saccharin, previously dissolved in water by the aid of one-half grain sodium bicarbonate, and finally the remainder of the water.

CHLORODYNES AND ANODYNES.

1822. Chandler's Chlorodyne.
Muriate of morphia ..... 8 grains.
Fl. ext. of cannabis indica. 30 minims.
Oil of peppermint ...... 10 drops.
Tincture of capsicum ... 15 drops.
Chloroform .... 2 drams.
Alcohol .... 1 ounce.
Glycerine .... 1 ounce.
Mix.
Dose: Ten to thirty drops in a wineglass of water.

1823. Chlorodyne Clear.
Chloroform .... 2 fl. ounces.
Ether .... ½ fl. ounce.
Alcohol (95 per cent)... 7 fl. ounces.
Essence of peppermint .. 6 fl drams.
Tinct. of capsicum ..... 6 fl drams.
Tinct. cardamom comp. .. 2 fl. ounces.
Fl. ext. of licorice ... 2 fl. ounces.
Hydrocyanic acid, diluted.. 1 fl. ounce.
Glycerine .... 16 fl. ounces.
Sulphate of morphia .... 40 grains.

1824. Chlorodyne.
The following formula is from Baily's Physician's Pharmacopoeia:
Hydrochlorate of morphia.. 4 grains.
Chloroform .... 48 minims.
Rectified ether .... 32 minims.
Rectified spirit .... 32 minims.
Dilute hydrocyanic acid. 32 minims.
Tincture of Indian hemp .. 32 minims.
Tincture of capsicum ... 24 minims.
Oil of peppermint, English. 3 minims.
Hydrochloric acid, pure. 4 minims.
Powdered tragacanth .... 2 grains.
Molasses, dark green ... 3 drams.
Distilled water, to .... 1 ounce.

1825. Dr. Brown's Chlorodyne.
Concentrated muriatic acid 5 parts.
Ether .... 10 parts.
Chloroform .... 10 parts.
Tincture of cannabis indica
(Indian hemp) .... 10 parts.
Tincture of capsicum ... 10 parts.
Morphine .... 2 parts.
Hydrocyanic acid .... 2 parts.
Oil of peppermint ...... 1 part.
Simple syrup .... 50 parts.
Tincture of hyoscyamus. 3 parts.
Tincture of aconite .... 3 parts.

1826. Chlorodyne.
Muriate of morphia ..... 64 grains.
Chloroform .... 4 ounces.
Glycerine .... 4 ounces.
Fl. ext. cannabis ind... 4 ounces.
Hydrocyanic acid dil. U. S. 2 drams.
Oil of peppermint ...... ½ dram.
Tinct. of capsicum ..... 6 drams.
Alcohol, 188 per cent to
make up to .... 16 fl. ounces.

1827. Anæsthetic Solution.
Hydrochlorate cocaine .. 2 drams.
Chloral hydrate .... 1 dram.
Carbolic acid .... ½ dram.
Chloroform .... ½ dram.
Glycerine .... 3 ounces.
Water .... 3 ounces.
Water for rinsing, filter.. ½ ounce.
Mix the carbolic acid and glycerine.
Mix the chloral hydrate and the chloroform.
Dissolve the cocaine in the water; mix all together and filter; after filtration has ceased, run half an ounce of distilled water through the filter. This solution contains 4 per cent of cocaine.

1828. Anodyne for Dentists. A
Cocaine .... 40 grains.
Sulph. ether conc. ..... 1 ounce.
Oil of peppermint ...... 1 ounce.
Dissolve the cocaine in the ether and add the oil of peppermint.

1829. Anodyne for Dentists. B

Cocaine	18 grains.
Menthol	60 grains.
Oil of cloves	2 drams.
Sulph. ether q. s. to make up to	1 fl. ounce.

1830. Dental Obtundent.

The following formula for a local obtundent has not the advantage of being a secret preparation; it has no one to publish quack certificates in its favor, and there is no liar, gifted as such by nature and perfected by constant practice, to vaunt its merits. In all other respects it is quite equal, if not superior, to any of the nostrums now offered by every alternate cross-roads dentists to a long-suffering profession.

Atropiae	1-10 grain.
Stropanthii	1-5 grain.
Cocaine mur.	50 grains.
Acidi carbolici	10 grains.
Ol. carophylli	3 minims.
Aquae destillatae	1 ounce.
M.	

Each of the ingredients is composed for a special purpose. The first is a narcotic and antispasmodic. The second is a heart tonic. The third is of course that on which the preparation solely depends for its anaesthetic action. The fourth is an antiseptic, preserves the preparation from decomposition, and perhaps adds to its anaesthetic properties. The fifth is also an antiseptic and slightly anaesthetic. It might be left out of the compound without seriously changing its character. The sixth is simply the diluent. The formula contains everything that can be useful in a cocaine preparation.—Dental Practitioner.

MISCELLANEOUS.

1831. Hall's Infant Colic Mixture.

Tincture of assafoetida	15 drops.
Tincture of cinnamon	½ ounce.
Soda carbonate	1 grain.
Aromatic syrup of rhubarb	3 drams.
Water	1½ ounces.
Mix.	

Dose: One teaspoonful.

1832. Children's Cough Syrup.

Ammonia muriate	32 grains.
Potash chlorate	1 scruple.
Tincture of aconite	15 drops.
Syrup of Dover's powder	2½ drams.
Syrup of tolu q. s. to make up to	2 ounces.
Mix.	

Dose: One teaspoonful every 3 hours.

1833. Dysentery Cure.

Claret wine, good quality.	1 bottle.
Rhubarb, ground	½ ounce.
Cassia bark, ground	½ ounce.
Allspice, ground	½ ounce.

Boil down to three-fourths; strain.
Adult dose: One wineglassful 3 times a day.

1834. Godfrey's Cordial.

Salts of tartar	2½ ounces.
Water	26 pints.
Molasses (sugar house)	2 gallons.
Oil of sassafras	½ ounce.
Alcohol, 188 per cent.	2 pints.
Laudanum	1½ pints.

Mix the oil with the alcohol, dissolve the salts of tartar in the water and add all the ingredients to the molasses. Mix well.

1835. Godfrey's Cordial (without Opium).

Sodii brom.	1 dram.
Sodii carb.	1 dram.
Ol. sassafras	4 minims.
Ol. anisi	3 minims.
Spt. chloroformi	2 drams.
Spt. rectificat.	½ ounce.
Tr. hyoscyam.	½ ounce.
Molasses	½ pound.
Aq. ad	16 ounces.

Dissolve the oils in the spirits, and add the tincture. Dissolve the soda salts in the water, and mix with the treacle. To this add the spirit mixture, shake well, and after four days decant the clear portion.

1836. Godfrey's Cordial.

There are various formulae for this preparation. Paris says the following was obtained from a wholesale druggist, who makes and sells many hundred dozen bottles a year:
Infuse

Sassafras	9 ounces.
Caraway	1 ounce.
Coriander	1 ounce.
Aniseed	1 ounce.
Water	6 pints.

Simmer till the liquid is reduced to 4 pints, add

Treacle	6 pounds.

And boil the whole for a few minutes; when cold add

Tincture of opium	3 ounces.

1837. Bateman's Drops. N. F.

Tincture of opium	320 minims.
Tincture of catechu co.	240 minims.
Spirit of camphor	300 minims.

Oil of anise .... 8 minims.
Caramel .... 120 minims.
Diluted alcohol q. s. to
 make .... 16 fl. ounces.
Mix.
Each fluid dram contains 2½ minims of tincture of opium.

1838. Paregoric.
Alcohol, 188 per cent ..... 1 gallon.
Oil of anise .... 1 ounce.
Gum camphor .... ¾ ounce.
Benzoic acid .... 1 ounce.
Water .... 1 gallon.
Laudanum .... 1 pint.
Caramel and red sanders, q. s.

1839. To Prepare Decoctions.
For making decoctions the substances, if dry, should be well bruised, or reduced to a very coarse powder, or, if fresh and soft, they should be sliced small. In the former case, any very fine powder or adhering dust should be removed with a sieve, as its presence would tend to make the product thick and disagreeable, and also more troublesome to strain. The vessel in which the boiling is conducted should be closely covered, the better to exclude the air; and the heat should be so regulated that the fluid may be kept simmering, or only gently boiling, as violent boiling is both unnecessary and injurious. In every case the liquor should be strained while hot, but not boiling; and the best method of doing this is to employ a fine hair sieve or a coarse flannel bag. In preparing compound decoctions, those ingredients should be boiled first which impart their active principles least readily, and those which most readily impart them should be added afterward. In many cases it will be proper simply to infuse the more aromatic substances in the hot decoctions of the other ingredients, by which means their volatile principles will be preserved. When the active principles of the principal ingredients are volatile, infusion should be had recourse to, instead of boiling.

Strength of.—Decoctions of substances not exerting a very powerful influence on the system may be made, as a general rule, by boiling an ounce, if dry, or a handful, if green, in a pint of water for ten or fifteen minutes.

Dose of.—The ordinary dose of decoctions thus prepared is a half to a wineglassful three or four times daily, or more frequently.

1840. Specific Gravity.
To Convert Degrees Baume into Specific Gravity.—1. For liquids heavier than water.—Subtract the degree of Baume from 145, and divide into 145. The quotient is the specific gravity.

2. For liquids lighter than water.—Add the degree of Baume to 130, and divide it into 140. The quotient is the specific gravity.

To Convert Specific Gravity into Degrees (Baume).—1. For liquids heavier than water.—Divide the specific gravity into 145, and subtract from 145. The remainder is the degree of Baume.

2. For liquids lighter than water.—Divide the specific gravity into 140, and subtract 130 from the quotient. The remainder will be the degree of Baume.

Comparison of Degrees Twaddell and specific Gravity.—In order to change degrees Twaddell into specific gravity, multiply by 5, add 1,000, and divide by 1,000.

Example.—Change 168° Twaddell into specific gravity.

$$\frac{168 \times 5}{840} $$
$$\frac{840}{1,000}$$
$$1,000) 1,840$$

1.84, specific gravity.

To change specific gravity into degrees Twaddell, multiply by 1,000, subtract 1,000, and divide by 5.

Example.—Change 1.84 specific gravity to degrees Twaddell.

$$1.84 \times 1,000$$
$$\frac{1,840}{1,000}$$
$$5) 840$$
$$168° \text{ Tw.}$$

1841. To Pack Chemicals and Drugs for Export.
The following suggestions will be found of practical value: 1. Salts should be put in stoppered glass bottles or packed in casks, if sent in large quantities. Casks used for hygroscopic salts should be lined with oil cloth or parchment paper. Salts should never be packed in tin boxes or in paper only.

2. The glass stoppers of all bottles containing either liquids or dry substances should be greased with a little vaseline in order to avoid any difficulty in removing them.

3. Parts of plants, such as leaves, roots, etc., should be packed in sacks, and these again in cases; very delicate drugs in tin boxes. Vegetable powders should be packed in hermetically closed glass bottles or tin boxes. Drugs which occupy much space should be pressed as much as possible before being packed, especially if the shipping

freight is calculated according to the bulk of the goods.

4. Boxes and cases should be lined with zinc, or where this is too expensive a strong and good oil cloth will usually be sufficient.

5. Although the utmost care is necessary in packing, yet packing materials, such as hay, straw, etc., should be used as sparingly as possible, as duty has usually to be paid for the weight of these as well as for the goods themselves.

6. Cases should be secured by iron bands, and it is always desirable that the weight and volume of cases should be as small as possible.

7. Acids, caustic or inflammable substances, must be packed according to the regulations of the different railways by which they are transmitted prior to shipment. As a rule stone bottles are best for acids and ammonia and glass or tin vessels for volatile substances. All these should be closed by corks saturated with paraffine, and then wrapped in sail cloth, which, with the string securing it, should also be soaked in paraffine.

8. Acetic acid may be safely conveyed from place to place in carboys of 5 to 10 gallons capacity.

9. Liquor ammonia should never be put into iron vessels.

10. Vessels containing volatile substances should never be quite filled.

11. As acids and caustic and inflammable substances are conveyed on the decks of sailing vessels only, the cases containing them should be well closed, and the address, mark, number, etc., be such as will resist sea water.

12. Liquids should not be packed in the same case with dry substances.

13. Valuable or expensive chemicals, such as ethereal oils and essences, should be packed in strong tin vessels and closed with corks saturated with paraffine as before described.

14. The weights and measures of the country to which the goods are sent should always be used, to avoid loss and inconvenience.

15. Besides observing these rules for packing, consignors of goods should be thoroughly acquainted with the customs, tariffs and regulations of the countries to which they are sending, as pecuniary loss and inconvenience may occur, from ignorance of them. For instance, if a case contains various substances, the duties on which are different, it is usual in some tariffs to calculate the duty of the whole of the contents of the case or at least of the packing materials at the highest rate. The importance of packing together goods upon which the customs tariffs are similar is self-evident from this.

16. In cases of urgency small quantities of any substance suitable for such transmission, e. g., quinine, antipyrine, salicylic acid, etc., may be sent as patterns without value, and thus avoid the delay caused by the customs office.

1842. Preserving Anatomical Specimens for a Private Museum.

Bones and skulls may be prepared by boiling them for some hours in water containing potash, which process, I know from experience gained in preserving specimens for my own museum, quickly causes the flesh to become detached. Another way is to carefully remove the flesh with dissecting apparatus, and then to place the specimens in weak brine, in order to draw away any blood from the bones; next wash them in fresh water, and lay them out to dry. Gullets, stomachs, windpipes and intestines may also be put into weak brine and then dried. At sea, in the case of the albatross, I have preserved these objects by simply cleaning them, blowing them out, making fast the ends with a clove hitch, and hanging up to dry. A coat of varnish will finish them off. All soft parts should be preserved in proof alcohol. Fishes and reptiles should be preserved whole in it, having first made very carefully an incision in the under part to facilitate the introduction of the spirit; or, if at its full strength, it would harden the exterior and not reach the entrails. Neglecting to make these incisions results, I have frequently found, in the putrefaction of the internals. With large specimens the natural juices quickly weaken the spirit, which should be added to until it keeps its strength. The one great advantage of alcoholic specimens is, that at any time they can be removed from the preserving jars and examined in their entirety. On no account should they be allowed to come into close contact with the sides of the glass or jar, and they should invariably be suspended by a strong thread, the end of which should not protrude above the cork or stopper.—C. L. Wragge, in English Mechanic.

1843. Preparations for Preserving Specimens.

1. Nearly saturate water with sulphurous acid and add a little creasote.

2. Dissolve chloride of lime, 4 parts, in water 100 parts, to which 3 per cent of hydrochloric acid has been added.

3. Dissolve corrosive sublimate, 1 part, and sodium chloride, 3 parts, in water, 100 parts, to which 2 per cent of hydrochloric acid has been added.

4. Babington's: 1 pint wood naphtha, 7 pints water.

5. Burnett's: 1 pound zinc chloride, 1 gallon water; immerse for 2 to 4 days, and then dry in the air.

6. Morrell's: 14 ounces arsenious acid, 7 ounces caustic soda, 20 fluid ounces water, and sufficient carbolic acid to produce opalescence when the mixture is stirred; add water to make up to 100 fluid ounces. Used for general disinfecting and embalming purposes.

7. Muller's: 2 to 2½ ounces bichromate of potash, 1 ounce soda sulphate; add water to make up to 100 fluid ounces.

8. Mix ammonia with 3 times its weight of water and rectified spirit.

9. Ammonium chloride, 1 part; water 10 or 11 parts. For muscular parts of animals: zinc sulphate, 1 part; water, 15 to 25 parts. Used for muscles and cerebral masses.

10. Passini's: 1 ounce mercury chloride, 2 ounces sodium chloride, 13 ounces glycerine, 113 fluid ounces distilled water.

11. Reboulet's: 1 ounce saltpeter, 2 ounces alum, 4 ounces calcium chloride, in 16 to 20 fluid ounces water; dilute according to need.

12. Seseman's: Dr. Seseman states that a corpse may be made to retain the natural form of expression for months by:

13. Injecting into it a solution consisting of 4 to 5 per cent of aluminum chloride dissolved in a mixture of 2 parts alcohol of 90 per cent and 1 part glycerine; or

14. Painting the entire epidermis with vaseline. The quantity of liquid required for injection is in the proportion of 1-10 to 1-7 of the weight of the corpse.

15. Thwaites': 1 ounce spirit of wine saturated with creasote, rubbed up with chalk into a thin paste, and 16 ounces water gradually added.

16. Von Vetter's: 7 ounces glycerine at 36° Tw. (22° B.), 1 ounce raw brown sugar, and ½ ounce niter; immerse for some days.

17. Gannel's: Sodium chloride and alum, of each ½ pound; niter, ½ pound; water, 1 gallon.

18. Goadsby's: Bay salt, 2 ounces; alum, 1 ounce; mercury bichloride, 1 grain; water, 1 pint, 4 ounces.

19. Bay salt, ¼ pound; bichloride of mercury, 1 grain; water, 20 fluid ounces.

20. Bay salt, ¼ pound; arsenious acid, 10 grains; water, 20 fluid ounces. Dissolve by heat.

21. To the last add 1 grain bichloride of mercury.

22. Stapleton's: Niter, 1 dram; alum, 2¼ ounces; water, 1 quart. For pathological specimens.

23. Beasley's (for feathers): Strychnia, 16 grains; rectified spirit, 1 pint.

1844. Preserving Natural History Specimens.

1. When ready, wipe the fish and place it in the following solution, and it will keep for years if good alcohol be used: Alcohol (95 per cent), 8 parts; distilled water, 2 parts.

2. If the fish are small, three or four days suffice to harden them and the following is a better solution for them, viz.: Alcohol, 6 parts, distilled water, 2 parts. Reptiles, rodentia, etc., can be also preserved in the same manner. The first alcoholic bath can be used over and over again for the same purpose, if strained.

3. Take of chloral, in crystals, one ounce, and dissolve it in five ounces of distilled water; alcohol (95 per cent), 1½ ounces; glycerine, 1½ drams; rock salt, 15 grains; saltpeter, 30 grains. Dissolve the glycerine, salt, and saltpeter in the alcohol, and when well mixed add to the chloral solution, shake well till thoroughly incorporated, filter, and it is ready for use.

4. The following solution for larvae of insects, spiders, and other small, delicate objects, will be found very valuable: Glycerine, 1 ounce, common salt, 1 dram; saltpeter, 1 dram; distilled water, 8 ounces. Mix well together. When wanted for use, take two ounces of pure alcohol, and add one ounce of the mixture; shake well and filter.

5. For the preservation of tadpoles, young frogs, salamanders, and similar objects, take 1 pound sulphate of zinc, 2 drams burnt alum and mix well together.—Sci. Am.

1845. Fluid for Anatomical Preparations.

(Objects of natural history, etc.)

1. Saturate water with sulphurous acid, and add a little creasote.

2. Dissolve 4 parts of chloride of tin in 100 parts of water, to which 3 per cent of muriatic acid has been added.

3. Dissolve 5 or 6 parts of corrosive sublimate in 100 of water, to which 2 per cent of muriatic acid has been added.

4. Mix together one part of ammonia water (strong) with three times its weight (each) of water and spirit of wine.

Remarks.—These fluids are used by immersing the objects therein, in close vessels. The third formula is apt to render animal substances very hard.—Cooley.

5. To preserve anatomical specimens, immerse in a saturated solution of 100 parts alum with 2 parts saltpeter. The article at first loses color, but regains it again in a few days, when it is removed from the liquid and kept in a saturated solution of alum and water only.

1846. To Preserve Soft and Delicate Animals.
(Carpenter.)
Glycerine, 1 part; alcohol, 1 part; 8 to 10 parts sea water.

1847. Preservative for Insects and Animal Tissues.
Glycerine, alcohol, distilled water, equal parts.

1848. To Preserve Insects.
1. Laboulbene recommends for the preservation of insects in a fresh state plunging them in a preservative fluid consisting of alcohol with an excess of arsenious acid in fragments; 1½ pints alcohol will take about 14 troy grains of arsenic. The living insect, put into this preparation, absorbs about 3-1000 of its own weight. When soaked in this liquor and dried, it will be safe from the ravages of moths, Anthrenus or Dermestes. This liquid will not change the colors of blue, green or red beetles if dried after soaking from twelve to twenty-four hours. Hemiptera and Orthoptera can be treated in the same way. The nests, cocoons, and chrysalids of insects may be preserved from injury from other insects by being soaked in the arseniated alcohol, or dipped into benzine or a solution of carbolic acid or creasote.

2. For spiders, puncture them and steep for several days in a strong alcoholic solution of pure phenol, and then in dilute alcoholic glycerine. Or use a saturated solution of salicylic acid in glycerine; dry carefully.

1849. Preparations for Taxidermy.
Arsenical soap. White arsenic, 2 pounds; white soap, 2 pounds; sugar in powder, 12 ounces; salt of tartar, 12 ounces; chalk in powder, 6 ounces; camphor, 5 ounces. Slice the soap and melt in an earthen vessel, with water, over a gentle fire, keeping it stirred with a wooden spatula. When melted, put in the sugar, salt of tartar, and chalk. Remove from the fire, and well stir and mix in the arsenic. This soap should be kept in a well closed glass or earthen vessel.

Corrosive Sublimate Solution.
Corrosive sublimate, 1 dram; spirit of salt, 2 drams; spirits of camphor, 6 ounces. Dissolve the sublimate in the spirits of camphor, and then add the hydrochloric acid. This solution is chiefly used for the skins of quadrupeds, to the inner side of which it is to be applied with a brush or sponge before stuffing.

Preservative Powder.
White arsenic, 2 drams; corrosive sublimate, 2 drams; nutgalls, 1 ounce; capsicum in powder, ½ ounce; sal. ammoniac, ½ ounce; camphor in powder, 6 drams. Well mixed together.

Dr. Richardson's Powder.
Nut galls coarsely powdered, 2 ounces; camphor powdered, 1 ounce; burnt alum, 1 ounce. Well mixed, and if used in a hot climate, with the addition of 2 drams of either oxymuriate of mercury or arsenic. One of these powders is generally used for dressing the skins of birds.

Preservative Compound.
Oak bark, powdered, 4 ounces; burnt alum, powdered, 3 ounces; sublimate of sulphur, 2 ounces; camphor, powdered, ½ ounce; oxymuriate of mercury, ½ ounce; well mixed. This compound is used for dressing the skins of reptiles and fishes before stuffing.

Preservative Baths.
Bay salt, 4 ounces; alum, 2 ounces; corrosive sublimate, ½ dram, dissolved in 1 quart boiling water, and when cold, strained through blotting paper. Or, one-half spirits of wine and one-half boiled water. These baths are for the immersion of small reptiles, such as lizards, snakes, etc., which may be kept in them for an unlimited length of time, in glass bottles or jars well stoppered, or corked and cemented down.

1850. Prescription for Offensive Breath.

Tinct. myrrhae	12 parts.
Tinct. lavandulae	12 parts.
Glycerin	30 parts.
Liq. sodae chloratae	30 parts.
Infus. salviae	250 parts.

M.
Sig.: Use as a gargle.

1851. Chemical Food.

Water	1 ounce.
Quinine	20 grains.
Citric acid	1 dram.
Hypophosphite sodium	½ ounce.
Glycerine	1 pint.
Simple syrup	3 pints.

1852.
Porous-plasters are generally made with a rubber base, various medicaments being added, according to purpose for which required. A formula for the base was published some years ago, viz.:

Indiarubber	2 parts.
Burgundy pitch	1 part.
Olibanum	1 part.

The rubber is well steeped in hot water, to soften, then passed through corrugated iron rollers, a stream of water being allowed to fall continuously upon it; it comes out in sheets. It is then left for some days, and passed through smooth rollers, when it becomes plastic and ready to incorporate with the other ingredients. This is done by passing between two rollers again, one revolving at double the speed of the other—at this stage the various substances used for medication are also added. The spreading is done by passing the thoroughly mixed mass through other rollers along with the cloth.—(C. and D.)

1853. Baby Powder (To Cure Severe Chafing).
Druggists' Circular.
Gum camphor............ ¼ ounce.
Carbolic acid............ 15 drops.
Oxide zinc............... ¾ ounce.
Eng. precip. chalk....... 2 ounces.
Oil of neroli............. 5 drops.
Oil of rose.............. 2 drops.

Rub the camphor to a fine powder in a mortar; use alcohol to reduce it, and mix the other components thoroughly. Sift through a bolting cloth of 100 meshes to the inch.

This powder is invaluable for healing raw and irritated surfaces and for curing sunburn. Mixed in the proportion of 3 parts of vaseline or cold cream it forms one of the most useful domestic remedies in the way of a general healing salve that can be suggested.

1854. Pilot's Infant Powder.
Fred J. Renner, Jr.—Era Prize.
Acid, carbolic........... 50 drops.
Acid, boracic............ 1½ ounces.
Powd. French chalk...... 14½ ounces.

Triturate the French chalk with the carbolic acid gradually added; then add the boracic acid and thoroughly mix them.

1855. Anti-Chafe Nursery Powder.
Hood & Co.—Era Competition.
Powd. fuller's earth...... 9 ounces.
Powd. boric acid......... 1½ ounces.
Powd. oxide zinc......... 3 ounces.
Powd. starch............ 9 ounces.
Powd. orris root......... 1½ ounces.
Oil bergamot............ 2 drams.

Mix the powders thoroughly, add the oil, and pass through a fine sieve.

1856. O. K. Baby Powder.
C. W. Moister.—Era Competition.
Oxide zinc............... ½ ounce.
Powd. starch............ 1½ ounces.
Boracic acid............. 20 grains.
Oil eucalyptus........... 10 drops.

Mix and rub very fine in a mortar.
Dust on parts affected, as occasion may require.

1857. Cutine or Nursery Powder.
W. D. Harnist.—Era Competition.
Talcum (purified)........ 8 ounces.
Fuller's earth (powd.).... 4 ounces.
Lycopodium............. 4 ounces.
Oil rose................. 5 drops.

Rub the oil of rose with the fuller's earth in a mortar until thoroughly incorporated; add the talcum and lycopodium, triturate thoroughly.

This makes a harmless and useful sprinkling powder and its cost will not exceed 25c per pound.

1858. Baby Powder.
Raynale.
Powd. French chalk...... 14 ounces.
Powd. boracic acid....... 2 ounces.
Ext. jasmine............. 1½ drams.
Ext. musk............... ½ dram.

Pass through fine sieve.

1859. Antiseptic Snuff Powder.
The following is a combination employed by Leonard A. Dessar:
Menthol 10.0
Tannic acid.............. 2.0
Boracic acid............. 30.0
Bismuth subnitrate....... 20.0
Starch 50.0
Cocaine 0.5
Aristol 0.5

Sig.: Make a fine powder.

1860. Ayer's Formula for Making Sarsaparilla.
(Sci. Am.)
Fluid extract sarsaparilla.. 3 ounces.
Fluid extract stillingia.... 3 ounces.
Fluid extract yellow dock. 2 ounces.
Fluid extract May apple... 2 ounces.
Sugar .... 1 ounce.
Potassium iodide......... 90 grains.
Iron iodide.............. 10 grains.

Mix them.

1861. British Cordial.
Gum opium.............. 1 ounce.
Gum asafoetida.......... 1½ ounces.
Gum benzoin............ ½ ounce.
Balsam tolu............. 2 drams.
Camphor................ ½ ounce.
Gum guiac .... 1½ ounce.
Alcohol, 188 per cent..... 1 pint.
Spts. ammon. arom...... 6 ounces.
Spts. of juniper.......... 5 ounces.

1862. Lemonade for Diabetics.

Aq. dest. .... 1,000 grams.
Glycerini pur. .... 20-30 grams.
Acid. citric. .... 5 grams.

To be drunk in small quantities during the twenty-four hours.

It can be prescribed for patients who prefer a sweet drink.—Journal des Practiciens.

1863. Cure for Morphinomania.

M. Comby reports a case of a woman who was cured of this vice by the use of the following mixture:

Sparteine sulph. .... 1¾ grains.
Caffeine .... 7¾ grains.
Sodium benzoate .... 7¾ grains.

The whole to be taken in the twenty-four hours.

The daily dose of morphine was gradually diminished, and in about a fortnight totally discontinued. The cure was complete in twenty-five days.

1864. Draught for Hysteria.

Spt. lavand. comp. .... 1½ drams.
Spt. ammon. arom. .... 1½ drams.
Spt. aetheris .... 1½ drams.
Aq. camph. .... 3½ ounces.
M.
Capt. 1 ounce ter in die.

1865. Antacid Draught.

Magnes. calc. .... ½ dram.
Aq. menth. pip. .... 1½ ounces.
Tr. aurant. .... 1 dram.
M. Ft. haust.

Suitable for heartburn and other cases of acidity in the stomach.

1866. For Inflammatory Earache.

Pulv. menthol. .... 20 grains.
Camphorae .... 20 grains.
Vaselin .... 6 ounces.
M. Ft. ung.

1867 To Relieve Cramps. A

Provide a good, strong cord—a long garter will do if nothing else is handy. When the cramp comes on, take the cord, wind it round the leg over the place that is cramped and take an end in each hand and give it a sharp pull—one that will hurt a little. The cramp will cease instantly, and the sufferer can go to bed assured that it will not come again that night.—Med. Fortnightly.

1868. To Relieve Cramps. B

I append a formula which some of my brethren may find useful. It is for what I think to be a specific for a common complaint, not dangerous, but very painful—viz.: cramp in the legs and feet at night. Relief comes five minutes after taking the following draught:

Tinct. aconiti. .... 5 minims.
Sodii bromid. .... 12 grains.
Tinct. chloroformi co. ..... 15 minims.
Aq. menthae pip. ad. ...... 1 ounce.

Repeat in an hour or two, if required. The draught also relieves an attack of stomach-spasm in a very few minutes.

1869. A Remedy for Seasickness.

Indian Medical Record.

An Indian medical officer writes after a stormy sea-voyage of the following as a "marvelous remedy for sea-sickness:"

Ext. hyoscyami. .... ½ grain.
Camphor .... 1 grain.
Asafoetidae .... ½ grain.

Ft. pil. One every four hours.

1870. Calisaya Tonic.

Cinchona, Loxa .... 100 grammes.
Bitter-orange peel .... 100 grammes.
Wild cherry bark .... 15 grammes.
Cinnamon .... 10 grammes.
Calamus .... 4 grammes.
Syrup .... 750 cc.
Alcohol ....
Water, of each sufficient to
make .... 2250 cc.

Reduce the solids to a No. 30 powder, and percolate with a menstruum consisting of 2 volumes of alcohol and 1 of water.

1871. Beef, Iron and Wine.

Chemist and Druggist.

Ammon. citrate of iron. ... 3½ ounces.
Water .... 20 ounces.
Aromatic elixir. .... 1 gallon.
Ext. of meat. .... 4 ounces.
Marsala wine, to. .... 5 gallons.

Dissolve and let stand in demijohn exposed to light, shaking occasionally, for seven days; filter through charcoal.

Few put the extract in, as it is argued that it gets precipitated along with some coloring-matter and iron. Sixteen ounce flat bottles sell at 75c.

NON-SECRET FORMULAS.

1872. Improved Wine of Beef and Iron.
J. R. Halley wins the Phar. Rec. prize for the following formula:
  Hydrated oxide of Iron.... 2 drams.
  Armour's fluid beef....... 384 minims.
  Tincture citrochloride of
    Iron. (N. F.)............. 256 minims.
  Alcohol .... 6 drams.
  California sherry wine,
    enough to make.......... 1 pint.
  Caramel, enough to color.
To the wine add the alcohol, the hydrated oxide of iron, the caramel and beef, in succession. Shake well together and allow to stand, with occasional agitation, for 48 hours; then filter and add the tincture citrochloride of iron. The addition of about 6 drams of simple syrup is considered an improvement by some pharmacists.

1873. Lithia and Potash Powders.
  Potash bicarb. powd....... 1 dram.
  Lithia carb., powd........ 2 grains.
    For the blue paper.
  Acid, citric, powd......... 40 grains.
    For the white paper.
Dissolve in separate tumblers filled one-third with cold water. Mix and drink while effervescing.

1874. Sweet Seidlitz Powders.
  Soda bicarb............... 480 grains.
  Saccharin .... 3 grains.
  Rochelle salts............ 1440 grains.
Mix thoroughly and divide into 12 powders; wrap in blue paper.
  Tartaric acid, powd....... 420 grains.
Divide in 12 equal parts; wrap in white paper.

1875. Caffeine Seidlitz Powders.
  Soda bicarb............... 480 grains.
  Rochelle salts............ 1440 grains.
Mix and make 12 powders in blue paper.
  Tartaric acid, powd....... 420 grains.
  Citrate of caffeine, powd... 24 grains.
Mix and make 12 powders in white paper.

1876. Neutralizing Cordial.
The following formula is given by Truscott:
  Essence peppermint....... 2 drams.
  Potassium bicarbonate..... 4 drams.
  Fluid extract rhubarb...... 4 ounces.
  Granulated sugar.......... 8 ounces.
  Soft water................ 2 pints.

1877. The Proper Time to Give Medicines.
Alkalies should be given before food. Iodine and iodides should be given on an empty stomach, when they rapidly diffuse into the blood. If given during digestion the acids and starch alter and weaken the action. Acids, as a rule, should be given between the digestive acts, because the mucous membrane of the stomach is in a favorable condition for the diffusion of the acid into the blood. Acids may be given before food when prescribed to check the excessive formation of the acids of the gastric juice. Irritating and dangerous drugs—such as the salts of arsenic, copper, zinc, and iron—should be given directly after food.

1878. Stimulating Liniment.
  Oleic acid................. 3 drams.
  Borax .... 20 grains.
  Water .... 4 drams.
  Ammonia .... 4 fl. ounces.
  Chloroform .... 1 fl. ounce.
  Oil turpentine............. 2 fl. ounces.
  Cottonseed oil, enough to
    make .... 16 fl. ounces.

1879. Orange Wine.
  Sugar .... 56 pounds.
  Juice of Seville oranges... 140
  Parings of the peel of same
  Water .... 15 gallons.
  Ferment, and add
  Brandy .... 2 pints.
Should the color not be sufficiently dark, add burnt sugar to give the required shade.

1880. Kola Wine.
The Bull. Med. gives this formula:
  Fluid extract kola......... 30 parts.
  Tincture nux vomica....... 10 parts.
  Malvoisie or sherry wine,
    sufficient to make....... 1,000 parts.

1881. Coca Wine.
  Claret .... 1 gallon.
  Cologne spt............... 16 ounces.
  White sugar............... 1 pound.
  Fl. ext. coca.............. 4 ounces.
  Tinct. cudbear............. q. s. to color.
Add the spirit to the claret to fortify it, as soon as it is opened; when all is ready, shake occasionally for seven days, and filter through charcoal.
Resembles vin. mariani, and is bottled after the same style.

1882. Kola Coca.

Bonham's Guide is authority for this formula:

Kola wine	8 ounces.
Coca wine	8 ounces.
Simple syrup	¾ gallon.
Albumen foam	2 ounces.

Color with caramel and cochineal.

1883. Compound Wine of Cinchona.
French Codex.

Yellow cinchona	10 parts.
Bitter orange peel	1 part.
Chamomile	1 part.
Alcohol	10 parts.
Stronger white wine	90 parts.

1884. Alterative Tonic.

The following, according to the Medical and Surgical Reporter, is said to be Dr. Goodell's favorite mixture:

Hydrarg. bichlor	1 grain.
Liq. arsen. chlor	1 dram.
Acidi mur. dil	
Tr. ferri. chlor., aa	2 drams.
Syr. zingib	2 ounces.
Aquae ad	6 ounces.

Sig.: One to two teaspoonfuls three times daily in water, after meals.

1885. Foot Powder.
(Chemist & Druggist.)

Bismuth subnitrate	45 parts.
Talcum	40 parts.
Potassium permanganate	3 parts.
Sodium salicylate	2 parts.

An excellent application for perspiring feet.

1886. Show Bottle Colors.

Blue:

Sulphate of copper	1 pound.
Water	1 gallon.

Dissolve and add liq. ammon. fort. until a clear liquid is obtained, then dilute to the shade desired.

Green: The above solution without ammonia, but add

Salt	2 pounds

to produce a green tint, or use solution of nitrate of copper. Sulphate of nickel makes a pretty and permanent solution, but is more expensive.

Red: Dissolve alizarine paste in liq. ammon. fort. and dilute to the color desired. This is a permanent color. Or

Iodine	2 drams.
Potassium iodide	2 drams.
Hydrochloric acid	3 drams.
Water cong	3

Orange: Solution of potass. bichrom.

Pink:

Nitrate of cobalt	1 pound.
Water	2 gallons.

Dissolve and add a solution of carbonate of ammonia until the precipitate formed is redissolved; dilute to 3 gallons (or as desired), and set aside in the sun for a month, then decant.

1887. Preston Salts.

William W. Bartlett, in a note read at the New Bedford meeting of the Massachusetts Pharmaceutical Association, gave the following formula for this "salt:"

Powdered chloride of ammonium	1½ ounces.
Powdered carbonate of potassium	1 ounce. 6 drams.
Powdered camphor	1 dram.
Coarsely powdered carbonate of ammonium	3 drams.
Oil of cloves	10 drops.
Oil of bergamot	10 drops.

Mr. Bartlett also gave a formula for a "menthol pungent," which he said was quite agreeable to the smell and a novelty for various kinds of headache and faintness. It is prepared by leaving out the essential oils in the above formula and substituting in their place

Menthol	1 dram.

1888. Smelling Salts.

The Seifensieder Zeitung gives the following directions for preparing a superior article of smelling salt:

Ammonium carbonate	120 grams.
Spirit of ammonia	60 grams.
Bergamot oil	12 drops.
Lavender oil	8 drops.
Oil of cloves	4 drops.
Neroli oil	4 drops.
Cinnamon oil	4 drops.

The ammonium carbonate, which should be quite fresh, and in lumps about the size of a hazelnut, is put into a wide-mouthed jar. The oils and ammonia are then mixed and poured into the jar and the stopper at once applied. Set aside for two days, at the end of which time the ingredients will be found to have united in a solid mass.

If it is desired to prevent this occurrence and have the substance in the shape of a dry salt, instead of letting the container remain quiet, shake it frequently and violently every day for a week. The salt thus obtained can be easily removed from the container, coarsely pulverized and put into little smelling bottles, should it be desirable so to do.

1889. Monocarbonate of Ammonia for Smelling Salts.

Ammon. carb.	2 pounds.
Liq. ammon. fort.	1 pound.
Ol. bergam	1 dram.
Ol. lavand	2 drams.
Ol. myrist	15 minims.
Ol. caryoph	15 minims.
Ol. cinnam	1 dram.

Break the ammon. carb. into small pieces, and in a large Wedgewood mortar pour over it the liq. ammon. fort., with which previously mix the perfumes. Cover the mortar, and let stand for a few days to effect the conversion of the ammon. carb. to monocarbonate. Reduce to coarse powder, and keep closely stoppered.

1890. Incense for Churches.

Benzoin	3 ounces.
Storax	3 ounces.
Olibanum	4½ ounces.
Myrrh	4½ ounces.
Cascarilla	2½ ounces.
Oil of lavender	20 minims.
Oil of bergamot	20 minims.
Oil of cinnamon	8 minims.
Oil of cloves	10 minims.

Mix well.

1891. Patent Insect Powder.

Powdered white helebore	1 pound.
Powdered borax	2 pounds.
Powdered angelica root	1 pound.
Insect powder true	6 pounds.

1892. Bed Bug Poison.

Corrosive sublimate	8 ounces.
Distilled water	4 pints.
Salt	8 ounces.
Sulphuric ether	1 ounce.

Mix.

1893. Death on Rats.

Fine corn meal	2 parts.
White arsenic, powdered	2 parts.

Mix thoroughly and color to suit the trade, either with burnt umber, charcoal, ultramarine, or vermilion, q. s.

1894. Cockroach Powder.

Equal parts of powdered borax, Persian insect-powder, and powdered colocynth, well mixed together, and thrown about such spots as are infested with these troublesome insects will prove an effectual means of getting rid of the scourge if used persistently.—C. & D.

1895. Fly Poison. A

A strong solution of white arsenic (say 1 dram to the pint) sweetened with moist sugar, molasses or honey. Poison.

1896. Fly Poison. B

Molasses, honey or moist sugar, mixed with about one-twelfth their weight of King's yellow or orpiment.

Both the above are dangerous preparations, and should never be employed where there are children.

1897. Fly Poison. C

(Redwood) quassia chips (small)	¼ ounce.
Water	1 pint.

Boil ten minutes, strain and add

Molasses	4 ounces.

Flies will drink this with avidity, and are soon destroyed by it.

1898. Fly Poison. D

Black pepper	1 teaspoonful.
Brown sugar	2 teaspoonfuls.
Cream	4 teaspoonfuls.

Fly powder. The dark gray colored powder (so called suboxide) obtained by the free exposure of metallic arsenic to the air. Mixed with sweets, it is used to kill flies. See also above.

1899. Insecticides. A

Scientific American Cyclo.

Kerosene Emulsion.—One of the most satisfactory formulas is as follows:

Kerosene	2 gallons, 67 per cent.
Common soap or whale oil soap	½ pound.
Water	1 gallon, 33 per cent.

Heat the solution of soap and add it boiling hot to the kerosene. Churn the mixture by means of a force pump and spray nozzle for five or ten minutes. The emulsion, if perfect, forms a cream which thickens upon cooling and should adhere without oiliness to the surface of glass. For use against scale insects dilute 1 part of the emulsion with 9 parts of water. For most other insects dilute 1 part of the emulsion with 15 parts of water. For soft insects like plant lice, the dilution may be carried to from 20 to 25 parts of water.

1900. Insecticides. B

The milk emulsion is produced by the same methods as the above.

1901. The Resin Washes. A

These insecticides act by contact, and also, in the case of scale insects, by forming an impervious coating which effectually smothers the insects treated. These resin washes vary in efficacy according to the insect treated. Experience has shown that the best formula for the red scale (Aonidia aurantii Maskell) and its yellow variety (A. citrinus Coquillett) is as follows:

Resin	18 pounds.
Caustic soda (70 per cent strength)	5 pounds.
Fish oil	2½ pints.
Water to make	100 gallons.

The necessary ingredients are placed in a kettle and a sufficient quantity of cold water added to cover them; they are then boiled until dissolved, being occasionally stirred in the meantime, and after the materials are dissolved the boiling should be continued about an hour, and a considerable degree of heat should be employed, so as to keep the preparation in a brisk state of ebullition, cold water being added in small quantities whenever there are indications of the preparation boiling over. Too much cold water, however, should not be added at one time, or the boiling process will be arrested and thereby delayed, but by a little practice the operator will learn how much water to add so as to keep the preparation boiling actively. Stirring the preparation is quite unnecessary during this stage of the work. When boiled sufficiently it will assimilate perfectly with water, and should then be diluted with the proper quantity of cold water, adding it slowly at first and stirring occasionally during the process. The undiluted preparation is pale yellowish in color, but by the addition of water it becomes a very dark brown. Before being sprayed on the trees it should be strained through a fine wire sieve, or through a piece of Swiss muslin, and this is usually accomplished when pouring the liquid into the spraying tank, by means of a strainer placed over the opening through which the preparation is introduced into the tank.

The preparing of this compound will be greatly accelerated if the resin and caustic soda are first pulverized before being placed in the boiler, but this is quite a difficult task to perform. Both of these substances are put up in large cakes for the wholesale trade, the resin being in wooden barrels, each barrel containing a single cake weighing about 375 lbs., while the caustic soda is put up in iron drums containing a single cake each, weighing about 800 lbs. The soda is the most difficult to dissolve, but this could doubtless be obviated by first dissolving it in cold water and then using the solution as required. This insecticide may be applied at any time during the growing season.

1902. The Resin Washes. B

A stronger wash is required for the San Jose scale (Aspidiotus perniciosus Comstock), and the following formula gives the best results:

Resin	30 pounds.
Caustic soda (70 per cent)	9 pounds.
Fish oil	4½ pints.
Water enough to make	100 gallons.

Place all the ingredients in a kettle and cover with water to a depth of 4 or 5 inches; boil briskly for about two hours or until the compound can be perfectly dissolved with water. When this stage is reached the kettle should be filled up with water, care being taken not to chill the wash by adding large quantities of cold water at once. It may be thus diluted to about 40 gallons, the additional water being added from time to time as it is used.

This preparation should only be applied during winter or during the dormant period. Applied in the growing season it will cause the loss of foliage and fruit.

In the application of both of these washes a very fine spray is not essential, as the object is not simply to wet the tree but to thoroughly coat it over with the compound, and this can be best accomplished by the use of a rather coarse spray, which can be thrown upon the tree with considerable force.

1903. For Subterranean Insects. A

For Subterranean Insects.—Recent experiments have shown the practical value of the resin compounds against the grape phylloxera, and they will also be applicable to the apple root louse and other underground insects. The cheapest and at the same time one of the most satisfactory compounds experimented with is the following:

Caustic soda, 77 per cent.	5 pounds.
Resin	40 pounds.
Water to make	50 gallons.

Dissolve the soda over fire with 4 gallons of water, add the resin, and after it is dissolved and while boiling add water slowly to make 50 gallons of compound. For use dilute in 500 gallons. Excavate basins about the vines 6 inches deep and about 2 feet in diameter and apply to each vine 5 gallons. The results will be more satisfactory if the treatment is made early in the spring, so that the rain of the season will assist in disseminating the wash about the roots.

1904. **For Subterranean Insects.** B

The kerosene emulsion made according to the formula given above is also applicable to certain underground insects in cases where it will not prove too expensive, as, for instance, the grape phylloxera or where white grubs are infesting a valuable lawn. It may then be used in the proportion of 1 part of the emulsion to 15 gallons of water, applied liberally to the soil, and afterward washed down at frequent intervals with large quantities of water for several days. This can be done only where there is plenty of water at hand, but will be found of great value in special cases.

1905. **For Subterranean Insects.** C

In other cases bisulphide of carbon may be used for specific and local underground forms. Nests of ants, for instance, may be destroyed by pouring 1 ounce of this substance into several holes, covering them with a wet blanket for ten minutes and afterward exploding the vapor at the mouth of the holes with a torch. Against onions, cabbage and radish maggots this substance may also be used by punching a hole with a sharp stick at the base of the plant and pouring in a teaspoonful of the liquid, covering afterward with earth.

1906. **The Arsenites—London Purple, Paris Green and White Arsenic.** A

The Arsenites.—London Purple, Paris Green and White Arsenic.—These poisons are of the greatest service against all mandibulate insects, as larvae and beetles, and they furnish the most satisfactory means of controlling most leaf feeders and the best wholesale remedy against the codling moth. Caution must be used in applying them on account of the liability of burning or scalding the foliage. The poisons should be thoroughly mixed with water at the rate of from 1 pound to 100-250 gallons water, and applied with a force pump or hand spray nozzle. In preparing the wash it will be best to first mix the poison with a small quantity of water, making a thick batter, and then dilute the latter and add to the reservoir or spray tank, mixing the whole thoroughly.

1907. **The Arsenites.** B

When freshly mixed, either London purple or Paris Green may be applied to apple, plum and other fruit trees except the peach, at the rate of 1 pound to 150-200 gallons, the latter amount being recommended for the plum, which is somewhat more susceptible to scalding than the apple. White arsenic does little if any injury at the rate of 1 pound to 50 gallons of water. As shown by Mr. Gillette, however, when allowed to remain for some time (two weeks or more) in water, the white arsenic acts with wonderful energy, scalding when used at the rate of 1 pound to 100 gallons, from 10 per cent to 90 per cent of the foliage. The action of the other arsenites remains practically the same, with perhaps, a slight increase in the case of London purple.

1908. **The Arsenites.** C

With the peach these poisons, when applied alone, even at the rate of 1 pound to 300 or more gallons of water, are injurious in their action, causing the loss of much of the foliage.

By the addition of a little lime to the mixture, London purple and Paris green may be safely applied at the rate of 1 pound to 125 to 150 gallons of water, to the peach or the tenderest foliage, or in much greater strength to strong foliage, such as that of the apple or most shade trees.

1909. **The Arsenites.** D

Whenever, therefore, the application is made to tender foliage or when the treating with a strong mixture is desirable, lime water, milky, but not heavy enough to close the nozzle, should be added at the rate of about 2 gallons to 100 gallons of the poison. Pure arsenic, however, should never be used with lime, as the latter greatly increases its action.

With the apple, in spraying for the codling moth, at least two applications should be made—the first on the falling of the blossoms, the apples being about the size of peas, and the second a week or ten days later; but the poison should never be applied after the fruit turns down on the stem, on account of the danger of the poison collecting and remaining permanently in the stem cavity.—Circular U. S. Depart. Agriculture.

1910. **To Destroy Insects.**

Hot alum water destroys red and black ants, cockroaches, spiders and chinch bugs.

1911. **Formula for Insect Bites.**

One of the very best applications for the bites of mosquitoes and fleas, also for other eruptions attended with intense itchings, is: Menthol in alcohol, one part to ten. This is very cooling and immediately effectual. It is also an excellent lotion for application to the forehead and temples in headache, often at once subduing the same.—Weekly Med. Review.

1912. To Discover Insects.

If the leaves of the plant turn reddish or yellow, or if they curl up, a close inspection will generally disclose that the plants are infested with a very small green insect, or else with the red spider, either of which must be destroyed. For this purpose, scald some common tobacco with water until the latter is colored to a yellow, and when cold sprinkle the leaves of the plants with it; but a better plan is to pass the stems and leaves of the plants between the fingers, and to then shake the plant and well water the bed immediately afterward. The latter operation destroys a large proportion of the insects shaken from the plant. This latter method is the only infallible one.

1913. Expelling Insects.

All insects dread pennyroyal; the smell of it destroys some and drives the others away. At the time that fresh pennyroyal cannot be gathered, get oil of pennyroyal; pour some into a saucer and steep in it small pieces of wadding or raw cotton and place them in corners, closet shelves, bureau drawers, boxes, etc., and the cockroaches, ants, or other insects will soon disappear. It is also well to place some between the mattresses and around the bed. It is also a splendid thing for brushing off that terrible little insect, the seed tick.

1914. Insects and How to Fight Them.

Cut Worms.—Where cut worms are troublesome in the field, a very old and at the same time a very good remedy is to entrap them in holes made near the plants, or hills, if in the cornfield. An old rake handle, tapered at the end so as to make a smooth hole five or six inches deep, or more, will answer very well for this purpose. In the morning the worms that have taken refuge in these holes may be crushed by thrusting the rake handle into them again, and the trap is set for the next night. It is always well in planting to make provisions for the loss of a stalk or two by cut worms or other causes, as it is easier to thin out than to replant.

1915. May Beetles.

May Beetles.—These are the perfect insects of the white grub, so destructive to lawns and sometimes to meadows. A French plan for destroying or rather catching the cockchafer, a very similar insect, is to place in the center of the orchard after sunset an old barrel, the inside of which has been previously tarred. At the bottom of the barrel is placed a lighted lamp, and the insects, circling around to get at the light, strike their wings and legs against the tarred sides of the barrel, and either get fast or are rendered so helpless that they fall to the bottom. Ten gallons of beetles have been captured in this way in a single night.

1916. Slugs.

Slugs.—English gardeners place handfuls of bran at intervals of eight or ten feet along the border of garden walks. The slugs are attracted to the bran, and in the morning each little heap is found covered with them. The ground is then gone over again, this time the operator providing himself with a dustpan and small broom and an empty bucket, and it is an easy matter to sweep up the little heaps and empty them, slugs and all, into the bucket. In this way many hundreds have been taken in a single walk, and if a little salt and water be placed on the bottom of the bucket the slugs coming in contact with it are almost instantly destroyed.

1917. Ants.

Ants.—When these insects are troublesome in the garden, fill small bottles two-thirds with water, and then add sweet oil to within an inch of the top; plunge these into the ground near the nest or hills to within half an inch of the rim, and the insects coming for a sip will get into the oil and perish, as it fills the breathing pores. The writer once entrapped in a pantry myriads of red ants in a shallow tin cover smeared with lard, the vessel having accidently been left in their track. Another means of entrapping them, suggested to me by Professor Glover many years ago, is to sprinkle sugar into a dampened sponge near haunts to attract the insects. When they have swarmed through the sponge it is squeezed in hot water, and the trap is reset until the majority of the insects are killed.

1918. Aphis.

Aphis.—A remedy for plant lice upon the terminal shoots of rose bushes (or similar hardy plants), said to work like a charm, is as follows: Take 4 ounces of quassia chips and boil for ten minutes in a gallon of soft water. Take out the chips and add 4 ounces of soft soap, which should be dissolved in it as it cools. Stir well before using, and apply with a moderate sized paint brush, brushing upward. Ten minutes after, syringe the trees with clean water to wash off the dead insects and the preparation, which would otherwise disfigure the rose trees.

1919. Scale.

Scale.—A French composition for destroying scale insects, plant lice, etc., on fruit and other trees, is as follows: Boil 2 gallons barley in water, then remove the grain (which may be fed to the chickens), and add to the liquid quicklime until it approaches the consistency of paint. When cold add 2 pounds of lampblack, mixing it for a long time, then add 1½ pounds flowers of sulphur and 1 quart alcohol.

The mixture is applied with a paint brush, first using a stiff bristle brush to remove moss, etc. It not only destroys the insects, but gives the bark greater strength.—Prairie Farmer.

A year or two ago the Ontario Agricultural College published a list of formulas for preparations useful in destroying the various insects and fungi injurious to plants, from which the following likely to prove most useful to druggists in agricultural districts are reproduced:

1920. Insecticides and Fungicides.

A good general fungicide is the Bordeaux mixture, the formula most used being the following:

Copper sulphate .... 6 pounds.
Lime .... 4 pounds.
Water .... 22 gallons.

Dissolve the copper compound in 16 gallons of water; slake the lime in 6 gallons of water, and, when the latter is cooled, pour it into the copper solution and mix thoroughly.

A modified form, known as eau celeste, consists of—

Copper sulphate .... 2 pounds.
Ammonia .... 1 quart.
Water .... 50 gallons.

Dissolve the copper sulphate in 2 gallons of hot water; as soon as cool add the 1 quart of ammonia, and dilute to 50 gallons.

The mixture should be sprayed over the infected parts.

The most useful insecticides are those containing, as a basis, Paris green. This substance, being insoluble, does not injure the foliage. A good formula is, 1 pound of Paris green to 200 gallons of water. This is very effective against leaf-eating insects. To destroy plant-lice and scale insects, the following emulsion should be used:

Soft soap .... 1 quart.
Boiling water .... 2 quarts.

Mix, and while hot add 1 pint of coal oil.

When using, dilute with twice the amount of either hard or soft water. Many other preparations are used, the chief being carbolic acid and tobacco dust; but the above emulsion is most useful. If a combined insecticide and fungicide be preferred, it may be made by adding 4 ounces of Paris green to the Bordeaux mixture.

1921. Precautions to be Adopted in Spraying.

1. Keep poison labeled, and out of the way of children.
2. Do not spray so far into the season as to affect the fruit.
3. In making emulsions remember the inflammable nature of coal oil.
4. Never spray trees in bloom.
5. Try solutions on a small scale if likely to injure foliage, and watch results.

As copper compounds act upon tin and iron, it is well to prepare such mixtures in earthen, wooden, or brass vessels.

For certain fungi and insects special mixtures must be used.

1922.

Pear-leaf Blight, which appears on both leaves and fruit, giving the leaves a spotted appearance and causing the fruit to crack.—Spray with ammonical solution of copper carbonate as soon as the leaves begin to open, and repeat two or three times at intervals of two weeks.

1923. Grape Black-rot.

Grape Black-rot.—Spray with ammoniacal solution of copper carbonate or Bordeaux mixture six times, every two weeks, commencing early in May. If the last two sprayings are with the copper carbonate the fruit will not be disfigured.

1924. Smut.

Smut.—(1) Immersing seed in hot water of 135° F. for five minutes will destroy the spores of smut; 5 degrees above or below that point will fail. (2) Put 1 pound of copper sulphate in 20 gallons of water and allow the seed to remain in this for about fifteen hours; then put the seed for ten minutes in lime water made by slaking the lime in ten times its weight of water.

1925. Cucumber Beetles.

Cucumber-beetles, which are often so troublesome, can only be kept away by covering the plants with netting.

1926. Strawberry Slugs.

Strawberry-slugs may be destroyed by the use of pyrethrum, either dry or mixed with water. If this fails to remove all, the Paris green mixture will finish them.

1927. Cabbage Worm.

Cabbage worm.—The same treatment (without using Paris green) will prove effective in destroying the common cabbage worm.

1928. To rid Trunks and Cupboards of Moths.

It frequently happens that in spite of care moths are discovered in the middle of the summer in trunks or closets supposed to have been so impregnated with preventives that their entrance would have been impossible. They hide in the crevices, and many attempts to dislodge them are futile. A simple and effective plan, according to a writer in Harper's Bazaar, is to heat stove lids or an iron shovel red hot, pour vinegar upon the iron, and let the fumes penetrate the cracks which could not be reached with a powder gun. Moths are particularly fond of new plaster, and the settling of the walls of houses affords them numberless hiding places which cannot well be reached except by fumigation. Burning sulphur is excellent for ridding walls of any sort of vermin, but the fumes of this are objectionable to many and they do not pass off so quickly as those of vinegar.

1929. Moth Pastilles.

Camphor	5
Black pepper	10
Absinthe	10
Patchouli	2
Oil lavender	2
Oil clove	1
Paraffin	100

Melt together, and make into pastilles.

1930. Bedbug Exterminator.

Soft soap	20
Water	65
Oil turpentine	5
Kerosene	10

Dissolve the soap in the water, with the aid of heat, add the turpentine, stir until the latter is thoroughly mixed, and finally add to the coal oil, continuing the heat and stirring until a homogeneous mixture is obtained.

Directions to go with the above: Wash the parts of the bedstead, let dry, and apply the mixture with a brush to all parts frequented by the bugs. The preparation may also be painted on walls, etc.

1931. Cockroach Exterminator.

Mix 3 pounds of oatmeal, or cornmeal, with a pound of white lead; add treacle to form a good paste, and put a portion down at night in the infested places. Repeat for a few nights alternately, and in the morning remove the paste and the corpses to a convenient place.

1932. Vermin Killer, for Rats and Mice.

Sulphate of strychnia	½ ounce.
Powdered sugar	1 ounce.
Wheaten flour	14½ ounces.
Oil of anise	½ dram.
Solution of aniline	q. s.

Drop the oil of anise on the flour and mix thoroughly with the other ingredients; spray with a solution of aniline of any color desired, before mixing.

1933. Sticky Fly Paper Mixture.

Yellow resin	2 pounds.
Boiled linseed oil	2 pounds.
Castor oil	1 pound.
Molasses	¼ pound.
Beeswax	⅛ pound.

Melt the resin and the beeswax in the oils by the heat from a water bath; whilst still hot mix in the molasses, and spread on sized parchment paper.

1934. Sizing for Fly Paper.

Glue	¼ pound.
Water	¾ pound.

Dissolve the glue in the water by the heat of a water bath; and while hot brush on to sheets of parchment paper; when the sizing has set on the paper, put on the sticky fly paper mixture (see preceding formula) with a varnish brush, using a metal edge to keep the margin of the paper free from the mixture.

1935. Fly Paint.

Arsenic powdered	1 ounce.
Sal soda	1 ounce.
Water	8 ounces.
Glycerine	8 ounces.

Dissolve the arsenic and sal soda in the water, using heat, when dissolved, filter and add the glycerine; mix well and apply with a brush to windows or other places infested with flies.

1936. Phosphorus Paste, for Exterminating Rats, Mice, Roaches and Ants.

Carbon bisulphide	1 pound.
Phosphorus	¾ ounce.
Oil of anise	½ ounce.
Wheaten flour	24 ounces.
Glucose	6 pints.

Dissolve the phosphorus in the carbon bisulphide, and add the oil of anise; set aside until needed; heat the glucose to 150° F., and stir in the flour when the temperature of the mixture has fallen to 100° (and not sooner); add the solution of phosphorus and mix well into the paste with a wooden stirring stick until thoroughly incorporated. A wide porcelain dish is the most suitable vessel to use for mixing the paste; be careful that no dry flour adheres to the side of the vessel whilst stirring in the solution of phosphorus. This paste will not ferment and will remain in good condition for a long time; when the oil of anise has been used for some time to perfume the paste with a change may be made to oil of rhodium; or oil of fennel, alternating the odors, as may seem fit.

1937. Fly Lotion.
(Ch. & Dr.)

Quillaia bark .... 1 ounce.
Boiling water .... 2 pints.
Infuse for an hour, strain and add
Corrosive sublimate ...... ½ ounce.
Hydrochloric acid .... ½ ounce.
Turpentine .... 5 ounces.
Oil of tar .... 5 ounces.

Directions for use:

To prevent the fly striking, and for maggot.—Mix two tablespoonfuls with a wine bottle of cold water.

To kill lice.—Mix three tablespoonfuls with a wine bottle of cold water, and rub on with a brush.

For mange.—Mix four tablespoonfuls with a wine bottle of cold water, and rub in the mixture with a brush every day until cured.

1938. Mosquito Oil.
Oil of eucalyptus .... 1 ounce.
Oil of pennyroyal .... 1 ounce.
Sweet oil .... 6 ounces.
Mix.

Anoint the hands and face with the oil.

1939. Nursery Insecticide.
Ch. and Dr.

Vinegar of cantharides....
  or
Vinegar of stavesacre..... 3 drams.
Glycerin .... 1 ounce.
Infusion of quassia (1 to 7)
  enough to make .... 1 pint.

1940. Fumigating Pastilles (Insecticide. A
Ch. and Dr.

Charcoal, in powder...... 500 parts.
Saltpetre .... 60 parts.
Carbolic acid .... 40 parts.
Insect powder .... 250 parts.

Make into a paste with tragacanth mucilage, and divide into suitable sized cones.

1941. Fumigating Pastilles. B
Charcoal powder.......... 500 parts.
Saltpetre .... 50 parts.
Insect powder .... 150 parts.
Benzoin .... 100 parts.
Tolu balsam .... 100 parts.

Make as above.

1942. Window-Polishing Paste.
Castile soap .... 2 ounces.
Boiling water .... 3 ounces.
Dissolve, and add the following in fine powder:
Precipitated chalk ...... 4 ounces.
French chalk .... 3 ounces.
Tripoli .... 2 ounces.

Mix, and reduce with water to the consistency desired.

1943. Invisible Writing on Glass.
Glass written upon with French chalk shows the design only when breathed upon. The glass is written on with a French-chalk pencil, cleaned with a handkerchief.

1944. To Destroy Ants.
Sci. Am. Cyc.

Flour of sulphur, ½ pound; potash, 4 ounces; set in an earthen vessel, over the fire, till dissolved and united. Afterward heat to powder; infuse a little of the powder in water, and sprinkle in places infested by ants.

1945. Black Ants.
A few leaves of green wormwood scattered among the haunts of black ants will drive them away.

1946. Red Ants.
Powdered borax sprinkled around the infested places will drive them away, as also will powdered cloves. Grease a plate with lard, they will leave sugar to go to it, and then turn them into the fire; cracked nuts will answer the same purpose. Oil of turpentine run into the cracks with a sewing machine oil can.

1947. Ant Poison.

Cape aloes	1 pound.
Water	1 gallon.

Boil together and add to the mixture

Camphor, in small pieces	6 ounces.

This can be used for other insects by diluting with water and sprinkling through a garden pump or watering can.

1948. To Exterminate Ants.

Sprinkle their haunts with quick lime containing a twentieth of its weight of powdered camphor.

1949. Caterpillars.

Rue	
Wormwood	Equal parts of each.
Tobacco	

Make a strong decoction in water and sprinkle it on the leaves and young branches every morning and evening during the time the fruit is ripening.

1950.

Artificial sea water for use in aquaria is made by fish dealers as follows:

Take of

Chloride of sodium	94 parts.
Sulphate of magnesium	7 parts.
Sulphate of potassium	2 parts.
Chloride of magnesium	9 parts.
Water	3328 parts.

It is claimed that the above mixture will make sea fish feel perfectly at home.

1951. Carbolized Sponges.

Carbolic acid	50.0 grams.
Alcohol	200.0 grams.
Water	750.0 grams.

Bleached sponges are allowed to remain in this solution for 24 hours, when an equal volume of water is added. The sponges remain in the fluid.

1952. Blackboard Paint.

Shellac	4 ounces.
Ivory black, in fine powder	2 ounces.
Emery	1 ounce.
Ultramarine	1 ounce.
Spirit	40 ounces.

Mix, and shake occasionally until the shellac is dissolved.

FERTILIZERS, ETC.

1953. Guano.

Dissolved bones	4 bushels.
Sulphate of ammon.	100 pounds.
Pearl ash	5 pounds.
Dry sulphate of soda	10 pounds.

Mix.

1954. Fertilizer for Gardens.
(Rev. Chem. Ind.)

Ammonium sulphate	10
Sodium nitrate	15
Ammonium phosphate	30
Potassium nitrate	45

1955. Fertilizer for Lawns.
(Rev. Chim. Ind.)

Potassium nitrate	30
Sodium nitrate	30
Calcium sulphate	30
Calcium superphosphate	30

1956. Fertilizer for Fruit Trees.
(Rev. Chem. Ind.)

Potassium chloride	100
Potassium nitrate	500
Potassium phospate	570

This total amount of 1170 grams to be used for one tree.

1957. Chemical Guano, Grandeau.
(Rev. Horticult.)

Calcium nitrate	100
Potassium nitrate	25
Potassium phosphate	25
Magnesium sulphate	25

Dissolve from 4 to 10 grams of this powder in 1 liter of water, and water each pot plant with this once or twice a month. The plants must be in full vegetation.

1958. Bottle Capping (Common).

Glue	4 ounces.
Whiting	2 ounces.
Glycerine	½ ounce.
Aqua	9 ounces.
Chinese vermilion	1 ounce.

1959. Bottle Capping (Best).

Gelatine	4 ounces.
Water	8 ounces.
Dry white lead	3 ounces.
Cochineal	q. s.
Glycerine	½ ounce.

Mix.

1960. Capsules for Bottles (Gelatine).

Soak
- Russian gelatine .... 7 pounds.
- Glycerine .... 10 ounces.
- Water .... 60 ounces.

Heat over a water-bath and add any desired color. Pigments may be used, and very beautiful tints obtained by the use of aniline colors. Store the substance in jars.

Modus operandi.—Liquify the mass and dip the cork and portion of neck of bottle into the liquid; it sets very quickly.

This capping is particularly applicable for varnishes, benzine, liquid glue, glycerine jelly, and other little odds and ends which we wish to make attractive on the shop counter, and it is at the same time a most "hermetical seal."

CEMENTS.

1961. Clarke's Anodyne Cement.

- Balsam, Canada .... 1 dram.
- Slaked lime q. s. to make a paste.

1962. Cement for Bicycle Tires.

- Asphalt .... 2 pounds.
- Gutta percha. .... 1 pound.

Melt together, apply to hot wheel, then slip on tire.

1963. Roman Cement.

- Ordinary clay............ 60 pounds.
- Calcine and mix with
- Lime .... 40 pounds.
- Recalcine the whole.

1964. Cement for Roofs. A

Roofs, Cement for.—Melt together in an iron pot two parts by weight of common pitch and one part gutta percha. This forms a homogeneous fluid much more manageable than gutta percha alone. To repair gutters, roofs or other surfaces, carefully clean out of the cracks all earthy matters, slightly warm the edges with a plumber's soldering iron, then pour the cement in a fluid state upon the cracks while hot, finishing up by going over the cement with a moderately hot iron, so as to make a good connection and a smooth joint. The above will repair zinc, lead or iron, and is a good cement for aquariums.

1965. Cement for Roofs. B

Take
- Rosin .... 4 pounds.
- Linseed oil............... 1 pint.
- Red Lead................. 2 ounces.

Stir in fine sand until the proper consistency is secured, and apply warm. This cement becomes hard, and yet possesses considerable elasticity, is durable and waterproof.

1966. Rubber Cement. A

Rubber Cements.—Rubber cements are very common and very useful, but great care should be taken in their preparation to guard against fire; they should not be prepared at night, as the carbon bisulphide, naptha, or chloroform is very inflammable. Vessels which are used to digest the rubber should be closed and if possible put out of doors. If heat is required, use a sand or hot water bath; on no account bring near a fire.

1967. Rubber Cement. B

Rubber Cement.—Digest caoutchouc, cut in fine shreds, with about 4 volumes of naphtha or carbon bisulphide in a well covered vessel for several days.

1968. Rubber Cement. C

Cement for sticking on leather patches and for attaching rubber soles to boots and shoes is prepared from virgin or native India rubber, by cutting it into small pieces or else shredding it up; a bottle is filled with this to about one-tenth of its capacity, benzine is then poured on till about three parts full, but be certain that the benzine is free from oil. It is then kept till thoroughly dissolved and of a thick consistency. If it turns out too thick or thin, suitable quantities must be added of either material to make as required.

1969. Rubber Cement. D

Cement used for repairing holes in rubber boots and shoes is made of the following solution:
- Caoutchouc .... 10 parts.
- Chloroform .... 280 parts.

This is simply prepared by allowing the caoutchouc to dissolve in the chloroform.
- Caoutchouc .... 10 parts.
- Resin .... 4 parts.
- Gum turpentine......... . 40 parts.

For this solution the caoutchouc is shaved into small pieces and melted up with the resin, the turpentine is then added, and all is then dissolved in the oil of turpentine. The two solutions are then mixed together. To repair the shoe with this cement first wash the hole over with it, then a piece of linen dipped in it is placed over it; as soon as the linen adheres to the sole, the cement is then applied as thickly as required.

1970. Rubber Cement. E

Good rubber cement for sheet rubber, or for attaching rubber material of any description or shape to metal, may be made by softening and dissolving shellac in ten times its weight of water of ammonia. A transparent mass is thus obtained, which, after keeping three or four weeks, becomes liquid, and may be used without requiring heat. When applied it will be found to soften the rubber, but when the ammonia is evaporated it forms a kind of hard coat, and causes it to become both impervious to gases as well as liquids.

1971. Rubber Cement. F

A cement for uniting India rubber is composed as follows:

Rubber, finely chopped.... 100 parts.
Resin .... 15 parts.
Shellac .... 10 parts.

These are dissolved in bisulphide of carbon.

1972. Rubber Cement. G

Another India rubber cement is made of

India rubber............ 15 grains.
Chloroform .... 2 ounces.
Mastic .... 4 drams.

First mix the India rubber and chloroform together, and when dissolved, the mastic is added in powder. It is then allowed to stand for a week or two before using.

1973. Rubber Cement. H

Rubber Cement to Mend Boots.—Dissolve 1 dram of gutta percha in 1 ounce of bisulphide of carbon; filter through coarse filter paper; add 15 grains of pure rubber; rub the whole smooth with a palette knife, taking care to do it quickly. If necessary, thin with bisulphide of carbon. Keep it away from fire or light, as it is volatile and inflammable.

1974. To Cement Hard Rubber.

Dissolve bleached gutta percha in carbon bisulphide. Cement, and when dry brush over carbon bisulphide in which sulphur has been dissolved.

1975. Cement to Mend Rubber.

Equal parts of pitch and gutta percha are melted together and linseed oil is added, which contains litharge. Melt until all are well mixed, use no more of the linseed oil than necessary. Apply warm.

1976. Cement for Rubber Shoes.

Cement for Rubber Shoes.—2½ parts India rubber are dissolved in 70 parts of chloroform by mastication. For the second solution melt 2½ parts India rubber with 1 part of resin, ½ part of Venice turpentine is added, and lastly 10 parts oil of turpentine. Mix the solutions.

1977. To Fasten Hard Rubber to Metal.

To Fasten Hard Rubber to Metal.—Make a thin solution of glue, and gradually add pulverized wood ashes till you have a stiff varnish. Use this cement hot.

1978. Cement for Mending Hard Rubber.

Rubber (Hard) Cement for Mending.—Fuse together equal parts of gutta percha and genuine asphaltum; apply hot to the joint, closing the latter immediately with pressure. See Ammonia and Shellac Cement. No. 1970.

1979. Oil and Sulphur.

Oil and Sulphur.—1 of sulphur to 12 of oil gives a substance like molasses; 4 to 12 of oil a stiff substance like rubber. To be successful in making this compound, take an iron ladle, such as is used for the melting of lead, and fill it not more than one-third full, and place it over a clear fire. Owing to a quantity of water being held in the oil by the vegetable matter, it will begin to seethe, and, if not closely watched, boil over into the fire. After a little time it will subside, the surface remaining quite placid, with now and then little flickers of smoke flitting across the surface. Your sulphur must be either roll brimstone or the crude sublimed, i. e., not washed or treated with acid. If the first, finely powder it, and mix by degrees in the oil, stirring all the time until incorporated.

1980. Cement to Fasten Rubber to Wood and Metal.

Rubber to Wood and Metal, Cement to Fasten.—As rubber plates and rings are now almost exclusively used for making connections between steam and other pipes and apparatus, much annoyance is often experienced by the impossibility or imperfectness of an air tight connection. This is obviated entirely by employing a cement which fastens equally well to the rubber and to the metal or wood. Such cement is prepared by a solution of shellac in ammonia. This is best made by soaking pulverized gum shellac in 10 times its weight of strong ammonia, when a slimy mass is obtained, which, in three or four weeks, will become liquid without the use of hot water. This softens the rubber, and becomes, after volatilization of the ammonia, hard and impermeable to gases and fluids.

1981. Rust Cement.

Rust Cement.—Rust Cements for Water and Steam Pipes, Steam Boilers, etc. 1. Make a stiff paste with

Sal ammoniac	2 parts.
Iron borings	35 parts.
Sulphur and water	1 part.

and drive it into the joint with a chisel; or, to

Sal ammoniac	2 parts.
Flowers of sulphur	1 part.

add

Iron chips	60 parts.

Mix the whole with water, to which one-sixth part vinegar or a little sulphuric acid is added. Another cement is made by mixing 100 parts of bright iron filings or fine chips or borings with 1 part powdered ammoniac, and moistening with urine; when thus prepared, force it into the joint. It will prove serviceable under the action of fire.

1982. Metallic Cement. A

Metallic Cement.—From 20 to 30 parts of finely divided copper, obtained by the reduction of oxide of copper with hydrogen, or by precipitations from solutions of its sulphate with zinc, are made into a paste with oil of vitriol, and 70 parts of mercury added, the whole being well triturated. When the amalgamation is complete the acid is removed by washing with boiled water, and the compound allowed to cool. In ten or twelve hours it becomes sufficiently hard to receive a brilliant polish, and to scratch the surface of tin or gold. By heat it assumes the consistence of wax, and, as it does not contract by cooling, it is recommended by a noted chemist for dentists' use for stopping teeth. This is a splendid cement for attaching to the surface of wood, glass, metal and porcelain.

1983. Metallic Cement. B

The following recipe for a metallic cement for repairing broken stone is given by Prof. Brune, of the School of Fine Arts. It was used in the restoration of the colonnade of the Louvre, of the Pont Neuf, and of the Conservatoire des Arts et Metiers. It consists of a powder and a liquid. The powder:

Oxide of zinc, (by weight)	2 parts.
Crushed limestone (of hard nature)	2 parts.
Crushed grit	1 part.

The whole intimately mixed and ground. Ocher in suitable proportions is added as a coloring matter. The liquid: A saturated solution of zinc in commercial hydrochloric acid, to which is added a part, by weight, of hydrochlorate of ammonia equal to one-sixth that of the dissolved zinc. This liquid is diluted with two-thirds of its bulk of water. To use the cement, 1 pound of the powder is to be mixed with 2½ pints of the liquid. The cement hardens very quickly and is very strong.

1984. Cement for Casein.

Casein, Cement for.—Mix with

Water quartz sand (elutriated)	5 parts.
Casein	4 parts.
Lime (slaked)	5 parts.

1985. To Cement Metals.

Any fibrous material can be stuck to metal, whether iron or other metal, by a mixture composed of good glue dissolved in hot vinegar with one-third of its volume of white pine pitch, also hot. This composition, it is said, will give a sure and certain result.

1986. Cement for Fastening Metal Letters on Glass, Marble, Wood, Etc.

Copal varnish	30 parts.
Linseed oil varnish	10 parts.
Oil of turpentine	10 parts.
Glue	10 parts.

Place the mixture in a water bath, to dissolve the glue, then add

Slaked lime	20 parts.

1987.

Copal varnish	15 parts.
Drying oil	5 parts.
Turpentine	3 parts.

Melt in a water bath, and add

Slacked lime	10 parts.

1988.

Into melted resin, 180 parts, are stirred

Burnt umber	30 parts.
Calcined plaster	15 parts.
Boiled oil	8 parts.

1989.

Rosin	4 to 5 parts.
Wax	1 part.
Colcothar	1 part.

The whole melted together. A little powdered plaster is often added.

1990.

Sandarac or galipot varnish	13 parts.
Boiled linseed oil	5 parts.
Turpentine	2½ parts.
Essence turpentine	2½ parts.
Marine glue	5 parts.
Pearl white	5 parts.
Dry carbonate of lead	5 parts.

Mixed.

1991.
Copal or lac varnish	15 parts.
Drying oil	5 parts.
India rubber or gutta percha	4 parts.
Coal oil	7 parts.
Roman cement	5 parts.
Plaster	5 parts.

1992.
Copal or rosin varnish	15 parts.
Turpentine	2½ parts.
Essence Turpentine	2½ parts.
Fish isinglass (in powder)	2 parts.
Iron filings	3 parts.
Ocher or rotten stone	10 parts.

These cements are much used for fixing metallic letters to glass, marble or wood. The two following are particularly good for uniting brass and glass:

1993.
Caustic soda	1 part.
Rosin	3 parts.
Plaster	3 parts.
Water	5 parts.

The whole is boiled. This compound hardens at the end of half an hour; the hardening may be retarded by replacing the plaster by zinc white, white lead, or slaked lime.

1994.
Fine litharge	2 parts.
White lead	1 part.
Copal	1 part.
Boiled linseed oil	3 parts.

The whole is triturated together. Dissolve by heat.

1995.
For joining metallic surfaces where soldering is inconvenient, recourse may be had to a composition formed in the following way: Pure and finely divided copper, such as that obtained by the reduction of sulphate of copper with zinc clippings, 20 to 36 parts, according to the degree of hardness desired in the cement, dissolved in a sufficient quantity of sulphuric acid to make a thick paste; with this is incorporated, by trituration in a mortar, mercury 70 parts. The mass is soft, but hardens at the end of some hours. For use it is heated to 212° F. (100° C.), and powdered in an iron mortar heated to 302° F. (150° C.); it then assumes the consistence of wax, and is harder in proportion, as it contains more copper.

1996. Cement for Metal.
Metal, Cement for.—Melt over a water bath
Copal varnish	30 parts.
Drying oil	10 parts.
Turpentine	6 parts.

When melted add
Slaked lime	20 parts.

1997. Cement for Metal and Rubber.
Metal and Rubber, Cement for.—Powdered shellac is softened in ten times its weight of strong water of ammonia, whereby a transparent mass is obtained, which becomes fluid after keeping some little time without the use of hot water. In three or four weeks the mixture is perfectly liquid, and when applied, it will be found to soften the rubber. As soon as the ammonia evaporates the rubber hardens again—it is said, quite firmly—and thus becomes impervious both to gases and to liquids. For cementing sheet rubber, or rubber material in any shape, to metal, glass, and other smooth surfaces, the cement is highly recommended.

1998. To Cement Thin Metal Sheets.
Metal Sheets, Thin, to Cement.—Dissolve isinglass, cut fine, in warm water, and add a little nitric acid. If more acid is used than is necessary the cement will not dry.

1999. Linseed Oil Cement for Metal.
Metal, Linseed Oil Cement for.—Linseed oil and well slaked lime are made into a paste. Great pressure must be used.

2000. Metal to Porcelain, Glass, Etc.
Metal to Porcelain, Glass, etc.—Dissolve good glue in water, heat and add one-half as much linseed and varnish and one-quarter as much Venice turpentine as the amount of glue used.

2001. Cement for Mica.
Mica, Cement for.—A colorless cement for joining sheets of mica is prepared as follows: Clear gelatine is softened by soaking it in a little cold water, and the excess of water is pressed out by gently squeezing it in a cloth. It is then heated over a water bath until it begins to melt, and just enough hot proof spirit (not in excess) stirred in to make it fluid. To each pint of this solution is gradually added, while stirring, one-quarter ounce of gum ammoniac and one and one-third ounces of gum mastic previously dissolved in 4 ounces of rectified spirit. It must be warmed to liquefy it for use and kept in stoppered bottles when not required. This cement, when properly prepared, resists cold water

2002. Microscope Cement.
Microscope Cement.—Put into a bottle
Isinglass .... 2 parts.
Gum arabic................ 1 part.

Cover them with proof spirit, cork the bottle loosely, and place it in a vessel of water, and boil it till a thorough solution is effected, when it must be strained for use. This is a highly valuable cement for many purposes, and is used for mounting opaque objects for the microscope.

2003. Minerals, Fossils, Etc. A
Use best fish glue (hot) and tie well.

2004. Minerals, Fossils, Etc. B
Starch .... ¼ ounce.
White sugar............... 1 ounce.
Gum arabic................ ¼ ounce.

Dissolve the gum in a little hot water, and the sugar and starch, and boil until the starch is cooked.

2005. Mohr's.
Mohr's.—Equal parts of pulverized brick and litharge are made into a paste with linseed oil. After application a little fine sand is dusted over the lute, and it is dried in the oven.

GLUES.

2006. Sci. Am. Cyclo.
Glue is a cement used for joining pieces of wood together and has for its chief constituent a substance called gelatine, obtained from the cuttings of hides, skins, tendons and other refuse parts of animals, as well as from cuttings of leather and parchment, which, after being well soaked in milk of lime, to dissolve any blood, flesh or fat, are thoroughly washed in a stream of water to remove the lime. The material is then boiled in water until the required adhesive strength is obtained, when the liquid is run off into a cistern and clarified with powdered alum, which precipitates in the form of sulphate any lime that may remain, as well as other impurities. Before cooling it is drawn off into moulds, and is then in the form of size, which, when cut into slices and dried in the air, hardens into glue.

2007. Hints About Glue.
Hints about Glue.—Good glue should be a light brown color, semi-transparent, and free from waves or cloudy lines. Glue loses much of its strength by frequent remelting; therefore, glue which is newly made is preferable to that which has been reboiled. The hotter the glue the more force it will exert in keeping the joined parts glued together. In all large and long joints it should be applied immediately after boiling. Apply pressure until it is set or hardened.

The following, translated from Des Ingenieurs Taschenbuch, contains a great deal of valuable information which will probably be acceptable to many of our readers.

Common Glue.—The absolute strength of a well glued joint is:

Pounds per square inch.

	Across the grain, end to end.	With the grain.
Beech	2,133	1,095
Elm	1,436	1,124
Oak	1,735	568
White wood....	1,493	341
Maple	1,422	896

It is customary to use from one-sixth to one-tenth of the above values, to calculate the resistance which surfaces joined with glue can permanently sustain with safety.

2008. Bank Note or Mouth Glue.
Bank Note or Mouth Glue.—Is made by dissolving 1 pound of fine glue or gelatine, in water, evaporating it till most of the water is expelled; adding one-half pound brown sugar, and pouring it into moulds. Some add a little lemon juice. It is also made with 2 parts of dextrine, 2 of water and 1 of spirit.

2009. Bookbinders' Glue.
Bookbinder's glue.—Use best carpenter's or white glue, to which, after soaking and heating, one-twentieth its weight of glycerine is added.

2010. Glue of Caseine.
Glue of Caseine.—1. (Braconnet.)—Dissolve caseine in a strong solution of bicarbonate of soda. 2. (Wagner.)—Dissolve caseine in a cold saturated solution of borax. Superior to gum, and takes the place of glue in many cases. May be used for backs of adhesive tickets.

2011. To Make Compound Glue.
Compound Glue, to Make.—Take very fine flour, mix it with white of eggs, isinglass and a little yeast; mingle the materials and beat them well together; spread them, the batter being made thin with gum water, on even tin plates and dry them in a stove, then cut them out for use. To color them tinge the paste with Brazil or vermilion for red; indigo or verditer, etc., for blue; saffron, turmeric or gamboge, etc., for yellow.

2012. To Prevent Glue from Cracking.

Cracking, to prevent Glue from.—Glue frequently cracks because of the dryness of the air in rooms warmed by stoves. An Austrian contemporary recommends the addition of a little chloride of calcium to glue to prevent this disagreeable property of cracking. Chloride of calcium is such a deliquescent salt that it attracts enough moisture to prevent the glue from cracking. Glue thus prepared will adhere to glass, metal, etc., and can be used for putting on labels without danger of their dropping off.

Add a very small quantity of glycerine to the glue. The quantity must be modified according to circumstances.

2013. Glue for Damp Wood. A

Damp Wood, Glue for.—Soak pure glue in water until it is soft; then dissolve it in the smallest possible amount of proof spirit by the aid of a gentle heat. In 2 ounces of this mixture dissolve 10 grains of gum ammoniacum, and while still liquid add one-half dram of mastic dissolved in 3 drams of rectified spirit. Stir well and keep the cement liquefied in a covered vessel over a hot water bath. It is essentially a solution of glue in mastic varnish.

2014. Glue for Damp Wood. B

Shellac, 4 ounces; borax, 1 ounce; boil in a little water until dissolved and concentrate by heat to a paste.

2015.

Elastic Glue, which does not spoil, is obtained as follows: Good common glue is dissolved in water, on the water bath, and the water evaporated down to a mass of thick consistence, to which a quantity of glycerine, equal in weight with the glue, is added, after which the heating is continued until all the water has been driven off, when the mass is poured out into the moulds or on a marble slab. This mixture answers for stamps, printer's rollers, galvano-plastic copies, etc.

2016. Ether Glue.

Ether Glue.—Dissolve glue in nitric ether. The ether will only dissolve a certain amount of glue, therefore the solution cannot be made very thick; it will be about the consistency of molasses, and is much more tenacious than glue made with hot water. It is improved by adding a few bits of India rubber, cut into pieces about the size of a buckshot. Let the solution stand a few days, stirring frequently.

2017. Fire-Proof Glue.

Fireproof Glue.—Mix a handful of quicklime in 4 ounces of linseed oil; boil to a good thickness; then spread on tin plates in the shade, and it will become exceedingly hard, but may be easily dissolved over the fire and used as ordinary glue.

2018. Glue for Cementing Labels on Flower Pots.

Flower Pots, Glue for Cementing Labels on.—Use thin paper for label and attach with white gelatine in solution, to which has been added one per cent of bichromate of potash. This must be done in a dark or obscure room. Then expose the labels to sunlight. After writing varnish with solution of shellac in alcohol.

2019. Frozen Glue.

Frozen Glue.—The glue while gelatinous is sliced, placed on nets and allowed to freeze by natural cold. Of course the process can only be conducted in cold weather. The product is porous and much more bulky than hard glue, but is a better article, as it dissolves more easily. It sells largely in New England, where it is preferred by buyers to the hard glue.

2020. Glue for Joining Glass to Wood.

Glass to Wood, Glue for Joining.—Finely sifted wood ashes are added to glue when hot; use immediately.

2021. Glue for Repairing Glass.

Glue for Repairing Glass.—Dissolve fine glue in strong acetic acid to form a thin paste.

2022. Hardening Glue.

Hardening Glue.—Try a little finely powdered brick dust, which will harden quickly in proportion to the quantity used.

2023. Isinglass Glue.

Dissolve isinglass in water and strain it through coarse linen. Then add a little alcohol and evaporate to such a consistency that when cold it will be dry and hard. This will be found to be more tenacious than common glue and therefore preferable in many cases.

2024. Glue for Ivory and Bone.

Isinglass is boiled in water until very thick, when enough zinc white is added to make the whole the consistency of molasses.

2025. To Glue Labels to Iron.

Labels, to Glue to Iron.—Make a paste of rye flour and glue. Add linseed oil varnish and turpentine, one-half ounce of each to the pound of the paste.

2026. Sticking Labels to Tinned Plate.

From the Chemists' and Druggists' Diary for 1879, p. 188, the following seven methods of making a cement for affixing paper to tin:

Add to ordinary paste a little honey or glycerine.

Add muriatic acid to the gum; this is apt to cause the metal to rust under and around the label.

Add a little ammonia, or

Tartaric acid to the starch paste or mucilage.

Add aluminum sulphate (not alum) to the mucilage.

The best plan is said to be to add 20 drops of a solution of chloride of antimony to 8 ounces of paste of mucilage.

2027. To Glue Leather to Iron.

There is a constant inquiry as to the best plan for fastening leather to iron, and there are many recipes for doing it. But probably the simplest mode, and one that will answer in a majority of cases, is the following: To glue leather to iron, paint the iron with some kind of lead color, say white lead and lamp black. When dry, cover with a cement made as follows: Take the best glue, soak it in cold water till soft, then dissolve it in vinegar with a moderate heat, then add one-third of the bulk of white pine turpentine, thoroughly mix, and by means of the vinegar make it of the proper consistency to be spread with a brush, and apply it while hot; draw the leather on quickly, and press it tightly in place. If a pulley, draw the leather round tightly, lap and clamp.

2028. Glue for Leather Goods.

This glue, though rather complex in composition, gives good results. Eight ounces of rye whisky are diluted with 8 ounces of water and the mixture is made into a paste with 2 ounces of starch, three-quarters of an ounce of good glue are dissolved in the same amount of water, an equal amount of turpentine is added and the mixture and the paste are combined.

2029. Leather, Etc., to Metals.

Leather, etc., to Metals.—One part crushed nut galls digested six hours with 8 parts distilled water and strained. Glue is macerated in its own weight of water for twenty-four hours, then dissolved. The warm infusion of nut galls is spread on the leather; the glue solution upon the roughened surface of the warm metal; the moist leather is then pressed upon it and dried.

2030. Liquid Glue. A

A liquid glue possessing great resisting power, recommended for wood and iron, is prepared, according to Hesz, as follows: Clear gelatine, 100 parts; cabinet-makers' glue, 100 parts; alcohol, 25 parts; alum, 2 parts; the whole mixed with 200 parts of 20 per cent acetic acid, and heated on a water bath for six hours. An ordinary liquid glue, also well adapted for wood and iron, is made by boiling together for several hours 100 parts glue, 260 parts water, and 16 parts nitric acid.—English Mechanic.

2031. Liquid Glue. B

An improved liquid glue, according to the Journal of Applied Chemistry, may be prepared by dissolving 3 parts of glue, broken into small pieces, in 12 to 15 parts of saccharate of lime. On warming, the glue dissolves rapidly, and remains liquid when cold, without losing its strength. Any desirable consistency may be secured by varying the amount of saccharate of lime.

2032. Liquid Glue. C

Two ounces gelatine, 4 ounces water; when the gelatine has fully swelled, add 2 ounces glacial acetic acid. It is capital for mending china, glass, etc.—A. Pumphrey.

2033. Liquid Glue Without Acid.

Liquid Glue Without Acid.—An excellent liquid glue is made thus: Take of best white glue, 16 ounces; white lead, dry, 4 ounces; rain water, 2 pints; alcohol, 4 ounces. With constant stirring dissolve the glue and mix the lead in the water by means of a water bath. Add the alcohol, and continue the heat for a few minutes. Lastly, pour into bottles while it is still hot.

2034.

Take a wide mouthed bottle, and dissolve in it 8 ounces best glue in one-half pint water, by setting it in a vessel of water, and heating until dissolved. Then add slowly 2½ ounces strong aquafortis (nitric acid), 36° Baume, stirring all the while. Effervesence takes place under generation of nitrous acid. When all the acid has been added, the liquid is allowed to cool. Keep it well corked, and it will be ready for use at any moment.

2035.
Take of best white glue, 16 ounces; white lead, dry, 4 ounces; rain water, 2 pints; alcohol, 4 ounces; with constant stirring, dissolve the glue and lead in the water by means of a water bath. Add the alcohol and continue the heat for a few minutes. Lastly pour into bottles while hot.

2036.
Take 1 pint of the common turpentine and mix in a quart bottle with 4 fluid ounces 98 per cent alcohol. Agitate well, and let stand until the two fluids separate. Decant the turpentine (which will form the lower layer) from the alcohol, and mix it with 1 pint clear water. Agitate thoroughly, and let stand until these two fluids separate, then from the water decant the turpentine (which this time will form the upper layer), and, finally, mix with the turpentine about 1 ounce powdered starch, and filter through paper.

2037.
Lehner publishes the following formula for making a liquid paste or glue from starch and acid. Place 5 pounds potato starch in 6 pounds water, and add one-quarter pound pure nitric acid. Keep it in a warm place, stirring frequently for forty-eight hours. Then boil the mixture until it forms a thick and translucent substance. Dilute with water, if necessary, and filter through a thick cloth. At the same time another paste is made from sugar and gum arabic. Dissolve 5 pounds gum arabic and one pound sugar in 5 pounds water, and add 1 ounce nitric acid and heat to boiling. Then mix the above with the starch paste. The resultant paste is liquid, does not mould, and dries on paper with a gloss. It is useful for labels, wrappers, and fine bookbinders' use. Dry pocket glue is made from 12 parts glue and 5 parts sugar. The glue is boiled until entirely dissolved, the sugar dissolved in the hot glue, and the mass evaporated until it hardens on cooling. The hard substance dissolves rapidly in lukewarm water, and is an excellent glue for use on paper.—Polytech. Notiz.; Pharm. Record.

2038.
Cut 6 parts glue in small pieces. Pour 16 parts water over it, allow it to stand for a few hours. Add 1½ part sulphate of zinc, 1 part hydrochloric acid gas. Keep the mixture at a temperature of 175° to 190° F. for ten or twelve hours. This glue may be used for joining all articles, even porcelain, glass, mother of pearl, etc. It does not congeal.

2039.
Take of best white glue, 16 ounces; white lead, dried, 4 ounces; rain water, 2 pints; alcohol, 4 ounces. Dissolve the glue and lead in the water by means of a water bath, stirring constantly. Add the alcohol, and continue the heat for a few minutes. Pour into bottles while it is hot.

2040. Very Strong Liquid Glue.
Very Strong Liquid Glue.—Glue 4½ parts; water, 12 parts. Let them stand several hours. To soften the glue: Add muriatic acid ¾ parts; sulphate of zinc, 1½ part. Heat the mixture to 185° F. for ten or twelve hours. This glue remains liquid after cooling. Used for sticking wood, crockery, and glass.

2041. Russian Liquid Glue.
Russian Liquid Glue.—Soften 50 parts best Russian glue in 50 parts warm water. Add slowly, from 2¾ to 3 parts aquafortis and 3 parts powdered sulphate of lead.

2042. Marine Glue. A
Although now far from new, the extremely valuable marine glue of Jeffrey, does not seem to be as well known in this country as it deserves. Prepared by dissolving 1 part India rubber in crude benzine, and mixing with 2 parts shellac by the aid of heat. The waterproof character of this cement, in connection with its slight elastic flexibility, the ease with which it is applied when warm, and the promptness with which it sets on cooling, make it a most useful substance in many applications to house construction and furniture, as well as on board ship, where it was originally intended to be chiefly employed.

2043. Marine Glue. B
Caoutchouc, 1 ounce; genuine asphaltum, 2 ounces; benzole or naptha, q. s. The caoutchouc is first dissolved by digestion and occasional agitation, and the asphaltum is gradually added. The solution should have about the consistency of molasses.

2044. Marine Glue. C
Take of coal naphtha, 1 pint; pure (not vulcanized) rubber, 1 ounce; cut in shreds; and macerate for ten or twelve days, and then rub smooth with a spatula on a slab; add at heat enough to melt, 2 parts shellac by weight, to 1 part of this solution. To use it, melt at a temperature of about 248° F.—E. H. H., of Mass.

2045. Elastic Marine Glue.

Elastic Marine Glue.—Dissolve unvulcanized rubber in chloroform, benzole or bisulphide of carbon. Ropes or other material exposed to the action of air and water are coated with this glue. Whiting or fine sand may be added.

2046. Hints in Melting and Using Glue.

Glue, Hints in Melting and Using.—The hotter the glue, the more force it will exert in keeping the two parts glued together. therefore, in all large and long joints, the glue should be applied immediately after boiling. Glue loses much of its strength by frequently remelting; that glue, therefore, which is newly made is much more preferable to that which has been reboiled.

2047. A Glue to Resist Heat or Moisture.

A Glue to Resist Heat or Moisture.—Mix a handful of quicklime in ¼ pound of linseed oil; boil them to a good thickness and then spread it on a slab to cool.

2048. Moisture Proof Glue.

Moisture proof glue is made by dissolving 16 ounces of glue in 3 pints of skim milk. If a still stronger glue be wanted, add powdered lime.

2049. Parchment Glue.

Parchment, 10 parts, is cut into small pieces and boiled in 128 parts water until the liquid is reduced to 80 parts. The decoction is filtered through linen, and evaporated over a gentle fire until it presents the required consistence.

2050. Dry Pocket Glue.

Dry pocket glue is made from 12 parts of glue and 5 parts of sugar. The glue is boiled until entirely dissolved, the sugar dissolved in the hot glue, and the mass evaporated until it hardens on cooling. The hard substance dissolves rapidly in lukewarm water, and is an excellent glue for use on paper.

2051. Portable or Mouth Glue.

Fine pale glue 1 pound, dissolve over a water bath in sufficient water; add brown sugar ¼ pound, continue the heat till amalgamation is effected; pour on a slab of slate or marble, and when cold cut into squares.

2052. Rice Glue.

The fine Japanese cement is made by mixing rice flour with a sufficient quantity of cold water, then boiling gently, with constant stirring.

2053. Spaulding's Glue.

Soak the glue in cold water, using only glass, earthern or porcelain dishes. Then by gentle heat dissolve the glue in the same water, and pour in a small quantity nitric acid, sufficient to give the glue a sour taste like vinegar, about 1 ounce to every pound of glue.

2054. Glue for Tablets.

For 50 pounds of the best glue (dry) take 9 pounds glycerine. Soak the glue for ten minutes and heat to solution and add the glycerine. If too thick, add water. Color with aniline.

2055. Tungstic Glue.

Tungstic glue has been suggested as a substitute for hard India rubber, as it can be used for all the purposes to which this latter is applied. It is thus prepared: Mix a thick solution of glue with tungstate of soda and hydrochloric acid. A compound of tungstic acid and glue is precipitated, which, at a temperature of 86 to 104 F., is sufficiently elastic to be drawn out into very thin sheets.

2056. Veneering Glue, Well Suited for Inlaying.

The best glue is readily known by its transparency. and being of a rather light brown, free from clouds and streaks. Dissolve this in water, and to every pint add a half gill of the best vinegar and one-half ounce of isinglass.

2057. Waterproof Glue. A

Glue may be rendered insoluble by tannic acid dissolved in a small quantity of soft water.

2058. Waterproof Glue. B

In order to render glue insoluble in water, even hot water, it is only necessary when dissolving the glue for use to add a little potassium bichromate to the water and to expose the glued part to light. The proportion of potassium bichromate will vary with circumstances: but for most purposes about one-fiftieth of the amount of glue used will suffice. In other words, glue containing potassium bichromate, when exposed to the light, becomes insoluble.

2059. Waterproof Glue. C

To make an impermeable glue, soak ordinary glue in water until it softens, and remove it before it has lost its primitive form. After this, dissolve it in linseed oil over a slow fire until it is brought to the consistence of a jelly. This glue may be used for joining any kinds of material. In addition to strength and hardness, it has the advantage of resisting the action of water.—Revue Industrielle.

2060. Fire and Waterproof Glue.

Fire and Waterproof Glue.—Mix a handful of quicklime with 4 ounces of linseed oil; thoroughly lixiviate the mixture. Boil until quite thick, and spread on tin plates. It will become very hard, but can be dissolved over a fire like common glue.

2061. Cheap Waterproof Glue.

Cheap Waterproof Glue.—Melt common glue with the smallest quantity of water possible. Add to this by degrees, linseed oil, rendered drying by boiling it with litharge. While the oil is added the ingredients must be well stirred, so as to mix them thoroughly.

2062. White Glue.

A writer in the Moniteur Scientifique says that to add oxalic acid and white oxide of zinc in the proportion of 1 per cent to glue gives a whiter and clearer product than any of the measures now in use. The glue should first be reduced with water and heated to a thick sirup, and the chemicals added while the mass is hot.

2063. Waterproof Glue for Wood. A

Very thick solution of glue, 100 parts; linseed oil varnish, 50 parts; and 10 parts of litharge. Boil for ten minutes and use while hot.

2064. Waterproof Glue. B

There is no glue for wood which must be kept in contact with water that is better than bichromated glue. Allow it to harden thoroughly.

2065. Waterproof Glue. C

Liquid glue for wood and iron is made, according to Hesz, as follows: Clear gelatine, 100 parts; cabinetmaker's glue, 100 parts; alcohol, 25 parts; alum, 2 parts; the whole mixed with 200 parts of 20 per cent acetic acid and heated in a water bath for six hours.

2066. Waterproof Glue. D

An ordinary glue for wood and iron is made by boiling together for several hours 100 parts glue, 260 parts water and 16 parts nitric acid.

2067. Waterproof Glue. E

Waterproof glue may be made by boiling 1 pound of common glue in 2 quarts of skimmed milk. This withstands the action of the weather.

2068. Waterproof Glue. F

Glue, 12 parts; water, q. s. to dissolve. Add yellow resin, 3 parts; and, when melted, turpentine, 4 parts. Mix thoroughly together in a water bath.

2069. Glue Which Stands Moisture Without Softening.

Dissolve in 8 fluid ounces of strong methylated spirit, ½ ounce each of sandarac and mastic; next add ½ ounce of turpentine. This solution is then added to a hot, thick solution of glue, to which isinglass has been added, and is next filtered while hot through cloth or a sieve.

2070. Glue Dressing for Wounds.

Cabinetmakers and woodworkers generally are familiar with the uses of glue in dressing tool cuts and other slight wounds incident to their calling. The addition of acetic acid to the glue and a little otto of roses will cover the odor of the glue and the acid. This compound spread on paper or muslin makes a good substitute for adhesive plaster for surgical use. It is easily and quickly prepared simply by putting into a vessel of boiling water a bottle containing 1 part of glue to 4 parts by measure of the acid, and letting the bottle remain in this bath until the glue is fully dissolved and mixed with the acid. Common glue may be used and officinal acetic acid, to be had at any drug store. The mixture should be kept in a wide mouthed bottle well stoppered by a long cork, which can always be removed by heating the neck of the bottle. Care should be taken to keep the mouth of the bottle clean by wiping it well with a cloth dipped in hot water. A bottle of this cheap and easily prepared dressing would be a good thing to have at home as well as at the workshop.

2071. Cement for China and Glass.

Russian glue .... 8 ounces.
Water .... 4 ounces.

Macerate for four hours; then dissolve in water bath and add strong acetic acid 6 ounces.

2072.   China Cement.
   Isinglass .... 1 ounce.
   Mastich (in powder) ...... 4 scruples.
   Water .... 2 ounces.
   Glacial acetic acid .... 4 ounces.

Soak the isinglass in the water, and when all has been absorbed, add the acid previously mixed with the mastich. Heat gently till a clear solution is formed.

2073.   Cold Liquid Glue.
To make glue liquid in the cold, nitric acid is generally added, thus we may take
   Glue .... 8 parts.
   Water .... 8 parts.
   Nitric acid .... 2½ parts.

The nitric acid may be replaced by acetic acid. Thus an excellent liquid gum is made by dissolving one part of glue in two parts of vinegar.

Another process consists in dissolving by the aid of heat:
   Glue .... 30 parts.
   Water .... 80 parts.
and immediately adding,
   Hydrochloric acid .... 5 parts.
   Zinc sulphate .... 7 parts.

A very strong liquid glue is obtained by the action of caustic soda upon glue. The following proportions are used:
   Glue .... 1000 parts.
   Water .... 1500 parts.
   Commercial caustic soda... 40 parts.

2074.   Liquid Glue.
   Chloral hydrate .... 2½ ounces.
   Gelatine .... 4 ounces.
   Water .... 10 ounces.
   Mix all together.

The solution is ready in forty-eight hours, and is said to be excellent for mounting photographs.

2075. Cement for Porcelain Letters.
   Boiled linseed oil .... 3 ounces.
   Litharge .... 2 ounces.
   White lead .... 1 ounce.
   Gum copal .... 1 ounce.

Free the surface from grease before applying.

2076. Cement for Mending Rubber Shoes and Tires.
Western Druggist.
   Caoutchouc in shavings.... 10
   Resin 4
   Gum turpentine 40
   Oil turpentine .... enough.

Melt together, first, the caoutchouc and resin, then add the gum turpentine, and when all is liquefied, add enough of oil of turpentine to preserve it liquid. A second solution is prepared by dissolving together:
   Caoutchouc 10
   Chloroform 280

For use these two solutions are mixed. First wash the hole in the rubber shoe over with the cement, then a piece of linen dipped in it is placed over it; as soon as the linen adheres to the sole, the cement is then applied as thickly as required.

2077. Waterproof Glue for Wood.
   Glue .... 12 parts.
   Water .... enough.

Soak the glue in water and liquefy by means of a water bath, then add:
   Resin .... 3 parts.
And when this is melted add
   Turpentine .... 4 parts.

2078.
To mend broken mortars or pestles, use a thick paste of either calomel or litharge with glycerine. It forms an excellent cement, although rather long in drying.

2079.   Mucilage Stick.
   Glue .... 5 ounces.
   Granulated sugar .... 1 ounce.
   Water .... 5 ounces.

Dissolve by the heat of a water bath; pour into molds and dry.

2080.   Acacia Mucilage.
   Gum acacia granld. .... 16 ounces.
   Water .... 32 ounces.
   Glycerine .... 2 ounces.
   Salicylic acid .... 90 grains.

Dissolve the gum in the water by the aid of heat; dissolve the salicylic acid in the glycerine and add.

COLORED FIRES.

2081.   Red Fire.
   Strontia nit. .... 10 ounces.
   Sulphur .... 3½ ounces.
   Chlor. pot. .... 2 ounces.
   Ant. sulph. .... 6 drams.
   Veg. black .... 10 drams.
   Mix.

2082.   Crimson Fire.
   Chlorate potash .... 1 dram.
   Sulphur .... 4 drams.
   Willow charcoal .... 1 dram.
   Nitrate of strontia........ 1½ ounces.
   Mix.

2083. Red Fire for Parades. Cheap.
Strontium nitrate 4
Potassium chlorate 1
Linseed meal 1

The proportion of linseed meal may be increased or decreased. This makes a slow-burning mixture. Green and blue fires cannot be produced in this manner.

2084. Green Fire.
Potassium chlorate 18
Barium nitrate 60
Sulphur 22

To get a mixture which will burn more quickly reduce the proportion of barium nitrate and increase that of potassium chlorate. For a slower burning fire adopt a reverse process.

2085. Red Fire.
Potassium chlorate 18
Strontium nitrate 60
Sulphur 21
Carbon 1

For quicker or slower burning fires proceed as above, reading strontium for barium.

2086. Violet Fire.
Potassium chlorate 51
Calcium carbonate 18
Malachite powdered 16
Sulphur 15

By increasing the calcium salt and reducing the malachite a slower burning flame is obtained, and vice versa.

2087. White Fire.
Druggists Circular.
Nitrate of potassa .... 18 parts.
Sulphur .... 10 parts.
Black sulphide of antimony 3 parts.
Powdered quicklime .... 4 parts.

The lime must not be slaked, but fresh and caustic.

2088. Red Fire.
Nitrate of strontia .... 13 parts.
Sulphur .... 1 part.
Powdered gunpowder .... 1 part.

2089. Blue Fire.
Nitrate of potassa .... 5 parts.
Sulphur .... 2 parts.
Metallic antimony .... 1 part.

2090. Green Fire.
Nitrate of baryta .... 60 parts.
Chlorate of potassa ...... 18 parts.
Sulphur .... 22 parts.

2091. Lilac Fire.
Chlorate of potassa ...... 49 parts.
Sulphur .... 25 parts.
Dry chalk .... 20 parts.
Black oxide of copper .... 6 parts.

2092. Yellow Fire.
Sulphur .... 6 parts.
Chlorate of potassa ...... 12 parts.
Bicarbonate of soda ...... 3 parts.
Sulphate of strontia ..... 3 parts.

2093. Dark Blue Fire.
Sulphur .... 6 ounces.
Copper sulphate .... 1¼ ounces.
Potassium chlorate .... 17 ounces.

2094. Light Blue Fire.
Sulphur .... 4 ounces.
Burnt alum .... 6 ounces.
Potassium chlorate .... 15 ounces.

2095. Caution.
Caution.—Competent druggists need no directions for properly mixing the chemicals of a colored fire, but as the compounding of fireworks is oftentimes the great ambition of beginners, a word of advice will not be amiss in regard to the dangers of the manipulation, and the way to avoid them. Each substance must be dried and powdered separately, and afterwards mixed together in small quantities with a card or a wooden spatula on a piece of paper. Sifting with a hair sieve is a good way also, but the use of a mortar and pestle is extremely dangerous.

2096. Butter Coloring.
Sal soda .... 2 pounds.
Carbonate of potash ...... 2 pounds.
Cold water .... 5 gallons.

Dissolve the soda and potash in the water and set aside.

Annatto .... 2 pounds.
Cold water .... 4 gallons.

Let stand one day stirring thoroughly meantime.

Mix the two preparations together; let stand for a week, stirring occasionally; use clear water and stone crocks for mixing purposes.

Directions: Use one teaspoonful of the coloring in 5 quarts of cream; add just before churning.

2097. Infants' Food. A
Best wheaten flour .... 24 ounces.
Fine oatmeal .... 12 ounces.
Fine lentil flour .... 6 ounces.
Powdered sugar of milk... 6 ounces.

Mix well in a mortar, pass through a sieve; place in a large dish and bake in a slow oven for two hours; when cool pass through a sieve and pack in air tight packages.

Directions: Mix one tablespoonful of the food with water or milk into a paste, then add half a pint of boiling milk (or milk and water according to age of child), and boil for a few minutes; if not sufficiently sweet add sugar to suit taste.

2098. Infants' Food. B

Baked wheaten flour	1 pound.
Soda bicarb.	30 grains.
Sugar of milk	½ ounce.

Mix.

2099. Hektograph Copying Pad.

Best glue	½ pound.
Clear soft water	12 ounces.
Granulated sugar	4 ounces.
Glycerin	16 fl. ounces.
Powd. precptd. chalk or oxide of zinc	2 ounces.
Soap, white castile	¼ ounce.

Dissolve the glue, sugar and soap in the water by the aid of water bath heat; when dissolved add the glycerine; when nearly cold stir in the oxide of zinc or the chalk, and pour into tins of the size desired. The tins should have a depth of at least ⅞ of an inch.

2100. Hektograph Copying Ink.

Purple aniline 3. B.	1 ounce.
Alcohol, 188 per cent	1 ounce.
Glycerine	1 ounce.
Gluocose	1 ounce.
Water, hot	7 ounces.

Dissolve the aniline in the alcohol add the glycerin, gluocose and hot water.

2101. Black Marking Ink for Linen.

Nitrate of silver crystals..	1 ounce.
Distilled water	10 ounces.
Acacia mucilage	4 ounces.
Nigrosine, black	30 grains.
Aqua ammonia	q. s.

Dissolve the silver in the water and add ammonia water until the precipitate first formed is dissolved (shake the solution after each portion of the ammonia water is added); then add the nigrosine and lastly the mucilage. Write on the linen (tightly stretched) with a gold pen, and pass a hot iron over the writing. A quill pen or a new steel pen may be used in place of a gold pen.

2102. Crimson Marking Ink for Linen.

Nitrate of silver crystals..	1 ounce.
Carmine	10 grains.
Distilled water	10 ounces.
Acacia mucilage	4 ounces.
Aqua ammon. q. s.	

Dissolve the silver in the water and add ammonia water until the precipitate first formed is dissolved (shake the solution after each portion of the ammonia water is added); then add the carmine in fine powder; and lastly add the mucilage; mix well. Write on the linen (tightly stretched) with a gold pen and pass a hot iron over the writing.

2103. Violet Stamp Ink.

Methyl violet 3B.	3 drams.
Distilled water	10 drams.
Dilute acetic acid	10 drams.
Rectified spirit	1½ ounces.
Glycerine	7 ounces.

Triturate the violet in a mortar with the water, add the glycerine gradually, then the acid and spirit.

2104. Cheap Blue-Black Ink.

Tannin	1 ounce.
Sulphate of iron	6½ drams.
Sulphuric acid	20 minims.
Methyl blue	1 scruple.
Spirit	½ ounce.
Water	25 ounces.

Dissolve the tannin in half of the water, and the sulphate of iron and acid in the rest. Dissolve the methyl blue in the spirit, and add to the iron solution; then add the tannin solution.

2105. Aniline Copying Ink.

The following is adapted for use without a press:

Nigrosin	1 ounce.
Hot water	1 ounce.
Glycerine	1 ounce.
Glucose	1½ drams.

Rub all these together, and dilute with as much water as will give the ink the necessary character—i. e., about 10 ounces.

2106. Ink Powder.

Tannin	1 ounce.
Dried sulphate of iron.	2½ drams.
Powdered gum arabic	4 scruples.
Sugar	2 scruples.
Aniline blue. B.	2 scruples.

Mix.

CLEANSING, RENOVATING AND PROTECTING.

Sci. Amer. Cyclo.

2107. To Remove Acid Stains. A
Chloroform will restore the color of garments, where the same has been destroyed by acids.

2108. To Remove Acid Stains. B
When acid has accidentally or otherwise destroyed or changed the color of the fabric, ammonia should be applied to neutralize the acid. A subsequent application of chloroform restores the original color.

2109. To Remove Acid Stains. C
Spots produced by hydrochloric or sulphuric acid can be removed by the application of concentrated ammonia, while spots from nitric acid can scarcely be obliterated.

2110. Acids, Vinegar, Sour Wine, Must, Sour Fruits.
White goods, simple washing, followed up by chlorine water if a fruit color accompanies the acid. Colored cottons, woolens, and silks are very carefully moistened with dilute ammonia, with the finger end. (In case of delicate colors, it will be found preferable to make some prepared chalk into thin paste, with water, and apply it to the spots.)

2111. To Clean Alabaster. A
The best method of cleaning these ornaments is to immerse them for some time in milk of lime, and then wash in clean water, and when dry dust them with a little French chalk. Milk of lime is made by mixing a little slaked lime in water. This has a "milky" appearance, whence its name. Benzol or pure oil of turpentine is very highly recommended.

2112. To Clean Alabaster. B
Use soap and water, with a little washing soda or ammonia, if necessary. Rinse it thoroughly.

2113. Alkali Stains.
To remove from garments. A mixture of acetic acid, diluted with a large quantity of water, will remove stains brought by soda, soap, boilers, lye, etc., if the solution is readily applied.

2114. To Remove Stains of Aniline from the Hands.
Wash with strong alcohol, or what is more effectual, wash with a little bleaching powder, then with alcohol.

2115. To Clean Stuffed Animals.
Give the animal a good brushing with a stiff clothes brush. After this warm a quantity of new bran in a pan, taking care it does not burn, to prevent which, quickly stir it. When warm, rub it well into the fur with your hand. Repeat this a few times, then rid the fur of the bran, and give it another sharp brushing until free from dust.

2116. Scouring Balls. A
Curd soap .... 8 ounces.
Oil of turpentine .... 1 ounce.
Oxgall .... 1 ounce.
Melt the soap, and when cooled a little, stir in the rest, and make it into cakes while warm.

2117. Scouring Balls. B
Soft soap .... 1 pound.
Fuller's earth .... 1 pound.
Beat them well together in a mortar, and form into cakes. To remove grease, etc., from cloth. The spot first moistened with water is rubbed with the cake, and allowed to dry, when it is well rubbed with a little warm water, and afterward rinsed or rubbed off clean.

2118. To Clean Barometer Tubes.
Try a small quantity of warm nitric acid. Then rinse with water, rinse with absolute alcohol, and finally with ether; warm to expel the vapor of ether.

2119. To Cleanse Barrels.
Put a few pounds unslaked lime in the barrel, add water, and cover. In a short time add more water and roll the barrel. Rinse with clean water.

2120. To Remove Grease from Blackboards.
Make a strong lye of pearlashes and soft water, and add as much unslaked lime as it will take up. Stir it together and let it settle a few minutes, bottle it and stopper close. Have ready some water to dilute it when used, and scour the part with it. The liquor must not remain long on the board, as it will draw the color with it. Hence use it with care and expedition.

2121. To Cleanse Blankets. A

Put two large tablespoonfuls of borax and a pint bowl of soft soap into a tub of cold water. When dissolved put in a pair of blankets, and let them remain over night. Next day rub and drain them out, and rinse thoroughly in two waters, and hang them up to dry. Do not wring them.

2122. To Cleanse Blankets. B

Scrape 1 pound of soda soap, and boil it down in sufficient water, so that when cooling you can beat it with the hand to make a sort of jelly. Add 3 tablespoonfuls spirit of turpentine and 1 tablespoonful of spirit of hartshorn, and with this wash the article well and rinse in cold water until all the soap is taken off. Then apply salt and water and fold between two sheets, taking care not to allow two folds of the article washed to lie together. Smooth with a cool iron. Only use the salt where there are delicate colors that may run. If you can get potash soap, it will be better, as woolen manufacturers do not use soda soap.

2123. To Remove Blood Stains. A

An accidental prick of the finger frequently spoils the appearance of work, and if for sale, decreases its value. Stains may be entirely obliterated from almost any substance by laying a thick coating of common starch over the place. The starch is to be mixed as if for the laundry, and laid on quite wet.

2124. To Remove Blood Stains. B

The free and early application of a weak solution of soda or potash, and the subsequent application of the solution of alum, is recommended.

2125. Blood and Albuminoid Matters.

Steeping in lukewarm water. If pepsine, or the juice of carica papaya, can be procured, the spots are first softened with lukewarm water, and then either of these substances is applied.

2126. To Clean and Prepare Bones and Ivory.

The curators of the anatomical museum of the Jardin des Plantes have found that spirits of turpentine is very efficacious in removing the disagreeable odor and fatty emanations of bones or ivory, while it leaves them beautifully bleached. The articles should be exposed in the fluid for three or four days in the sun, or a little longer if in the shade. They should rest upon strips of zinc, so as to be a fraction of an inch above the bottom of the glass vessel employed. The turpentine acts as an oxidizing agent, and the product of the combustion is an acid liquor which sinks to the bottom, and strongly attacks the ivory if allowed to touch it.

2127.

Make a thick paste of common whiting in a saucer. Brush well with a toothbrush into the carved work. Brush well out with plenty of clean water. Dry gently near the fire. Finish with a clean dry hard brush, adding one or two drops (not more) of alcohol.

2128.

Mix about a tablespoonful of oxalic acid in ½ pint of boiling water. Wet the ivory over first with water, then with a toothbrush apply the acid, doing one side at a time and rinsing, finally drying it in a cloth before the fire, but not too close.

2129.

Take a piece of fresh lime, slake it by sprinkling it with water, then mix into a paste, which apply by means of a soft brush, brushing well into the interstices of the carving; next set by in a warm place till perfectly dry, after which take another soft brush and remove the lime. Should it still remain discolored, repeat the process, but be careful to make it neither too wet nor too hot in drying off, or probably the article might come to pieces, being most likely glued or cemented together. If it would stand steeping in lime water for twenty-four hours, and afterward boiling in strong alum water for about an hour and then dried, it would turn out white and clean. Rubbing with oxide of tin (putty powder) and a chamois leather will restore a fine gloss afterward.

2130.

Clean well with spirits of wine, then mix some whiting with a little of the spirits, to form a paste, and well brush with it. It is best to use a rubber of soft leather where there are no delicate points; put a little soap on the leather, and dip into the paste and rub the ivory until you get a brilliant polish, finish off with a little dry whiting; the leather should be attached to a flat wood surface and rub briskly.

2131.

When ivory ornaments get yellow or dusky looking, wash them well in soap and water, with a small brush to clean the carvings, and place them while wet in full sunshine; wet them two or three times a day for several days with soapy water, still keeping them in the sun; then wash them again, and they will be beautifully white. To bleach ivory, immerse it for a short time in water containing a little sulphurous acid, chloride of lime or chlorine.

2132.

Soda ash	1 pound.
Lime (burned)	½ pound.
Hot water	3 quarts.

Mix, and soak the bones for twenty-four hours in the liquid; wash them thoroughly and bleach them.

2133.

Put the bones in a strong warm alcoholic solution of caustic potash for a short time, then immerse in running water.

2134.   To Clean Straw.

Wash in warm soap liquor, well brushing them both inside and out, then rinse in cold water, and they are ready for bleaching.

2135.   To Bleach Straw.

To bleach.—Put a small quantity of salts of sorrel or oxalic acid into a clean pan, and pour on it sufficient scalding water to cover the bonnet or hat. Put the bonnet or hat into this liquor, and let it remain in it for about five minutes; to keep it covered hold it down with a clean stick. Dry in the sun or before a clear fire. Or, having first dried the bonnet or hat, put it, together with a saucer of burning sulphur, into a box with a tight-closing lid. Cover it over to keep in the fumes, and let it remain for a few hours. The disadvantage of bleaching with sulphur is that the articles so bleached soon become yellow, which does not happen to them when they are bleached by oxalic acid.

2136.   To Finish or Stiffen Straw.

To Finish or Stiffen.—After cleaning and bleaching, white bonnets should be stiffened with parchment size. Black or colored bonnets are finished with a size made from the best glue. Straw or chip plaits, or leghorn hats and bonnets, may also be cleaned, bleached and finished as above.

2137.   Removal of Stains from and Cleaning Books.

Dust can be removed by using bread or very soft rubber.

2138.

Water stains are removed by boiling water and alum. It will be necessary to float the sheet on this bath for some hours. Dry between clean blotting paper. The amount of alum is immaterial.

2139.

Damp stains are treated the same way, but with less chance of success.

2140.   Mud.

Mud.—Very little can be done. Wash in cold water, then in dilute hydrochloric acid and afterward in a weak solution of chloride of lime. Rinse and dry.

2141.   Fox Marks.

Fox Marks.—Use very dilute hydrochloric acid or Javelle water.

2142.   Finger Marks.

Finger Marks.—Very difficult to erase. Apply a jelly of white or curd soap, then wash with a brush in cold water.

2143.   Blood Stains.

Blood Stains.—Soak in cold water, wash with soap and rinse.

2144.   Writing Ink Stains.

Ink stains (of writing ink) usually try oxalic acid followed by chloride of lime. Wash well.

2145.   Marking Ink Stains, Etc.

Ink Stains (Marking Ink, etc.).—Apply tincture of iodine. The silver in the ink forms silver iodide, which is removed by weak solution of potassium cyanide (deadly poison).

2146.   Grease Spots.

Grease Spots.—Put over the spot a piece of blotting paper, apply a hot iron.

Or, apply Fr. chalk, put a piece of paper over it and apply the iron.

Or, try ether or benzine, put blotting paper above and below the spot.

2147.   To Clean Ink Bottles.

For cleaning ink bottles, the best and quickest agent is oxalic acid, but it is a violent poison. Try shaking small nails, with water or vinegar in them, and if this does not answer, use hydrochloric acid, carefully washing out two or three times after its application.

2148. To Clean Oily or Greasy Bottles.

Pour into them a little strong sulphuric acid; after they have been allowed to drain as much as possible, the bottle is then corked, and the acid caused to flow into every portion of it, for about five minutes. It is then washed with repeated rinsings of cold water. All traces of oil or grease left will be removed in a very expeditious manner, and no odor whatever will be left in the bottle after washing.

2149. To Clean Brass. A

There are many substances and mixtures which will clean brass. Oxalic acid, muriatic acid, and several other acids will clean brass very effectively; oxalic acid is the best, but the acids must be well washed off, the brass dried, and then rubbed with sweet oil and tripoli, otherwise it will soon tarnish again. Mixture to clean brass is:

Soft soap .... 1 ounce.
Rotten stone .... 2 ounces.

2150. To Clean Brass. B

Oxalic acid .... 1 ounce.
Rotten stone .... 2 ounces.
Sweet oil .... 1½ ounces.

Spirits of turpentine enough to make a paste.

When used, a little water is added and friction applied. If brass is very dirty, it requires a strong acid to make it bright; such is chromic acid, best prepared by mixing bichromate of potassa, sulphuric acid, and water, equal parts of each. This makes the dirtiest brass bright and clear at once, but it must be immediately washed off with plenty of water, rubbed dry, and polished with rotten stone. There are no patents on any of these proceedings; and if there were, the patentees would not be sustained in their claims.

2151. To Clean Brass. C

Wash with rock alum, boiled in a strong lye in the proportion of 1 ounce to 1 pint; polish with dry tripoli.

2152. To Clean Brass. D

The government method prescribed for cleaning brass, and in use at all the United States arsenals, is claimed to be the best in the world. The plan is to make a mixture of 1 part common nitric acid and ½ part sulphuric acid, in a stone jar, having also ready a pail of fresh water and a box of sawdust. The articles to be treated are dipped into the acid, then removed into the water, and finally rubbed with sawdust. This immediately changes them to a brilliant color. If the brass has become greasy, it is first dipped in a strong solution of potash and soda in warm water; this cuts the grease, so that the acid has free power to act.

2153. To Clean Brass. E

Rub the surface of the metal with rotten stone and sweet oil, then rub off with a piece of cotton flannel, and polish with soft leather. A solution of oxalic acid rubbed over tarnished brass soon removes the tarnish, rendering the metal bright. The acid must be washed off with water, and the brass rubbed with whiting and soft leather. A mixture of muriatic acid and alum dissolved in water imparts a golden color to brass articles that are steeped in it for a few seconds.

2154. To Clean Brass. F

First boil your articles in a pan with ordinary washing soda, to remove the old lacquer; then let them stand for a short time in dead nitric acid; then run them through bright dipping nitric acid. Swill all acid off in clean water, and brighten the relieved parts with a steel burnisher, replace in clean water, and dry out in beech sawdust. Next place your work on the stove till heated, so that you can with difficulty bear your hand on articles, and apply pale lacquer with brush, the work will burn if heated too much or too rapidly.

2155. To Clean Brass. G

Put a coat of nitric acid over the part you want cleaned, with a piece of rag; as soon as it turns a light yellow, rub it dry and the brass will present a very clean appearance; if not satisfactory, repeat.

2156. To Clean Brass. H

Oxalic acid and whiting mixed and applied wet, with brush, and brushed again when dry with soft plate brush to polish with dry whiting.

2157. Brass Instruments. A

Brass Instruments.—If the instruments are very much oxidized, or covered with green rust, first wash them with strong soda and water. If not so very bad, this first process may be dispensed with. Then apply mixture of 1 part common sulphuric acid and 12 parts of water, mixed in an earthen vessel, and afterward polish with oil and rotten stone, well scouring with oil and rotten stone, and using a piece of soft leather and a little dry rotten stone to give a brilliant polish. In future cleaning, oil and rotten stone will be found sufficient.

2158.   Brass Instruments.   B

Take a strip of coarse linen, saturate with oil and powdered rotten stone, put round the tubing of instrument, and work backward and forward; polish with dry rotten stone. Do not use acid of any kind, as it is injurious to the joints. To hold the instrument, get a piece of wood turned to insert in the bells; fix in a bench vise. The piece of wood will also serve for taking out any dents you may get in the bells.

2159.   Brass Instruments.   C

Oil and rotten stone for this purpose, though very efficacious, are objectionable on account of dirt, the oil finding its way to the pistons, and because the instrument cleaned in this manner so soon tarnishes. Dissolve some common soda in warm water, shred into it some scraps of yellow soap, and boil it till the soap is all melted. Then take it from the fire, and when it is cool add a little turpentine and sufficient rotten stone to make a stiff paste. Keep it in a tin box covered from the air, and if it gets hard, moisten a small quantity with water for use.

2160.   Brass Instruments.   D

If very much oxidized or covered with green rust, first wash it with strong soda and water. If not so very bad, this first process may be dispensed with. Then apply a mixture of 1 part of common sulphuric acid and 12 parts of water, mixed in an earthen vessel; wash well, first with clear water, and then with water containing some ammonia, afterward scouring well with oil and rotten stone, and using a piece of soft leather and a little dry rotten stone to give a brilliant polish. In subsequent cleaning oil and rotten stone will be found sufficient.

2161.

Brass work that is so dirty by smoke and heat as not to be cleaned with oxalic acid, should be thoroughly washed or scrubbed with soda, or potash water, or lye. Then dip in a mixture of equal parts of nitric acid, sulphuric acid, and water; or, if it cannot be conveniently dipped, make a swab of a small piece of woolen cloth upon the end of a stick, and rub the solution over the dirty or smoky parts; leave the acid on for a minute, and then wash clean and polish.

2162.   Paste for Cleaning Brass.

Paste for Cleaning Brass.
Starch .... 1 part.
Powdered rotten stone ... 12 parts.
Sweet oil .... 2 parts.
Oxalic acid .... 2 parts.
Water to mix.

2163.

Soft soap .... 2 ounces.
Rotten stone .... 4 ounces.
Beat them to a paste.

2164.

Rotten stone made into a paste with sweet oil.

2165.

Rotten stone .... 4 ounces.
Oxalic acid .... 1 ounce.
Sweet oil .... 1½ ounces.
Turpentine enough to make a paste.

2166.

Oxalic acid .... 1 part.
Iron peroxide .... 15 parts.
Powdered rotten stone.... 20 parts.
Palm oil .... 60 parts.
Petrolatum .... 4 parts.

See that solids are thoroughly pulverized and sifted, then add and thoroughly incorporate oil and petrolatum.

2167.   Cleaning Brass Inlaid Work.

Mix tripoli and linseed oil, and dip felt into the preparation. With this polish; if the wood be rosewood or ebony, polish it with finely powdered elder ashes, or make a polishing paste of rotten stone, a pinch of starch, sweet oil, and oxalic acid, mixed with water.

2168.   To Restore Brass Gas Fixtures.

Have the water clean and boiling in two vessels. Dip in one water and then in the next as soon as taken from the nitric acid bath, so that there shall be no traces of acid on the fittings. Dry in box-wood sawdust while hot, and place upon a piece of hot sheet iron over a stove. As soon as all traces of water have left, quickly lacquer with very thin shellac varnish, using a camel's hair brush. You can make the lacquer, by dissolving shellac in best alcohol. Do not touch the metal with the fingers before lacquering.

2169.   To Clean Brass Gun Shells.

For such as have been used, boil in a strong solution of caustic soda, rinse in hot water, then dip in a hot pickle of sulphuric acid, 1 part; water, 4 parts; and rinse in hot water.

2170. To Clean Britannia Metal.

Use finely powdered whiting, 2 tablespoonfuls of sweet oil and a little yellow soap. Mix with spirits of wine to a cream. Rub on with a sponge, wipe off with a soft cloth, and polish with a chamois skin.

2171. To Remove Stains from Broadcloth.

Grind fine 1½ ounces pipe clay; mix with 18 drops of alcohol and the same quantity spirits of turpentine. Moisten a little of this mixture with alcohol and rub on the stains. When dry, rub off with a woolen cloth.

2172. To Cleanse Bronze.

Clean the surface, first of all, with whiting and water, or crocus powder, until it is polished; then cover with a paste of plumbago and crocus, mixed in the proportions that will produce the desired color. Heat the paste over a small charcoal fire. Perhaps the bronzing has been produced by a corrosive process; if so, try painting a solution of sulphide of potassium over the cleaned metal.

2173. To Clean Bronze Statuary.

Use weak soap-suds or aqua ammonia.

2174. To Wash Brushes.

Dissolve a piece of soda in some hot water, allowing a piece the size of a walnut to a quart of water. Put the water into a basin, and after combing out the hair from the brushes, dip them, bristles downward, into the water and out again, keeping the backs and handles as free from the water as possible. Repeat this until the bristles look clean; then rinse the brushes in a little cold water; shake them well, and wipe the handles and backs with a towel, but not the bristles, and set the brushes to dry in the sun, or near the fire; but take care not to put them too close to it. Wiping the bristles of a brush makes them soft, as does also the use of soap.

2175. To Clean Calico and Linen.

When linen or calico is discolored by washing, age, or lying out of use, the best method of restoring the whiteness is by bleaching in the open air, and exposure on the grass to the dews and winds. There may occur cases, however, where this may be difficult to accomplish, and where a quicker process may be desirable, and the following is the best:

Lay the linen for twelve hours in a lye formed of 1 pound soda to a gallon of boiling hot soft water; then boil it for half an hour in the same liquid. Then make a mixture of chloride of lime with 8 times its quantity of water, which must be well shaken in a stone jar for three days, then allowed to settle, and being drawn off clear, the linen must be steeped in it thirty-six hours, and then washed out in the ordinary way. This will remove all discoloration.

2176. To Renovate Cane seated Chairs.

Clean the articles with a solution of oxalic acid. Their color will be restored.

2177.

Wash with hot water and a sponge, using soap if necessary. Dry in a current of air.

2178. To Renovate Canvas.

Coat it with a black leather varnish, such as the following:

Digest shellac .... 12 parts.
White turpentine .... 5 parts.
Gum sandarac .... 2 parts.
Lampblack .... 1 part.
Spirits of turpentine...... 4 parts.
Alcohol .... 96 parts.

2179. To Clean Carpets.

If brooms are wet with boiling suds once a week, they will become very tough, will not cut a carpet, and will last much longer. A handful or so of salt sprinkled on a carpet will carry the dust along with it and make the carpet look bright and clean. A very dusty carpet may be cleaned by dipping the broom in cold water, shaking off all the drops, and sweeping a yard or so at a time. Wash the broom and repeat until the entire carpet has been swept.

2180.

Use 1 pint oxgall to a pailful of water; after washing apply cold water to rinse out the oxgall, and finally sponge as dry as possible.

2181. Dry Cleaning.

Dry Cleaning.—Have ready a number of dry coarse cotton or linen cloths, some coarse flannels and one or more large pieces of coarse sponge; two or more hard scrubbing or scouring brushes, some large tubs or pans, and pails, and also a plentiful supply of both hot and cold water. First take out all grease spots; this may be effected in several ways. Well rub the spot with a piece of hard soap and wash out with a brush and cold water, and well dry each spot before leaving it.

2182.

Or use, instead of the soap, a mixture of fuller's earth, gall and water, well rinsing and drying each spot as before. When this has been done, the carpet may be cleaned by one of the three following methods:

2183. How to Sweep Carpet.

It is not an easy matter to sweep well, at any rate, if we may judge by experience; for when a broom is put into the hands of the uninitiated, more harm than good generally results from the use of it. Without the greatest care and some little knowledge, furniture and paint, by being knocked about with the broom, may soon receive an irreparable amount of damage. Before sweeping rooms, the floors should be strewed with a good amount of dry tea leaves, which should be saved for the purpose; these will attract the dust and save much harm to other furniture, which as far as possible, should be covered up during the process. Tea leaves also may be used with advantage upon druggets and short piled carpets. Light sweeping and soft brooms are here desirable. Many a carpet is prematurely worn out by injudicious sweeping. Stiff carpet brooms and the stout arms of inexperienced servants are their destruction. In sweeping thick piled carpets, such as Axminster and Turkey carpets, the servant should be instructed to brush always the way of the pile; by so doing they may be kept clean for years; but if the broom is used in a different way, all the dust will enter the carpet and soon spoil it. Salt sprinkled upon the carpet before sweeping will make it look bright and clean. This is also a good preventive against moths.

2184. To Remove Grape Stains from Carpet.

Wash out with warm soap-suds and a little ammonia water.

2185. To Preserve Carriages.

Ammonia cracks varnish and fades the colors both of painting and lining. A carriage should never, under any circumstances, be put away dirty. In washing a carriage, keep out of the sun, and have the lever end of the "setts" covered with leather. Use plenty of water, which apply (where practicable) with a hose or syringe, taking care that the water is not driven into the body to the injury of the lining. When forced water is not attainable, use for the body a large soft sponge. This, when saturated, squeeze over the panels, and by the flow down of the water the dirt will soften and harmlessly run off, then finish with a soft chamois leather and oil silk handkerchief. The same remarks apply to the under works and wheels, except that when the mud is well soaked, a soft mop, free from any hard substance in the head, may be used. Never use a "spoke brush," which, in conjunction with the grit from the road, acts like sandpaper on the varnish, scratching it, and of course effectually removing all gloss. Never allow water to dry itself on the carriage, as it invariably leaves stains. Be careful to grease the bearings of the fore carriage so as to allow it to turn freely. Examine a carriage occasionally, and whenever a bolt or slip appears to be getting loose, tighten it up with a wrench, and always have little repairs done at once. Top carriages should never stand with the head down, and aprons of every kind should be frequently unfolded or they will soon spoil.

2186. To Whiten Celluloid Collars and Cuffs.

If the coloring does not disappear when the affected portions are rubbed with a woolen cloth and a little tripoli, and then polished with a clean woolen rag, the injury is a permanent one.

Cream of tartar is excellent. Use with a little water.

2187. To Clean Celluloid Covered Mountings.

Rub the covered parts with a woolen cloth and a little tripoli, and polish with a clean woolen rag.

2188. To Clean China.

Use a little fuller's earth and soda or pearlash with your water.

2189. To Clean Chromos.

Keep a wet towel lying on its face till the dirt is thoroughly softened, say 3 or 4 days, occasionally rubbing off carefully with a sponge; then rub with clear nut or linseed oil.

2190. To Clean Clocks and Watches.

In cleaning clock and watch movements take 1 quart water, about 1 teaspoonful or 5 grains liquid ammonia or alkali; into this liquid should be grated or scraped fine 5 grains common soap. These proportions can be varied as desired, if the following remarks are kept in view: The articles to be cleaned should be plunged into this bath, where they should be allowed to remain at least ten minutes. Twenty or thirty minutes is better, especially for clocks. The articles should be wiped dry when removed from the bath, or polished up with a brush dipped in some polishing powder. Rectified benzine is preferable, as ammonia is apt to turn the movement black if in excess. Use great care in using benzine, as it is very inflammable and never should be used at night.

2191. To Clean Black Cloth.

Dissolve
Bicarbonate of ammonia... 1 ounce.
Warm water .... 1 quart.

With this liquid rub the cloth, using a piece of flannel or black cloth for the purpose. After the application of this solution, clean the cloth well with clear water, dry and iron it, brushing the cloth from time to time in the direction of the fiber.

2192. Cloth Cleaning Compound.

Glycerine .... 1 ounce.
Sulphuric ether .... 1 ounce.
Alcohol .... 1 ounce.
Ammonia .... 4 ounces.
Castile soap .... 1 ounce.

Mix together and add sufficient water to make 2 quarts. Apply and rinse.

2193. To Brush Clothes.

Brushing clothes is a very simple but very necessary operation. Fine clothes require to be brushed lightly, and with rather a soft brush, except where mud is to be removed, when a hard one is necessary, being previously beaten lightly to dislodge the dirt. Lay the garment on a table, and brush it in the direction of the nap. Having brushed it properly, turn the sleeves back to the collar, so that the folds may come at the elbow joints; next turn the lapels or sides back over the folded sleeves, then lay the skirts over level with the collar, so that the crease may fall about the center, and double one-half over the other, so that the fold comes in the center of the back.

2194. To Clean Coins, Medals, Etc.

If the coins are silver, clean with potassium cyanide. This is a deadly poison, and should be handled with care.

2195.

Dip in strong hot solution of potash or soda, rinse and dip for a moment in nitric acid, after which rinse quickly in running water.

2196.

Coins can be quickly cleansed by immersion in strong nitric acid, and immediate washing in water. If very dirty, or corroded with verdigris, it is better to give them a rubbing with the following:

Pure bichromate of potash. ½ ounce.
Sulphuric acid .... 1 ounce.
Nitric acid .... 1 ounce.

Rub over, wash with water, wipe dry, and polish with rotten stone or chalk.—Lyle.

2197. To Restore Color.

When color on a fabric has been accidentally or otherwise destroyed by acid ammonia is applied to neutralize the same, after which an application of chloroform will, in almost all cases, restore the original color. The application of ammonia is common, but that of chloroform is but little known.

2198. To Revive the Color of Faded Black Cloth or Leather.

Take of the best quality of
Blue galls .... 4 ounces.
Logwood .... 1 ounce.
Clean sulp. iron (copperas) 1 ounce.
Clean iron filings .... 1 ounce.
Sumac leaves .... 1 ounce.

Put the galls, logwood and sumac berries into 1 quart of the best white wine vinegar and heat to nearly the boiling point in a sand bath, then add the iron filings and copperas; digest for twenty-four hours and strain for use. Apply with a sponge.

2199. To Clean Combs.

If it can be avoided, never wash combs, as the water often makes the teeth split and the tortoiseshell or horn of which they are made rough. Small brushes, manufactured purposely for cleaning combs, may be purchased at a trifling cost; with this the comb should be well brushed, and afterward wiped with a cloth or towel.

2200. To Clean Copper.

Take
Oxalic acid .... 1 ounce.
Rotten stone .... 6 ounces.
Gum arabic .... ½ ounce.
All in powder,
Sweet oil .... 1 ounce.

And sufficient of water to make a paste. Apply a small portion, and rub dry with a flannel or leather.

2201.

Use soft soap and rotten stone, made into a stiff paste with water, and dissolved by gently simmering in a water bath. Rub on with a woolen rag, and polish with dry whiting and rotten stone. Finish with a leather and dry whiting.

2202.

Copper plates are cleaned by laying them on the hob near the fire, and pouring on them some turpentine, and then rubbing them with a small soft brush.

2203. To Clean and Bleach Coral.

The secret in cleaning coral is to turn the mass bottom upward and suspend it by means of a piece of wire in the saucepan, so that the dirt, as it boils off, may drop into the water, instead of down the septa. A strong solution of ordinary washing soda, or better, oxalic acid, is to be used to boil it in. The mass is to be boiled at least three hours. This is not only to clean the coral, but to bleach it also.

2204.

Apply a mixture of hydrochloric acid and water, or wash the coral with a stiff brush in cold salt and water, with a little soap powder, a little chloride of lime will improve it, then put in the sun to dry and bleach.

2205. To Restore Crape.

Skimmed milk and water, with a little bit of glue in it, made scalding hot, is excellent to restore rusty Italian crape. If clapped and pulled dry like muslin, it will look as good as new; or, brush the veil till all the dust is removed, then fold it lengthwise, and roll it smoothly and tightly on a roller. Steam it till it is thoroughly dampened, and dry on the roller.

2206. To Clean Crape.

Crape is cleansed by rinsing it in oxgall and water to remove the dirt, afterward in pure water to remove the gall, and lastly in a little gum water to stiffen and crisp it. It is then clapped between the hands until dry.

2207. To Wash Curtains.

Shake every curtain, or hang them on a line and brush them down with a soft haired brush. Prepare a soaking liquid by melting a small quantity of borax in warm water, soak for an hour or two, then squeeze between the hands to remove the superfluous water. Take some good soap and chip it in hot water, stir until all the soap is melted, and a fine lather produced. By this time the water will be moderately warm. Immerse the curtains in this, pass them repeatedly through the lathered water, or work them up and down. Rubbing should be avoided; when absolutely necessary, do it gently and without a brush. Squeeze out the soapy water, and rinse in plenty of soft warm water. Wring carefully. Curtains should be dried quickly. If in the country, they may be spread to dry on clean grass. Otherwise curtains are always better for being stretched and pinned to wooden frames while drying.

It is advisable to use cooked starch for curtains. Use good starch, mix it thoroughly in warm water, which should be made to boil for fifteen or twenty minutes. While cooling add a very little indigo blue. This is only to be used for pure white curtains. The starch should be decidedly thick. Draw the curtains through the starch, squeeze out gently, and dry rapidly.

2208. Coloring Curtains.

Many persons prefer tinted curtains to pure white ones. If they have to be colored, do not put any blue in the starch, but use water that has been slightly tinted with coffee (for ecru curtains), tea for a more decided hue, or saffron (for yellow tint) for preparing the starch. A decoction of logwood may be used if you wish to give the curtains a delicate pink hue.

2209. How to Prepare Special Coloring Starches for Curtains.

The basis of these coloring starches is thus prepared:

Soak 1 pound of good white glue for twelve hours, using just enough water to make it into a jelly; dissolve this with boiling water adding about 18 to 19 pounds of Paris white; add more water until the compound is diluted to the consistency of milk. This starch may be colored to taste. A little Prussian blue and vermilion (in the proportions of 2 to 1) gives a fine lilac. Raw umber and a pinch of lamp-black gives a gray. Vermilion and red lead (in the proportion of 3 to 1) produce a tender rose. Indigo blue just tinted with vermilion gives a lavender. Chrome yellow and a pinch of Spanish brown gives lemon yellow. Indian yellow and burnt sienna (in the proportion of 2 to 1) gives a buff hue. Experiments should be tried, as some of the colors look very badly if they are dark.

2210. To Clean Diamonds.

Clean all diamonds and precious stones by washing them with soap and water with a soft brush, adding a little ammonia in the water, and then dry in fine boxwood sawdust. A little potash or pearlash put in the water will answer the same purpose.

2211. To Clean Drawing Instruments.

If the lacquering is badly spotted, clean it off with strong alcohol, and then polish the brass or German silver with the following paste by means of flannel and a little water, and polish off with clean chamois leather or cotton cloth and a little whiting, after which you might re-varnish with shellac dissolved in alcohol, colored with a little dragon's blood, which can be got from any apothecary:

Soft soap	3 ounces.
Sweet oil	½ ounce.
Turpentine	¼ ounce.
Powdered rotten stone	4 ounces.
Finest flour emery	1 ounce.
Fine powd. crocus of antimony	½ ounce.

Melt the soap, oil and turpentine together, add the powders, a little water to make a stiff paste and mix well.

2212. To Clean Engravings.

Presuming these to be mounted, proceed in the following manner: Cut a stale loaf in half, with a perfectly clean knife; pare the crust away from the edges. Place the engravings on a flat table, and rubbing the surface with the fresh cut bread, in circular sweeps, lightly but firmly performed, will remove all superficial markings. Soak the prints for a short time in a dilute solution of hydrochloric acid, say 1 part acid to 100 of water, and then remove them into a vessel containing a sufficient quantity of clear chloride of lime water to cover them. Leave them here until bleached to the desired point. Remove, rinse well by allowing to stand an hour in a pan in which a constant stream of water is allowed to flow, and finally dry off by spreading on clean cloths. Perhaps they may require ironing between two sheets of clean paper.

2213.

Put the engraving on a smooth board, cover it thinly with common salt finely powdered; squeeze lemon juice upon the salt so as to dissolve a considerable proportion of it; elevate one end of the board, so that it may form an angle of about 45° or 50° with the horizon. Pour on the engraving boiling water from a tea kettle until the salt and lemon juice be all washed off; the engraving will then be perfectly clean, and free from stains. It must be dried on the board, or on some smooth surface, gradually. If dried by the fire or the sun, it will be tinged with a yellow color.

2214.

Hydrochloric acid, oxalic acid, or eau de Javelle may be employed, weakened by water. After the leaves (if it be a book) have by this means been whitened, they must be bathed again in a solution of sulphate of soda, which will remove all the chlorine, and leave the leaves white and clean. They will, however, have lost all firmness of texture, owing to the removal of the size from the paper. It will, therefore, be advisable to give a bath of gelatine and alum made with boiling water, to which may be added a little tobacco, or any other simple substance to restore the tint of of the now too white paper.

2215.

Immerse each mildewed sheet separately in a solution made in the proportions of one-half pound chloride of lime to 1 pint of water. Let it stand, with frequent stirring, for 24 hours, and then strain through muslin, and finally add 1 quart water. Mildew and other stains will be found to disappear very quickly, and the sheets must then be passed separately through clear water, or the chloride of lime, if left in the paper, will cause it to rot. Old prints, engravings, and every description of printed matter may be successfully treated in the same manner.

2216.

"I have in my time cleaned many hundreds. The plan which I adopt is as follows: I place them, one or two at a time, in a shallow dish, and pour water over them until they are completely soaked or saturated with it. I then carefully pour off the water, and pour on to the prints a solution of chloride of lime (1 part liquor calcis chloratae to 39 parts of water). As a general rule, the stains disappear as if by magic, but occasionally they are obstinate. When that is the case, I pour on the spot pure liquor calcis chlorate, and if that does not succeed, I add a little dilute nitro-muriatic acid. I have never had a print which has not succumbed to this treatment—in fact, as a rule, they become too white. As soon as they are clean they must be carefully washed with successive portions of water until the whole of the chlorine is got rid of. They should then be placed in a very weak solution of isinglass or glue, and many collectors color this solution with coffee grounds, etc., to give a yellow tint to the print. They should be dried between folds of blotting paper, either in a press or under a heavy book, and finally ironed with an ordinary flat iron to restore the gloss, placing clean paper between the iron and the print. Grease stains are much more difficult. I find benzine best. Small grease spots may be removed by powdered French chalk being placed over them, a piece of clean blotting paper over the chalk, and a hot iron over that."—F. Andrews.

2217.

Mildew often arises from the paste used to attach the print. Take a solution of alum of medium strength and brush on back and face of the engraving 2 or 3 coats, then make the frame air-tight by pasting a strip of paper all round the inside of glass, leaving about one-half inch overlapping (taking care not to paste the paper on the glass so as to be seen from the front), then place your glass in frame, take the overlapping piece and paste to side of rabbet; place your picture in position, spring back board in, and then place a sheet of strong paper (brown) on the table, damp it, and paste round back of frame, lay it on to the paper, leave to dry, cut level. If this does not answer, there will be no help for it, but dust off as the mould accumulates. Do not brush on surface with the alum if the engraving is colored, but several coats on the back.

2218.

It has been found that ozone bleaches paper perfectly without injuring the fibre in the least. It can be used for removing mildew and other stains from engravings that have been injured by hanging on the walls of damp rooms. The engraving should be carefully moistened and suspended in a large vessel partially filled with ozone. The ozone may be generated by putting pieces of clean phosphorus in the bottom of the vessel partially covered with water; or by passing electric sparks through the air in the vessel.

2219.

If the engravings are very dirty, take two parts of common salt and one part common soda, and pound them together until very fine. Lay the engraving on a board, and fasten it with drawing pins, and then spread the mixture dry equally over the surface to be cleaned. Moisten the whole with warm water and a little lemon juice, and, after it has remained about a minute, or even less, tilt the board up on its end, and pour over it a kettleful of boiling water, being careful to remove all the mixture, and avoid rubbing. If the engraving is not very dirty, the less soda used the better, as it has a tendency to give the engraving a yellow hue.

2220. To Cleanse Emery after using.

Boil with caustic potash, stirring constantly, then wash with acid, dilute and dry.

2221. To Remove Grease from Emery Wheels.

Wash with bisulphide of carbon.

2222. Lightning Eradicator.

Strong ammonia water, 4 ounces; water, 2 quarts; saltpeter, 1 ounce; mottled soap, 2 ounces; the soap must be finely shaved. Mix thoroughly and allow the preparation to stand for several days before using. Cover any grease spot with this preparation, rub well and rinse with clean water.

2223. To Clean Feathers.

To clean feathers from their own animal oil, steep them in 1 gallon of water mixed with 1 pound of lime; stir them well, and then pour off the water, and rinse the feathers in cold spring water. To clean feathers from dirt, simply wash them in hot water with soap. Rinse them in hot water.

2224.

To Clean White Ostrich Feathers.—4 ounces white curd soap cut small, dissolved in 4 pints water, rather hot, in a basin. Make the solution into a lather by beating it with birch rods or wires. Introduce the feathers and rub well with the hands for five or six minutes. After the soaping, wash in clean water as hot as the hand can bear. Shake until dry.

2225.

Slightly soften the soiled feathers with warm water, using a camel's hair brush. Next raise each feather with a flat piece of wood or paper knife, and clean them with spirits of wine. Dry with plaster of Paris, and afterward brush them carefully with a dry camel's hair brush.

2226.

Make a strong solution of salt in water, saturate a large and thick cloth with it. Wrap the bird up in the damp cloth in as many folds as you can, not disarranging the plumage. Look at the bird in six hours, and if not long dried on the blood will be soft; if not soft, keep it in the cloth longer, and rewet it. When soft, rub out with gentle pressure, putting something hard under each feather with blood on, and rubbing with the back of a knife. Of course each feather must be done separately.

2227.

Col. Wragge treated the soiled plumage of albatrosses, Cape petrel, etc., by simply washing the feathers in rain water, after the process of skinning, and then laying a thick mixture of starch and water over the portion to be cleansed. Next he laid the birds aside, and left them till the plastering of starch had become thoroughly dry. He then removed the dry plaster by tapping it, and found that the feathers had become much cleaner. Old specimens may be cleaned in this way. Feathers may be set by just arranging them naturally with a needle or any pointed instrument.

2228.

White.—Dissolve 4 ounces of white soap in 2 quarts of boiling water, put it into a large basin or small pan, and beat to a strong lather with a wire egg beater or a small bundle of birch twigs; use while warm. Hold the feather by the quill with the left hand, dip it into the soap liquor and squeeze it through the right hand, using a moderate degree of pressure. Continue this operation until the feather is perfectly clean and white, using a second lot of soap liquor if necessary. Rinse in clean hot water to take out the soap, and afterward in cold water in which a small quantity of blue has been dissolved. Shake well, and dry before a moderate fire, shaking it occasionally, that it may look full and soft when dried. Before it is quite dry, curl each fibre separately with a blunt knife or ivory paper folder.

2229. To Purify Feathers for Beds, Pillows, Etc.

Prepare a quantity of lime water in the following manner: Well mix 1 pound of quicklime in each gallon of water required, and let it stand until all the undissolved lime is precipitated, as a fine powder, to the bottom of the tub or pan, then pour off the clear liquor for use. The number of gallons to be prepared will, of course, depend on the quantity of feathers to be cleaned. Put the feathers into a clean tub, pour the lime water on them, and well stir them in it until they all sink to the bottom. There should then be sufficient of the lime water to cover them to a depth of 3 inches. Let them stand in this for three or four days, then take them out, drain them in a sieve, and afterward well wash and rinse them in clear water. Dry on nets having a mesh about the same size as a cabbage net; shake the net occasionally, and the dry feathers will fall through. When they are dried, beat them well to get rid of the dust. It will take about three weeks to clean and dry a sufficient quantity for a bed. This process was awarded the prize offered by the Society of Arts.

2230. To Render Feathers White and to Remove the Gray Color.

Feathers must be cleansed by immersing for a short time in naphtha or benzine. Rinse in a second dish of the same and dry in the air. Then bleach by exposing in a box to the vapor of burning sulphur in a moist atmosphere.

2231. To Wash Flannels.

Shave a little white soap into a pail; and pour on it water nearly boiling hot to dissolve it, adding, if you choose, a tablespoonful of spirits of ammonia. Pour the hot suds upon the flannels in a tub, and use a good pounder or a machine, as the water needs to be of too high a temperature for the hands. Wring the flannels, and put them into a second water, like the first, except with less soap, and use again the pounder or machine. Rub the soiled spots in the suds as hot as you can bear, but never rub soap on the spots. Wring the flannels as dry as you can with a good wringer, and put them on a line in a brisk, drying air. The hotter they are when wrung and the sooner they dry the better. Their color may be improved by a little bluing; and if they are well ironed before getting quite dry, fulling is prevented.

2232. Flannel Shrinking.

All flannel ought properly to be shrunk before it is cut out and made up into garments. The process is quite simple. Soak the flannel for a few minutes in warm water, then rub some good laundry soap over every inch of it, dip it in the water and knead it, or shake it up and down; do not scrub. After the washing, let the flannel be thoroughly rinsed in warm water. It must be remembered that boiling or hot water should never touch flannel. Wring carefully and dry slowly. On no account allow flannel to be dried in an overheated drying closet or before a fire.

2233. Flannel Washing.

To wash flannel or flannel garments, prepare a good lather in hot water; when just warm throw in your flannel and work it up and down, backward and forward. Scrubbing must be avoided, and no soap should be actually rubbed on it, as this will induce further shrinkage. Rinse in warm water, twice if necessary. Never wash or rinse in hot or cold water, as they both cause the flannel to shrink suddenly.

2234. To Wash Flannel Blankets.

Put the soiled blankets to soak for fifteen minutes in plain soft warm water. Prepare a soft jelly with first-class laundry soap and boiling water, 1 pound of soap for every blanket. Pour this into a tub of warm water, let it melt and lather it up well with the hand. Wring the blankets from the soaking tub, and throw them into the lather; stir them about and leave to soak ten minutes, then hand rub every inch of the blankets, paying especial attention to stains. Take them out and wring, then rinse in warm water twice. Dry well, but do not expose them to great heat. When dry stretch them in every direction, and rub all over with a piece of clean rough flannel. This makes them fluffy and soft. If very dirty, a little borax may be added to the water, but no soda or bleaching powder should ever be used.

2235. To Iron Flannels.

Most flannels are the better for not being ironed, but in some cases it is necessary to do so. The proper way is to dry the flannels, then spread them on an ironing board, cover them with a slightly damp cloth, and iron over this, pressing down heavily. The iron must not be too hot.

2236. Fleckenwasser.
Bronner.

Cleansing fluid (literally spot or stain water) for the removal of grease and dirt spots. Benzine only.

2237. Englisches Fleckenwasser.

English cleansing fluid for removing acid, resin, wax, tar, and grease spots. A mixture of 95 per cent alcohol, 100 grammes; liq. ammon. sp. gr. 875, 30 grammes; benzine, 4 grammes.—Artus.

2238. To Scour Floors.

Clean sand, 12 parts; soft soap, 8 parts; lime, 4 parts. Use a scrubbing brush and rinse.

2239. To Remove Fly Specks from Brass, Etc.

If you cannot wash off the fly specks with soap and warm water on a cloth, there is no way that an amateur can refinish lampwork with any satisfaction. To do this the lamp must be taken apart and the brasswork boiled in caustic soda to remove all oil and varnish; then rinse in hot water and dip in strong nitric acid for a few seconds only, when it will come out clean and bright; then rinse clean in boiling water. Dry in sawdust, brush off, and lacquer with thin shellac varnish. The metal must be warm and perfectly free from grease.

2240. To Remove Fly Specks from Bronze.

Lavender oil, 1 dram; alcohol, 1 ounce; water 1½ ounces. Use a soft sponge and proceed quickly with little rubbing.

2241. To Remove Fly Specks from Gilding.

Old ale is a good thing to wash any gilding with, as it acts at once on the fly dirt. Apply it with a soft rag.

2242. To Renovate Frames.

You may improve them by simply washing them with a small sponge moistened with spirits of wine or oil of turpentine, the sponge only to be sufficiently wet to take off the dirt and fly marks. They should not be wiped afterwards, but left to dry of themselves.

2243. Fruit and Wine Stains.

White cotton or linen, fumes of burning sulphur, warm chlorine water. Colored cottons or woolens, wash with tepid soapsuds of ammonia. Silks the same, with very gentle rubbing.

2244.

First rub the spot on each side with hard soap and then lay on a thick mixture of starch and cold water. Rub this mixture of starch well into the spot, and afterward expose it to the sun and air. If the stain has not disappeared at the end of three or four days, repeat the process.

2245.

Stains of wine may be quickly and easily removed from linen, by dipping the parts which are stained into boiling milk. The milk to be kept boiling until the stain disappears.

2246.

Most fruits yield juices which, owing to the acid they contain, permanently injure the tone of the dye; but the greater part may be removed without leaving a stain, if the spot be rinsed in cold water in which a few drops of aqua ammonia have been placed before the spot has dried. Wine stains on white materials may be removed by rinsing with cold water, applying locally weak solution chloride of lime, and again rinsing in an abundance of water. Some fruit stains yield only to soaping with the hand, followed by fumigation with sulphurous acid; but the latter process is inadmissible with certain colored stuffs. If delicate colors are injured by soapy or alkaline matters, the stains must be treated with colorless vinegar of moderate strength.

2247.

To remove fruit and wine stains from table linen moisten with dilute sulphuric acid and then rub with aqueous solution of sulphite or hyposulphite of soda in water.

2248.

Spread the stained part over a bowl or basin, and pour boiling water through it; or rub on salts of lemon and pour boiling water through until the stain disappears or becomes very faint.

2249. How to Improve the Appearance of Furniture.

Mr. G. J. Henkels, of Philadelphia, Pa., suggests that when the polish on new furniture becomes dull it can be renewed by the following process: Take a soft sponge, wet with clean cold water, and wash over the article. Then take a soft chamois skin and wipe it clean. Dry the skin as well as you can by wringing it in the hands, and wipe the water off the furniture, being careful to wipe only one way. Never use a dry chamois on varnished work. If the varnish is defaced and shows white marks, take linseed oil and turpentine in equal parts; shake them well in a phial and apply a very small quantity on a soft rag until the color is restored; then with a clean soft rag wipe the mixture entirely off. In deeply carved work the dust cannot be removed with a sponge. Use a stiff haired paint brush instead of a sponge. The cause of varnished furniture becoming dull, and the reason why oil and turpentine restore its former polish, it will be appropriate to explain. The humidity of the atmosphere and the action of gas cause a bluish white coating to collect on all furniture, and show conspicuously on bright polished surfaces, such as mirrors, pianos, cabinet ware, and polished metal. It is easily removed as previously directed. The white scratches on furniture are caused by bruising the gum of which varnish is made. Copal varnish is composed of gum copal, linseed oil, and turpentine or benzine. Copal is not soluble in alcohol, as other gums are, but is dissolved by heat. It is the foundation of varnish, as the oil is used only to make the gum tough, and the turpentine is required only to hold the other parts in a liquid state, and it evaporates immediately after its application to furniture. The gum then becomes hard and admits of a fine polish. Thus, when the varnish is bruised, it is the gum that turns white, and the color is restored by applying the oil and turpentine. If the mixture is left on the furniture, it will amalgamate with the varnish and become tough. Therefore the necessity of wiping it entirely off at once. To varnish old furniture, it should be rubbed with pulverized pumice stone and water to take off the old surface, and then varnish with varnish reduced, by adding turpentine, to the consistency of cream. Apply with a stiff haired brush. If it does not look well, repeat the rubbing with pumice stone, and when dry, varnish it again.

For a crack, a worm eaten hole, or a deep flaw, prepare the proper dust, by the admixture of brick dust in flour (also kept ready), or whiting or ocher, or any required tint. Then take well-cooked glue, and on a house plate stir it in slowly while hot, with sufficient powder for your work. Dab the hole or crack with your glue brush, then with a putty knife stir about the mixture on the plate, taking care you have the right color. When sure on this point, take some of the cement on the end of the knife and insert it in the desired place. Then use as much pressure as you possibly can with the blade, and keep smoothing at it. Sprinkle a little of the dry powder on the spot. When thoroughly dry, sand paper the surface with an old used piece, so as not to abrade the joint. You can then varnish the mending. Where weevil and wood worms have devoured the furniture, cautiously cut out the part till a sound place be reached. Poison the wood with a solution of sulphate of copper injected into the hollow. Let it dry. Cut an angular piece of same wood from your board, and with a sharp chisel make a suitable aperture for its reception. Fix it with glue. When thoroughly dry, work with carving tools or rasp and glass, scraping till the new bit of work exactly matches the old.

2250. Polish for Removing Stains from Furniture.

One pint of 98 per cent alcohol, ground resin one-half ounce, gum shellac 1½ ounces. After the resin and shellac cut in the alcohol, mix in 1 pint of linseed oil, and give the whole a good shaking. Apply with a cloth or newspaper and polish with a flannel after applying the solution.

2251. To Clean Dark Furs.

Sable, chinchilla, squirrel, fitch, etc. Heat a quantity of new bran in a pan, taking care that it does not burn, stir constantly. When well heated rub thoroughly into the fur. Repeat two or three times. Shake the fur and brush briskly until free from dust.

2252. To Clean Light Furs.

White furs, ermine, etc., may be cleaned in the following way: Lay the fur on a table and rub with bran, moistened with warm water. Rub until dry, then rub with dry bran. Use flannel for rubbing with the wet bran and book muslin for the dry. After using the bran, rub with magnesia. Dry flour may be used instead of wet bran. Rub against the way of the fur.

2253. To Clean Gilt Picture Frames.

Fly marks can be cleaned off with soap and water used sparingly on end of finger covered by piece of rag. When all cleared off, rinse with cold water, and dry with chamois leather; next buy a pound of common size and two penny paint pans. Boil a little of the size in one of the pans with as much water as will just cover it. When boiled, strain through muslin into clean pan, and apply thinly to frames with camel hair brush (called technically a "dabber"). Take care you do not gives the frames too much water and "elbow grease." On no account use gold size, as it is used only in regilding, and if put on over the gold would make it dull and sticky.

2254.

Dissolve a very small quantity of salts of tartar in a wine bottle of water, and with a piece of cotton wool soaked in the liquid dab the frames very gently, no rubbing on any account or you will take off the gilt, then stand up the frames so that water will drain away from them conveniently, and syringe them with clean water. Care must be taken that the solution is not too strong.

2255.

If new gold frames are varnished with the best copal varnish it improves their appearance considerably, and fly marks can then be washed off carefully with a sponge. The frames also last many times longer. It also improves old frames to varnish them with it.

2256.

Gilt frames may be cleaned by simply washing them with a small sponge, moistened with hot spirits of wine or oil of turpentine, the sponge only to be sufficiently wet to take off the dirt and fly marks. They should not afterward be wiped, but left to dry of themselves.

2257.

Old ale is a good thing to wash any gilding with as it acts at once upon the fly dirt. Apply it with a soft rag; but for the ins and outs of carved work, a brush is necessary; wipe it nearly dry, and don't apply any water. Thus will you leave a thin coat of the glutinous isinglass of the finings on the face of the work, which will prevent the following flies' faeces from fastening to the frame, as they otherwise would do.

2258. To Clean Gilt Mountings.

Gilt mountings, unless carefully cleaned, soon lose their luster. They should not be rubbed, if slightly tarnished, wipe them off with a piece of Canton flannel, or what is better, remove them if possible, and wash in a solution of one-half ounce of borax dissolved in 1 pound of water, and dry them with a soft linen rag; their luster may be improved by heating them a little and rubbing with a piece of Canton flannel.

2259. Glass Cleaning Preparation.

Photographers will find the following a useful glass-cleaning preparation: Water, 1 pint; sulphuric acid, one-half ounce; bichromate of potash, one-half ounce. The glass plates, varnished or otherwise, are left for 10 or 12 hours, or as much longer as desired, in this solution, then rinsed in clean water and wiped dry with soft white paper. The liquid quickly removes silver stains from the skin without any of the attendant dangers of cyanide of potassium.

2260. To Clean Glass.

To clean glass in frames, when the latter are covered or otherwise so finished that water cannot be used, moisten tripoli with brandy, rub it on the glass while moist, and when dry rub off with a silk rag; to prevent the mixture injuring the cloth on the frame, use strips of tin bent to an angle, set these on the frame with one edge on the glass; when the frames are of a character that will not be injured by water, rub the glass with water containing a little liquid ammonia and polish with moist paper.

2261.

Glass Bottles.—If vessels are oily or otherwise greasy, they should not be washed with water, but wiped with dry tow, or a dry dirty cloth, so as to remove as much grease as possible. By changing the cloth for one that is clean, the vessel can be wiped until all traces of grease disappear.

2262.

A strong solution of an alkali such as pearl-ash may be used, whereby the removal of the grease is materially facilitated.

2263.

If a vessel be soiled by resin, turpentine, resinous varnishes, etc., it should be washed with a strong alkaline solution, and rubbed by means of the wire and tow.

2264.

If the alkali fail to act, a little sulphuric acid acid may be employed with advantage. The latter acid will also be found advantageous in removing pitch and tar from vessels of glass. Nitric or sulphuric acids may be employed to clean flasks which have contained oil.

2265.

A correspondent of the Philadelphia Photographer says: "To clean a silver bottle, pour in a strong solution of cyanide; shake a few times, pour out, and rinse with water io or three times, and your bottle is perfectly clean. Keep the solution, and filter and strengthen when required. By doing this you can sun your bath better in two hours than in a week's exposure in the dirty black bottles, photographers appear to delight in."

2266.

It would be easy for a practical brush maker to construct a brush in the form of a hollow cone, which would reach the bottom of bottles; but the difficulty would be to get it into the bottle without spoiling it (the brush). A brush composed of a single bundle of long hairs, something like a painter's sash tool, with the bristles cut somewhat tapering, should answer the purpose. The bottle must, of course, be turned round with the hand, to bring every part into contact with the brush.

2267.

Lead shot, where so used, often leave carbonate of lead on the internal surface, and this is apt to be dissolved in the wine or other liquids afterward introduced, with poisonous results; and particles of the shot are sometimes inadvertently left in the bottle. Fordos states that clippings of iron wire are a better means of rinsing. They are easily had, and the cleaning is rapid and complete. The iron is attacked by the oxygen of the air, but the ferruginous compound does not attach to the side of the bottle, and is easily removed in washing. Besides, a little oxidized iron is not injurious to health. Fordos found that the small traces of iron left had no apparent effect on the color of red wines; it had on white wines, but very little; but he thinks it might be better to use clippings of tin for the latter.

2268.

Take a small piece of the very finest and softest flannel without crease or seam, or a few inches of superfine broadcloth, dip this in powder blue, and with it clean your plate glass, polishing with a rag of soft silk or fine chamois leather.

2269. To Cleanse Laboratory Glassware.

Laboratory flasks which have contained oil or fatty matter may be easily cleansed by a solution of permanganate of potassa. To remove turpentine, petroleum, photogene, etc., wash with an ounce or so of sulphuric acid and rinse with water.

2270. To Clean Discolored Glass.

Apply dilute nitric acid. Water of ammonia is also good.

2271. To Clean Gloves.

Ganteine.—A composition used to clean kid and other leather gloves. 1. Curd soap (in small shavings), 1 part; water, 3 parts; mix with heat, and stir in essence of citron, 1 part. —M. Buhan.

2272.

2. Saponine.—Duvignau soap in powder, 250 parts; water, 155 parts; dissolve with heat, cool, and add of eau de Javelle, 165 parts; solution of ammonia, 10 parts, and rub the whole to a smooth paste. A small portion of either of the above is rubbed over the glove with a piece of flannel (always in one direction) until it is sufficiently clean.

2273. To Clean Kid Gloves.

Put them together with a sufficient quantity of pure benzine in a large stoppered vessel, and shake the whole occasionally, with alternate rest. If, on removing the gloves, there remain any spots, rub them out with a soft cloth moistened with ether or benzole. Dry the gloves by exposure to the air, and then place smoothly between glass plates at the temperature of boiling water until the last traces of benzine are expelled. They may then be folded and pressed between paper with a warm iron. Another way is to use a strong solution of pure soap in hot milk beaten up with the yelk of one egg to a pint of the solution. Put the glove on the hand, and rub it gently with the paste, to which a little ether may be added, then carefully lay by to dry. White gloves are not discolored by this treatment, and the leather will be made thereby clean and soft as when new.

2274.

Damp them slightly, stretch them gently over a wooden hand of appropriate size, and clean them with a sponge dipped in benzole, recently rectified oil of turpentine, or camphine. As soon as they are dry, withdraw them gently from the stretcher, and suspend them in a current of air for a few days, or until they cease to smell of the cleaning liquid used. Heat must be avoided. The cleaning liquid should be used liberally, and the first dirty portion should be sponged off with clean liquid.

2275.

Make a strong lather with curd soap and warm water; lay the glove flat on a board, the bottom of a dish, or other unyielding surface; dip a piece of flannel in the lather, and well rub the glove with it till all the dirt is out, turning it about so as to clean it all over. Dry in the sun or before a moderate fire. When dry they will look like old parchment and should be gradually pulled out and stretched.

2276.

Have a small quantity of milk in a cup or saucer, and a piece of brown Windsor or glycerine soap in another saucer. Fold a clean towel or other cloth three or four times thick, and spread the glove smoothly on the cloth. Dip a piece of flannel in the milk, and rub it well on the soap. Hold the glove firmly with the left hand, and rub it with the flannel toward the fingers. Continue this operation until the glove, if white, appears of a dirty yellow; or if colored, until it looks dirty and spoiled, and then lay it to dry. Gloves cleaned by this method will be soft, glossy and elastic.

2277.

French Method.—Put the gloves on your hands, and wash them in spirits of turpentine until they are quite clean, rubbing them exactly as if washing your hands; when finished, hang them in a current of air to dry and to take off the smell of the turpentine.

2278.

Eau de javelle............ 135 parts.
Ammonia.................. 8 parts.
Powdered soap........... 200 parts.
Water..................... 150 parts.

Make a soft paste, and use with a flannel.

2279.

Wash them with soap and water; then stretch them on wooden hands, or pull them into shape without wringing them; next rub them with pipe clay or yellow ocher, or a mixture of the two in any required shade, made into a paste with beer; let them dry gradually, and when about half dry rub them well, so as to smooth them and put them into shape; then dry them, brush out the superfluous color, cover them with paper, and smooth them with a warm iron. Other colors may be employed to mix with the pipe clay besides yellow ocher.

2280. Glove Cleaner.

Castile soap, white........ 3 troy ounces.
Javelle water............. 2 fl. ounces.
Water..................... 2 fl. ounces.
Water of ammonia........ 1 dram.

Dissolve the soap by the aid of heat in the water, and when nearly cold, add the Javelle water and the water of ammonia. The preparation should form a paste, to be rubbed on the soiled part of the glove with a piece of flannel. This recipe is in use in many large cleaning establishments, and can be recommended.

2281. To Clean Kid Gloves without Wetting.

Stale bread is sometimes used for this purpose. The gloves are put on and the softer part of the bread is broken up into crumbs and the hands are rubbed one over the other as in the act of washing, the crumbs being thus rubbed over all parts of the gloves. Spongy rubber is often used for glove cleaning. It is applied in the same manner as in cleaning drawings, i. e., it is rubbed over the soiled parts of the glove.

2282.

Lay the gloves upon a clean board, make a mixture of dried fuller's earth and powdered alum, and pass them over on each side with a stiff brush. Then sweep the dust off and sprinkle them well with dry bran and whiting and dust them well. This, if the gloves be not exceedingly soiled, will effectually cleanse them; but if they are much soiled, take out the grease with crumbs of toasted bread and powder of burnt bone, then pass them over with a woolen cloth, dipped in fuller's earth or powdered alum.

2283. Doeskin, Wash Leather (Chamois) and Undressed Kid.

Wash them in luke warm soft water, with a little castile or curd soap, oxgall or bran tea; then stretch them on wooden hands; or pull them into shape without wringing them; next rub them with pipe clay, yellow ocher, or umber, or a mixture of them in any required shade, made into a paste with ale or beer; let them dry gradually, and when about half dry rub them well so as to smooth them, and put them into shape; when they are dry brush out the superfluous color, cover them with paper and smooth them with a warm (not hot) iron.

2284.
Take out the grease spots by rubbing them with magnesia or with cream of tartar. Then wash them with soap dissolved in water as directed for kid gloves, and afterward rinse them, first in warm water and then in cold. Dry in the sun, or before the fire. All gloves are better and more shapely if dried on glove trees or wooden hands.

2285.
Stretch them on a hand or lay them flat on a table, and rub into them a mixture of finely powdered fuller's earth and alum; sweep it off with a brush, sprinkle them with a mixture of dry bran and whiting, and lastly dust them off well. This will not do if they are very dirty.

2286. To Clean Gold Bronze.
Boil in a weak alkali prepared from an infusion of wood ashes. Then clean with a solution composed of equal parts nitric acid, water and alum.

2287. Gold Detergent.
(Upton.)
Quicklime, 1 ounce; sprinkle it with a little hot water to slake it, then gradually add 1 pint boiling water, so as to form a milk. Next dissolve pearlash, 2 ounces, in boiling water, 1½ pints. Mix the two solutions, cover up the vessel, agitate occasionally for an hour, allow it to settle; decant the clear, put it into flat ½ pint bottles, and cork them well. Use to clean gilding either alone or diluted with water. It is applied with a soft sponge, and then washed off with clean water. It is essentially a weak solution of potassa and may be extemporaneously prepared by diluting solution of potassa with about five times its volume.

2288. Cleaning Dull Gold.
A solution of 80 grams chloride of lime, 80 grams bicarbonate of soda, and 20 grams common salt in 3 liters distilled water is prepared and kept in well-closed bottles. The article to be cleaned is allowed to remain some short time in this solution (which is only to be heated in the case of very obstinate dirt), then taken out, washed with spirit, and dried in sawdust.

2289. Removing Stains from Gold and Silver.
Immerse for some time in a solution of ½ ounce cyanide of potassium to 1 pint rain water and brush off with prepared chalk.

2290. To Wash Gold Lace.
It is placed over night in urine or wine and washed. Take 1½ pints water and 1½ pints whisky, and a little ground gum arabic and saffron. Apply with a brush when the laces are stretched on a table.

2291. Removal of Stains from Granite.
A paste of 1 ounce oxgall, 1 gill of strong solution of caustic soda, 1½ tablespoonfuls of turpentine, with enough pipe clay to make it thick and consistent, scour well.

2292.
Mix together ¼ pound whiting, ¼ pound soft soap, 1 ounce washing soda, and a piece of sulphate of soda as big as a walnut. Rub it over the surface you propose to treat, let it stand twenty-four hours, and then wash off. If it succeeds, try another portion.

2293.
Smoke and soot stains can be removed with a hard scrubbing brush and fine sharp sand, to which add a little potash.

2294.
Use strong lye, or make a hot solution of 3 pounds of common washing soda dissolved in 1 gallon of water. Lay it on the granite with a paint brush.

2295. To Remove Grass Stains.
Wash the stained places in clean, cold, soft water, without soap, before the garment is otherwise wet.

2296. Removal of Grease.
Fatty oils have a greater surface tension than oil of turpentine, benzole or ether. Hence, if a grease spot on a piece of cloth be moistened on the reverse side with one of these solvents, the tension on the greasy side is larger, and therefore the mixture of benzole and fat or grease will tend to move toward the main grease spot. If we were to

to moisten the center of this spot with benzole, we should not remove it, but drive the grease upon the clean portion of the cloth. It is, therefore, necessary to distribute the benzole first over a circle surrounding the grease spot, to approach the latter gradually, at the same time having blotting paper in contact with the spot to absorb the fat immediately.

2297.

Another method, namely, to apply a hot iron on one side, while blotting paper is applied to the other, depends upon the fact that the surface tension of a substance diminishes with a rise of temperature. If, therefore, the temperature at different portions or sides of the cloth is different, the fat acquires a tendency to move from the hotter parts toward the cooler.—The Pharmacist.

2298.

Grease and Oil.—For white linen or cotton goods, use soap or weak lye. For colored calicoes, warm soapsuds. For woolens, soapsuds or ammonia. For silks, benzine, ether, ammonia, magnesia, chalk, yolk of egg with water.

2299.

Dissolve 1 ounce pearlash in 1 pint water, and to this solution add a lemon cut into thin slices. Mix well, and keep the mixture in a warm state for two days, then strain and bottle the clear liquid for use. A small quantity of this mixture poured on stains, occasioned by either grease, oil or pitch, will speedily remove them. Afterward wash in clear water.

2300.

Carbonate of magnesia—magnesia that has been previously calcined is best—is dried in an oven and mixed with sufficient benzine to form a soft, friable mass. In this state it is put into a wide mouthed glass bottle, well stoppered and kept for use. It is spread pretty thickly over the stains, and rubbed well to and fro with the tip of the finger. The small rolls of earthy matter so formed are brushed off, and more magnesia is laid on and left until the benzine has evaporated entirely. Materials that will bear washing are then cleaned with water; on silks, alcohol or benzine should be used instead. The process may be applied to textile fabrics of every description, except those containing very much wool, to which the magnesia adheres very tenaciously. It may also be used for stains, old or new, on all sorts of fancy woods, ivory, parchment, etc., without risk of injury. Ordinary writing ink is not affected by it, but letterpress quickly dissolves, owing to the absorption of the fatty matter in the ink.

2301.

A method of cleansing greasy woolen or cotton rags and waste. The rags are thrown into a closed revolving drum, with a quantity of perfectly dry and finely powdered plaster of Paris; when the plaster has absorbed all the grease, the whole is transferred to another revolving drum, pierced with holes, by which means the greater portion of the greasy plaster is got rid of. The operation is finished by beating the rags on a kind of wooden sieve.

2302.

In the removal of grease from clothing, with benzol or turpentine, people generally make the mistake of wetting the cloth with the turpentine and then rubbing it with a sponge or piece of cloth. In this way the fat is dissolved, but is spread over a greater space and is not removed; the benzol or turpentine evaporates, and the fat covers a greater surface than before. The way is to place soft blotting paper beneath and on top of the grease spot, which is to be first thoroughly saturated with the benzol, and then well pressed. The fat is then dissolved and absorbed by the paper, and entirely removed from the clothing.

2303.

Castile soap in shavings..	4 ounces.
Carbonate of soda.........	2 ounces.
Borax.....................	1 ounce.
Aqua ammonia.............	7 ounces.
Alcohol...................	3 ounces.
Sulphuric ether...........	2 ounces.

Soft water enough to make 1 gallon. Boil the soap in the water until it is dissolved, and then add the other ingredients. Although it is not apparent what good 2 ounces of ether can do in 1 gallon of liquid, the mixture is said to be very efficient.

2304.

Make a weak solution of ammonia by mixing the ordinary "liquor ammoniae" of the druggist with its own volume of cold water, and rub it well into the greasy parts, rinsing the cloth in cold water from time to time until the grease is removed. The ammonia forms a soap with the fatty acids of the grease, which is soluble in water.

2305.

On Paper.—Press powdered fuller's earth lightly upon the greasy spot, and allow it to soak out the grease.

2306.

Hannett says the spots may be removed by washing the part with ether, chloroform or benzine, and placing between white blotting paper, then passing a hot iron over.

2307.

A more expeditious and thought by some the best way is to scrape fine pipe clay, magnesia, or French chalk on both sides of the stain, and apply a hot iron above, taking great care that it is not too hot.

2308.

After gently warming the paper, take out all the grease you can with blotting paper and a hot iron, then dip a brush into essential oil of turpentine, heated almost to ebullition, and draw it gently over both sides of the paper, which must be kept warm. Repeat the operation until all is removed, or as often as the thickness of the paper may render necessary. When all the grease is removed, to restore the paper to its former whiteness, dip another brush in ether, chloroform, or benzine, and apply over the stain, especially the edges of it. This will not affect printer's or common writing ink.

2309.

Lay on a coat of India rubber solution over the spot, and leave it to dry. Afterward remove with a piece of ordinary India rubber. Any operation with ether, chloroform, or benzine should never be conducted by candle light, as their vapor is apt to kindle even at several feet from the liquid. No. 2308 will remove grease from colored calf. Even if the spot be on the under side of the leather, it may thus be clearly drawn right through.

2310.

Apply a solution of pearlash (in the proportion of 1 ounce pearlash to 1 pint water) to oil-stained drawing paper.

2311.

Grease can be removed from billiard or other cloths by a paste of fuller's earth and turpentine. This should be rubbed upon the fabric until the turpentine has evaporated, and a white powder remains. The latter can be brushed off, and the grease will have disappeared.

2312.

To Remove from Silk.—Use chloroform and a cotton cloth, finishing with a dry cloth. Benzine can also be used as well as French chalk. If chalk is used, place a hot iron over the spot until the grease is removed.

2313.

Spots of Grease.—On white goods, soap water or alkalies; on dyed tissues of cotton, hot soap water; dyed tissues of wool, soap water or ammonia; on silk, benzine, ether, ammonia, magnesia, chalk, yolk of egg.

2314. Grease Extractor.
Fuller's earth............. 15 parts.
French chalk............. ½ part.
Yellow soap............... 10 parts.
Pearlash.................. 8 parts.

Mix thoroughly and make it into paste with spirits of turpentine. Color if desired, with yellow ocher. Form into cakes.

2315.

An earthy compound for removing grease spots is made as follows: Take fuller's earth free it from all gritty matter by elutriation with water; mix with ½ pound of the earth so prepared ½ pound of soda, as much soap, and 8 yolks of eggs well beaten up, with ½ pound of purified oxgall. The whole must be carefully triturated upon a porphyry slab, the soda with the soap in the same manner as colors are ground, mixing in gradually the eggs and the oxgall previously beaten together. Incorporate next the soft earth by slow degrees, till a uniform thick paste be formed, which should be made into balls or cakes of a convenient size and laid out to dry. A little of this detergent being scraped off with a knife, made into a paste with water and applied to the stain, will remove it.

2316. To Remove Grease from Crocks and Jars.

Use hot water and sal soda.

2317. To Clean Gutta Percha.

This can be done by using a mixture of soap and powdered charcoal, polishing afterward with a dry cloth with a little charcoal on it.

2318. To Clean White Manilla Hats.

Sprinkle with water and expose to the fumes of burning sulphur in a tight box.

2319. To Clean Felt Hats.

Clean with ammonia and water; if greasy, wash with fuller's earth. Size with glue size, and block while warm. Glue size made by diluting hot glue with hot water. Apply inside, not outside the hat. The thicker the glue, the stiffer the hat.

2320.

The stains of grease and paint may be removed from hats by means of turpentine or benzine, and if the turpentine leaves a mark, finish with a little spirits of wine.

2321.

To remove grease stains from silk hats, use first turpentine and then alcohol.

2322. Cleaning Panama Hats.

To renovate white straw hats the following method has been recommended. Prepare two solutions as given:

I.—Sodium hyposulphite...	10 grams.
Glycerine................	5 grams.
Alcohol..................	10 grams.
Water....................	75 grams.
II.—Citric acid..........	2 grams.
Alcohol..................	10 grams.
Water....................	90 grams.

First sponge the straw hat with solution No. I, and lay aside in a moist room (cellar) for twenty-four hours; then apply solution No. II and treat similarly as before. Finally the hat should be gone over with a flat-iron, not too hot. If very dirty, the hat must be cleaned with some detergent and dried before beginning the bleaching operation.—Western Druggist.

2323. Alizarine Inks.

White goods, tartaric acid, the more concentrated the older are the spots. On colored cottons and woolens, and on silks, dilute tartaric acid is applied, cautiously.

2324. To Remove Ink and Iron Mould.

Equal parts of cream of tartar and citric acid, powdered fine, and mixed together. This forms the salts of lemon as sold by druggists.

Directions for using: Procure a hot dinner plate, lay the part stained in the plate, and moisten with hot water; next rub in the above powder with the bowl of a spoon until stains disappear; then rinse in clean water, and dry.

2325.

Place the stained part flat in a plate or dish, and sprinkle crystals of oxalic acid upon it, adding a little water; the stains will soon disappear, when the linen should be well wrung out in two or three changes of clean water.

2326.

Dip the part in boiling water, and rub it with crystals of oxalic acid, then soak in a weak solution of chloride of lime—say 1 ounce to the quart of water. Under any circumstances, as soon as the stain is removed, the linen should be thoroughly rinsed in several waters.

2327.

The Journal de Pharmacie d'Anvers recommends pyrophosphate of soda for the removal of ink stains. This salt does not injure vegetable fiber, and yields colorless compounds with the ferric oxide of the ink. It is best to first apply tallow to the ink spot, then wash in a solution of pyrophosphate until both tallow and ink have disappeared.

2328.

Thick blotting paper is soaked in a concentrated solution of oxalic acid and dried. Laid immediately on a blot, it takes it out without leaving a trace behind.

2329.

Tin. chloride.............	2 parts.
Water....................	4 parts.

To be applied with a soft brush, after which the paper must be passed through cold water.

2330.

Hydrochloric acid and hot water, in the proportion of 8 of hot water to 1 of acid; if not strong enough, add more acid; when clear of stain, wash well and boil, to remove all traces of acid.

2331.

A weak solution of chloride of zinc.

2332.

To remove from clothes use a mixture of 4 parts of tartar and 2 parts of powdered alum. This is not injurious to clothes. Other stains may be removed with it.

2333.

To remove a blot, dip a camel hair brush in water, and rub over the blot, letting the water remain on a few seconds; then make as dry as you can with blotting paper, then rub carefully with India rubber. Repeat the operation if not all removed. For lines, circles, etc., dip the ink leg of your instruments in water, open the pen rather wider than the line, and trace over, using blotting paper and India rubber, as for a blot. Applicable to drawing paper, tracing paper, and tracing linen. If the surface is a little rough after, polish with your nail.

2334. To Remove Printer's Ink.

Put the stained parts of the fabric into a quantity of benzine, then use a fine, rather stiff brush, with fresh benzine. Dry and rub bright with warm water and curd soap. The benzine will not injure the fabric or dye.

2335. Iron Spots and Black Ink.

White goods, hot oxalic acid, dilute muriatic acid, with little fragments of tin. On fast-dyed cottons and woolens, citric acid is cautiously and repeatedly applied. Silks, impossible.

2336. Iodine Stains on Paper.

Apply solution of pure sodium hyposulphite, and then strong ammonia water, by means of blotting paper; remove excess by pressing between sheets of bibulous paper moistened with water, and dry between clean warm (dry) blotting pads.

Iodine stains may be removed by alcohol.

2337. Iron and Steel.

Take a spongy piece of fig tree wood and well saturate it with a mixture of sweet oil and finely powdered emery, and with this well rub all the rusty parts. This will not only clean the article, but will at the same time polish it, and so render the use of whiting unnecessary.

2338.

Bright iron or steel goods (as polished grates and fire irons) may be preserved from rust in the following manner: Having first been thoroughly cleaned, they should be dusted over with powdered quicklime, and thus left until wanted for use. Coils of piano wire are covered in this manner, and will keep free from rust for many years.

2339.

Dissolve ½ ounce camphor, and 1 pound hog's lard, and take off the scum; then mix with the lard as much black lead as will give the mixture an iron color. Rub the articles all over with this mixture, and let them lie for twenty-four hours; then dry with a linen cloth, and they will keep clean for months.

2340.

Table knives which are not in constant use should be put in a case containing a depth of about 8 inches of quicklime. They are to be plunged into this to the top of the blades, but the lime must not touch the handles.

2341.

Steel bits that are tarnished, but not rusty, can be cleaned with rotten stone, common hard soap, and a woolen cloth.

2342. To Clean Iron.

To clean iron parts of machinery, tools, etc., two to three cents worth of paraffine chipped fine are added to one liter petroleum in a stoppered bottle, and during two or three days from time to time shaken up until the paraffine is dissolved. To apply it, the mixture is well shaken, spread upon the metal to be cleaned by means of a woolen rag or brush, and on the following day rubbed off with a dry woolen rag.

2343.

Yellow stains, commonly called iron mould, are removed from linen by hydrochloric acid or hot solution of oxalic acid. Wash well in warm water afterward.

2344. To Remove Iron Rust.

This may be removed by salt mixed with a little lemon juice.

2345.

Salts of lemon, mixed with warm water and rubbed over the mark, will, most probably, remove the stains.

2346.

Throw on the stain a small quantity of the dry powder of magnesia, rubbing it slightly in with the finger, leaving it there for an hour or two, and then brushing it off, when it will be found that the stain has quite disappeared.

2347.

Fresh ink and the soluble salts of iron produce stains which, if allowed to dry, and especially if afterward the material has been washed, are difficult to extract without injury to the ground. When fresh, such stains yield rapidly to a treatment with moistened cream of tartar, aided by a little friction, if the material or color is delicate. If the ground be white, oxalic acid, employed in the form of a concentrated aqueous solution, will effectually remove fresh iron stains.

2348. Removal of Smoke Stains from Ivory.

Immerse in benzine; if burned, there is no remedy.

2349. To Clean Jet.

Remove all dust with a very soft brush, touch the jet with a bit of cotton, moistened with a little good oil, polish with wash leather. Clean with great care, as the jet is often brittle.

2350. To Remove Kerosene Oil from Carpets.

Spread over the stain above and below warm pipe clay, and allow it to remain twenty-four hours; then brush it off and beat out the carpet.

2351. To Remove Stains from Knives.

Cut a solid potato in two, dip one of the pieces in brick dust, such as is usually used for knife cleaning, and rub the blade with it.

2352. To Wash Lace.

Cover an ordinary wine bottle with fine flannel, stitching it firmly round the bottle. Tack one end of the lace to the flannel, then roll it very smoothly round the bottle and tack down the other end, then cover with a piece of very fine flannel or muslin. Now rub it gently with a strong soap liquor, and, if the lace is very much discolored or dirty, fill the bottle with hot water and place it in a kettle or saucepan of suds and boil it for a few minutes, then place the bottle under a tap of running water to rinse out the soap. Make some strong starch, and melt in it a piece of white wax and a little loaf sugar. Plunge the bottle two or three times into this and squeeze out the superfluous starch with the hands; then dip the bottle in cold water, remove the outer covering from the lace, fill the bottle with hot water and stand it in the sun to dry the lace. When nearly dry take it very carefully off the bottle and pick it out with the fingers. Then lay it in a cool place to dry thoroughly.

2353.

First rip off the lace, carefully pick out the loose bits of thread, and roll the lace very smoothly and securely round a clean black bottle, previously covered with old white linen, sewed tightly on. Tack each end of the lace with a needle and thread to keep it smooth, and be careful in wrapping not to crumple or fold in any of the scallops or pearlings. After it is on the bottle, take some of the best sweet oil, and with a clean sponge wet the lace thoroughly to the inmost folds. Have ready in a wash kettle a strong, cold lather of clear water and castile soap. Fill the bottle with cold water, to prevent its bursting, cork it well and stand it upright in the suds, with a string round the neck secured to the ears or handle of the kettle, to prevent its knocking about and breaking while over the fire. Let it boil in the suds for an hour or more, till the lace is clean and white all through. Drain off the suds and dry it on the bottle in the sun. When dry, remove the lace from the bottle and roll it round a wide ribbon block, or lay it in long folds; place it within a sheet of smooth white paper, and press it in a large book for a few days.

2354. To Clean Gold and Silver Lace.

Sew the lace in a clean linen cloth, boil it in 1 quart of soft water, and ¼ pound of soap, and wash it in cold water. If tarnished, apply a little warm spirits of wine to the tarnished spots.

2355.

A weak solution of cyanide of potassium cleans gold lace well.

2356. To Revive Black Lace.

Make some black tea about the strength usual for drinking and strain it off the leaves. Pour enough tea into a basin to cover the quantity of lace, let it stand ten or twelve hours, then squeeze it several times, but do not rub it. Dip it frequently into the tea, which will at length assume a dirty appearance. Have ready some weak gum water, and press the lace gently through it; then clap it for a quarter of an hour; after which, pin it to a towel in any shape which you wish it to take. When nearly dry, cover it with another towel and iron it with a cool iron. The lace, if previously sound and discolored only, will after this process look as good as new.

2357.
Wash the lace thoroughly in some good beer; use no gum water; clap the lace well, and proceed with ironing and drying, as in the former recipe.

2358. To Cleanse Wash Leather.
(Chamois Skin.)
A German optical journal recommends washing soiled polishing leather in a weak solution of soda and warm water, then rubbing a good deal of soap in the leather and letting it soften for two hours. It is afterward thoroughly washed until perfectly clean, and rinsed in a weak solution of warm water, soda, and yellow soap. It must not be washed in clean water, or it will become so hard when dry that it cannot be used again. It is the small quantity of soap remaining in the leather which penetrates its smallest particles and makes the leather as soft as silk. After the rinsing it is wrung out in a coarse hand towel and dried quickly. It is then pulled in every direction and well brushed, after which it is softer and better than most wash leather when first bought. If rough leather is used to finish highly polished surfaces, it will often be observed that the surface is scratched or injured. This is caused by particles of dust and even grains of hard rouge that were left in the leather. As soon as they are removed with a clean brush and rouge, a perfectly bright and beautiful finish can be obtained.

2359.
Use a weak solution of soda and warm water, rub plenty of soft soap into the leather, and allow it to remain in soak for two hours, then rub it sufficiently, and rinse in a weak solution of warm water, soda, and yellow soap. If rinsed in water only, it becomes hard when dry and unfit for use. After rinsing, wring out in a rough towel, and dry quickly, then pull it about and brush it well.

2360. To Clean Leather.
Mix well together 1 pound of French yellow ocher and a dessertspoonful of sweet oil; then take 1 pound pipe clay and ¼ pound starch. Mix with boiling water; when cold lay on the leather; when dry, rub and brush well.

2361. Removing Rust from a Lens.
A lens sometimes acquires a brown, rusty stain on the surface, which no amount of rubbing or cleaning will remove. By applying a paste composed of putty powder, or very fine rouge, and water to the stains, and then rubbing briskly with either the point of the finger or the side of the hand, every spot of rust or stain will be removed in a few minutes. This applies to photographic or other lenses, except the object glass of a telescope, which would be irreparably damaged by such treatment.

2362. To Clean Lenses.
A very soft chamois skin is best; if greasy, wipe with a little tissue paper wet with weak alkali. Lenses should be cleaned as rarely as possible; use old linen, not silk.

2363. Lime, Lyes, Alkalies.
On white goods, simple washing in water. On dyed tissues of cotton and wool, and on silk, weak nitric acid poured drop by drop, and rub with the finger the spot previously moistened.

2364. To Prevent Blistering in Linen.
Blistering is almost always due to bad starching, but occasionally to ironing the articles when too wet. Each article must be well starched through, and when about to iron damp it evenly, but do not wet it. Use a hot iron. Collars and cuffs that have to be turned down should be fixed in the proper shape immediately after each one is ironed, for then the starch is still flexible.

2365. To Restore Whiteness to Scorched Linen.
One-half pint of vinegar, 2 ounces of Fuller's earth, 1 ounce of dried fowl's dung, one-half ounce soap, the juice of 2 large onions. Boil all these ingredients together to the consistency of paste; spread the composition thickly over the damaged part, and if the threads be not actually consumed, after it has been allowed to dry on, and the place has subsequently been washed once or twice, every trace of scorching will disappear.

2366. To Polish Linen.
Put 2 drams of powdered wax, 2 drams of of powdered soap, and 4 drams of powdered Frenh chalk in each pint of starch.

2367. To Clean Machinery.
To clean iron parts of machinery, tools, etc., about 10 grammes paraffin chipped fine are added, to 1 liter petroleum in a stoppered bottle, and during two or three days from time

to time shaken up until the paraffin is dissolved. To apply it the mixture is well shaken, spread upon the metal to be cleaned by means of a woolen rag or brush, and on the following day rubbed off with a dry woolen rag.

2368. Spots on Mahogany.
Stains and spots may be taken out of mahogany with a little aquafortis and water, or oxalic acid and water, rubbing the part by means of cork, till the color is restored, observing afterward to wash the wood well with water, and to dry and polish as usual.

2369. To Remove Grease from Marble.
Apply a little pile of whiting or fuller's earth saturated with benzine, and allow it to stand some time.

2370.
Or apply a mixture of 2 parts washing soda, 1 part ground pumice stone, and 1 part chalk, all first finely powdered and made into a paste with water; rub well over the marble, and finally wash off with soap and water.

2371 To Clean Marble
Mix with water 5 parts soda, 2½ parts powdered chalk, 2½ parts pumice stone (powdered). Wash the spots with this mixture; then wash off with soap and water.

2372.
To extract oil from marble or stone, soft soap, 1½ parts; fuller's earth, 3 parts; potash, 1½ part, boiling water to mix. Apply to the grease spots and let it remain two or three hours.

2373.
Marble, to Remove Oil Stains in.—Stains in marble caused by oil can be removed by applying common clay saturated with benzine. If the grease has remained long enough it will become acidulated, and may injure the polish, but the stain will be removed. Boil one-half pound soft soap in 1 quart water, very slowly, until the water is reduced to 1 pint. Apply this in the same manner as the preceding.

2374.
Take 2 parts common soda, 1 part pumice stone, and 1 part finely powdered chalk; sift it through a fine sieve and mix with water; then rub it well all over the marble, and the stains will be removed; then wash the marble over with soap and water, and it will be as clean as it was at first.

2375.
A bullock's gall, 1 gill soap lees, one-half gill turpentine. Mix into a paste with pipe clay. Apply to the marble, allow it to remain two or three days, then rub off.

2376.
Cover the soiled part with a paste of quicklime, moistened with a strong aqueous solution of sal soda for several hours; then remove the paste, wash the parts thoroughly, and polish if necessary.

2377.
Common soda, 3 parts; pumice stone, 1½ part; finely powdered chalk 1½ part; sift very fine, and mix with water. Rub all over the marble. Wash well with soap and water.

2378.
If the marble is white, coat it with gum arabic and expose to the sun. When it peels off wash with water, or make a paste with fuller's earth and hot water, cover the spots therewith, let it dry on, and next day scour off with soft soap. The luster can be restored by rubbing with a dry cloth.

2379.
Be sure that the dust is all brushed from the marble. Rub with the following: Whiting, 6 ounces; soft soap, 6 ounces; soda, 1½ ounces; a piece of stone blue size of a large walnut. Mix and rub on the marble with a flannel cloth. Let it remain for twenty-four hours. Wash off and polish with a piece of flannel.

2380.
To take Stains from White Marble.—Turpentine, 2¼ tablespoonfuls; lye, 1½ gills; ox-gall, 1½ ounces; pipe clay, q. s. to make a paste. Apply the paste to the stain and let it remain for several days. Iron mould or ink spots may be taken out by dissolving in 1½ pints rainwater, 1½ ounces oxalic acid, three-quarters ounce butter antimony, flour sufficient to make the mixture of a proper consistency. Put on with a brush, let it remain a few days, wash off. Grease spots may be removed by applying common clay saturated with benzine.

2381.
Ink Stains on Marble.—Dissolve 1 ounce antimony trichloride and 2 ounces oxalic acid in 1 quart of water. Add flour enough to make a paste. Leave on the spot for a few days until the spot is removed.

2382.

Iron Stains on Marble.—Boil your marble in a strong solution of caustic soda, then take out, and rub well. Soon all the stains will come out.

2383.

Matches, to Remove Marks Made by.—Spots from sulphur and phosphorus caused by lucifer matches can be extracted from marble by carbon disulphide; or take 2 parts of common soda, 1 part of pumice stone and 1 part of finely powdered chalk; sift it through a fine sieve and mix it with water; then rub it well all over the marble, and the stains will be removed, then wash the marble over with soap and water, and it will be as clean as it was at first.

2384. To Clean Matting.

Wash with water in which bran has been boiled, or in weak salt and water. Dry it well with a cloth.

2385. Mildew.

Well mix together a spoonful of table salt, 2 of soft soap, 2 of powdered starch, and the juice of a lemon. Lay this mixture on both sides of the stain with a painter's brush, and then lay the article on the grass, day and night, until the stain disappears.

2386.

Get a piece of flannel, dip it into whisky, and well rub the place marked; then iron on the wrong side, taking care to put a piece of damp cotton cloth between the iron and silk, and iron on the cotton cloth, which will prevent the silk assuming a shiny glazed appearance.

2387.

Wash clean and take every particle of soap off, then put the linen into a galvanized bath or tub full of clean cold water, procure a little chloride of lime, and tie it up in a muslin bag or piece of muslin, dissolve the lime in lukewarm water by squeezing the bag, then pour the water among the clothes. Stir and leave them for 24 hours, but do not put too much lime in, or you will rot the clothes; then well rinse in clean cold water.

2388.

Hypochlorite of alumina is said to be one of the best remedies. Moisten with water, rub well into the cloth, moisten again with dilute sulphuric acid (1 to 20), and after half an hour, rinse thoroughly in soft water and then in water containing about an ounce to the gallon of sulphite or hyposulphite of soda. A stiff brush may be advantageously employed in applying the hypochlorite.

2389.

Mildew, to Prevent.—Housekeepers are often greatly troubled and perplexed by mildew from damp closets and from rust. By putting an earthen bowl or deep plate full of quicklime into the closet, the lime will absorb the dampness and also sweeten and disinfect the place. Rats, mice, and many bugs that are apt to congregate in damp places have a dislike to lime. As often as the lime becomes slaked throw it on the compost heap if in the country, or into the ash barrel if in the city.

2390.

Mildew, to Prevent in Canvas, etc.—Dissolve 1 pound zinc sulphate in 40 gallons water, and then add 1 pound sal soda. When dissolved, 2 ounces tartaric acid are added. This holds the partially separated zinc carbonate without neutralizing the excess of alkali used. The canvas, etc., should be soaked in this solution for 24 hours, and then dried without wringing.

2391.

Mildew, to Remove from Brickwork.—Builders' acid (hydrochloric acid) is often used for removing white stains from brickwork. Its efficacy in the case of mildew would be doubtful. A coat of linseed oil on the perfectly dry brick would have a good preventive tendency. Melted paraffin applied hot, and worked in with a paint burner would also be efficacious. Perhaps either of the last named applications would destroy the mildew or white stain also. Acid used by an experienced man would not injure the joints.

2392.

Canvas, Rendering it Mildew-proof.—Saturate the cloth in a hot solution of soap (one-quarter pound to a gallon of water); wring out and digest it for twelve hours in solution of one-half pound alum to 1 gallon of water.

2393.

Use the following: Alum, 2 pounds, dissolved in 60 pounds water; blue vitriol, 2 pounds, dissolved in 8 pounds of water, to which is added gelatine, 1 pound, dissolved in 30 pounds water; lead acetate, one-half pound dissolved in 30 pounds water. The solutions are all hot, and separately mixed, with the exception of the vitriol, which is added.

2394.

Treatment with strong aqueous solution of alum or lead acetate answers very well.

2395.

To Remove from Canvas.—Wash with solution of calcium hypochlorite (bleaching powder) in cold water or vinegar. Use plenty of cold water afterward.

2396.

Cotton Goods, to Remove from.—If the goods are colored, soak for twenty-four hours or more in sour milk or buttermilk, then rinse in water, and wash in strong soapsuds. If the goods are white, moisten the spots repeatedly with Javelle water diluted with volumes of water, rinse well, then wash in strong soapsuds, not too hot.

2397.

Gold Lace, to Remove Mildew from.—For this purpose no alkaline liquors are to be used; for while they clean the gold, they corrode the silk, and change or discharge its color. Soap also alters the shade, and even the species of certain colors. But spirit of wine may be used without any danger of its injuring either color or quality, and in many cases proves as effectual for restoring the luster of the gold as the corrosive detergents. But though the spirit of wine is the most innocent material employed for this purpose, it is not in all cases proper. The golden covering may be in some places worn off, or the base metal, with which it has been alloyed, may be corroded by the air, so as to have the particles of gold disunited, while the silver underneath, tarnished to a yellow hue, may continue of a tolerable color; so it is apparent that the removal of the tarnish would be prejudicial, and make the lace less like gold than it was before.

2398.

Linen, Mildew from.—Take soap and rub it well; then scrape some fine chalk, and rub that also in the linen, lay it on the grass as it dries, wet it a little, and it will come out at once.

2399.

Two tablespoonfuls of soft soap and the juice of a lemon. Lay it on the spots with a brush, on both sides of the linen. Let it lie a day or two till the stains disappear.

2400.

Nets, to Prevent from Rotting.—The following treatment is said to preserve nets for a long time in a good condition: Soften 1 pound good glue in cold water; then dissolve it in 10 gallons of hot soft water, with one-half pound curd soap. Wash the nets in soft water, then boil them in this for two hours, press out excess of the liquid and hang up overnight. The second bath consists of alum, 2 pounds; water, 5 gallons; heat nearly to boiling, and immerse the nets in this for about three hours, then press and transfer to a strong decoction of oak bark or a solution of sumac in warm water (water, 5 gallons, sumac, 8 pounds), and let them remain immersed in this for forty-eight hours, or longer, if convenient.

2401. To Remove Mildew from Paper.

Soak one ounce of gelatine for some hours in 1 pint of water, and 1 ounce of white soap scraped, in the same quantity of water; mix the two solutions and boil till dissolved. Dissolve 1 dram of alum in 2 ounces of water, and add it to the above. When the mixture is cold, decant the solution from all sediment. Spread the above over the damaged paper with a stout feather. If the paper be in a very bad state, a second coat may be applied. A little spirits of wine added to the solution tends to keep it good.

2402. The Preservation of Ropes.

The ropes should be dipped, when dry, into a bath containing 20 grammes of sulphate of copper per liter of water, and kept in soak in this solution for four days, afterward being dried. The ropes will thus have absorbed a certain quantity of sulphate of copper, which will preserve them from the attacks of animal parasites and from rot. The copper salt may be fixed in the fiber by a coating of tar or by soapy water. For tarring the rope it is best to pass it through a bath of boiled tar, hot, drawing it through a thimble to press back the excess of tar, and suspending it afterward on a staging to dry and harden. In the second method, the rope is soaked in a solution of 100 grammes of soap per liter of water. The copper soap thus formed in the fiber of the rope preserves it from rot even better than the tar, which acts mechanically to imprison the sulphate of copper, which is the real preservative. It is not stated whether the copper treatment is equally serviceable with dressed as with plain hemp ropes.

2403.

Ropes, to Prolong the Life of.—To prolong the duration of ropes, steep them in a solution of sulphate of copper, 1 ounce to 1 quart of water, and then tar them.

2404.
Stone, Mildew or Mould, to Remove from.—Try a little strong aqueous solution of caustic soda. It should remain ten minutes in contact with the stone, which, after washing with water, should be well rubbed with a stiff brush or broom.

2405. To Remove Milk and Coffee Stains.
These stains are very difficult to remove, especially from light colored and finely finished goods. From woolen and mixed fabrics they are taken out by moistening them with a mixture of 1 part glycerine, 9 parts water, and one-half part aqua ammonia. This mixture is applied to the goods by means of a brush, and allowed to remain for twelve hours, occasionally renewing the moistening. After this time, the stained pieces are pressed between cloth, and then rubbed, with a clean rag. Drying, and if possible a little steaming, is generally sufficient to thoroughly remove the stains.

2406.
Stains on silk garments which are dyed with delicate colors, or finely finished, are more difficult to remove. In this case 5 parts glycerine are mixed with 5 parts water, and one-fourth part of ammonia added. Before using this mixture it should be tried on some part of the garments where it cannot be noticed, in order to see if the mixture will change the color. If such is the case, no ammonia should be added. If, on the contrary, no change takes place, or if, after drying, the original color is restored, the above mixture is applied with a soft brush, allowing it to remain on the stains for six or eight hours, and is then rubbed with a clean cloth. The remaining dry substance is then carefully taken off by means of a knife. The injured places are now brushed over with clean water, pressed between cloths and dried. If the stain is not then removed, a rubbing with dry bread will easily take it off. To restore the finish, a thin solution of gum arabic, or in many cases beer is preferred, is brushed on, then dried, and carefully ironed. By careful manipulation these stains will be successfully removed.

2407. To Remove Nitric Acid Stains.
According to Reimann's Faerber Zeitung, these yellow stains, so familiar to the chemist and druggist, can be removed either from the skin or from brown or black woolen garments by moistening the spots for a while with permanganate of potash and rinsing with water. A brownish stain of manganese remains, which may be removed from the skin by washing with aqueous solution of sulphurous acid. If the spots are old, they cannot be entirely removed.

2408.
Nitric Acid Stains, to remove from the Hands.—Touch the stains with solution of permanganate of potassium; wash, rinse in dilute hydrochloric acid, and wash again.

2409. To Renovate Oil Cloths.
Dissolve 2½ pounds paraffin and 1 gallon oil of turpentine by the aid of a gentle heat, and apply with a sponge or piece of flannel, while warm. Let it remain on the oil cloth twenty-four hours; then polish with flannel. This solution not only renovates but preserves the cloth. It has been used on oil cloths which have been down four years, and they look as good as new. The same preparation may also be used on painted floors. When rubbed with flannel, it will have a beautiful gloss, equal to varnish.

2410. To Clean Oil Cloth.
Wash with a large soft woolen cloth and lukewarm or cold water, dry thoroughly with a soft cloth, and afterward polish with milk, or a weak solution of beeswax, in spirits of turpentine. Never use a brush, or hot water, or soap, as either will be certain to bring off the paint.

2411.
Wash with equal quantities of milk and water. Once in several months a little linseed oil may be used. It must be well rubbed in and polished with a piece of silk.

2412. Oil Colors, Varnish and Resins.
On white or colored linens, cottons, or woolens, use rectified oil of turpentine, alcohol lye, and their soap. On silks, use benzine, ether, and mild soap, very cautiously.

2413. Oil Stains on Paper.
Use pipe clay mixed with water. Allow it to remain on the spot for several hours.

2414. To Remove Oil Stains from Floors.
Use oxalic acid and water, then wash well with soda and soap.

2415. To Clean Paint Brushes.
When a paint brush is stiff and hard through drying with paint on it, put some turpentine in a shallow dish and set it on fire. Let it burn for a minute until hot, then smother the flame and work the pencil in the fingers, dipping it frequently into hot spirits. Rinse all paint brushes, pencils, etc., in turpentine, grease with a mixture of sweet oil and tallow, to prevent them from drying hard, and put them away in a close box.

2416.

To soften brushes that have become hard, soak them twenty-four hours in raw linseed oil, and rinse them out in hot turpentine, repeating the process till clean; or wash them in hot soda and water and soft soap.

2417. To Clean Paint.

To clean paint, provide a plate with some of the best whiting to be had; have ready some clean warm water and a piece of flannel, which dip into the water and squeeze nearly dry; then take as much whiting as will adhere to it, and apply it to the painted surface, when a little rubbing will instantly remove any dirt or grease. After which, wash the part well with clean water, rubbing it dry with a soft chamois. Paint thus cleaned looks as well as when first laid on, without any injury to the most delicate colors. It is far better than using soap, and does not require more than half the time and labor.

2418.

To clean paint, take 1 ounce pulverized borax, 1 pound small pieces best brown soap, and 3 quarts water; let simmer till the soap is dissolved, stirring frequently. Do not let it boil. Use with a piece of old flannel, and rinse off as soon as the paint is clean. This mixture is also good for washing clothes.

2419.

Dissolve one-half ounce glue and a bit of soft soap the size of a walnut in about 3 pints of warm water, and with a well-worn whitewash brush well scrub the work, but not sufficient to get off the paint, and rinse with plenty of cold clean water, using a wash leather; let dry itself. Work done in this manner will often look equal to new.

2420.

First take off all the dust with a soft brush and a pair of bellows. Scour with a mixture of soft soap and fuller's earth, and use lukewarm water. If there are any spots which are extra dirty, first remove these by rubbing with a sponge dipped in soap and water. Commence the scouring at the top of the door or wainscot, and proceed downward; and dry with a soft linen cloth. When cleaning paint, it is always better to employ two persons, one to scour and the other to rub dry.

2421. To Remove Paint.

Scraping or burning it off is extremely laborious, and too slow for general purposes. A more thorough and expeditious way is by chemical process, using for that purpose a solution of soda and quicklime in equal proportions. The solution may be made as follows: The soda is dissolved in water, the lime is then added, and the solution is applied with a brush to the old paint. A few moments are sufficient to remove the coats of paint, which may be washed off with hot water. The oldest paint may be removed by a paste of the soda and quicklime. The wood should be afterward washed with vinegar or an acid solution before repainting to remove all traces of the alkali.

2422.

Wet the place with naphtha, repeating as often as required; but frequently one application will dissolve the paint. As soon as it is softened rub the surface clean. Chloroform, mixed with a small quantity of spirit ammonia, composed of strong ammoniac, has been employed very successfully to remove the stains of dry paint from wood, silk, and other substances.

2423.

To Remove from Floors.—Take 1 pound American pearlash, 3 pounds quick stone lime, slake the lime in water, then add the pearlash, and make the whole about the consistence of paint. Lay the mixture over the whole body of the work which is required to be cleaned, with an old brush; let it remain for 12 or 14 hours, when the paint can be easily scraped off.

2424. To Soften Putty and Remove Old Paint.

Take 3 pounds of quick stone lime, slake the lime in water, and then add 1 pound of American pearlash. Apply this to both sides of the glass, and let it remain for twelve hours, when the putty will be softened, and the glass may be taken out without being broken. To destroy paint apply it to the whole body of the work which is required to be cleaned; use an old brush, as it will spoil a new one; let it remain about twelve or fourteen hours and then the paint may be easily scraped off.

2425.

To remove paint from old doors, etc., and to soften putty in window frames, so that the glass may be taken out without breakage or cutting, take 1 pound of pearlash and 3 pounds of quicklime; slake the lime in water, and then add the pearlash, and make the whole about the consistence of paint. Apply it to both sides of the glass, and let it remain for twelve hours, when the putty will be so softened that the glass may be taken out of the frame without being cut and with the greatest facility. To destroy paint lay the above over the whole body of the work which is required to be cleaned, using an old brush (as it will spoil a new one); let it remain for twelve or fourteen hours, when the paint can be easily scraped off.

2426.

Paint Stains on Glass.—American potash, 3 parts; unslaked lime, 1. Lay this on with a stick, letting it remain for some time, and it will remove either tar or paint.

2427.

Common washing soda dissolved in water. Let it soak awhile—if put on thick, say 30 minutes—and then wash off. If it does not remove, give it another application.

2428. Paint, Varnish and Resin Stains on Clothes.

For white or colored cotton and woolen goods, oil of turpentine or benzine, followed by soapsuds. For silk, benzine, ether, soap; hard rubbing is to be avoided. For all kinds of fabrics chloroform is best, but must be carefully used.

2429.

Stains of paint or varnish, after being softened with olive oil or fresh butter, may generally be removed by the same means as ordinary grease spots.

2430.

Saturate the spots with a solution of equal parts turpentine and spirits of ammonia; wash out with strong soapsuds.

2431.

Paint stains that are dry and old may be removed from cotton or woolen goods with chloroform. First cover the spot with olive oil or butter.

2432. To Clean Paintings.

Dissolve a little common soda in urine, then add a grated potato and a little salt; well rub this over the paintings till clean. Wash off in spring water and dry with a clean cloth.

2433.

First rub the picture well with good whisky, which will make the varnish come off in froth, then wash well with cold water, and when dry varnish again; this will restore the picture to its original color unless very old. Keep the picture covered from dust until the varnish is dry.

2434. Renovation of Papier Mache Goods.

One-half pint linseed oil, one-half pint old ale, the white of an egg, 1 ounce spirits of wine, 1 ounce hydrochloric acid; well shake before using. A little to be applied to the face of soft linen pad, and lightly rubbed for a minute or two over the article to be restored, which must afterward be polished off with old silk handkerchief. This will keep any length of time if well corked. Invaluable for delicate cabinet work.—Dustpan.

2435.

Wash with water, dredge with flour, and polish with a dry flannel cloth.

2436. To Extract Paraffin Oil from Floor.

A strong hot solution of oxalic acid applied, and by the after use of the scrubbing brush, you will remove all the stains from your boards.—A. E. B. Smith.

2437. To Clean Parchment.

Immerse the parchment in a solution of acetic acid, and gently rub the stained parts while wet on a flat board with lump pumice, then bleach it with chloride of lime. This process was recommended in the English Mechanic. It is not very successful, but it makes it white enough for bookbinding. It has, however, the objectionable qualities of not making the parchment flexible, and when dried it is as hard as a board, and it has no gloss like the virgin parchment. On no account must the parchment be washed in very hot water, or held before a fire, as it will shrivel up in a most provoking manner.

2438. To Clean Pearls.

Soak them in hot water in which bran has been boiled, with a little cream of tartar and alum, rubbing gently between the hands when the heat will admit of it. When the water is cold renew the application till any discoloration is removed, rinse in lukewarm water; lay them on white paper in a dark place to cool.

2439. Piques and Colored Muslins.

French method: Make a strong lather with best white soap dissolved in soft water, and use while rather warm, but not hot. Wash the dress in this, but do not soak it previously. As soon as the lather appears soiled squeeze out the dress, throw away the lather, and wash the dress again in a second lot, and so continue until the dress is thoroughly clean. Then well rinse it in cold water, and afterward in cold water slightly blued. Squeeze all the water out of the dress, but do not wring it, and hang in a shady place to dry, or, if the weather be wet, dry it before the fire. When dry they are to be starched. It is in this operation that the failures in getting up muslins and piques more often occur than in the washing. Use a large basin and have plenty of starch, and dissolve in the starch, according to the quantity of it, 3 or

4 in. of composite or wax candle. Squeeze the starch well out of the dress, and while it is still wet put it between some old sheets or table cloths, and pass it between the rollers of a wringing machine or under a mangle; by this means all lumps of starch will be removed. Finish by ironing. Piques should be ironed on the wrong side, as lightly as possible.

2440. To Renovate Plush.

To restore the plush, hold the wrong side over steam arising from boiling water, until the pile rises; or dampen lightly the wrong side of the plush, and hold it over a pretty hot iron, not hot enough to scorch, however, or make a clean brick hot; place upon it a wet cloth, and hold the plush over it, and the steam will raise it.

2441. To Clean Iron Pots.

Put a few ounces of washing soda (sodium carbonate) into the pot, fill wth water, and boil until the inside looks clean.

2442. Lightning Renovator.

Castile soap 4 oz.; hot water, 1 qt. When the soap is dissolved, add water, 4 qt.; water of ammonia, 4 fl. oz.; sulphuric ether, 1. fl. oz.; glycerine, 1 fl. oz.; alcohol, 1 oz. Medical Brief states that this is an excellent preparation for removing grease.

2443. To Clean Goatskin Rugs.

One washing with warm (not hot) suds will not materially hurt the skin itself. The skin may not seem quite so soft after the washing, but if the washing is done quickly, the skin well rinsed in cold water, and dried with only moderate warmth, being frequently turned and shaken, the difference will hardly be perceptible.

2444. To Remove Rust Spots.

By adding 2 parts cream of tartar to 1 part oxalic acid ground fine and kept dry in a bottle, you will find, by applying a little of the powder to rust stains while the article is wet, that the result is much quicker and better. Wash out in clear warm water to prevent injury to the goods.

2445. Rust, Black Ink.

On white goods, warm solution oxalic acid; weak muriatic acid. On dyed tissues of cotton, repeated washings with citric acid if the color is well dyed. Ditto of wool, same; weak muriatic acid if the wool is of the natural color. On silk, no remedy.

2446. To Clean Satins.

Satins may be cleansed with a weak solution of borax or benzine when greasy. Care should be taken to sponge moderately and lengthwise, not across, the fabric; iron on the wrong side only. White, cream, and pink satins may be treated in the same way as cream-colored silks.

2447.

To Clean Black.—Boil 3 lb. potatoes to a pulp in a quart of water; strain through a sieve, and brush the satin with it on a board or table. The satin must not be wrung, but folded down in cloths, for three hours, and then ironed on the wrong side.

2448. Scouring Liquid.

M. LeClerc.

For scouring and removing grease from tissues of all kinds and worn clothes. To take out spots the liquid is used pure, but for general scouring it is mixed with 4 or 5 times its own quantity of water. In 22 gal. hot water dissolve 15½ lb. white Marseilles soap; 1 3/10 lb. carbonate of potash; or 15 or 18 lb. soft soap. To the solution add extract of Panama, 1 1/10 lb. In another vessel mix ox or sheep gall, 15 qt.; and ammonia at 22°, 3 pt. Heat this mixture, skim it, let it cool, and then add alcohol at 90°, 3 3/10 gal.; decant and filter. Take 1/3 part of the soap mixture and 2/3 part of the gall mixture, and add some aromatic essence.

2449. Scouring Preparations for Removing Grease.

One ounce camphor dissolved in 3 oz. alcohol. Add 4 oz. essence of lemon.

Camphine, 8 oz.; alcohol, 1 oz.; sulphuric ether, 1 oz.; essence of lemon, 1 dram.

Alcohol, 8 oz.; white soap, 1½ oz.; oxgall, 1¼ oz.; essence of lemon, ⅛ to ¼ oz.

2450. Scouring Paste.

Oxalic acid, 1 part; iron peroxide, 15 parts; powdered rotten stone, 20 parts; palm oil, 60 parts; petrolatum, 4 parts. Pulverize the oxalic acid and add rouge and rotten stone, mixing thoroughly, and sift to remove all grit; then add gradually the palm oil and petrolatum, incorporating thoroughly. Add oil of myrbane or oil of lavender to suit. By substituting your red ashes from stove coal, an inferior representative of the foregoing paste will be produced.

2451.   **Removal of Stains and Grease Spots.**

The following table gives at a glance the best means of cleansing all kinds of fabrics from any stain whatever.

KIND OF STAIN.	FROM LINENS.	FROM COLORED GOODS. COTTON.	WOOLEN.	FROM SILKS.
Sugar, glue, blood and albumen.	Simple washing with water			
Grease	Soapsuds, alkaline lyes.	Lukewarm soap suds.	Soapsuds, ammonia.	Benzine, ether, ammonia, pot ash, magnesia, chalk, yolk of egg.
Varnish and oil paints.	Turpentine, or benzine, and soap.			Benzine, ether, soap; rub carefully.
Stearine.	Very strong alcohol, 95°.			
Vegetable colors, red wine, fruit, red ink.	Sulphur vapors; warm chlorine water.	Wash out with warm soapsuds or ammonia water.		The same; rub gently and carefully.
Alizarine ink.	Tartaric acid; the older the stain the stronger the solution.	Dilute tartaric acid if the stuff will bear it.		The same; with care.
Iron rust and ink made of galls.	Warm oxalic acid solution; dilute hydrochloric acid, then tin turnings.	Repeated washings with a solution of citric acid, if the colors will bear it.	The same, dilute hydrochloric acid if the wool is dyed naturally.	Nothing can be done, and all attempts only make it worse.
Lime, lye or alkalies.	Simply wash with water.	Drop dilute nitric acid upon it. The stain previously moistened can be rubbed off with the finger.		
Tannin, green nut shells.	Javelle water, warm chlorine water, concentrated solution of tartaric acid.	Alternate washing with water and with more or less dilute chlorine water according to the colors.		
Coal tar, wagon grease.	Soap, oil of turpentine, alternating with a stream of water.	Rub with lard, then soap it well. After a time wash alternately with water and turpentine.		The same, but use benzine instead of turpentine, and the water must fall on it from some height.
Acids.	Red acid stains are destroyed by ammonia, followed by thorough washing with water. Brown stains of nitric acid are permanent.			

With the above table, a few simple chemicals, and a good deal of care and perseverance, any one may set up a chemical cleaning establishment. Great pains must be taken when ether and benzine are employed to avoid their taking fire, the vapor of which when mixed with air is highly explosive. An open bottle of ether will take fire at a distance of several feet from an open flame, as a heavy invisible vapor issues from the bottle; when the vapor reaches the flame of a lamp the whole mass of vapor takes fire.—*Muster Zeit.*

2452. Scouring Bricks.

Scouring brick may be made by mixing sand with a small percentage of clay and baking. The quantity and heat required may be easily ascertained by trial. Mucilage and gums may be used, but they are not equal to clay as a cement for scouring brick. A very small portion of Portland cement might be made available, to avoid the baking process.

2453. To Clean Shawls.

White woolen shawls will not always stand washing successfully. A safe way to clean such an article is to brush all the dust out, spread it on a table, then sprinkle over it a quantity of finely ground white starch (rice or potato, not wheat); fold up the shawl into a square, powdering liberally between each fold. The shawl should be put away for several hours, and then be opened and dusted. The starch will have absorbed all the grease that may have been present and collected the dust. If such shawls are very dirty, they may be pressed between two damp blankets before the starch is put on. Gray and light blue woolen shawls may be treated in the same way, only using slightly blued starch instead of pure white starch. The shawls must be well shaken to get rid of the powder.

2454. Laundrying of Shirts. A
(Chinese Method.)

A rather thick starch paste is prepared by first beating up a handful of raw starch, usually corn starch, and a teaspoonful of fine rice flour, with about 1 quart of water, making a liquid of creamlike consistency. A certain quantity (determined alone by personal experience) is poured into a quantity of boiling water, while the latter is violently stirred with a short wooden spatula. With this the portions of the linen to be dressed are well smeared, the linen moist from wringing and the starch quite hot. Thus smeared the pieces are laid aside for a few minutes, then rubbed well between the hands, so that the paste is well distributed in the fabric. The linen is then usually dried by artificial heat. When ready for ironing, the starched portions are dampened by means of a cloth dipped in raw starch water, to which has been added a small quantity—about ½ an ounce to the quart of blood albumen—clarified serum of bullock's blood. The proportion of starch in this water is usually about as 1 to 50 of water. In ironing the irons are first made very hot, and cooled somewhat externally just before using by momentarily plunging them into a pail of water. The irons, commonly employed are what are termed polishing irons—they have the posterior edge rounded instead of angular, as in the ordinary smoothing or sadiron. Much of the fine gloss observed on shirts laundried by Chinamen is accomplished by the skillful manipulation of this "rounded edge" over the work—a manipulation very difficult to describe in words. It is most laborious work for those not accustomed to it. It not only renders the surface glossy, but imparts easy flexibility to the heavily starched fabric otherwise not attainable. Custom made shirts are usually laundried before delivery in trade at the factory, the ironing in these cases being largely performed by steam mangles, though some are hand finished. The following recipe for a laundry starch is said to produce a very fine and lasting gloss on linen without the expenditure of the amount of labor in ironing usually requisite to produce a fair appearance:

Corn starch	1	ounce.
Water, boiling	1 7-8	pints.
Bluing	q. s.	

To this when it has cooled somewhat is added and thoroughly mixed in about half an ounce of the following preparation:

Gum arabic	8 3-5	parts.
Sugar, loaf	2½	parts.
Soap, white curd	¼	part.
Water glass ("A" syrup)	1	part.
Egg albumen	4	parts.
Water, warm	20	parts.

In preparing this the first three ingredients are dissolved together in the water at boiling heat, the water glass is then added, and when the mixture has cooled down to about 150° Fah. the egg albumen is put in and the whole well beaten together.

2455. Laundrying of Shirts. B

Starch	1	ounce.
Paraffin	3 drams (about).	
White Sugar	1 tablespoonful.	
Table salt	1 tablespoonful.	
Water	q. s.	

Rub up the starch with soft water into a thick smooth paste. Add nearly or quite a pint of boiling water, with the salt and sugar dissolved in it, and, having dropped in the paraffin, boil for at least half an hour, stirring to prevent burning. Strain the starch and use while hot. Sufficient bluing may be added to the water, previous to the boiling, to overcome the yellowish cast of the starch, if necessary. Spermaceti may be used in place of paraffin. Starched linen can only be properly finished by hard pressure applied to the iron.

2456. Glossed Shirt Bosoms. A

Take 2 ounces of fine white gum arabic powder, put it in a pitcher and pour on a pint or more of water, and then, having covered it, let it stand all night. In the morning, pour it carefully from the dregs into a clean bottle, cork, and keep it for use. A teaspoonful of gum water stirred in a pint of starch, made in the usual way, will give to lawns, white or printed, a look of newness, when nothing else can restore them, after they have been washed.

2457. Glossed Shirt Bosoms. B

Melt 2½ pounds of the very best paraffin wax over a slow fire. When liquefied remove from the fire and stir in 100 drops oil of citronella. Have some new round pie tins; place them on a level table, coat them slightly with sweet oil, and pour about six tablespoonfuls of the enamel into each tin. The pan may be floated in water to cool the contents sufficiently to permit the mixture to be cut or stamped out with a tin cutter into small cakes about the size of a peppermint lozenge. Two of these cakes added to each pint of starch will cause the smoothing iron to impart the finest possible finish to muslin or linen, besides perfuming the clothes.

2458. Glossed Shirt Bosoms. C

Take of white wax, 1 ounce; spermaceti, 2 ounces; melt them together with a gentle heat. When you have prepared a sufficient amount of starch, in the usual way, for a dozen pieces, put into it a piece of the polish about the size of a large pea; using more or less, according to large or small washings. Or thick gum solution (made by pouring boiling water upon gum arabic) may be used. One tablespoonful to a pint of starch gives clothes a beautiful gloss.

2459. To Clean Shoes.

Defaced kid boots will be greatly improved by being rubbed well with a mixture of cream and ink.

2460. To Clean White Satin Shoes.

Put in the shoe something which will fill it out. Then rub the shoe gently with a piece of muslin dipped in spirits of wine. Do this several times. Then wipe the shoe carefully with a piece of dry muslin.

2461. To Clean Show Windows.

A good cleaning powder for show windows and mirrors is prepared by moistening calcined magnesia with pure benzine, so that a mass is formed sufficiently moist to let a drop form when pressed. The mixture has to be preserved in glass bottles with ground stoppers, in order to retain the easily volatile benzine. A little of the mixture is placed on a wad of cotton and applied to the glass plate. Do not use near a fire or light, as the benzine vapor is very inflammable and explosive.

2462. Silk Cleaner.

Soft soap	½ pound.
Brandy	2 teaspoonfuls.
Proof spirit	1 pint.
Water	1 pint.

Mix well together.

Apply with a sponge on each side of the silk, taking care not to crease the silk. Rinse 2 or 3 times and iron on the wrong side, putting a piece of thin muslin between the silk and the iron.

2463. To Clean Silk.

No silks look well after washing, no matter how carefully it may be done, and, therefore, it should never be resorted to without absolute necessity. It is recommended to sponge faded silks with warm water and soap, and then to rub them with a dry cloth on a flat board, after which, to iron them on the inside with a smoothing iron. Sponging a little with spirits will also improve old black silks. The ironing may be done on the right side, with thin paper spread over them to prevent glazing.

2464. To Clean White Silk.

White silk is best cleaned by dissolving curd soap in water as hot as the hand can bear, and passing the silk through and through, handling it gently, and rubbing any spots till they disappear. The silk should then be rinsed in lukewarm water, and stretched by pins to dry.

2465. To Clean Black Silk.

To bullock's gall add boiling water sufficient to make it warm, and with a clean sponge rub the silk well on both sides; squeeze it well out, and proceed in like manner. Rinse it in spring water, and change the water until perfectly clean. Dry it in the air, and pin it out on a table; but first dip the sponge in glue water, and rub it on the wrong side; then dry before a fire.

2466. To Renovate Black Silk.

The French process is to use a weak solution of coffee water. Do not wet the silk too much, and restore the luster by careful rubbing with a soft silk handkerchief. White silks can be cleaned with a dry powder formed of fine starch and a little laundry blue. Rub over the tissue and dust out thoroughly. Bread crumbs or chalk should be used for pink or cream colored silks. Silks may be ironed on the wrong side with a moderately hot iron, or on the right side (to give the fine luster) if well protected by two folds of slightly damped muslin.

2467. To Clean Silver. A
Silver articles discolored by sulphureted hydrogen may be cleaned by rubbing them with a boiling saturated solution of borax. Another good preparation is a solution of caustic potash with some bits of metallic zinc.

2468. To Clean Silver. B
Silver which has become much tarnished may be restored by immersion in a warm solution of 1 part cyanide of potassium to 8 parts of water. (This mixture is extremely poisonous.) Washing well with water, and drying, will produce a somewhat dead-white appearance, which may be quickly changed to a brilliant luster by polishing with a soft leather and rouge.

2469. To Clean Silver. C
Wash in hot soapsuds (use the silver soap if convenient); then clean with a paste of whiting and whisky. Polish with buckskin. If silver was always washed in hot suds, rinsed well, and wiped dry, it would seldom need anything else.

2470. To Clean Silver. D
A fresh concentrated solution of hyposulphite of soda will dissolve at once the coat of sulphide of silver, which is the cause of the blackness produced by mustard, eggs, etc., or anything containing sulphur.

2471. To Clean Silver. E
Add gradually 8 ounces of prepared chalk to a mixture of 2 ounces of spirits of turpentine, 1 ounce of alcohol, ½ ounce of spirits of camphor, and 2 drams of aqua ammonia. Apply with a soft sponge, and allow it to dry before polishing.

2472. Silver Cleaning Compound. A
Ammonium carbonate .... 1 ounce.
Water .... 4 ounces.
Paris white .... 16 ounces.
Mix well, and apply by means of soft leather.

2473. Silver Cleaning Compound. B
Rouge (very fine) and prepared chalk, equal parts; use dry.

2474. Silver Cleaning Compound. C
Whiting (fine)............ 2 parts.
White oxide of tin .... 1 part.
Calcined hartshorn .... 1 part.

2475. To Remove Yellow Coating from Silver Spoons.
Dissolve 1 ounce cyanide of potassium in 1 quart of soft water and you will have a dip in which you can wash your spoons and instantly remove the sulphide of silver. The solution must be kept in a bottle that is tightly corked and labeled "poison."

2476.
Egg spoons get tarnished by the sulphur in the egg uniting with the silver. This tarnish is a sulphuret of silver, and may be removed by rubbing with wet salt or ammonia.
It may be exposed to uniform heat, and then boiled in strong alum water.

2477. To Remove Ink Stains from Silver
Make a paste of chloride of lime and water and rub upon the stains.

2478. To Restore the Color of Filigree Silver Jewelry.
How can the original white color of silver filigree jewelry be restored when tarnished by wear or shop worn? A. First wash the articles in a solution of 1 fluid ounce of liquid potassa in 20 of water, rinse and then immerse in a mixture of salt, 1 part; alum, 1 part; saltpeter, 2 parts; dissolved in 4 parts water. Let them remain for five minutes; wash in cold water and dry with chamois leather.

2479. To Prepare and Bleach Skeletons.
It is impossible to extract the oily material from the bones except by a very slow process. Boiling in any amount of alkali, say washing soda, will not accomplish it, and all the oil must be absolutely removed before you can do anything toward the bleaching. Very long maceration in water alone or in soda and water will eventually effect it, but a much better material is benzine. Make a tin box into which you pack your skeleton, solder on the cover, leaving only a round hole for filling. Pour in benzine till the box is filled, stop the hole closely, and leave it undisturbed for three months. The skeleton will come out

clean, and can be bleached perfectly by sunlight. Chlorine will do the bleaching quicker, but it injures the bones; never use it. Any shorter process will give you a skeleton that is always nasty.

2480. To Remove Silver Nitrate Stains.

In the manipulation of the nitrate of silver bath solutions in photography, the operator frequently receives stains of the salt upon his clothing, which are not very attractive in appearance. Stains or marks of any kind made with the above silver solution or bath solution may be promptly removed from the clothing by simply wetting the stain or mark with a solution of bichromate of mercury. The chemical result is the change of the black-looking nitrate of silver into chromate of silver, which is whiter or invisible on the cloth. Bichromate of mercury can be obtained at the drug stores.

2481.

Sodium sulphite .... 1 ounce.
Chloride of lime .... ½ ounce.
Water .... 2 ounces.
Mix.
Use a nail brush.

2482.

Dip the fingers into a strong solution of cupric chloride. In about a minute the silver will be converted into a chloride, and may then be washed off with hyposulphate of soda solution.

2483.

The immediate and repeated application of a very weak solution of cyanide of potassium (accompanied by thorough rinsings in clean water) will generally remove these without injury to the colors.

2484.

How to Remove Nitrate of Silver Stains from the Fingers.—Paint the blackened parts with tincture of iodine; let remain until the black becomes white. The skin will then be red, but by applying ammonia the iodine will be bleached, leaving white instead of black stains of nitrate of silver.

2485.

Nitrate of silver stains may be removed by rubbing them with a weak solution of sulphydrate of ammonium or strong solution of iodide of potassium.

2486. Soap for Removing Stains.

Take 22 pounds of the best white soap and reduce it to thin shavings. Place it in a boiler, together with water, 8.8 pounds; oxgall, 18.25 pounds. Cover up and allow to remain at rest all night. In the morning heat up gently and regulate it so that the soap may dissolve without stirring. When the whole is homogeneous and flows smoothly, part of the water having been vaporized, add turpentine, 0.55 pounds; benzine, best clear, 0.44 pounds; and mix well. While still in the state of fusion color with green ultramarine and ammonia, pour into moulds and stand for a few days before using. The product will be found to act admirably, and the yield is very good indeed.—Moniteur de la Teinture.

2487. To Clean Sponges.

"In a large basin mix about a pint of water and 2 tablespoonfuls of sulphuric acid (common oil of vitriol), then steep the sponge about two hours, wring it out several times in the acid, and finally well wash out the acid in clean water; it was then just like new, having regained its former size, color and elasticity, with not the slightest trace of its former sliminess. It was a large bath sponge, and in an extremely bad condition."—English Mechanic.

2488. To Remove Spots and Stains.

Taking out grease and other spots from clothes is an application of chemistry which has a practical interest for everybody. It demands a certain acquaintance with solvents and reagents, even though we may not understand the laws of chemical affinity on which their action depends. The general principle is the applying to the spot a substance which has a stronger affinity for the matter composing it than this has for cloth, and which shall render it soluble in some liquid, so that it can be washed out. At the same time it must be something that will not injure the texture of the fabric or change its color. The practical hints we shall give are condensed from a variety of foreign sources.

2489.

The best substances for removing grease or oil are: 1. Benzine. 2. Soap. 3. Chalk, fuller's earth, steatite, or "French chalk." These should be merely diffused through a little water to form a thin paste, which is spread upon the spot, allowed to dry, and then brush out. 4. Oxgall and yolk of egg which have the property of dissolving fatty bodies without affecting perceptibly the texture or colors of cloth. The oxgall should be purified to prevent its greenish tint from degrading the brilliancy of dyed stuffs or the purity of whites. Thus prepared it is the most effective of all substances known for removing this kind of stains, especially from woolen cloths. It is to be diffused through its own bulk of water, applied to the spots, rubbed well into them with the hands till they disappear, after which the stuff is to be washed with soft water. 5. The volatile oil of turpentine. This will take out only recent stains; for which purpose it ought to be previously purified by distillation over quicklime.

2490.

The following recipes deal especially with the garment dyer: 1. Steam has the property of softening fatty matters, and thus facilitating their removal by reagents.

2. Sulphuric acid may be employed in certain cases, especially to brighten and raise greens, reds, and yellows; but it must be diluted with at least 100 times its weight of water and more, according to the delicacy of the shades.

3. Muriatic acid is used with success for removing spots of ink and iron mould upon a great number of colors which it does not sensibly affect.

4. Sulphurous acid is only used for bleaching undyed goods, straw hats, etc., and for removing fruit stains upon white woolen and silk tissues. The fumes of burning sulphur are also employed for this object, but the liquid acid (or a solution of the bisulphite—not bisulphate—of soda or magnesia) is safer.

5. Oxalic acid serves for removing spots of ink and iron and the residues of mud spots, which do not yield to other cleansing agents. It may also be employed for destroying the stains of fruit and of astringent juices, and stains of urine which have become old upon any tissue. Nevertheless, it is best confined to undyed goods, as it attacks not merely fugitive colors, but certain of the lighter fast colors. The best method of applying it is to dissolve it in cold or lukewarm water, and to let a little of the solution remain upon the spot before rubbing it with the hands.

6. Citric acid serves to revive and raise certain colors, especially greens and yellows; it destroys the effect of alkalies and any bluish or crimson spots which appear upon scarlets. In its stead acetic acid may be employed.

7. Liquid ammonia is the most energetic and useful agent employed for cleaning tissues and silk hats, and for quickly neutralizing the effects of acids. In the latter case it is often sufficient to expose the goods to the fumes of this alkali in order to remove such spots entirely. Ammonia gives a violet cast to all shades produced with cochineal, lac, the redwoods or logwood, and all colors topped with cochineal. It does not deteriorate silks, but at elevated temperatures it perceptibly attacks woolens. It serves to restore the black upon silks damaged by damp.

8. The carbonate of soda (soda crystals) serves equally in most of the cases where ammonia is employed. It is good for hats affected by sweat.

9. Soda and potash only serve for white goods, of linen, hemp, or cotton; for these alkalies attack colors and injure the tenacity and suppleness of woolen and silk. For the same reason white soap is only to be recommended for cleaning white woolen tissues.

10. Mottled soaps serve for cleaning heavy stuffs of woolen or cotton, such as quilts; for such articles which do not require great suppleness or softness of feel the action of the soap may be enhanced by the addition of a small quantity of potash.

11. Soft potash soaps may be usefully employed in solution, along with gum arabic or other mucilaginous matters, for cleaning dyed goods, and especially self-colored silks. This composition is preferable to white or marbled soaps, as it removes the spots better and attacks the colors much less.

12. Oxgall, which can be obtained from the butchers in a sort of membraneous bag (the so-called gall bladder), has the property of dissolving the majority of fatty bodies without injuring either the color or the fiber. It may be used preferably to soap for cleaning woolens; but it should not be employed for cleaning stuffs of light and delicate colors, which it may spoil by giving them a greenish yellow, or even a deep green tint. It is mixed also with other matters, such as oil of turpentine, alcohol, honey, yelk of egg, clay (fuller's earth), etc., and in this state is used for cleaning silks.

13. To obtain a satisfactory result gall ought to be very fresh. To preserve it a simple method is to tie the neck of the gall bladder well with a string, and hold the bladder in boiling water for some time. This being done, it is taken out and let dry in the shade.

14. Yelk of egg possesses nearly the same properties as oxgall, but is much more costly. It must be used as quickly as possible, for it losses its efficacy with keeping. It is sometimes mixed with an equal bulk of oil of turpentine.—*Moniteur de la Teinture.*

2491. To Remove Spots made by Stearin Sperm Candles.

1. For all kinds use 95 per cent alcohol.
2. Scrape off as much as possible with a knife then lay a thin, soft white blotting paper upon the spots and press with a warm iron. By repeating this the spermaceti will be drawn out. Afterward, rub the cloth where the spots have been with some very soft, brownish paper.

2492. To Clean Stones.

To remove grease from stone steps or passages, pour strong soda and water boiling hot over the spot, lay on it a little fuller's earth made into a thin paste with boiling water, let it remain all night, and if the grease be not removed, repeat the process. Grease may sometimes be taken out by rubbing the spot with a hard stone—not hearthstone—using sand and very hot water, with soap and soda.

2493. Spots of Sugar, Glue, Blood, Albumen.

On white goods, on dyed tissues of cotton and wool, and on silk, simple washing with water.

2494. To Cleanse and Bleach Tallow.

Dissolve 1 pound of alum in 2 gallons of water; the water should be boiling. Now add 20 pounds of tallow and continue to boil for about an hour, skimming frequently. Strain through stout muslin and allow it to harden.

2495. Jackman's Washing Compound.

Six pounds sal soda, 1 pound borax, dissolve in 1 gallon boiling water. When cold, add 1-3 pound potassium carbonate, 3 ounces liquid ammonia, 4 spoonfuls alcohol. Boil for five minutes ¾ pound fresh, unslaked lime in 1 gallon water. Draw off the clear fluid when thoroughly settled. Add to this the other ingredients with 9 gallons cold water. Directions for using: Soak the clothes over night, after rubbing soft soap on the dirty places. In the morning add ½ pint of the compound, ½ pint soft soap, and 4 gallons hot water. Boil not more than five minutes, and turn into a tub, putting into your boiler the same mixture as before. Wring the clothes into this and boil again ten minutes, suds, blue, and hang them out to dry. Should the wristbands or parts that are very dirty need a little rubbing, it should be done while the mixture is boiling.

2496. Wash Mixture. A

Wash Mixture.—Take 5 pounds bar soap, shave fine, add 1 quart lye, ¼ ounce pearlash, dissolved over a slow fire. When dissolved, put into a vessel prepared for it to stand in; then add ¼ pint turpentine, 1 gill hartshorn; stir well, and it is ready for use.

2497. Wash Mixture. B

Dissolve ½ pound soda in 1 gallon boiling water, and pour upon it ¼ pound lime. After this has settled, cut up 10 ounces of common bar soap, and strain the solution upon it and mix perfectly. Great care must be taken that no particles of lime are poured upon the soap. Prepare the mixture the evening before washing.

Directions: To 10 gallons water add the above preparation when the water is boiling. Each lot of linen must boil half an hour, and the same liquid will answer for three batches of clothes. The white clothes must be put in soak over night, and if the collars and wristbands are soaped and rubbed slightly, so much the better. Clean cold water may be used for rinsing. Some prefer boiling them for a few moments in clean bluing water, and afterward rinse in cold water.

2498. Wash Mixture. C

The following compound is said greatly to facilitate the washing of clothes: Dissolve 2 pounds bar soap in about 3 gallons of water as hot as the hand can bear. Add 1 tablespoonful of turpentine and 3 of ammonia. Stir, and steep the clothes in this for three hours, keeping the vessel tightly covered. Then wash the clothes in the usual way. The soap and water may be used a second time, in which case a teaspoonful of turpentine and the same amount of ammonia must be added. This treatment is calculated to save much labor in cleansing summer clothes stained by fruit, etc.

2499. Wash Mixture. D

The German washerwomen use a mixture of 2 ounces turpentine and 1 ounce spirits of ammonia well mixed together. This is put into a bucket of warm water in which one-half pound soap has been dissolved. The clothes are immersed for twenty-four hours and then washed. The cleansing is said to be greatly quickened, and two or three rinsings in cold water remove the turpentine smell.

2500. Wash Mixture. E

Borax is valuable for laundry use, instead of soda. Add a handful of it, powdered, to about 10 gallons of boiling water, and you need use only half the ordinary allowance of soap. For laces, cambrics, etc., use an extra quantity of the powder. It will not injure the texture of the cloth in the least.

2501. Washing Powders.

Hager, in Phar. Centralhalle, gives the following analyses:

1. The so-called English Washing Crystal is an impure, half efflorescent crystallized soda, containing a large proportion of sulphate of soda and common salt.

2. Under the name of Washing Crystals simply a filtered solution of borax and soda has been introduced.

3. The English Patent Cleansing Crystal Washing Powder is a half efflorescent soda, containing about 25 per cent of Glauber's salts.

4. The Washing and Cleansing Crystals (Harper Twelvetrees & Sons), are pure crystallized soda, with 1 to 2 per cent of borax.

5. Krimmelbein's Wool Washing Composition is a mixture of 35 parts of dried soda, 10 parts of soap powder, and 10 parts of sal ammoniac.

6. Ward's Wool Washer is a mixture of 90 parts of effloresced soda crystals with 10 parts of soap powder.

7. The Universal Washing Powder (Henkel's) is a water glass containing soda, with a small percentage of tallow soap and starch powder.

8. Hudson's Soap Extract is a mixture of crystallized soda and soda soap, containing water (soap 14:3, anhydrous soda 30, and water 55).

9. A washing powder for the finest white linen is a powdery mixture of 90 parts of effloresced soda with 10 parts of hyposulphite of soda and 2 parts of borax.

10. The so-called Finest Brilliant Elastic Starch is a mixture of about 7 to 8 parts of stearine, with 100 parts of wheaten starch (melted stearine is mixed with about fifteen times its weight of starch, and after cooling powdered and combined with the rest of the starch).

11. The Berlin Prepared Brilliant Dressing Starch is good wheaten starch, mixed with 2 to 2½ per cent of borax.

2502. Benzine Jelly.

White castle soap	12 parts.
Ammonia water	4 parts.
Benzine	65 parts.
Water	20 parts.

Dissolve the soap in the water by the aid of heat, remove from the fire and add the ammonia water; stir until nearly ready to set, and then incorporate the benzine.

2503. Kid-Reviving Cream.

White wax	2 parts.
Tallow	1 part.
Linseed oil	2 parts.
Turpentine	4 parts.
Curd-soap	1 part.
Water to	20 parts.

Dissolve the soap in the water with the aid of heat; mix and dissolve other ingredients; then add gradually, while warm, the soap solution, so as to form a thickish cream; add any cheap essential oil.

The above, colored with any suitable aniline dye, or with fine lampblack and a trace of indigo, will give a suitable polish.

2504. General Cleaning Powder.

Soft soap	8 ounces.
Washing soda	4 ounces.
Borax	1 ounce.
Strong solution of ammonia	10 ounces.
Methylated spirit	2 ounces.
Water to	1 gallon.

Add any cheap essential oil to the spirit before mixing with the ammonia and solution of soap, etc., in the water.

2505. Bijou Cleaning Fluid.

Ether	1 dram.
Chloroform	1 dram.
Alcohol	2 drams.
Methyl. salicylate	½ dram.
Deodorized benzine, to	32 ounces.

Directions same as benzine.

2506. Deodorized Benzine.

Benzine	1 gallon.
Conc. sulphuric acid	½ pound.

Let stand a few days, shaking cautiously, pour off benzine and to it add 4 ounces dried slaked lime; shake this up in it occasionally for twelve hours, decant and bottle; or deodorize by shaking with a small quantity of plumbate of sodium which can be made by dissolving freshly precipitated oxide of lead in caustic soda.

2507. Gloss for Starch. A

French chalk	3 ounces.
Powdered white soap	1 ounce.

Directions: Take a piece of new dry flannel and dip it into the glaze-powder, rub it well over the right side of the starched article, then proceed to iron in the usual way, when a beautiful gloss will be obtained. Put in a little borax in making the starch to give stiffness as usual.

2508. Gloss for Starch. B

Powdered borax	1 dram.
Powdered spermaceti	1 dram.
Powdered French chalk	6 drams.

Mix and sift.

2509. Labarraque's Solution of Soda.

　　Sal soda .... 4 pounds.
　　Chlor. lime .... ½ pound.
　　Water .... 1 gallon.

Dissolve the sal soda in a vessel in 1 gallon boiling water; let it boil for 10 or 15 minutes, then add the chloride lime; let settle and decant.

2510.　Soaps and Soap Making.

On the manufacture of soap in small quantities without boiling, Mr. W. J. Menzies, in the course of a paper on the above subject, printed in the Chemist and Druggist of August 4, gives the following practical recipe:

Take exactly 10 pounds of double refined 98 per cent caustic soda powder (Greenbank), put it in any can or jar with 45 pounds of water, stir it once or twice, when it will dissolve immediately and become quite hot; let it stand until the lye thus made is cold. Weigh out and place in any convenient vessel for mixing, exactly 75 pounds of clean grease, tallow, or oil (not mineral oil). If grease or tallow be used, melt it slowly over the fire until it is liquid and just warm—say, temperature not over 100° F. If oil be used, no heating is required. Pour the lye slowly into the melted grease or oil in a small stream continuously, at the same time stirring with a flat wooden stirrer about three inches broad; continue gently stirring until the lye and grease are thoroughly combined and in appearance like honey. Do not stir too long, or the mixture will separate itself again. The time required varies somewhat with the weather and the kind of tallow, grease or oil used; from fifteen to twenty minutes will be enough. When the mixing is completed, pour off the liquid soap into any old square box for a mould sufficiently large to hold it, previously dampening the sides with water so as to prevent the soap sticking. Wrap up the box well with old blankets, or, better still, put it in a warm place until the next day, when the box will contain a block of 130 pounds of soap, which can afterward be cut up with a wire. Remember the chief points in the above directions, which must be exactly followed. The lye must be allowed to cool. If melted tallow or grease be used, it must not be more than warm. The exact weights of double refined 98 per cent powdered caustic soda and tallow or oil must be taken; also the lye must be stirred into the grease, not grease or oil added to the lye. If the grease or tallow used be not clean or contains salt it must be rendered, or purified, previous to use, that is to say, boiled with water, and allowed to become hard again to throw out the impurities. Any salt present will spoil the whole operation entirely, but discolored or rancid grease or tallow is just as good as fresh for soap making purposes.

If the soap turn out streaky and uneven it has not been thoroughly mixed. If very sharp to the taste too much soda has been taken. If soft, mild and greasy, too little soda has been used. In either case it must now be thrown into a pan and brought to a boil with a little more water. In the first case boiling is all that is necessary; in the other instances a very little oil or a very little more of the double refined powdered caustic soda must be added to the water. These things will never happen, however, if the directions are exactly followed, and after the soap has been made several times with the experience thus gained the process is extremely easy and the result will be always a good batch of soap. Beef tallow makes the hardest soap, mutton fat a rather softer soap; of oils, cotton seed is the cheapest and best, but the soap is much softer, lathering very freely indeed. Ordinary household fat or dripping will make a nice soap and in many places can be obtained at a very trifling cost, and in exchange for goods sold. Such grease, however, must be carefully examined for salt, which it often contains. It will be evident that any smaller quantity of soap can be made at a time, according to the above directions, by taking the ingredients in exact proportion. It is not advisable to make more than double the quantity prescribed, as it is difficult to work more by hand. By making successive batches, however, a single person can make two tons of soap in a day simply with apparatus (pans, etc.), obtainable in any household.

By adding a few drops of essential oil just when the mixing is completed a toilet soap is produced. Oil of mirbane (artificial almond oil) is the cheapest, but the perfume is not nearly so pleasant as real almond oil, citronella or oil of cloves. If made with clean grease or tallow or light colored oil, the soap produced is quite white.

Sometimes a little coloring matter will make the soap sell better, although of no better quality. Half an ounce of bichromate of potash ash dissolved in the lye will give a green: 1 pound palm oil melted with the tallow or oil, a yellow color; or a good brown can be got by burning ½ pound of sugar in a saucepan until black, then dissolving it in a pint of water, and adding it to the melted tallow before mixing.

A very cheap and good jelly soft soap can be made with the above soap. Take 5 pounds of the hard soap, crush it down or cut it up into as small pieces as possible; put this into a pan or boiler with 10 gallons of water if a strong hard tallow soap; if an oil soap only half the quantity of water (five gallons); just bring it to a boil, and stir well, to thoroughly dissolve all the pieces of hard soap; pour or ladle it into any can, tub or barrel that is tight, and leave it to cool for two or three days. This will give about 80 pounds of jelly soft soap, at an exceedingly small cost. Of course, if made from colored and scented hard soap it will be a colored and scented jelly soap. This is a good way of working up the scraps and bits of soap after cutting up. It can be sold with a good profit at a very low figure and often as a substitute for regular soft soap. It is a very different article, however, to a real potash soft soap, which should invariably be used for washing woolens. It is possible to produce this real potash soft soap in the cold by a somewhat similar process to the above.

2511. Washing Powder Compound.

Sal. soda, dried .... 4 ounces.
Muriate of ammonia, powd. 4 ounces.
Soda ash .... 4 pounds.

The ingredients should be well dried before mixing.

Directions: Put the clothes to soak over night in clear water. Then put the boiler on the stove half full of cold water and dissolve one tablespoonful of compound in a little water and add to the boiler. Stir well. Now put in the clothes and boil twenty minutes, then take them out and rub lightly and rinse and hang out to dry, and you will be surprised to see how much labor is saved. Will not injure the clothes. It saves one-half the labor. Try it, &c.

2512. Wash Bluing.

Ferrocyanuret of iron..... 6 ounces.
Oxalic acid .... 1½ ounces.
Water distilled.......... 2 gallons.

Dissolve the iron and acid in a quart of the water, and add the remaining 1¾ gallons. This makes a good article of bluing.

2513. Indigo Wash Bluing.

Best bengal indigo....... 5 pounds.
Strong sulphuric acid .... 30 pounds.

After 5 days, place mixture in a tub and pour on 40 gallons boiling water.

2514. Bluing for Laundry Use.

Sci. Am. Cyclo.

1. Dissolve indigo sulphate in cold water and filter.
2. Dissolve good cotton blue (aniline blue 6 B) in cold water.
3. Dissolve fine Prussian or Berlin blue with ⅛ part of oxalic acid in water; or use ferrocyanide of potassium (1/12 part) in place of oxalic acid.
4. Dissolve 7 oz. of yellow prussiate of potash in 2.1 pints of water. Make a solution of sesquichloride of iron which shall contain 1 part of the solid salt by weight to every 10 parts of water by weight. Take equal volumes of the two solutions, and add to each twice its volume of cold concentrated solution of sulphate of soda. Finally, mix the two solutions thus obtained. The solid Prussian blue will immediately precipitate. This may be put upon a filter and washed, being kept exposed to the air for perhaps fifteen or twenty days. The excess of soluble salts will first be washed away, and then the latter washings will dissolve the blue, forming a deep-blue liquid, which may be used for preparations of bluing for clothing. It is, however, better to buy the soft Prussian blue than to attempt to prepare it on a small scale. 1 oz. of the soft Prussian blue powdered, and put into a bottle with 1 qt. of clear rain water, acidulated by ¼ of an oz. of oxalic acid, is a good preparation. A very small portion suffices for a large amount of clothing.

2515. A Disinfective Laundry Blue.

Mix together 16 parts of Prussian blue, 2 parts of carbolic acid, 1 part of borax, and 1 part of gum arabic into a stiff dough. Roll it out into balls as large as hazel nuts, and coat them with gelatine or gum to prevent the carbolic acid from escaping.

2516. A Liquid Washing Blue.

Water 15 parts; dissolve in this 1½ parts indigo-carmine. Add ¾ part gum arabic.

2517. Silverine.

We have found the following silver-cleaning preparation excellent:

Precipitated chalk......... 1 ounce.
Solution of ammonia...... 1 ounce.
Wood alcohol............. 1½ ounces.
Water to................. 10 ounces.

Mix:

The following label is a suitable one:

SILVERINE.
A New Preparation.

For cleansing and restoring Gold, Silver, Gilt, Plated or Parcel-gilt Jewelry, Electro or Nickel-plated Wares, Polished Brass, &c., &c.

WARRANTED FREE FROM MERCURY.

Instructions for Use.—Well shake up, and use on a piece of cotton wool, sponge, or soft cloth; then rub off perfectly dry with wool, soft leather, or cloth. If for fancy work, apply as above and lightly polish off with a soft cloth. For gold, gilt, and brass articles, dilute to half strength by adding water.

To be kept tightly corked when not in use.

TO CLEAN BRASS.

The Government method prescribed for cleaning brass, and in use at all the United States arsenals, is claimed to be the best in the world. The plan is to make a mixture of 1 part common nitric acid and one-half part sulphuric acid, in a stone jar, having also ready a pail of fresh water and a box of sawdust. The articles to be treated are dipped into the acid, then removed into the water, and finally rubbed with sawdust. This immediately changes them to a brilliant color. If the brass has become greasy, it is first dipped in a strong solution of potash and soda in warm water; this cuts the grease, so that the acid has free power to act.

2518.   Brass Paste.   A
Rotten stone.............. 2 pounds.
Soft soap................. 1 pound.
Oil of amber.............. 1 ounce.

2519.   Brass Paste.   B
Oxalic acid............... 2 ounces.
Soft soap................. ½ pound.
Sweet oil................. ½ pound.
Turpentine .... 1 ounce.
Rotten stone.............. 4½ pounds.
Boiling water............. 16 ounces.

Dissolve the acid in the water, add the rotten stone, and, finally, the other ingredients.

2520.   Gilding Powder.
For gilding such metals as copper and silver the following powder is said by Martin to give good results:
Gold chloride............. 20 parts.
Potassium cyanide......... 60 parts.
Cream of tartar........... 5 parts.
Precipitated chalk........ 100 parts.

Before using, the powder is to be mixed with 100 parts of water, and rubbed upon the metal with a pad of cotton-wool.

**2521.   Lacquers Not Requiring Heat
            for Metals.   A**
Shellac .... 5 ounces.
Gamboge .... 5 drams.
Pyro-acetic ether (acetone). 30 ounces.
S. V. M................... 3 pints.

2522.   B
Shellac .... 1 ounce.
Dragon's blood .... 1 dram.
Annatto .... 1 dram.
Saffron .... 4 drams.
Gamboge .... 2 ounces.
Sandarac .... 1 ounce.
S. V. M................... 2 pints.

2523.   C
Shellac .... 2 ounces.
Dragon's blood .... 1 dram.
Annatto .... 8 drams.
Turmeric .... 4 ounces.
Sandarac .... 8 ounces.
S. V. M................... 2 pints.

These give: A, pale yellow; B, fine pale; C, pale gold. Cold lacquers are like the cold-water starches—it greatly depends upon the directions for success in their use. The lacquering-room must be sufficiently warm to ensure absence of moisture from the surface of the metal, and to prevent blistering and scaling off of the varnish. Cold lacquers require at least two days before they are sufficiently hard; longer should be given if possible.

2524.   D
Gold, green, and light blue. The following is a good basis. Use aniline colors; for gold, turmeric or gamboge.
Turpentine .... 8 ounces.
Linseed oil (boiled)...... 4 ounces.
Fused amber............... 4 ounces.
Shellac .... 1 ounce.
Dissolve with heat.

2525.   Brass Paste.   C
Rotten stone in finest powder .... 4 ounces.
Oxalic acid............... 1 ounce.
Sweet oil................. 1½ ounces.
Turpentine....q. s. to make a paste.
Coloring matter may be added if desired.

2526.   Silver Plating Paste.
Nitrate of silver......... ½ ounce.
Common salt............... ½ ounce.
Cyanide of potassium...... 1 ounce.
Chalk .... a sufficiency.

Dissolve the silver nitrate in a pint of water, and add the salt-dissolved in as much water. Mix the solutions, and collect the precipitate on a piece of cotton cloth. Transfer the moist precipitate to a mortar containing the cyanide (in powder), and dissolve by adding more water if necessary; then make the solution into a spreadable paste with prepared chalk.

To silver any tarnished article spread some of the paste upon the spot, and leave for a few hours; then brush it off. Repeat if necessary. The result is not so good as by electro-deposition, but home-made things are never so good as those produced by experts.

2527. Polishing Paste for Brass.
Tripoli .... 1 pound.
Spanish whiting........... 1 pound.
Pumice (finest powder)..... ½ pound.
Oleic acid................. 4 ounces.
Petrolatum....q. s. to make a soft paste.
The oleic acid and petrolatum to be the crude commercial articles.

2528.
The red polishing-paste for metals is made according to the following formula:
Peroxide of iron........... 6 ounces.
Kieselguhr .... 1 ounce.
Paraffin oil............... 1½ ounces.
The powders are to be in as fine a state of division as possible. Mix them, add the paraffin oil, then make into a paste with equal parts of lard and crude vaseline, and perfume with oil of mirbane.

2529. Silverine Solution.
Cyanide of potassium...... 2 ounces.
Nitrate of silver........... q. s. or 1 oz.
Distilled water............ 12 ounces.
Precipitated chalk......... 2 ounces.
Dissolve the cyanide in the water and add to it a concentrated solution of nitrate silver as long as the precipitate found at first is redissolved, and lastly mix in the chalk.

This liquid is applied with a soft bit of linen. The piece when silvered is well washed with water and the surface dried and gently polished with chamois skin.

For gilding substitute chloride of gold for nitrate of silver.

2530. Stove Blacking.
(Sci. Am. Cyclo.)

Mix 2 parts of black lead, 4 parts of copperas, and 2 parts of bone black, with water, so as to form a creamy paste. This is an excellent polish, as the copperas produces a jet black enamel, causing the black lead to adhere to the iron.

2531.
Plumbago, 2 lb.; water, 8 oz.; turpentine, 8 oz.; sugar, 2 oz. Knead thoroughly and keep in tin boxes. Apply with a brush.

2532.
Plumbago, make into a thin paste with sodium silicate or water glass. This makes an excellent stove polish and should be brushed thoroughly.

2533.
Pulverized black lead, 2 lb.; spirits of turpentine, 2 gal.; water, 2 oz.; sugar, 2 oz. Mix.

2534.
Mix 5 parts black lead, 5 parts bone black and 10 parts of iron sulphate. Use water q. s. to form a paste. This is an excellent preparation and the coating is very permanent.

2535.
Reduce graphite to an impalpable powder by grinding in a mill with water, dry; use with water first, then dry and polish. This is the base of nearly all commercial stove polishes.

2536.
Turpentine and black varnish, put with any good stove polish, is the blacking used by hardware dealers for polishing heating stoves. If properly put on, it will last throughout the season.

2537. Paste Stove Polish.
Pulverized black lead, 2 lb.; spirits of turpentine, 2 gal.; water, 2 oz.; sugar, 2 oz.; mix.

2538. Liquid Stove Polish.
Bone black, 2½ parts; pulverized graphite, 2½ parts; copperas, 5 parts, water, q. s. to form a creamy paste.

2539. Liquid Black Lead Polish.
Pulverized black lead, 1½ lb.; turpentine, 1½ gill; water, 1½ gill; sugar, 1½ oz.

2540. Bone Black Polish.
Mix 2 parts copperas, 1 part powdered bone black, and 1 part black lead with enough water to give proper consistency, like thick cream. Two applications are to be recommended.

2541. Brunswick Black for Grates, Etc.
Asphaltum, 5 lb.; melt and add boiled oil, 2 lb.; spirits of turpentine, 1 gal.; mix.

2542. Paste Black Lead for Stoves.
Black lead in powder..... 20 ounces.
Treacle .... 1 ounce.
Water .... a sufficiency.
Make into a paste, and perfume if desired with a drop or two of oil of mirbane.

2543. Artistic Enamel Black.

Asphaltum	8 ounces.
Black resin	4 ounces.
Sugar of lead (powdered)	¾ ounce.
Drop black (powdered)	¾ ounce.
Oil of cassia	½ ounce.
Boiled linseed oil	4 ounces.
Turpentine	32 ounces.

Powder the asphaltum and resin; place in an iron saucepan with the sugar of lead; drop black and linseed oil and apply heat until liquefied. Withdraw from heat and gradually add the turpentine; stirring well; then add the oil of cassia and mix well. Keep the bottles well corked.

2544. Paste Blacking for Shoes.

Ivory-black	16 ounces.
Lamp-black	16 ounces.
Treacle	16 ounces.
Sperm oil	4 ounces.
Vinegar	5 ounces.

Mix and add gradually

Sulphuric acid	4 ounces.

When action ceases add

Sulphate of iron	½ ounce.
Gum arabic	6 drams.
Hot water	5 ounces.

Previously mixed to form a solution. Work well until the paste is brought to a proper consistency.

2545. Brown Leather Paste Dressing.

Oil of turpentine	3 ounces.
Dark-yellow wax	1 ounce.
Palm oil	1 ounce.
Oil of mirbane	15 minims.

Make a paste sec. art. If not of the right shade add a few drops of solution of tincture of catechu.

2546. Brown Shoe Polish Paste.

Yellow wax	4 ounces.
Spirit of turpentine	8 ounces.

Melt on a water-bath, strain, stir occasionally until the paste turns creamy, then add

Nankin brown	15 grains.
Phosphine	5 grains.
Water	½ ounce

previously dissolved. Stir constantly until the mixture is perfect.

2547. Polish.

Yellow wax	6 ounces.
Linseed oil	10 ounces.
Spirit of turpentine	30 ounces.

Dissolve by means of a water-bath in a closed vessel, and add

Primrose soap	4 ounces.

previously dissolved in

Water	2 pints.

Stir continually till cold. Then with each 1 oz. of cream mix thoroughly

Nankin brown	5 grains.

dissolved in

Rectified spirits	½ dram.

The resulting polish is applied to leather with a rag, allowed to dry, and then lightly polished with a soft duster.

2548. Liquid Shoe Polish, Like Brown's.

Water	4½ gallons.
Solid ext. of logwood	4 ounces.
Bichromate of potash	2 ounces.
Prussiate of potash	¼ ounce.
Lump borax	1¾ pounds.
Gum shellac	4½ pounds.
Ammonia water	1 pint.

Dissolve the logwood in the water by the aid of direct heat; when the logwood is dissolved, add the bichromate and prussiate of potash, then the lump borax. When the borax is dissolved and the solution is at the boiling point, add the shellac, a portion at a time, stirring constantly until the latter is dissolved; add the ammonia and continue the boiling until the smell of the ammonia has disappeared. When cold strain through cheese cloth.

2549. Furniture Polish.

Acid acetic	1 ounce.
Raw linseed oil	1 ounce.
Alcohol, 188 per cent	2 ounces.
Turpentine	2 ounces.

Shake well before using.

The polish may be colored, if desired, by adding a little aniline brown. If made in large quantities keep well stirred while bottling.

2550. Mahogany Stain.

Dragon's blood	8 ounces.
Benzine	6 pints.

Dissolve.

2551. Patent Knot Filler.

Powdered shellac	2 pounds.
Benzine	3¼ pints.

Dissolve.

2552. French Polish.

Gum benzoin	6 ounces.
Gum shellac	2 pounds.
Resin. nig.	2 ounces.
Alcohol, 188 per cent	1¼ gallons.

2553. French Polish. B
Shellac	2 ounces.
Gum sandrac	2 drams.
Gum benzoin	2 drams.
Naptha, rect.	½ pint.

2554. Furniture Cream. A
Ch. and Dr.
Castile soap	1 ounce.
Yellow wax	1 pound.
White wax	1 ounce.
Turpentine	2 pints.
Boiling water	2 pints.

Melt the waxes on a water-bath and add turpentine, stirring until the mixture is quite liquid. Separately dissolve the soap in the boiling water, and pour the two mixtures simultaneously into a hot earthenware jug or jar. Stir for five minutes, and pour into wide mouthed bottles for sale.

2555. Furniture Cream. B
Pearlash	2 ounces.
Soft soap	4 ounces.
Pure yellow wax	12 ounces.
Water	20 ounces.

Boil together until a uniform cream is obtained, adding a little more water from time to time, and stirring all the while; then transfer to a 2-gallon jar containing 2 pints of warm water. Cautiously add with shaking 30 oz. of oil of turpentine, and enough water to make 1 gallon.

2556. Furniture Paste.
Yellow wax	8 ounces.
Resin	2 ounces.
Turpentine	16 ounces.
Alkanet	1 ounce.

Put the wax and resin in a 2-lb. or 3-lb. covered jar, and put the jar in a pan of water (with a layer of tow at the bottom). Heat until the wax and resin are melted; add the alkanet, and simmer for an hour or more. Then remove from the fire, add the turpentine, with constant stirring, and strain.

Should the mixture not be hot enough for straining, heat carefully on the water-bath again.

2557. Taylor's Solution of Four Chlorides, Disinfectant.
H. S. Taylor (Era Prize).
Alum	10 ounces.
Sal soda	10 ounces.
Sal ammoniac	2 ounces.
Common salt	2 ounces.
Chlor. zinc	1 ounce.
Muriatic acid, com'l	q. s.
Water	q. s. to 1 gal.

Dissolve the alum in one-half gallon of boiling water; then add the sal soda, which gives a precipitate of aluminum hydrate; muriatic acid is then added in sufficient quantity to dissolve this precipitate, thereby forming aluminum chloride. The other salts are then dissolved in the remainder of the water and added to the first solution.

The advantages claimed for this preparation are cheapness, ease of preparation, odorless, non-poisonous, and its adaptability for general use. Its freedom from iron in the disinfection of clothing is an important point in so much that it will not injure the fabric in any way. It commends itself for the disinfection of rooms by saturating a sheet with the diluted solution and hanging up in any convenient place. This diluted solution may be made by mixing one pint of the concentrated solution with 1 gallon of water.

2558. Salicylic Acid Preservative Powder.
For meat use water containing 5 grains in the pint; add 5 grains to the pint of milk; for preserved fruits add 3 or 4 grains to 1 lb., and cover with parchment paper steeped in a solution of the acid containing about 20 grains to the pint.

2559. Meat Preservative Powder.
The following is one of the most used:
Nitrate of potash	15.5 parts.
Chloride of sodium	73.5 parts.
Boric acid	9.5 parts.

2560. Lemon Sugar.
Granulated sugar	12 pounds.
Tartaric acid (powdered)	12 ounces.

Mix well and put into 12-ounce cans; put a half an ounce vial of soluble essence of lemon into each can.

Directions: Dissolve 3 or 4 teaspoonfuls of the lemon sugar in a tumblerful of cold water; add a few drops of the essence of lemon and mix well.

2561. Custard Powder.
Gum tragacanth (powdered)	2 ounces.
Powdered starch	1 pound.
Powdered turmeric	150 grains.
Oil of bitter almonds (sine poison)	30 minims.
Essence of lemon	1 dram.

Put up in 1-ounce packages for 1 pint of milk.

Directions: One packet to be rubbed in a dish with 2 tablespoonfuls of milk; boil the remainder of the milk with 2 ounces of sugar and while boiling pour gradually into the dish, stirring briskly. Bake as a custard.

NON-SECRET FORMULAS.

2562. Curry Powder.
Powdered cardamom...... 1 ounce.
Powdered curcuma......... 1 ounce.
Powdered capsicum........ 1 ounce.
Powdered foenugreek..... 4 ounces.
Powdered ginger........... 1 ounce.
Powdered coriander....... 1 ounce.

2563. Mixed Spices. A
Powdered turmeric .... 1 ounce.
Powdered liquorice .... 1 ounce.
Powdered coriander .... ½ ounce.
Powdered caraway .... 2 drams.
Powdered fenugreek ..... 1 dram.
Powdered anise .... 1 dram.
Caraways .... 2 drams.
Mix.

2564. Mixed Spices. B
Powdered ginger .... 1 ounce.
Powdered nutmegs .... ¼ ounce.
Powdered cloves .... ½ ounce.
Powdered mace .... ¼ ounce.
Powdered cinnamon ...... 1 ounce.
Powdered allspice........ 1 ounce.
Mix.

2565. Pickle Spice.
Black pepper............. 1 pound.
White pepper............. ½ pound.
Ginger .... ½ pound.
Mustard seeds............ ½ pound.
Capsicums................ 2 ounces.

2566. Tomato Catsup. A
Tomato pulp.............. 20 gallons.
Vinegar .... 2 gallons.
Salt .... 4½ pints.
Cloves (powdered)........ ½ pound.
Allspice (powdered)...... ½ pound.
Black pepper (powdered).. ¼ pound.
Red pepper (powdered)... 1 ounce.
Mix.

2567. Tomato Catsup. B
Bruised tomatoes......... 1 gallon.
Common salt............. 8 ounces.
Stand for three or four days. Squeeze out the juice, and to every one-half gallon add black pepper 1 ounce. Boil half an hour, strain and add
Allspice .... ½ ounce.
Ginger .... ½ ounce.
Mace .... ½ ounce.
Cochineal .... ¼ ounce.
Simmer gently half an hour, strain, cool, and bottle. A little brandy may be added, and shallots, if the flavor be liked, may be boiled along with the black pepper.

2568. Scotch Marmalade.
Seville orange juice....... 2 pints.
Seville orange peel cut small .... 2 pounds.
Yellow honey............. 2 pounds.
Cook to proper consistency.

2569. Universal Seasoning.
Salt .... ½ pound.
Mace .... ½ ounce.
White pepper .... 1 ounce.
Cloves .... ½ ounce.
Cayenne .... 2 drams.
Nutmegs .... 1 dram.

2570. Celery Salt.
Salt (finely powdered)..... 8 ounces.
Starch (powdered)........ 1 ounce.
Celery seed (powdered)... 2 ounces.
Mix.

2571. Brown Gravy Salt.
Salt (finely powdered)...... 8 ounces.
Gran'd sugar............. 4 ounces.
Cayenne (powdered)...... 10 grains.
Mix and fry in a frying pan until brown; rub through a sieve whilst hot.

2572. Kitchener's Soup Herb Powder.
Dried parsley............. 2 ounces.
Winter savory............ 2 ounces.
Sweet marjoram.......... 2 ounces.
Lemon thyme............. 2 ounces.

2573. Sausage Flavor. A
Sage .... ½ pound.
Pepper .... 1 pound.
Allspice................. 1 pound.

2574. Sausage Flavor. B
Sage .... 1 pound.
Marjoram .... 1 pound.
Thyme................... 1 pound.
Pepper .... 1 pound.
Ground nutmeg.......... 1 ounce.
Mix.

2575. Sausage Flavor. C
Allspice................. 1 pound.
Cloves .... ½ pound.
White pepper............ ½ pound.
Sage .... ½ pound.
Mix.

2576. Ham Sausage Seasoning.

Cardamon (powdered)	1 dram
Mace	½ dram
White pepper	2 ounces
Salt	4 ounces
Coriander	¼ ounce

Mix.

2577. Savory Spices.

Powdered white pepper	8 ounces
Powdered mace	1 ounce
Powdered cloves	2 ounces
Powdered allspice	2 ounces
Powdered cardamom	¼ ounce

2578. Pork Flavoring.

Sage (powdered)	4 ounces
Marjoram	1 ounce
White pepper	2 ounces
Ginger (powdered)	¼ ounce
Cayenne (powdered)	⅛ ounce

2579. Croft's Fine Table Sauce.

Vinegar	50 gallons
Tamarinds	40 pounds
Anchovies (ground)	6 pounds
Cayenne pepper	3 pounds
Onions (ground)	12 pounds
Garlic (ground)	2 pounds
Cloves (ground)	3 pounds
Nutmegs (ground)	½ pound
Mace (ground)	1 pound
Salt	14 pounds
Crude pyroligneous acid	1 pint
Salicylic acid	1 ounce
Canton soy	4 gallons
Brown N. O. Sugar	25 pounds

Put the vinegar in an 80-gallon cask (having a wide bung hole); add the tamarinds, sugar, salt and spices; grind the fish, onions and garlic in a cider mill and add—let stand (with occasional agitation) for two months; strain through hair cloth sieve and add the acids and soy; mix well. If color is not dark enough add burnt sugar coloring; stir well when bottling. In making this sauce a combination cider mill with press will be found useful for grinding the materials and pressing the marc. For making small quantities bruise the materials in an iron mortar.

2580. Delmonico Sauce, Cheap.

Vinegar	50 gallons
Cayenne pepper	4 pounds
Onions (ground)	8 pounds
Garlic (ground)	2 pounds
Tamarinds	20 pounds
Cloves (ground)	3 pounds
Nutmegs (ground)	1 pound
Crude pyroligneous acid	1 pint
Salicylic acid	1 ounce
Salt	14 pounds
Brown N. O. sugar	25 pounds
Canton soy	4 gallons
Burnt sugar coloring	½ gallon

Put the pressed marc from the Croft's sauce into an 80-gallon cask with the vinegar and proceed according to directions in preceding formula for making Croft's sauce.

Sugar house molasses may be substituted for canton soy by adding an additional 2 pounds of salt for each gallon of molasses used; but the flavor is not so good. When bottling sauces stir well to equalize the sediment in each bottle.

2581. Digestive Relish.

Jamaica ginger (ground)	2 ounces
Black pepper	1 ounce
Capsicum (ground)	1 ounce
Pimento (ground)	1 ounce
Mustard (ground)	1 ounce
Coriander seed (ground)	1 ounce
Mace (ground)	½ ounce
Nutmegs (ground)	½ ounce
Cloves (ground)	½ ounce
Cardamon seed (ground)	3 drams
Garlic	4 ounces
Shallots (young onions)	4 ounces
Tartaric acid	1 ounce
Vinegar (best)	5 quarts

Bruise the onions and garlic; boil with the spices for 15 minutes, then add

Mushroom catsup	3 pints
Canton soy	2 pints

Again boil for 15 minutes; pour into a keg; add

Salt	½ pound

Let stand for two weeks (agitate occasionally) strain.

Always use a porcelain lined vessel for boiling acid preparations.

2582. East India Sauce, Cheap.

Vinegar	25 gallons
Canton soy	4 gallons
Sugar coloring	½ gallon
Salt	14 pounds
Cayenne pepper	1½ pounds
Ginger (ground)	3 pounds
Cloves (ground)	1 pound
Tamarinds	10 pounds
Onions	10 pounds
Garlic	4 pounds
Salicylic acid	4 ounces
Borax	8 ounces
Water, sufficient to make up to	60 gallons

Process for making: Put the spices in a pan of cold water and boil for half an hour; boil the onions and garlic until soft; soak the tamarinds in water for 12 hours and wash out the pulp; dissolve the borax and salicylic acid in boiling water; mix all the ingredients together in a large cask; stir occasionally for two weeks and strain. Stir well when bottling so as to equalize the sediment in each bottle.

2583. Yorkshire Relish.

Curcuma (powdered)	4	ounces.
Coriander seed (powdered)	2	ounces.
Cayenne (powdered)	2	ounces.
Cardamom seed (powdered)	1	ounce.
Black pepper (powdered)	2	ounces.
Mustard seed (powdered)	4	ounces.
Cinnamon (powdered)	1	dram.
Mace (powdered)	1	dram.
Cloves (powdered)	5	drams.
Allspice (powdered)	2	ounces.
Assafoetida (powdered)	1	ounce.
Acetic acid (strong)	4	ounces.
Brown sugar	24	ounces.
Sugar coloring	1	pint.
Canton soy	2	pints.
Salicylic acid	1	dram.
Vinegar	1	gallon.
Salt	½	pound.
Mushroom catsup	½	gallon.

Dissolve the assafoetida in the strong acetic acid; boil the spices in the vinegar for 15 minutes; pour into a keg; add the other ingredients; stir occasionally for a month and strain. Always use a porcelain lined vessel for boiling vinegar.

2584. North of England Sauce.

Powdered pimento	6	pounds.
Powdered cloves	3	pounds.
Powdered black pepper	3	pounds.
Powdered assafoetida	4	ounces.
Cayenne pepper	½	pound.
Acetic acid	2	gallons.
Malt vinegar	4	gallons.
Water	6	gallons.

Macerate together for three days, then strain, and wash the marc with 4 gallons of water. Reserve the strained portion, then boil the marc for ten minutes with 24 gallons of water, add

Molasses	12	pounds.
Salt	12	pounds.
Burnt sugar	2	pounds.
Soy	6	gallons.

Boil for another quarter of an hour, and strain. When cold mix the strained liquors, and add salicylic acid one-half ounce dissolved in spirit of chloroform 2 ounces.

2585. Barsaloux Sauce.

New Orleans sugar	3¾	pounds.
Salt	15	ounces.
Garlic	15	ounces.

Grind the garlic in a meat cutter or mill; put into a frying pan with the sugar and salt and fry brown. Take

Cayenne pepper	2	ounces.
Ginger (ground)	7	ounces.
Cloves	7	ounces.
Black pepper	7	ounces.

Soak in water (one-half gallon) over night and boil for three-quarters of an hour. Mix all together and add

Vinegar	5	pints.
Water	7	pints.

Let stand for a week and strain.

2586. Alum Baking Powder, One Spoon.

Burnt alum (powdered)	16	pounds.
Soda bicarb	17	pounds.
Starch (powdered)	25	pounds.

2587. Alum Baking Powder, Two Spoons.

Burnt alum (powdered)	16	pounds.
Soda bicarb	17	pounds.
Starch (powdered)	50	pounds.

2588. Phosphate Baking Powder, One Spoon.

Acid phosphate of calcium	20	pounds.
Burnt alum	20	pounds.
Soda bicarb	29	pounds.
Starch (powdered)	30	pounds.

2589. Phosphate Baking Powder, Two Spoons.

Acid phosphate of calcium	20	pounds.
Burnt alum	20	pounds.
Soda bicarb	29	pounds.
Starch (powdered)	60	pounds.

2590. Slow Rising Cream Tartar Baking Powder, Two Spoons.

Cream of tartar	8	pounds.
Soda bicarb	6	pounds.
Starch powdered	14	pounds.

Mix.

2591. Quick Rising Baking Powder, Two Spoons.

Tartaric acid	15	pounds.
Soda bicarb	17	pounds.
Starch powdered	64	pounds.

Mix.

2592. Salt Rising Baking Powder, Two Spoons.

Tartaric acid	5 pounds.
Soda bicarb.	6 pounds.
White sugar powdered	4 pounds.
Dried powdered salt	4 pounds.
Magnesia carb., light	½ pound.
Starch powdered	8 pounds.

Mix.

2593. Self-Raising Flour.

Cream of tartar	10 ounces.
Soda bicarb.	6 ounces.
Best flour	100 pounds.

2594. General Directions for Mixing Baking Powder.

The ingredients should be sifted separately into a mixing trough; sift the starch or flour first; then the acid, mix well and then sift the soda, mix again well using preferably a flat wooden paddle. Then put the powders into a mixing machine; or sift them well at least three times so as to ensure thorough mixing; if you have no mixing machine, you can mix the powders in one of those keg-shaped rectangular churns kept for sale by leading hardware dealers; be careful to have all your materials quite dry; moisture is detrimental to the keeping properties of all baking powders especially so to those made with tartaric acid or cream of tartar. The starch in baking powders tends to preserve the quality unimpaired by preventing the acids from attacking the soda.

2595. Fruit Juices.

I give instructions by which all confectioners may extract and preserve their own fruit essences, and so guard the health and add to the pleasure of all for whom they provide. Among the juicy fruits are strawberries, raspberries, blackberries, cherries and currants; among non-juicy fruits are the apples, pears, peaches, quinces, apricots, and plums.

Mash the juicy fruits in a basin to a pulp. Place on the fire and make scalding hot. Now pour into a hair sieve and allow the juice to strain through. Put into bottles and securely tie down. Place these bottles in a caldron of cold water and boil for twenty minutes. Remove from the fire and allow to remain in the caldron until cold. Then set away for use.

In the case of non-juicy fruits, such as apples, pears, peaches, etc., put the fruit into a basin. Cover with water and boil to a pulp. Now place on a hair sieve and allow to drain without any pressing. Observe now that it is only the liquor which passes through the sieve without pressing which is to be used for flavoring purposes. What remains in the form of pulp is not adapted for these uses. Now put the juice obtained as above into bottles, and proceed to treat as already laid down for the juicy fruits.

The foregoing processes are to be gone through with in the case where the extracts are to be kept transparent and clear, as for syrups, cordials and beverages.

In case where the flavorings are to be used for any purpose where transparency or clearness is not desirable, such as for ice creams, fruit ices, or bonbons, then I would use not only the clear fluid, but the pulp of the fruit also. I would for these opaque purposes save and utilize everything of the fruit except the skins and seeds. This pulp is to be treated as already laid down.

As thus obtained and preserved our confectioners can supply themselves with a quantity of perfectly pure extracts of all their favorite fruits, and which can always be at hand, for flavoring every description of pastry, cakes, pies, tarts, puddings, creams, ices and beverages, and at any season of the year. Especially when there is any one in the house who is sick or feverish, cordials may be flavored with these delightful sub-acids—these remedies and restoratives of kind mother Nature herself—such as will shoot through all the veins of the most debilitated and infirm the most delicious sensations of happiness and hope.—James W. Parkinson, in Confectioners' Journal.

2596. Lemon Extract.

Oil of lemon	8 ounces.
Cologne spirits, 188 per cent	96 ounces.
Water	24 ounces.
Tincture of turmeric q. s. to color.	

Dissolve the oil in the spirits; shake well, and slowly add the water color and filter.

Always use cologne spirits (deodorized and purified alcohol) for the manufacture of flavoring extracts the cost is very little more, the product is much finer than can be made from common alcohol.

2597. Lemon Extract, Soluble.

Oil of lemon	2½ ounces.
Cologne spirits, 188 per cent	16 ounces.
Water	48 ounces.
Magnesia carb.	1 ounce.
Tincture of turmeric	q. s.

Put the magnesia into a mortar; rub in the oil; stir in the spirits slowly; pour into a gallon bottle and set aside for two days, then add the water; a portion at a time, shaking well; let stand a week before filtering; when filtered add the tincture of turmeric.

2598. Orange Extract, Soluble.

May be made in the manner directed for lemon extract soluble; by substituting oil of orange for oil of lemon, and by making the color a darker tinge by using a few drops of caramel in addition to the tincture of turmeric.

2599. Extract of Vanilla No. 1.

Vanilla beans .... 2½ pounds.
Granulated sugar .... 2½ pounds.
Cologne spirits, 188 per
  cent .... 2½ gallons.
Water .... 2 gallons.

Cut the beans lengthwise, then crosswise into small pieces; bruise in an iron mortar with the sugar (adding the sugar a portion at a time); place in a covered vessel with the spirits and water and macerate for 7 days; then place in a percolator; percolate and press the marc. Save the marc for second quality goods.

2600. Extract of Vanilla, Cheap.

Tonka beans .... 8 ounces.
Marc left from the No. 1
  extract ....
Hot water .... 1½ gallons.
Simple syrup .... 1 pint.
Cologne spirits, 188 per
  cent .... 3 quarts.
Sugar coloring .... 1 pint.

Cut the tonka beans, and bruise in a mortar; pour half a gallon of boiling water on them, cover up; when cold skim off any fat that may rise to the surface; strain and set aside.

Stew the marc left from the No. 1 extract for half an hour with a gallon of water; in a tightly closed vessel; when cold strain; add 3 quarts of spirits, 188 per cent, 1 pint of simple syrup, 1 pint of sugar coloring and the tonka extract. Mix well and filter.

2601. Extract of Vanilla from Vanilline.

Vanilline crystals .... ½ ounce.
Cologne spirits, 188 per
  cent .... 1 quart.
Distilled water........... 2 quarts.
Simple syrup .... 1 quart.

Some confectioners prefer a colorless extract as above; when color is required add caramel (burnt sugar) 4 ounces.

Dissolve the vanilline in the alcohol; then add the water, shake well and add the syrup.

2602. Extract of Vanilla from Vanilline and Coumarin.

Vanilline crystals .... ½ ounce.
Coumarin crystals .... 1 dram.
Cologne spirits, 188 per
  cent .... 1 quart.
Distilled water .... 2 quarts.
Simple syrup .... 1 quart.
Caramel (burnt sugar).... 6 ounces.

Dissolve the vanilline and coumarin in the alcohol; then add the water; shake well and add the syrup then add the coloring.

2603. Vanilla Sugar.

Vanilline .... ½ ounce.
Cologne spirits, 188 per
  cent .... 2 ounces.
Powdered sugar .... 32 ounces.

Dissolve the vanilline in the alcohol; put 4 ounces of the sugar in a porcelain lined or granite-ware pan, and pour on the solution of vanilline; mix well; then mix in the remainder of the sugar and dry by a very gentle heat; the ordinary summer temperature will do; when dry pack in tin cans.

2604. Vanilla Syrup.

Vanilline .... ¼ ounce.
Alcohol .... 8 ounces.
Simple syrup .... 7 pints.
Caramel .... 8 ounces.

Dissolve the vanilline in the alcohol, and add to the syrup; then add the coloring.

2605. Lemon Syrup Without Acid.

Lemon extract soluble..... 8 ounces.
Simple syrup .... 1 gallon.
Color with tincture of turmeric.

2606. Lemon Syrup With Acid.

Lemon extract soluble..... 8 ounces.
Tartaric acid .... 1 ounce.
Water .... 8 ounces.
Simple syrup .... 7 pints.

Dissolve the acid in the water and add to the syrup; then add the soluble lemon extract.

Color with turmeric.

2607. Raspberry Extract, Artificial.

Butyrate of amyl	1 ounce.
Oenanthic ether	½ ounce.
Formic ether	¼ ounce.
Aldehyde	¼ ounce.
Acetate of amyl	2 ounces.
Tincture of orris root	4 ounces.
Oil of rose	5 drops.
Glycerin	8 ounces.
Cologne spirits, 188 per cent	48 ounces.
Water, clear	16 ounces.
Solution of cochineal	q. s.
Caramel	q. s.

Mix the ethers with the spirits; add the tincture of orris and oil of rose.

Mix the water and glycerine together and in this mixture add enough solution of cochineal and caramel to give the desired shade; and add slowly with continuous shaking to the spirituous solution.

2608. Strawberry Extract, Artificial.

Butyric ether	4 ounces.
Acetate of amyl	2 ounces.
Formic ether	1 dram.
Aldehyde	1 dram.
Extract of orris	8 ounces.
Oil of rose	5 drops.
Oenanthic ether	1 ounce.
Cologne spirits, 188 per cent	48 ounces.
Water, clear	16 ounces.
Solution of cochineal	q. s.
Caramel	q. s.

Mix the ethers with the spirits, add the tincture of orris and oil of rose.

Mix the water and glycerine together and in this mixture add enough solution of cochineal and caramel to give the color desired; and add slowly with continuous shaking to the spirituous solution.

Make the color of a lighter shade than the raspberry extract. The exact proportions of color for the above cannot be given here on account of the varying strengths of caramel and cochineal solutions.

2609. Cinnamon Extract.

Oil of cinnamon	2 ounces.
Cologne spirits, 188 per cent	64 ounces.
Water	32 ounces.

Color with tincture of red saunders.

For cheap trade use oil of cassia instead of oil of cinnamon and add 32 ounces more of water and carb. magnesia 1 ounce; for filtering see directions for lemon extract soluble.

2610. Clove Extract.

Oil of cloves	2 ounces.
Cologne spirits, 188 per cent	64 ounces.
Water	32 ounces.

Dissolve the oil in the spirit; add the water slowly; filter if necessary. Color with tincture of red saunders.

2611. Peppermint Extract.

Oil of peppermint	2 ounces.
Cologne spirits, 188 per cent	64 ounces.
Water	32 ounces.
Color with chlorophyll	q. s.

Filter with carbonate of magnesia. The cheap extracts of cloves, peppermint, cinnamon, etc., are made by proceeding as directed in formula for lemon extract soluble.

2612. Banana Extract.

Acetate of amyl	4 ounces.
Butyrate of amyl	4 ounces.
Aldehyde	½ ounce.
Chloroform	¼ ounce.
Butyric ether	½ ounce.
Cologne spirits	48 ounces.
Water	16 ounces.
Tincture of turmeric	q. s.

2613. Pine Apple Extract.

Aldehyde	½ ounce.
Chloroform	½ ounce.
Butyrate of amyl	2½ ounces.
Acetate of amyl	5 ounces.
Butyric ether	½ ounce.
Cologne spirits	48 ounces.
Water	16 ounces.
Tincture of turmeric	q. s.

2614. Coloring for Extracts.

Dealers in aniline colors sell yellow, red, green, crimson and brown colors, for coloring extracts; the goods are made from anilines freed from arsenic and are generally described as vegetable colors; they are extensively used by manufacturers of flavoring extracts and perfumers, instead of turmeric, chlorophyll, red saunders, cudbear, etc.

2615. Extract of Rose.

Otto of rose	2 drams.
Oil of rose geranium	1 dram.
Cologne spirits, 188 per cent	64 ounces.
Water, warm	64 ounces.

Dissolve the oils in the spirits; shake well; and add the warm water (temperature of 130° F.) a portion at a time. Color pink with cochineal.

NON-SECRET FORMULAS.

2616. Extract of Apple.
Chloroform .... ½ ounce.
Spirits of nitrous ether... 1 ounce.
Valerianate of amyl ...... 5 ounces.
Acetate of ethyl .... 1 ounce.
Aldehyde .... 2 ounces.
Glycerin .... 8 ounces.
Cologne spirits .... 48 ounces.
Water .... 30 ounces.
Color yellow with turmeric.

2617. Extract of Celery.
Celery seed, ground....... 8 ounces.
Cologne spirits, 188 per cent .... 5 pints.
Water q. s. to make up to 1 gallon.
Macerate the celery with 1 pint of spirits and ½ pint of water for 3 days; place in a percolator. Mix the remaining 4 pints of spirits with 2 pints of water and pour upon the drug; when percolation has ceased, run water through until the product measures one gallon. Color with turmeric tincture.

2618. Extract of Peach.
Oil of bitter almonds (without prussic acid)... ½ ounce.
Cologne spirits, 188 per cent .... 64 ounces.
Banana extract, No. 2612. 32 ounces.
Water .... 32 ounces.
Dissolve the oil of bitter almonds in the cologne spirits; add the banana extract (see preceding formula for making same); shake well, and then add the water.

2619. Extract of Ginger.
Jamaica ginger ground.... 8 pounds.
African ginger ground.... 1 pound.
Cayenne .... 1¼ ounces.
Cologne spirits, 188 per cent .... 3¼ gallons.
Water .... 1½ gallons.
Red saunders .... 1 ounce.
Macerate the ginger, cayenne and red saunders, with a portion of the spirits and water mixed; percolate with the remainder of the menstruum, after 3 days maceration.

2620. Extract of Ginger, Aromatic.
Jamaica ginger ground.... 3 pounds.
African ginger ground.... 1 pound.
Grains of paradise, ground 4 ounces.
Cloves ground .... 4 ounces.
Cassia ground .... 2 ounces.
Macerate with 1 gallon of 75 per cent alcohol for 7 days; percolate and run alcohol 75 per cent through until the product measures 3 gallons.

2621. Extract of Ginger, Soluble.
Extract of ginger......... 12 fl. ounces.
Magnesia carb. .... 2 ounces.
Water .... 12 ounces.
Rub the magnesia and ginger together in a mortar; slowly add 12 ounces of water; when well mixed, put into a bottle and let stand for 3 days (shaking occasionally); filter.

2622. Aromatic Extract of Ginger, Soluble.
Extract of ginger aromatic 12 fl. ounces.
Magnesia carb. .... 2 ounces.
Water .... 12 ounces.
Rub the magnesia and extract of ginger together in a mortar; slowly add 12 ounces of water; when well mixed, put into a bottle and let stand for 3 days (shaking occasionally); filter.

2623. Ginger Ale Extract.
Ext. of ginger arom. soluble .... 12 ounces.
Extract of rose .... 2 ounces.
Extract of lemon soluble.. 2 ounces.

2624. Ginger Ale Syrup.
Ginger ale extract .... 8 ounces.
Tartaric acid .... ½ ounce.
Water .... 8 ounces.
Simple syrup .... 7 pints.
Caramel .... q. s.
Dissolve the acid in the water and filter, if necessary; add to the syrup; then add the ginger ale extract and color with caramel q. s.

2625. Extract of Mead, Soluble.
Oil of lemon .... 1 ounce.
Oil of sassafras .... 1 dram.
Oil of cassia .... 1 dram.
Oil of cloves .... 2 drams.
Oil of nutmegs .... 1 dram.
Oil of coriander .... 1 dram.
Magnesia carb. .... 1 ounce.
Cologne spirits .... 32 ounces.
Water .... 48 ounces.
Put the magnesia into a mortar; rub in the mixed oils; stir in the spirits slowly; pour into a gallon bottle and set aside for two days; then add the water, a portion at a time, shaking well; let it stand a week before filtering; when filtered add caramel q. s. to color brown.

2626. Mead Syrup.
Extract of mead soluble... 16 ounces.
Tartaric acid .... ¼ ounce.
Water .... 4 ounces.
Caramel .... 8 ounces.
Simple syrup q. s. to make up to .... 1 gallon.

Dissolve the acid in the water, add to half a gallon of simple syrup; add the other ingredients and make up to 1 gallon with simple syrup.

2627. Extract of Soap Bark for Foam.
Soap bark, crushed........ 8 ounces.
Alcohol .... 16 ounces.
Glycerine .... 16 ounces.
Water .... 32 ounces.

Macerate the soap bark for 2 days in a portion of alcohol, glycerine and water mixed; place in a percolator and percolate with the remainder of the menstruum; run water through the percolator until the product measures 4 pints.

For making a foam on beverages use from one-half to one ounce for each gallon of syrup.

2628. Extract of Malt, Genuine.
Malt, coarse ground....... 4 pounds.
Hot water .... 12 pints.

Place the malt in a percolator and pour on 6 pints of hot water (temperature 175° F.); macerate for an hour. Then commence to percolate and run through the remaining 6 pints of hot water; press out the malt, add to the percolate and evaporate by the heat of a water-bath, at a temperature not exceeding 130° F. to a syrupy consistence.

2629. Extract of Malt, Factitious.
Glucose .... 2 gallons.
New England rum......... 4 ounces.
Fluid extract of hops..... 3 ounces.
Caramel .... 2 ounces.

Heat the glucose in a water-bath; stir in the other ingredients and bottle whilst the mixture is warm. By substituting muriatic acid two ounces and water 14 ounces for the rum, hops and caramel, you will have a predigested food.

2630. Solution of Salicylic Acid for Fruit Preserving.
Salicylic acid .... 1 ounce.
Glycerine .... 2 pints.
Saccharin .... 1 dram.
Sugar white granld....... 8 pounds.
Water, clear q. s. to make up to .... 2 gallons.

Dissolve the saccharin and salicylic acid in the glycerine; use a gentle heat; dissolve the sugar in the water; mix together and strain.

Take fresh sound clean fruit, pack tightly in jars and fill the jars to the top with the extract, keep the fruit in a cool place.

2631. Vegetable Preservative.
Salicylic acid .... 1 ounce.
Common salt .... 1 pound.
Boiling water .... 2 gallons.

Dissolve the acid and salt in the boiling water; when cold filter. Pack the vegetables tightly in glass jars and fill up with the preservative.

2632. Extract of Tolu, Soluble.
Balsam of tolu .... 3 ounces.
Alcohol, 188 per cent.... 8 ounces.
Carbonate of magnesia.... 4 ounces.
Water q. s. to make up to 1 quart.

Dissolve the tolu in the alcohol with heat from a water-bath. Put the magnesia into a mortar and rub the solution of tolu into it thoroughly; add gradually to this 1 quart of boiling water, rubbing the mixture well; transfer to a bottle and let stand for 3 days, shaking occasionally; then filter through filtering paper, letting enough water run through the filter to make the product measure one quart.

2633. Syrup of Tolu.
Extract of tolu soluble.... 2 ounces.
Simple syrup............. 14 ounces.

2634. Glycerine Jelly. A
Glycerine .... 1 fl. ounce.
Corn starch .... 1 dram.
Water .... 1½ drams.
Otto of rose ....
or
White rose extract........ q. s.

Mix the starch, glycerine and water, bring to the boiling point; when cold add the perfume and color with solution of red aniline or cochineal.

2635. Glycerine Jelly. B
(Ch. and Dr.)
Gelatini .... 2 ounces.
Glycerini .... 4 ounces.
Aq. bullient. .... 9 ounces.

Put the gelatine in the water contained in a jug, and continue to heat on a water-bath until it is soft; then add the glycerine, and when solution is effected the following:
Liq. cocci. .... ½ dram.
Ol. rosae .... 12 minims.
Fill into bottles.

2636. Glycerine and Honey Jelly.
Gelatine .... 2½ parts.
Honey .... 10 parts.
Glycerine .... 60 parts.
Water .... 27½ parts.

Mix the glycerine and water, and dissolve in the mixture, by the aid of heat, first the honey, then the gelatine. Perfume as required.

2637. Arnica Jelly.

Glycerine .... 8 fl. ounces.
Water .... 2 fl. ounces.
Starch .... 1 ounce.
Tincture of arnica .... 1 ounce.
Otto of rose ....
  or
White rose extract......... q. s.

Make it the desired color with solution of cochineal.

2638. Oxide of Zinc Jelly.
Ch. and Dr.

Gelatine .... 4 ounces.
Oxide of zinc .... 3 ounces.
Glycerine .... 5 ounces.
Water .... 9 ounces.

Soak the gelatine in the water for an hour or so, add the glycerine, and melt with a gentle heat; rub this up smoothly with the zinc in a warm mortar, strain through fine muslin, if necessary; stir until it begins to cool.

When required for use it should be melted, and applied with a brush.

2639. Simple Syrup.

Granulated sugar .... 16 pounds.
Distilled water, cold ...... 1 gallon.

Dissolve the sugar in the cold water, stirring occasionally, until dissolved; select the best granulated sugar free from ultramarine or other adulteration.

2640. Syrup of Squills.

Vinegar of squills (1 to 6).. 12 ounces.
Water .... 5 ounces.
Sugar .... 32 ounces.

Dissolve the sugar with a gentle heat in the mixture of vinegar of squills and water.

2641. Syrup of Saffron. A

Saffron, crushed .... 1 ounce.
Alcohol, 188 per cent....... 4 ounces.
Water .... 14 ounces.
Sugar .... 2 pounds.

Make a tincture and dissolve 2 pounds of granulated sugar in it.

2642. Syrup of Saffron. B

Saffron .... 1 ounce.
Glycerine .... 5 ounces.
Boiling water .... 20 ounces.

Infuse 4 hours; strain and add
Sugar .... 40 ounces.
Make a syrup and add
Alcohol, 188 per cent....... 4 ounces.

2643. Syrup of Tar, U. S.

Tar .... 3 ounces.
Cold water .... 5 ounces.
Boiling water .... 20 ounces.
Granulated sugar .... 1¾ pounds.

Pour the cold water upon the tar, and stir frequently during 24 hours; then pour off the water and throw it away. Pour the boiling distilled water upon the residue, stir briskly for 15 minutes, and set aside for 36 hours, stirring occasionally. Decant the solution, and filter. Lastly, in seventeen fluid ounces of the filtered solution dissolve the sugar by agitation without heat.

2644. Tasteless Syrup of Quinine.
(Two grains to teaspoonful.)

Cinchonine alkaloid .... 1½ ounces.
Soda bicarb. .... ¼ ounce.

Rub in mortar with simple syrup q. s. until perfectly smooth. Add 2 ounces soluble essence lemon, uncolored, and enough simple syrup to measure 328 ounces.

2645. Tasteless Syrup of Quinine.
(3 grains to teaspoonful.)

Cinchonine alkaloid .... 1½ ounces.
Soda bicarb. .... ¼ ounce.

Rub in mortar with simple syrup q. s. until perfectly smooth; add 2 ounces soluble essence lemon and enough simple syrup to measure 131 ounces.

Cinchonine alkaloid or cinchonia alkaloid is the basis of sulphate cinchonia. U. S. P., p. 114, Rev. of 1870, it is a tasteless preparation.

Dose is about the same as sulph. quinia. It is manufactured by Powers & Weightman and other makers of cinchona salts.

2646. Syrup of Iodide of Iron, U. S.

Iron wire, cut small .... 266 grains.
Iodine .... 2 ounces av.
Granulated sugar .... 14 ounces av
Distilled water q. s. to
  make .... 1 pint.

Introduce the iron into a flask of thin glass of suitable capacity, add to it 5 fluid ounces of distilled water and afterward the iodine. Shake the mixture occasionally until the reaction ceases and the solution has acquired a green color and has lost the odor of iodine. Place the sugar in a porcelain capsule and filter the solution of iodide of iron into the sugar. Rinse the flask and iron wire with two fluid ounces of distilled water and pass the washings through the filter into the sugar. Stir the mixture with a porcelain or wooden spatula; heat it to the boiling point on a sand bath and having strained the syrup through linen into a tared bottle; add enough distilled water to make the product measure 16 ounces. Lastly shake the bottle and transfer its contents to small vials which should be completely filled, securely corked and kept in a cool dark place.

2647. Syrup of Iodide of Iron, Tasteless, N. F.

Iodine	400 grains.
Iron wire, fine bright and finely cut	200 grains.
Citrate of potassium	620 grains.
Sugar	10 troy oz.
Distilled water q. s. to make	16 fl. ounces.

Mix the iron with four fluid ounces of distilled water in a flask; add 267 grains of the iodine and apply a gentle heat until the iodine is combined and the solution has acquired a greenish color. Then heat the contents of the flask to boiling; filter the liquid and wash the filter with one-half a fluid ounce of hot distilled water. To the hot filtrate add the citrate of potassium and afterwards the remainder of the iodine and agitate until the liquid has assumed a greenish color; pour this upon the sugar contained in a bottle; agitate until solution has been affected and when the liquid is cold add enough distilled water to make 16 fluid ounces. Each fluid dram contains an amount of iron corresponding to about 3.6 grains of ferric iodide. The officinal syrup of iodide contains about 8 grains of ferrous iodide (protiodide of iron), in each fluid dram. The above preparation contains the iron in a ferric condition.

2648. Syrup of Iodide of Iron.

Syrup of iodide of iron can be extemporaneously prepared, says Miss Austa Worthrop in Pac. Drug. Rev., by placing 480 grains iodine in a flask adding 2½ ounces water and by degrees 150 grains reduced iron. When reaction has ceased, and the liquid has become green filter the solution into sufficient hot syrup (heated nearly to boiling point) to make 10 fluid ounces. Finally add a 50 per cent solution of citric acid containing 10 grains of the acid. The syrup keeps well, and the method of preparation is a rapid one.

2649. Solution of Iodide of Iron, N. F.

(For syrup of iodide of iron.)

Iron wire, fine, bright and finely cut	3 troy oz.
Iodine	4718 grains.
Hypophosphorus acid (N. F.)	180 minims.
Distilled water enough to make	16 fl. ounces.

Mix the iron with 12 fluid ounces of distilled water in a flask, add about one-half of the iodine, agitate continuously until the liquid becomes hot. Then moderate the reaction by placing the flask in cold water or by allowing cold water to flow over it, meanwhile, keeping up the agitation. When the reaction has moderated, add one-half of the remaining iodine at a time and carefully moderate the reaction each time, in the manner above directed. Finally raise the contents of the flask to boiling and filter immediately through moistened, pure filtering paper (the point of the filter being supported by a pellet of absorbent cotton), into a bottle containing the hypophosphorus acid. When all the liquid has passed through, rinse the flask with ½ an ounce of boiling distilled water and pass this through the filter. Cork the bottle and set it aside to cool. Finally add enough distilled water to make the product measure 16 fluid ounces.

Each fluid dram contains about 45 grains of iodide of iron (ferrous). On mixing 1 volume of this solution of iodide of iron with 5 volumes of simple syrup the product will contain about 60 grains of iodide of iron (ferrous) in each fluid ounce and will be practically identical measure for measure, but not weight for weight with the officinal syrup of iodide of iron.

2650. Solution of Iodide of Iron, Br.

(For syrup of iodide of iron.)

Iron wire, fine and bright.	1 ounce.
Iodine	2 ounces.
Water	2 ounces.

Cut the wire and add it to the water and iodine contained in the flask. Start chemical action by heating slightly, then set aside until action ceases and all the iodide has disappeared. Decant, add 1 dram of hypophosphorus acid, and filter, making up to 4 ounces with water which has been used to wash out the flask. One part of this solution to 7 parts of syrup makes syr. ferri iod.

MEDICINAL SYRUPS.

2651. Syrup of Acacia Gum.
Gum arabic .... 2½ ounces.
Granulated sugar .... 17½ ounces.
Oil wintergreen .... 5 minims.
Oil cloves .... 10 minims.
Water distilled .... 26 ounces.

Dissolve the gum arabic in 8 ounces of the water.

Dissolve the sugar in the remainder of the water by the aid of heat; whilst still hot add the oils, and shake well; then add the mucilage of acacia.

2652. Syrup of Allii.
Garlic, fresh peeled .... 3½ ounces.
Granulated sugar .... 16 ounces.
Acetic acid, diluted .... 20 ounces.

Bruise the garlic in a mortar and macerate in the acetic acid for seven days; press out and filter; in the filtrate dissolve the sugar. Keep the syrup in a cool place, and in well stoppered bottles.

2653. Syrup of Apomorphine Hydrochlorate.
Br. Form.
Apomorphine hydrochlorate 4 grains.
Alcohol .... 5½ fl. drams.
Water distilled .... 5½ fl. drams.
Hydrochloric acid .... 1½ fl. drams.
Simple syrup .... 14½ fl. ounces.

Mix the alcohol and water; add the apomorphine and dissolve by agitation; add the acid and the syrup.

2654. Syrup of Asafetida.
Asafetida gum .... 240 grains.
Alcohol .... 1 ounce.
Water .... 7 ounces.
Granulated sugar .... 13 ounces.

Rub the asafetida in a mortar with the alcohol; heat the water to 150 F. and add to the alcohol and asafetida; pour into a quart bottle and let stand for 3 days; filter and dissolve the sugar in the filtrate by aid of gentle heat.

2655. Syrup of Aurantii.
Orange peel recent ...... 3 ounces.
Alcohol, 188 per cent.... 6 ounces.
Carbonate of magnesia ... ¼ ounce.
Granulated sugar .... 28 ounces.
Water .... 2 pints.

Cut the orange peel into small pieces and macerate in the alcohol for 7 days; press out the tincture, and add to it the magnesia; rub to a smooth cream in a mortar, gradually adding a pint of the water; filter, and run the remainder of the water through the filter in this dissolve the sugar and strain.

2656. Syrup of Blackberry Arom. N. F.
Blackberry root, powdered 2¼ ounces.
Cinnamon, powdered ...... 120 grains.
Nutmeg, powdered .... 120 grains.
Cloves, powdered .... 60 grains.
Allspice, powdered ...... 60 grains.
Sugar granulated......... 11 ounces.
Alcohol diluted .... q. s.
Blackberry juice .... q. s.

Percolate the drugs with diluted alcohol until 4 fl. ounces are obtained. To this add 7 fluid ounces of blackberry juice and dissolve the sugar in the liquid by agitation. Lastly add enough blackberry juice to make sixteen fluid ounces.

2657. Syrup of Buckthorn Bark.
Fl. ext. of frangula..... 3 ounces.
Simple syrup .... 13 ounces.
Mix.

Syrup Blood and Liver.
Syrup blood and liver, see Formula 25.

2658. Syrup of Calcium Lactophosphate.
Phos. calcium, precipitated 1 ounce.
Lactic acid .... 9½ fl. drams.
Orange flower water...... 3 fl. ounces.
Sugar granulated .... 28 ounces.

Hydrochloric acid, water of ammonia, water, each a sufficient quantity to make 2 pints.

Mix the precipitated phosphate of calcium with 13 fl. ounces of cold water and add enough hydrochloric acid to dissolve it. Filter the solution and add to the filtrate 3 pints of cold water and water of ammonia, until after standing a few moments the odor of ammonia may be distinguished. Transfer the mixture at once to a fine wetted muslin strainer.

As soon as the liquid has run off return the magma to the vessel, pour on more water, agitate, and repeat until the precipitate is thoroughly washed and again transfer to the strainer. When it is drained, mix the magma at once with the lactic acid and stir until dissolved. Then add the orange flower water and enough water to make the solution weigh about three hundred and fifty parts (or measure 15 fl. ounces), filter and pass enough water through filter to measure in all seventeen fluid ounces. Lastly, add to this the sugar, dissolve it by agitation, without heat; strain.

2659. Syrup of Calcium Phosphate. A
(Wiegand's.)

Calcium phos., precipitated	1¼ ounces.
Hydrochloric acid	4½ drams.
Sugar	14½ ounces.
Water	8 ounces.

Dissolve the calcium phosphate in the acid previously mixed with 12 fluid ounces of water, filter, add the sugar and the remainder of the water, dissolve by agitation and strain.

2660. Syrup of Calcium Phosphate. B

Calcium phos., precipitated	256 grains.
Phosphoric acid, glacial	240 grains.
Sugar	15 ounces av.
Distilled water	8 fl. ounces.
Spirit of lemon	24 drops.

Mix the calcium phosphate with the water, heat moderately, gradually add the acid until all the calcium salt is dissolved, replace the water lost by evaporation, filter, dissolve the sugar in the filtrate, strain, if necessary, and add the spirit.

2661. Syrup of Cascara.

Cascara cordial, Formula No. 57	8 ounces.
Simple syrup	8 ounces.

Mix.

2662. Syrup of Castanea.
(For whooping cough.)

Fl. ext. of chestnut leaves.	1 ounce.
Tincture of belladonna	2 drams.
Tincture of hyoscyamus	2 drams.
Syrup of wild cherry to make	16 ounces.

Dose: One teaspoonful.

2663. Syrup of Chloral Hydrate Br.

Chloral hydrate	320 grains.
Distilled water	6 fl. drams.
Simple syrup, q. s. to	4 fl. ounces.

Dissolve the chloral in the water and add the syrup.

Syrup of Figs.

Syrup of figs, see Formula 726.

Syrup of Ginger Ale.

Syrup of ginger ale, see Formula 2615.

2664. Syrup of Glycyrrhizin.

Ammoniated glycyrrhizin	½ ounce.
Glycerine	2 ounces.
Hot water	2 ounces.
Simple syrup	12 ounces.

Dissolve the glycyrrhizin by rubbing in a mortar with the hot water; add the glycerine and syrup.

2665. Syrup of Hypophosphites. (U. S. P.)
(Churchill's.)

Calcium hypophosphite	345 grains.
Sodium hypophosphite	115 grains.
Potassium hypophosphite	115 grains.
Dil. hypophosphorous acid	15 minims.
Granulated sugar	8¾ ounces.
Spirit of lemon	1¼ drams.
Water enough to make	16 fl. ounces.

Triturate the hypophosphites with 7 fluid ounces of water until dissolved; add the spirit and acid and filter. In the filtrate dissolve the sugar by agitation or percolation and add enough water through the filter to make 16 fluid ounces. Strain, if necessary.

Syrup of Hypophosphites Compound.

Syrup of hypophosphites, compound, see also Formula 1261.

2666. Syrup of Hypophosphites, Co.(N. F.)

Calcium hypophosphite	256 grains.
Potassium hypophosphite	128 grains.
Sodium hypophosphite	128 grains.
Iron hypophosphite	16 grains.
Manganese hypophosphite	16 grains.
Potassium citrate	40 grains.
Citric acid	15 grains.
Quinine hydrochlorate	8 grains.
Tincture of nux vomica	160 minims.
Sugar	13 ounces.
Water	q. s.

Rub the hypophosphites of iron and manganese with the potassium citrate and citric acid to powder, add 1 fluid ounce of water, and warm the mixture a few minutes until a clear greenish solution is obtained. Introduce the other hypophosphites and the quinine hydrochlorate, previously triturated together, into a bottle, next add the sugar, the iron and manganese solution first prepared, the tincture of nux vomica, and, lastly, enough water to make up the volume, as soon as the sugar is saturated by the liquid, to 16 fluid ounces. Agitate until solution has been effected, and strain, if necessary.

2667. Parrish's Syrup of Hypophosphites.

Calcium hypophosphite	288 grains.
Sodium hypophosphite	96 grains.
Potassium hypophosphite	96 grains.
Sugar	12½ ounces.
Distilled water, hot	9 fl. ounces.
Orange flower water	4 fl. drams.

Make a solution of the hypophosphites in the hot water, filter, dissolve the sugar in the filtrate, strain, and to the whole add the orange flower water.

2668. Compound Syrup of Hypophosphites with Iron, Nonprecipitating.

Calcium hypophosphite	256 grains.
Sodium hypophosphite	128 grains.
Potassium hypophosphite	128 grains.
Manganese hypophosphite	16 grains.
Tinct. citro-chloride of Iron, N. F.	1 ounce.
Tinct. nux vomica	160 minims.
Quinine hydrochlorate	8 grains.
Sugar	12 ounces.
Water, enough to make	16 ounces.

The hypophosphites are dissolved in 6 ounces of water previously boiled, which is easily done by triturating the salts in successive portions of the water, the addition of an acid not being required. The quinine is dissolved in ½ ounce of warm water. These solutions are mixed and poured over the sugar. Shake well and add the tinctures of iron and nux vomica, then add enough water to make 16 fluid ounces. Shake until the sugar is dissolved, let stand for 24 hours and filter.

The substitution of the chloride for the hypophosphite of iron cannot well be urged against this preparation, since the amount of the original formula is comparatively insignificant and one of the causes of precipitation.

2669. Syrup of Hypophosphites of Calcium. (N. F.)

Calcium hypophosphite	256 grains.
Citric acid	10 grains.
Sugar	13½ ounces.
Water, enough to make	16 fl. ounces.

Dissolve the calcium hypophosphite and citric acid in 8 fluid ounces of water, filter the solution, add the sugar to the filtrate, and pass enough water through the filter to make the product, after the sugar has been dissolved by agitation, measure 16 fluid ounces. Each fluid dram contains 2 grains of calcium hypophosphite.

2670. Syrup of Hypophosphites of Calcium, Manganese and Potassium. (N. F.)

Calcium hypophosphite	256 grains.
Manganese hypophosphite	128 grains.
Potassium hypophosphite	128 grains.
Distilled water, boiling	3¼ fl. ounces.
Simple syrup enough to make	16 fl. ounces.

Triturate the hypophosphites with the water, filter, and add the syrup.

2671. Syrup of Hypophosphites of Calcium and Sodium. (N. F.)

Calcium hypophosphite	256 grains.
Sodium hypophosphite	256 grains.
Citric acid	10 grains.
Sugar	13½ ounces.
Water, enough to make	16 fl. ounces.

Dissolve the two hypophosphites and citric acid in 8 fluid ounces of water, filter the solution, add the sugar to the filtrate and pass enough water through the filter to make the product, after the sugar has been dissolved by agitation, measure 16 fluid ounces. Each fluid dram contains 2 grains each of calcium and sodium hypophosphites.

2672. Syrup of Hypophosphites, with Iron (U. S. P.)

Ferrous lactate in crusts	72 grains.
Potassium citrate	72 grains.
Syrup of hypophosphites, enough to make	16 fl. ounces.

Triturate the two salts with a small quantity of syrup gradually added, until they are dissolved, then add the remainder of the syrup.

This preparation should be freshly made when wanted.

2673. Syrup of Hypophosphite of Iron (N. F.)

Iron hypophosphite	128 grains.
Potassium citrate	160 grains.
Orange flower water	1 fl. ounce.
Simple syrup q. s. to make	16 fl. ounces.

Dissolve the iron hypophosphite with the aid of the potassium citrate in the orange flower water, and add the syrup.

Each fluid dram contains 1 grain of hypophosphite of iron (ferric).

2674. Syrup of Hypophosphites, Manganese (N. F.)

Manganese sulphate	120 grains.
Calcium hypophosphite	80 grains.
Sugar	13 ounces.
Orange flower water	2 fl. drams.
Water	q. s.

Dissolve the hypophosphite and sulphate in separate portions of water, mix the two solutions, filter, washing the precipitate in the filter with fresh distilled water; evaporate the filtrate to 8 fluid ounces, dissolve the sugar in the filtrate, strain, and add the orange flower water.

Each fluid ounce contains 2 1-3 grains of manganese hypophosphite.

2675. Syrup of Hypophosphite of Sodium. (N. F.)

Sodium hypophosphite....	256 grains.
Citric acid	10 grains.
Sugar	13 ounces.
Water, enough to make...	16 fl. ounces.

Dissolve the sodium hypophosphite and the citric acid in 8 fluid ounces of water, and filter the solution. In this dissolve the sugar by agitation, and pass the remainder of the water through the filter. Each fluid dram contains 2 grains of sodium hypophosphite.

2676. Syrup of Iron and Sodium Albuminate.

Whites of eggs...........	4 only.
Sugar	2 ounces.
Tincture chloride of iron..	2 fl. ounces.
Solution of soda	q. s.
Water	q. s.

Mix the whites of eggs with the sugar and add enough water to effect complete solution; add the tincture of iron, and then enough of the solution of soda to dissolve the coagulated albumen; finally make up to 16 fluid ounces with water.

Syrup of Iodide of Iron.

Syrup of Iodide of iron, see Formulas, 2637, 2638, 2639, 2640, 2641.

2677. Syrup of Iron Ferric Chloride. A (Codex.)

Solution of iron chloride...	2 fl. drams.
Simple syrup, q. s. to make up to	16 fl. ounces.

2678. Syrup of Iron Ferric Chloride. B (Codex.)

Tincture of chloride of iron	1 fl. ounce.
Sodium citrate	2 ounces.
Water	6 fl. ounces.
Sugar	10 ounces.
Syrup enough to make.....	16 fl. ounces.

Mix the tincture of ferric chloride with the water and dissolve in this mixture the sodium citrate and the sugar with the aid of heat; when cold add sufficient syrup to make 16 fl. ounces.

2679. Syrup of Iron and Ammonium Phosphate.

Iron sulphate	635 grains.
Sodium phosphate	820 grains.
Glacial phosphoric acid, C. P.	900 grains.
Ammonia water	q. s.
Sugar	13½ ounces.
Distilled water	q. s.

Dissolve the sodium phosphate and the iron sulphate separately in distilled water, mix the solutions; wash the resulting precipitated iron phosphate. Then to one-half of the phosphoric acid, dissolved in 2¼ fluid ounces of water, add ammonia water until exactly neutral. To the remainder of the phosphoric acid, dissolved in a like quantity of water, add the moist iron phosphate and dissolve by the aid of gentle heat; then add the solution of ammonium phosphate and the sugar, dissolve the whole, strain and evaporate to 16 fluid ounces. Each fluid dram contains 4½ grains iron phosphate, 4¾ grains ammonium phosphate, and 3½ grains of phosphoric acid.

2680. Syrup of Iron and Ammonium Tartrate (Codex.)

Tartrate of iron and ammonium	225 grains
Distilled water, hot.......	4 fl. drams.
Simple syrup, q. s. to make up to	16 fl. ounces.

Dissolve the iron salt in the water and add the syrup.

2681. Syrup of Iron and Potassium Tartrate (Codex.)

Tartrate of iron and potassium	225 grains.
Distilled water, hot	4 fl. drams.
Simple syrup, enough to make	16 fl. ounces.

Dissolve the iron salt in the water and add the syrup.

2682. Syrup of Iron and Quinine Iodides (Bouchardat.) A

Iodine	42 grains.
Iron in powder............	17 grains.
Simple syrup	15½ fl. ounces.
Quinine sulphate	8 grains.
Diluted sulphuric acid.....	q. s.
Distilled water	4½ fl. drams.

Digest the iodine, iron and 3 fluid drams of the water until the red-brown color of the iodine has disappeared; filter into the syrup. Then dissolve the sulphate of quinine in 2 fluid drams of water with the aid of diluted sulphuric acid and mix this solution with the prepared syrup.

2683. Syrup of Iron Citrate (Codex.)
Iron citrate soluble........ 240 grains.
Distilled water, hot...... 4 fl. drams.
Simple syrup, q. s. to make
up to .... 16 fl. ounces.

2684. Syrup of Iron and Quinine Iodides. B
Quinine sulphate .... 20 grains.
Hypophosphorus acid dil.. q. s.
Potassium iodide .... 8 grains.
Simple syrup enough to
make .... 8 fl. ounces.
Syrup of iron iodide (U. S.) 8 fl. ounces.

To the quinine sulphate add about 10 drops of commercial solution of hypophosphorus acid and then a small amount of syrup; when the quinine salt is dissolved, add the remainder of the syrup and afterwards the potassium iodide dissolved in a few drops of water; mix well. Now add the syrup of iron iodide and mix. Should any cloudiness appear, clear it up by a few drops of the hypophosphorus acid.

A fluid dram of this syrup contains about 4 grains of dry iodide of iron and about 6 grains of hydriodide of quinine.

2685. Syrup of Iron Pyrophosphate (Codex).
Iron pyrophosphate soluble 90 grains.
Distilled water .... 4 fl. drams.
Simple syrup, enough to
make .... 16 fl. ounces.

Syrup of Lemons.
Syrup of lemons, see Formulas, 2605, 2606.

2686. Syrup Lobelia (Eclectic).
Vinegar of lobelia .... 8 fl. ounces.
Sugar .... 16 ounces.
Dissolve by aid of heat; strain while hot.

2687. Syrup of Lobelia, Thompsonian.
Lobelia seed .... 1 ounce.
Water .... 16 fl. ounces.
Acetic acid dilute .... 1 fl. ounce.
Sugar .... 13 ounces.
Tincture of lobelia ...... 4 fl. ounces.

Boil the lobelia with the water and vinegar for one-half hour, occasionally replacing the water lost by evaporation, then strain, add the sugar, dissolve and when cool add to the tincture of lobelia.

2688. Syrup of Manganese Iodide.
Manganese sulphate ...... 480 grains.
Potassium iodide .... 570 grains.
Sugar .... 6 ounces.
Distilled water .... q. s.

Dissolve the two salts each in 2 fluid ounces of water; mix them; dissolve and filter; add the sugar and enough water to make up to 8 ounces; strain.

2689. Syrup of Manganese Phosphate.
Manganese sulphate....... 920 grains.
Sodium phosphate .... 3½ ounces.
Hydrochloric acid .... 5 fl. drams.
Sugar .... 13¾ ounces.
Water, enough to make. ... 16 fl. ounces.

Dissolve the salts separately in 5 fluid ounces of water each, and add the solution of sodium phosphate to the solution of manganese sulphate as long as it produces a precipitate, which wash with cold water, and then dissolve the magma by adding the hydrochloric acid; dilute with water until it measures 9 fluid ounces, and in this dissolve the sugar; strain.

Each fluid dram contains 5 grains of manganese phosphate.

Syrup of Mead.
Syrup of mead, see Formula, 2626.

2690. Syrup of Mercury Iodide (Gibert).
Red iodide of mercury.... 3 grains.
Potassium iodide .... 120 grains.
Water .... 3 fl. drams.
Simple syrup, enough to
make ... . 10 fl. ounces.

Dissolve the mercuric and potassium iodides in the water and add the syrup.

2691. Syrup of Mitchella Compound. (Eclectic.)
(Mother's Cordial.)
Squaw vine .... 960 grains.
Helonias root .... 240 grains.
Cramp bark .... 240 grains.
Blue cohosh .... 240 grains.
Oil of sassafras .... 4 drops.
Sugar .... 3½ ounces.
Alcohol dilute .... q. s.

Mix the oil with the drugs and percolate with diluted alcohol until 14 ounces are obtained. In this dissolve the sugar and strain.

The above is known as uterine tonic. Compound syrup of partridge berry and mother's cordial.

2692. Syrup Opiated (Codex).
Extract of opium .... 19½ grains.
Water, hot .... ½ ounce.
Simple syrup, enough to
  make .... 16 fl. ounces.

Dissolve the extract in the hot water and add the syrup.

2693. Syrup of Opium and Ipecac (N. F).
(Syrup of Dover's Powder.)
Fluid ext. ipecac. ...... 64 minims.
Tincture of opium ..... 670 minims.
Sugar .... 12 troy ounces.
Cinnamon water q. s. to
  make .... 16 fl. ounces.

Mix the fluid extract and tincture with 6 fluid ounces of cinnamon water and filter the liquid. To this add the sugar and enough cinnamon water to make the product, after the sugar has been dissolved by agitation, measure 16 fluid ounces.

Each fluid dram represents 5 grains of Dover's Powder or ½ grain each of ipecac and opium.

In place of the above directed quantities of fluid extract of ipecac and tincture of opium, 640 minims of the officinal tincture of ipecac and opium may be taken.

2694. Syrup of Phosphates Compound.
(Chemical Food.)
Calcium phosphate ...... 256 grains.
Iron phosphate .... 128 grains.
Sodium phosphate .... 128 grains.
Potassium phosphate ..... 64 grains.
Solution of acid phosphate 1 ounce.
Orange flower water...... 1 ounce.
Simple syrup, q. s. to make 1 pint.

Dissolve the salts in the solution of acid phosphate and orange flower water; add the syrup.

Syrup of Quinine, Tasteless.
See Formulas Nos. 2644, 2645.

2695. Syrup of Rhubarb and Potassium.
(Neutralizing Cordial.)
Rhubarb .... 240 grains.
Hydrastis .... 120 grains.
Cinnamon .... 120 grains.
Potassium carbonate ..... 240 grains.
Oil of peppermint........ 5 drops.
Sugar .... 14 ounces.
Alcohol .... 8 ounces.
Water .... 16 ounces.

Dissolve the potassium carbonate in a portion of the water and mix in a suitable sized container with the rhubarb, hydrastis and cinnamon, the last three being in fine powder. Now add the alcohol and the remainder of the water and allow to stand for 48 hours, agitating the whole briskly at frequent intervals. Decant the clear portion, and filter the remainder through absorbent cotton, adding sufficient water through the filter to make the whole measure 24 fluid ounces. In this dissolve the sugar by agitation, and add the oil of peppermint.

2696. Syrup of Tolu, U. S. P.
Tincture of tolu.............. 2 fl. ounces.
Magnesium carbonate .... 120 grains.
Sugar .... 28½ ounces.
Water..................... 16 fl. ounces.

Triturate the tincture with the magnesium carbonate and 2 ounces of sugar to a smooth paste, gradually add the remainder of the sugar, stirring constantly meanwhile, filter, and in the filtrate dissolve the remainder of the sugar by agitation or percolation.

2697. Syrup of Rhubarb Aromatic.
(Spiced Syrup of Rhubarb.)
Rhubarb, powdered ...... 600 grains.
Cloves, powdered .... 60 grains.
Cinnamon, powdered .... 60 grains.
Nutmeg, powdered .... 60 grains.
Syrup .... 3 pints.
Diluted alcohol .... q. s.

Mix the powders, and having moistened the mixture with diluted alcohol place in a conical percolator and pour diluted alcohol upon it, until 8 fluid ounces are obtained; add this to the syrup previously heated and mix.

The aromatic tincture of the U. S. P. of 1870 is identical with that used in making this syrup.

The U. S. P. Formula for 1880 is:
Aromatic tinct. of rhubarb 2 fl. ounces.
Syrup .... 14 fl. ounces.

Mix the aromatic tincture of rhubarb with the syrup.

The substitution of glycerin for one-half of the syrup would certainly be an improvement.

2698. Syrup of Saccharin.
Saccharin .... 150 grains.
Sodium carbonate, pure... 165 grains.
    or
Sodium bicarbonate, pure.. 180 grains.
Distilled water .... 32 fl. ounces.

Dissolve by the aid of a gentle heat.
May be employed as a substitute for simple syrup.

Syrup of Saffron.
See Formulas 2641, and 2642.

Syrup of Sarsaparilla.
See Formulas 1, 2, 3, 8.

2699. ### Syrup of Senna with Manna.
(Syrupus Mannatus.—Compound Syrup of Manna.)

Syrup of senna, U. S. P.... 4 fl. ounces.
Syrup of manna, N. F..... 4 fl. ounces.

Syrup Simple.
See Formula 2639.

Syrup of Squills.
See Formula 2640.

2700. ### Syrup of Squills Compound.
(Hive Syrup, U. S. P.)

Squills, powdered .... 2½ ounces.
Senega, powdered .... 2½ ounces.
Tartrate of antimony and
  potassium .... 28 grains.
Sugar .... 26 ounces.
Precipitated phosphate of
  calcium .... 90 grains.
Diluted alcohol ....
Water....aa q. s. to make 2 pints.

Mix the squill and senega and moisten with diluted alcohol; macerate for 24 hours; pack in conical percolator and gradually pour upon it diluted alcohol until 1½ pints of tincture are obtained. Boil and evaporate by means of a water-bath to half a pint; triturate the mixture with the precipitated phosphate of calcium; filter, and add through the filter enough warm water to make the whole measure one pint. In this dissolve the sugar. Dissolve the tartar emetic in one ounce of water and mix thoroughly with the syrup.

Syrup of Tar.
See Formula 2643.

Syrup of Tolu.
See Formula 2633.

Syrup of Trifolium.
See Formula 7.

Syrup of Vanilla.
See Formula 2604.

2701. ### Syrup of Violets.

Ionone solution (1 to 10)... 2 drams.
Cologne spirits, 188 per
  cent.................... 6 drams.
Simple syrup q. s. to make. 1 pint.
Color with chlorophyll.

Syrup of White Pine Expectorant.
See Formulas No. 583, 584.

2702. ### Syrup Wild Cherry (U. S).
1880.

Wild cherry, powdered.... 5½ ounces.
Sugar granulated .... 28 ounces.
Glycerine .... 2 fl. ounces
Water q. s. to make up to.. 2 pints.

Moisten the wild cherry thoroughly with water and macerate for 24 hours. Pack firmly in a cylindrical glass percolator and gradually pour water upon it until 15 ounces of percolate are obtained. Dissolve the sugar in the liquid by agitation without heat, add the glycerine and strain.

A syrup may be readily made if desired by adding to 2 ounces fluid ext. wild cherry soluble, 12 ounces simple syrup (2639) and 2 ounces of glycerin.

2703. ### Syrup of Yerba Santa, Aromatic (N. F.)
(Aromatic Syrup of Eriodictyon.)

Fl. ext. of yerba santa..... 4 fl. drams.
Solution of potassa .... 3 fl. drams.
Comp. tinct. of cardamom. 1 fl. ounce
Oil of sassafras .... 4 drops.
Oil of lemon .... 4 drops.
Oil of cloves .... 8 drops.
Alcohol .... 4 fl. drams.
Sugar .... 14 ounces av.
Water, enough to make... 16 fl. ounces.

Mix the fluid extract and solution of potassa, then add 12 fluid drams of water previously mixed with the compound tincture of cardamom, and afterwards add the oils dissolved in the alcohol. Shake the mixture thoroughly, then filter it, and pour enough water through the filter to obtain 6 fluid ounces of filtrate. Pour this upon the sugar contained in a bottle, and dissolve it by placing the bottle in hot water, frequently agitating. Lastly, cool the product and add enough water, passed through the filter previously used, to make 16 fluid ounces.

TINCTURES.

2704. Tincture of Aconite Root.
Aconite root, powdered.... 5½ ounces.
Tartaric acid .... 24 grains.
Alcohol, 188 per cent, q. s.
   to make .... 1 pint.

Moisten the aconite root with 4 ounces of the alcohol in which the tartaric acid has been previously dissolved and macerate for 24 hours. Then percolate with alcohol until one pint is obtained.

2705. Tincture Aloes.
U. S. 1880.
Purified aloes, powdered... 3¼ ounces.
Ext. of glycyrrhiza, powd.. 3¼ ounces.
Dil. alcohol q. s. to make.. 2 pints.

Mix the powders with one pint and a half of diluted alcohol and macerate for seven days in a well closed vessel; then filter through paper, adding through the filter enough diluted alcohol to make the tincture measure 2 pints.

2706. Tincture of Aloes and Myrrh. (Elixir Proprietatis). U. S 1880.
Purified aloes, powdered.... 3 ounces.
Myrrh, powdered.......... 3 ounces.
Alcohol, q. s. to make..... 2 pints.

Mix the powdered drugs; moisten with alcohol, q. s., and macerate for a week in a well closed vessel; then filter through paper adding through filter alcohol sufficient to make tincture measure two pints.

2707. Tincture of Arnica Flowers.
Arnica flowers............ 3⅛ ounces.
Alcohol, diluted, q. s. to
   make .... 1 pint.

Rub the arnica flowers through a coarse sieve. Then moisten with a portion of the dilute alcohol, and macerate in a closely covered vessel for two days; place in a percolator; pack firmly and run diluted alcohol through until 1 pint is obtained.

2708. Tincture of Arnica Root.
Arnica root, powdered..... 3⅛ ounces.
Alcohol diluted, q. s. to
   make .... 1 pint.

Moisten the arnica root with a portion of the dilute alcohol and macerate in a closely covered vessel for two days; place in a percolator; pack firmly and run diluted alcohol through until 1 pint is obtained.

2709. Tincture of Asafetida Compound. Am. Dis.
Asafetida .... 200 grains.
Lupulin .... 200 grains.
Stramonium seed .... 200 grains.
Valerian root .... 200 grains.
Alcohol .... 20 fl. ounces.

Mix the drugs, reduce to coarse powder, add the alcohol, macerate for 14 days, strain, express and filter.

2710. Tincture of Avena Sativa Homeopathic (Tincture of Oats).
Oats, unhusked .... 8 ounces.
Potassium carbonate ..... q. s.
Water .... q. s.
Alcohol.................. q. s.

Grind the oats to moderately fine powder, moisten with a five per cent aqueous solution of potassium carbonate, first warmed to 113° F., macerate for three hours, pack in a percolator and add alcohol until 16 fluid ounces of product are obtained.

2711. Tincture of Aurantii Amara.
(Tincture of Bitter Orange Peel.)
Bitter orange peel, powd. 3⅛ ounces.
Alcohol dil. q. s. to make.. 1 pint.

Moisten the orange peel with a portion of the diluted alcohol and macerate for two days. Then percolate with diluted alcohol until 1 pint is obtained.

2712. Tincture of Aurantii Dulcis.
(Tincture of Sweet Orange Peel.)
Sweet orange peel, recent,
   and deprived of the inner
   white layer .... 3⅛ ounces.
Alcohol, 188 per cent q. s
   to make .... 1 pint.

Cut the orange peel into small pieces; macerate with 8 ounces of the alcohol for 7 days in a tightly closed vessel; remove to a percolator and pack firmly; run alcohol through until one pint is obtained.

2713. Tincture of Belladonna.
Belladonna leaves, powdered, 4¾ ounces; diluted alcohol q. s. to make 2 pints. Moisten the powder with six ounces diluted alcohol and macerate for 24 hours; then pack firmly in cylindrical percolator, and pour sufficient diluted alcohol upon it until two pints of tincture are obtained.

2714. Tincture of Benzoin.
U. S. 1880.

Benzoin, powdered, 6 ounces; alcohol q. s. to make 2 pints. Mix the powder with sufficient alcohol and macerate for seven days in a closed vessel; then filter through paper, adding enough alcohol to make the tincture measure 2 pints.

2715. Tincture of Benzoin Compound.
(Turlington's Balsam.)

Benzoin, powdered	3½ ounces.
Purified aloes, powdered	260 grains.
Storax	2½ ounces.
Balsam of tolu	1¼ ounces.
Alcohol q. s. to make	2 pints.

Mix the powders and gums in one and a half pints of alcohol and macerate for a week or ten days, in a closed vessel; then filter through paper, adding enough alcohol through the filter to measure, in all, 2 pints.

2716. Tincture of Black Cohosh Compound.
Am. Dis.
(Co. Tincture of Cimcifuga.)

Tincture of black cohosh	8¼ fl. ounces.
Tincture of blood root, U. S. P.	6 fl. ounces.
Tincture of poke root	1¾ fl. ounces.

Mix.

2717. Tincture of Blood Root Compound
(Eclectic).

Blood root	1 ounce.
Lobelia herb	1 ounce.
Skunk cabbage	1 ounce.
Diluted alcohol	sufficient.

Extract the drug by percolation with alcohol, so as to obtain 16 fluid ounces of tincture.

2718. Tincture of Blue Cohosh. (Am. Dis.)

Blue cohosh, fine powder	3¼ ounces.
Alcohol	q. s.

Extract the drug by percolation with alcohol, so as to obtain 16 fluid ounces of tincture.

2719. Tincture of Blue Cohosh Co. (Am. Dis.)

Blue cohosh, fine powder	640 grains.
Ergot, fine powder	320 grains.
Water pepper, fine powder	320 grains.
Oil of savin	2½ fl. drams.
Alcohol	q. s.

Extract the mixed drugs by percolation with alcohol, so that the percolate, with the oil added, will make 16 fluid ounces.

2720. Tincture of Blue Flag.

Blue flag, fine powder	3¼ ounces.
Alcohol	q. s.

Extract the mixed drugs in fine powder by percolation, with diluted alcohol, so as to obtain 16 fluid ounces of tincture.

2721. Tincture of Buchu.

Buchu, coarse powder	2 ounces.
Diluted alcohol	sufficient.

Extract the drug by percolation, so as to obtain 16 fluid ounces of product.

2722. Tincture of Burdock Seed.

Burdock seed, ground	4½ ounces.
Water; alcohol; of each	sufficient.

Mix the liquids in the proportion of 1 by measure of the water to 3 of the alcohol, and percolate the drug in the usual way, until 16 fluid ounces of percolate are obtained.

2723. Tincture of Bryonia.

Bryonia, recent, No. 40, powder	2¾ ounces.
Alcohol q. s. to make	2 pints.

Moisten the powder with 3 ounces of alcohol and macerate for 24 hours; put in percolator and gradually pour on sufficient alcohol, until two pints of tincture are obtained.

2724. Tincture of Cacao.
(Tincture of Theobroma.)

Cacao beans, freshly roasted	16 ounces.
Cinnamon	2 ounces.
Tincture of vanilla, U. S. P.	2½ fl. ounces.
Diluted alcohol, enough to make	16 fl. ounces.

Reduce the cacao beans and the cinnamon to moderately fine powder; add 16 fluid ounces of diluted alcohol; macerate for 7 days, agitating occasionally; transfer to a percolator and percolate, adding sufficient of the diluted alcohol to make the percolate measure one pint.

2725. Tincture of Cactus Grandiflorus.
(Eclectic.)

Fresh flowers and stems of cactus grandiflorus	4½ ounces.
Alcohol	16 fl. ounces.

Macerate for 14 days, occasionally agitating; express and filter.

2726. Tincture of Calamus.
(Ger. Phar.)
Calamus, coarse powder... 3 ounces.
Water .... 4½ fl. ounces.
Alcohol .... 13 fl. ounces.

Mix, macerate for 7 days, agitating occasionally, strain with expression and filter.

2727. Tincture of Calendula.
Calendula, rough ground, 6 ounces; alcohol, diluted q. s. to make 2 pints. Macerate the calendula with a portion of the diluted alcohol for 2 days; then place in a percolator and run through enough menstruum to obtain 2 pints.

2728. Tincture of Calumba.
Calumba, rough ground, 3 ounces; alcohol and water q. s. to make 2 pints. Mix alcohol and water in the proportion of 1½ pints of alcohol to 12 fluid ounces of water, and moisten the powder with a portion. Macerate for 24 hours, then pack in a percolator and pour the menstruum upon it, until 2 fluid pints are obtained.

2729. Tincture of Cannabis Indica.
(Indian Hemp.)
Indian Cannabis powder, 5½ ounces; alcohol q. s. to make 2 pints. Moisten the powder with 6 ounces of alcohol, and macerate for 24 hours; then pack in a cylindrical percolator and gradually pour alcohol upon it until two pints of tincture are obtained.

2730. Tincture of Capsicum.
Capsicum, powdered...... 1¼ ounces troy.
Alcohol .... 2 pints.

Mix alcohol and water in the proportion of 19 parts of alcohol to 1 part of water; and having moistened the powder with half a fluid ounce of the mixture pack it firmly in a percolator. Then run menstruum through until 2 pints are obtained.

2731. Tincture of Cardamom Co.
Cardamom, powdered..... 280 grains.
Cinnamon, powdered...... 280 grains.
Caraway, powdered....... 140 grains.
Cochineal, powdered...... 70 grains.
Glycerine .... 1½ fl. ounces.
Diluted alcohol q. s. to
  make .... 2 pints.

Mix the drugs; moisten with 2 ounces of diluted alcohol; pack them firmly in a cylindrical percolator and gradually pour the menstruum upon them until 30½ fluid ounces, of the tincture are obtained. Then add the glycerine and mix them thoroughly. This is a pleasant aromatic tincture, a favorite addition to bitters or other stomachics. Used occasionally as a carminative. Dose, a teaspoonful.

2732. Tincture of Carduus Mariana.
(Tincture of Mary Thistle.)
Carduus Mariae fruit whole 10 ounces.
Alcohol, 188 per cent....?.. 12 fluid ounces.
Distilled water........... 10 fluid ounces.
Macerate for 8 days, then filter.

2733. Tincture Carminative.
(Brit. Form.)
Cardamom seeds, bruised.. 480 grains.
Tincture of ginger........ 2½ fl. ounces.
Oil of cinnamon........... 80 minims.
Oil of cloves............. 80 minims.
Oil of caraway............ 80 minims.
Alcohol, enough to make... 16 fl. ounces.

Macerate the cardamoms with 12 fluid ounces of alcohol for 7 days; decant the liquid; express the residue, filter; add the oils to the filtrate, and finally add the remainder of the alcohol.

2734. Tincture of Cascara Sagrada. (Codex.)
Cascara sagrada, in coarse
  powder .... 3 ounces.
Water .... 5¾ fl. ounces.
Alcohol .... 11¼ fl. ounces.

Mix, macerate for 10 days, agitating occasionally, express, and filter.

2735. Tincture of Castor.
(Am. Dis.)
Castor (Russian preferred). 1¼ ounces.
Alcohol .... q. s.

Reduce the castor to as fine a condition as possible. Macerate with the alcohol for 14 days, occasionally agitating; express, and filter, adding enough alcohol through the filter to make the liquid measure 16 fluid ounces.

2736. Tincture of Castor—Ammoniated.
Castor .... 480 grains.
Asafetida .... 240 grains.
Spirit of ammonia .... 16 fl. ounces.

Reduce the drugs to coarse powder, add the spirit, macerate for 7 days, agitating occasionally, and express.

2737. Tincture of Catechu Co.
Catechu, No. 40 powder.... 4 ounces.
Cinnamon, No. 40 powder.. 2½ ounces.
Diluted alcohol q. s. to
  make .... 2 pints.

Mix the powders and having moistened the mixture with 4 fluid ounces of diluted alcohol, macerate for 24 hours; then pack firmly in percolator and gradually pour diluted alcohol upon it until 2 pints of tincture are obtained. This is a grateful astringent tincture. The dose is ½ to 2 teaspoonfuls. It may be advantageously added to diarrhoea mixtures astringent washes; and similar preparations.

2738. Tincture of Celandine.
(Rademacher's.)
Fresh herb of chelidonium. 10 ounces.
Alcohol, 188 per cent....... 12 fluid ounces.

Contuse the herb to a pulp, add the alcohol; macerate for 8 days, express, and filter.

2739. Tincture of Chloroform Co.
(Brit. Phar.)
Chloroform .... 1 fluid ounce.
Alcohol .... 4 fluid ounces.
Com. tincture of cardamon. 5 fluid ounces.
Mix.

2740. Tincture of Cimicifuga.
(Black Cohosh.)
Cimicifuga No. 60, powder.. 5½ ounces.
Alcohol, q. s. to make.... 2 pints.

Macerate the cimicifuga for 48 hours; then transfer to a percolator, and pour alcohol upon it until 2 pints of tincture are obtained. Dose a fluid dram to one half a fluid ounce.

2741. Tincture of Cinnamon Co.
(Eclectic.)
Cinnamon .... 240 grains.
Cardamon .... 90 grains.
Prickly ash berries........ 90 grains.
Ginger .... 90 grains.
Diluted alcohol .... sufficient.

Extract the mixed drugs in fine powder by percolation so as to obtain 16 ounces of tincture.

2742. Tincture of Cochineal.
(Brit. Pharm.)
Cochineal powdered........ 2 ounces.
Diluted alcohol, enough to
  make .... 16 fluid ounces.

Extract the drug by percolation or maceration.

The product may be used for coloring elixirs and other preparations.

2743. Tincture of Cochineal.
(Rademacher's.)
Cochineal in coarse powder. 1 ounce.
Alcohol .... 11 fl. ounces.

Macerate for 3 days, agitating occasionally, and filter.

2744. Tincture of Colchicum Co.
(Eclectic.)
Tinct. of colchicum seed. 8 fluid ounces.
Tincture of black cohosh. 8 fluid ounces.
Mix.

2745. Tincture of Colchicum.
Colchicum seed, 30 powder. 4⅝ ounces.
Alcohol, dilute q. s. to make 2 pints.

Moisten the colchicum with 5 ounces of alcohol; dilute; macerate for 3 days; percolate with diluted alcohol until 2 pints are obtained.

2746. Tincture of Colocynth.
(Ger. Phar.)
Colocynth, with seeds, cut
  coarse .... 1½ ounces.
Alcohol .... q. s.

Percolate alcohol through the drug so as to obtain 16 fluid ounces of tincture.

2747. Tincture of Colocynth Seed.
(Rademacher's.)
Colocynth seed............ 3 ounces.
Alcohol, 188 per cent...... q. s.

Wash the seeds with water, dry and reduce to coarse powder, add 16½ fluid ounces of alcohol. Macerate for 14 days, agitating; express, filter, and add enough of the alcohol to the filtrate to make 16 fluid ounces.

2748. Tincture of Conium.
(U. S. P., 1880.)
Conium seed, powder...... 2¼ ounces.
Diluted hydrochloric acid.. ½ fluid dram.
Diluted alcohol .... sufficient.

Extract the drug by percolation so as to obtain 16 fluid ounces of product, adding the acid to that portion of the diluted alcohol which is used for moistening the drug.

2749. Tincture of Convallaria.
(Brit. Form.)
(Tincture of Lily of the Valley.)
Lily of the valley flowers
  and stalks, dried, coarse
  powder .... 2 ounces.
Diluted alcohol .... sufficient.

Extract the drug by percolation, so as to make 16 fluid ounces of tincture.

2750. Tincture of Copper Acetate. A
Copper sulphate, pure...... 675 grains.
Lead acetate, pure .... 840 grains.
Distilled water .... 8½ fl. ounces.
Alcohol, 188 per cent...... 7½ fl. ounces

Triturate the two salts together until a smooth paste is formed, transfer this to a copper vessel, add the water, heat to boiling, allow to cool, add the alcohol, set aside for 4 weeks, agitating frequently, and filter.

2751. Tincture of Copper Acetate. B
Copper acetate crystallized 480 grains.
Distilled water .... 9 fl. ounces.
Alcohol, 188 per cent...... 7 fl. ounces.

Dissolve the acetate in the water previously warmed and filter.

2752. Tincture of Corydalis—Eclectic.
(Tincture of Turkey Corn.)
Turkey corn, fine powd.... 3¼ ounces.
Diluted alcohol .... q. s.

Extract the drug by percolation with diluted alcohol so as to obtain 16 fluid ounces of tincture.

2753. Tincture of Cubeb.
Cubeb No. 30, powder..... 4 ounces.
75 per cent alcohol q. s.
to make .... 2 pints.

Moisten the powder with 3 ounces of 75 per cent alcohol and macerate for 24 hours; then pack it firmly in a percolator, and gradually pour 75 per cent alcohol upon it until 2 pints of tincture are obtained.

2754. Tincture of Culvers Root—Eclectic.
(Tincture of Leptandra.)
Culvers root .... 3¼ ounces.
Diluted alcohol .... q. s.

Extract the drug in moderately fine powder by percolation so as to obtain 16 fluid ounces of product.

2755. Tincture of Digitalis—Ethereal.
Digitalis, cut fine .... 1¼ ounces.
Spirit of ether .... 16 fl. ounces.
Mix, macerate for 7 days, and filter.

2756. Tincture of Ergot.
(Brit. Pharm.)
Ergot, powdered .... 4 ounces.
Diluted alcohol .... q. s.

Percolate the drug so as to obtain 16 fluid ounces of tincture.

2757. Tincture of Eucalyptus.
(Brit. Form.)
Eucalyptus, powdered .... 3¼ ounces.
Alcohol .... q. s.

Extract the drug by percolation so as to obtain 16 fluid ounces of tincture.

2758. Tincture of Gelsemium.
Gelsemium in fine powder. 4¼ ounces.
Alcohol, 188 per cent, q. s.
to make .... 2 pints.

Moisten the gelsemium with 4 fluid ounces of alcohol; percolate with alcohol until 2 pints of tincture are obtained.

2759. Tincture of Gentian.
G. P.
Gentian, powdered.......... 3¼ ounces.
Diluted alcohol........... 1 pint.

Moisten the powder with sufficient menstruum; and macerate for 24 hours; then place in a filter and pour on diluted alcohol until 1 pint of tincture is obtained.

2760. Tincture Gentian Compound.
Gentian .... 2¼ ounces.
Bitter orange peel.......... 1¼ ounces.
Cardamom .... 280 grains.
Diluted alcohol........... 4 pints.

Mix the gentian, orange peel and cardamom and reduce them to a coarse powder; moisten the powder with 6 ounces of diluted alcohol; macerate for 24 hours, then pack firmly in percolator and pour diluted alcohol upon it until 4 pints of tincture are obtained.

2761. Tincture of Ginger.
(U. S. P.)
Ginger in No. 40 powder.. 5¾ ounces.
Alcohol q. s. to make..... 2 pints.

Moisten the ginger with 2 ounces of alcohol and macerate for 24 hours; percolate with menstruum until 2 pints of tincture are obtained.

2762. Tincture of Golden Seal Co.
(Eclectic.)
Tincture of Golden Seal
 (U. S. P.) .... 9½ fl. ounces.
Tincture of lobelia .... 6½ fl. ounces.
Mix.

2763. Tincture of Henbane.
(Tincture of Hyoscyamus.)
Hyoscyamus leaves........ 4¾ ounces.
Alcohol diluted, q. s. to
  make .... 2 pints.
Moisten the hyoscyamus with 4 fluid ounces of diluted alcohol and macerate for 24 hours; percolate with diluted alcohol until 2 pints of tincture are obtained.

2764. Tincture of Hips.
(Rademacher's.)
(Tincture Cynosbati.)
Fresh rose hips, cut fine.. 2 ounces.
Alcohol .... q. s.
Macerate the hips with 12 fluid ounces of alcohol, agitating frequently, express, filter, and add enough alcohol to the filtrate to make 12 fluid ounces.

2765. Tincture of Iodine.
Iodine resublimed .... 510 grains.
Alcohol .... 1 pint.
Dissolve the iodine in the alcohol.
This tincture is seldom given internally, but is used for outward application as an absorbent, alone, or combined with other substances.

2766. Tincture of Iodine Co.
(U. S. P. 1870.)
Iodine .... 240 grains.
Potassium Iodide .... 480 grains.
Alcohol .... 16 fl. ounces.
Mix and dissolve.
This must not be confused with the compound solution of iodine of the present pharmacopoeia.

2767. Tincture of Iron Co.
Tincture of ferrated extract of apples, N. F.... 8 fl. ounces.
Vinous tincture of rhubarb 8 fl. ounces.
Tincture of nux vomica... 1 fl. ounce.
Mix.

2768. Tincture of Iron.
(Athenstaedt.)
Compound Aromatic Tincture of Iron—Athenstaedt's Tincture.
Soluble oxide of iron..... 330 grains.
Distilled water .... 19 fl. ounces.
Simple syrup .... 6 fl. ounces.
Alcohol .... 6½ fl. ounces.
Citric acid .... 30 grains.
Tincture of orange peel... 50 minims.
Aromatic tincture........ 12 drops.
Tincture of cinnamon .... 12 drops.
Tincture of vanilla ..... 12 drops.
Acetic ether .... 1 drop.

Dissolve the iron salt in the water; then add the other ingredients and filter. The iron oxide used for the above should represent 10 per cent of metallic iron. If it be weaker, a proportionately larger amount should be employed, and slightly decreasing the amount of syrup subsequently added.

2769. Tincture of Iron Acetate. A
(Rademacher's.)
Iron sulphate, pure....... 656 grains.
Lead acetate, pure .... 684 grains.
Diluted acetic acid ...... 3 fl. ounces.
Distilled water .... 3 fl. ounces.
Alcohol .... 6 fl. ounces.
Triturate the two salts together to a pasty mass, introduce this into an iron vessel, add the water and acid, heat to boiling, allow to cool; transfer to a large flask, add the alcohol; set the flask, loosely stoppered, aside for several months, agitating occasionally until the liquid has acquired a light red tint, and filter.

2770. Tincture of Iron Chloride.
Solution of chloride of iron 4 ounces.
Alcohol, 188 per cent .... 12 ounces.
Mix; let stand for 3 months; keep in glass stoppered bottles.

2771. Tincture of Iron. B
Solution of iron tersulphate .... 2½ fl. ounces.
Distilled water .... 2½ fl. ounces.
Lead acetate, pure........ 1¼ ounces.
Diluted acetic acid ...... 5 fl. ounces.
Alcohol .... 5 fl. ounces.
Dissolve the lead acetate in the acid; add the iron solution previously mixed with the water; then gradually add the alcohol; set aside for two weeks and decant the clear liquid.

2772. Tincture of Jaborandi.
(Brit. Pharm.)
Jaborandi, powder .... 4 ounces.
Diluted alcohol .... q. s.
Extract by percolation so as to obtain 16 fluid ounces of tincture.

2773. Tincture of Kalmia—Eclectic.
(Tincture of Sheep Laurel or Mountain Mint.)
Sheep laurel leaves, grd... 3¼ ounces.
Diluted alcohol .... q. s.
Extract the drug by percolation so as to obtain 16 fluid ounces of product.

2774. Tincture of Kino.

Kino	360 grains.
Glycerine	1 fl. ounce.
Alcohol	q. s. to make
Water	½ pint.

Mix the glycerine with 6 ounces of alcohol, and 1¼ ounces of water. Rub the kino in a mortar, adding gradually 3 ounces of this menstruum until a smooth paste is made; transfer this to a bottle add the remainder of the menstruum and macerate for 24 hours, occasionally shaking the bottle; then filter through paper, adding through the filter enough of a mixture of alcohol and water, made in the proportion of 5 drams of alcohol to 1 dram of water, to make half a pint of tincture.

2775. Tincture of Lobelia Co.—Eclectic.
(King's Expectorant Tincture.)

Lobelia (herb)	120 grains.
Bloodroot	120 grains.
Skunk cabbage	120 grains.
Canada snake root	120 grains.
Pleurisy root	120 grains.
Water	q. s.
Alcohol	q. s.

Mix the drugs and reduce to fine powder; mix the alcohol and water in the proportion of 3 of the former to 1 of the latter, and extract the mixed drugs by percolation with this menstruum so as to obtain 16 fluid ounces of product.

2776. Tincture of Lobelia and Capsicum Co.—Eclectic.
(Anti-spasmodic Tincture, Eclectic.)

Lobelia	1 ounce.
Capsicum	1 ounce.
Skunk cabbage	1 ounce.
Diluted alcohol	q. s.

Mix the drugs in moderately fine powder, and extract by percolation with diluted alcohol so as to obtain 16 fluid ounces.

2777. Tincture of Lupulin—Eclectic.

Lupulin	2¾ ounces.
Alcohol	16 fl. ounces.

Macerate for 7 days, shaking occasionally, and filter, adding enough alcohol through the filter to make 16 fluid ounces.

2778. Tincture of Myrrh.

Myrrh, No. 30, powder	5½ ounces.
Alcohol, sufficient to make	2 pints.

Mix the powder with 1½ pints alcohol; macerate for seven days in a well stoppered vessel, agitating occasionally; then filter through paper, adding through the filter enough alcohol to make the tincture measure 2 pints.

2779. Tincture of Opium—Ammoniated.
(Brit. Pharm.)

Opium	80 grains.
Spanish saffron	144 grains.
Benzoic acid	144 grains.
Oil of anise	50 minims.
Stronger water of ammonia	3¼ fl. ounces.
Alcohol	q. s.

Mix the first five ingredients with 13 fluid ounces of alcohol, macerate for 7 days, agitating occasionally, express, filter, and add enough alcohol to the filtrate to make 16 fluid ounces.

2780. Tincture of Opium—Camphorated.
(Paregoric) From Laudanum.

Laudanum	1¾ ounces.
Benzoic acid	1 dram.
Oil of anise	1 dram.
Camphor	2 scruples.
Alcohol dilute	30 ounces.
Glycerine	1 ounce.
Caramel to color	q. s.

Dissolve the benzoic acid, camphor and oil of anise in the alcohol; mix the glycerine, laudanum and water, and add gradually to the first solution; after standing a few hours; filter through paper.

The dose for an infant is from five to twenty drops.

2781. Tincture of Opium—Camphorated.
U. S. 1880.

Opium, powdered	35 grains.
Benzoic acid	35 grains.
Camphor	35 grains.
Oil of anise	37 minims.
Glycerine	5 fl. drams.
Diluted alcohol q. s. to make	20 fl. ounces.

Add eighteen ounces of diluted alcohol to the other ingredients and macerate for seven days in a well covered vessel; then filter through paper, adding through the filter sufficient diluted alcohol to measure in all twenty fluid ounces.

2782. Tincture of Poke Root Co.

Fluid extract of poke root	3 fl. ounces.
Fluid extract of cardamom	1 fl. dram.
Diluted alcohol, enough to make	16 fl. ounces.

Mix and filter.

2783. Tincture of Prickly Ash Berries.
(Eclectic.)
Prickly ash berries in fine powder .... 4½ ounces.
Diluted alcohol .... q. s.

Extract the drug by percolation with diluted alcohol so as to obtain 16 fluid ounces of tincture.

2784. Tincture of Pulsatilla.
Pulsatilla herb, fresh..... 8½ ounces.
Strong alcohol .... q. s.

Cut the herb into small pieces and add strong alcohol enough so that the product will measure 16 fluid ounces; macerate for 14 days, express, and filter.

2785. Tincture of Quinine.
(Brit. Pharm.)
Quinine sulphate .... 128 grains.
Tinct. of bitter orange peel 16 fl. ounces.

2786. Tincture of Quinine—Ammoniated.
(Brit. Pharm.)
Quinine sulphate .... 128 grains.
Water of ammonia.......... 4 fl. ounces.
Diluted alcohol .... 14 fl. ounces.

Dissolve the sulphate of quinine in the alcohol with the aid of a gentle heat and add the ammonia.

2787. Tincture of Rhubarb—Aromatic.
Rhubarb, coarse ground... 6¾ ounces.
Cinnamon, coarse ground. 1¼ ounces.
Cloves, coarse ground..... 1¼ ounces.
Nutmeg, coarse ground.... 275 grains.
Alcohol dilute q. s. to make 2 pints.

Mix the drugs and moisten with 10 ounces of dilute alcohol; macerate for 3 days; percolate and run menstruum through until 2 pints of product are obtained.

2788. Tincture of Rhubarb—Sweet.
Rhubarb, coarse ground... 2½ ounces.
Licorice root, coarse grd... 1¼ ounces.
Anise seed, coarse ground. 1¼ ounces.
Cardamom seed coarse grd. 136 grains.
Diluted alcohol q. s. to make .... 2 pints.

Mix the drugs and moisten with 5 ounces of diluted alcohol; macerate for 3 days; percolate and run through menstruum until 2 pints are obtained.

2789. Tincture of Opium and Saffron.
(Germ. Pharm.)
(Sydenham's Laudanum Compound Wine of Opium.)
Opium, powdered........... 1½ ounces.
Spanish saffron .... ½ ounce.
Cloves, bruised .... 90 grains.
Cassia bark, coarse powder 90 grains.
Alcohol .... 6¾ fl. ounces.
Water .... 9¼ fl. ounces.

Mix all; macerate for 7 days, agitating occasionally, and filter.

2790. Tincture of Phosphorus Co..
(Brit. Pharm.)
Phosphorus .... 8 grains.
Chloroform .... 14 fl. drams.
Alcohol, enough to make.. 10 fl. ounces.

Place the phosphorus in a stoppered bottle, apply the heat of a water-bath until dissolved, and then add the alcohol, then shake well.

This tincture should be protected from the light, in well stoppered bottles. Each fluid dram contains 1-10 grain of phosphorus.

2791. Tincture of Poison Oak—Eclectic.
(Tincture of Poison Ivy.)
Fresh leaves of rhus toxicodendron .... 9 ounces.
Alcohol .... 6 fl. ounces.

Macerate for 14 days; express and filter in a well-covered funnel.

2792. Tincture of Podophyllum—Eclectic.
Podophyllum, fine powder. 3¼ ounces.
Alcohol .... q. s.

Extract the drug by percolation with alcohol so as to obtain 16 fluid ounces of tincture.

2793. Tincture of Quillaia.
(Tincture of Soap Bark.)
Quillaia, coarse powder... 3¼ ounces.
Alcohol, 188 per cent...... 5¾ fl. ounces.
Water .... q. s.

Boil the quillaia with 13 fluid ounces of water for 15 minutes; strain; wash the residue on the strainer, with 1½ fluid ounces of water, boil the strained liquid down to 10 fluid ounces; allow to cool; add the alcohol, filter, and through the filtrate add enough water to make the filtrate measure 16 fluid ounces.

2794. Tincture of Poke Root—Eclectic.

Poke root, fine powder.... 3½ ounces.
Diluted alcohol .... q. s.

Extract the drug by percolation with diluted alcohol so as to obtain 16 fluid ounces of tincture.

2795. Tincture of Rhubarb Co.—Eclectic.

Rhubarb .... 384 grains.
Dogsbane .... 192 grains.
Golden seal .... 192 grains.
Gentian .... 192 grains.
Prickly ash berries..... 192 grains.
Diluted alcohol .... q. s.

Mix the drugs, reduce to fine powder, and extract with diluted alcohol by percolation, so as to obtain 16 fluid ounces of tincture.

2796. Tincture of Rhubarb—Koelreuter's.

Rhubarb, cut fine .... 2½ ounces.
Bitter orange peel, cut fine 360 grains.
Centaury, cut fine ...... 180 grains.
Fennel, crushed.......... 110 grains.
Distilled water .... 9 fl. ounces.
Alcohol, 188 per cent ... 7½ fl. ounces.

Mix and macerate for 8 days; strain and filter.

2797. Tincture of Saffron.
(Tincture of Crocus.)

Saffron .... 1¾ ounces.
Diluted alcohol .... q. s.

Macerate the saffron for 3 days in a portion of the diluted alcohol; percolate with menstruum until 16 ounces are obtained.

2798. Tincture of Savin.
(Brit. Pharm.)

Savin, coarse powder .... 2 ounces.
Diluted alcohol .... q. s.

Extract the drug by percolation so as to obtain 16 fluid ounces of tincture.

2799. Tincture of Savin, Compound—Eclectic.

Fluid extract of savin.... 1 fl. ounce.
Tincture of castor .... 7½ fl. ounces.
Tincture of myrrh .... 7½ fl. ounces.

Mix.

2800. Tincture of Senna, Compound—Eclectic.
(Elixir Salutis—Elixir of Health.)

Alexandria senna, cut..... 480 grains.
Jalap, finely powdered.... 240 grains.
Coriander .... 120 grains.
Raisins deprived of seeds. ½ ounce.
Diluted alcohol .... 16 fl. ounces.

Macerate for 7 days, shaking occasionally, and filter.

2801. Tincture of Serpentaria Co.—Eclectic.
Sudorific Tincture.)

Serpentaria .... 160 grains.
Ipecac .... 160 grains.
Spanish saffron .... 160 grains.
Camphor .... 160 grains.
Opium .... 160 grains.
Diluted alcohol .... 16 fl. ounces.

Macerate the finely powdered drugs with the diluted alcohol for 7 days, agitating occasionally, and filter.

2802. Tincture of Shepherd's Purse.
(Rademacher's.)
(Tincture Bursæ Pastoris.)

Shepherd's purse herb freshly gathered .... 10 ounces.
Alcohol .... 12 fl. ounces.

Contuse the herb to pulp, add the alcohol; macerate for 7 days, express and filter.

2803. Tincture of Skunk Cabbage.—Eclectic.

Skunk cabbage, recently dried .... 3½ ounces.
Diluted alcohol .... q. s.

Extract the drug in fine powder by percolation with diluted alcohol so as to obtain 16 fluid ounces.

2804. Tincture of Stavesacre—Eclectic.

Stavesacre seed, fine powd. 11 ounces.
Absolute alcohol .... q. s.

Percolate the drug with the absolute alcohol so as to obtain 16 fluid ounces of product.

2805. Tincture of Stillingia—Eclectic.

Stillingia, fine powder..... 3 ounces.
Diluted alcohol .... q. s.

Extract the drug by percolation so as to obtain 16 fluid ounces of product.

2806. Tincture of Strychnine.
(Brit. Pharm.)

Strychnine (alkaloid)....... 12 grains.
Alcohol .... 4 fl. ounces.

Agitate occasionally until dissolved.

2807. Tincture of Strychnine, Co.—Eclectic.

Strychnine (alkaloid)...... 16 grains.
Acetic acid .... 4 fl. drams.
Comp. tinct. cardamom.... 4 fl. drams.
Water .... 7½ fl. ounces.
Alcohol .... 7½ fl. ounces.

Dissolve the strychnine in the alcohol and acetic acid, add the remaining ingredients and filter.

2808. Tincture of Sulphur.
(Hager.)
Washed sulphur .... 290 grains.
Alcohol, 188 per cent..... 16 fl. ounces.
Mix; macerate for 4 days, agitating occasionally, and filter.

2809 Tincture of Sulphur—Homeopathic.
Washed sulphur .... 1½ ounces.
Alcohol, 188 per cent...... 16 fl. ounces
Mix; macerate for 8 days, shaking twice a day, decanting the clear liquid, and filtering. This is considered equal to the first centesimal potency.

2810. Tincture of Tolu.
(U. S. P.)
Tolu .... 1¾ ounces.
Alcohol, enough to make.. 16 fl. ounces
Mix: agitate occasionally, until dissolved, and filter.

2811. Tincture of Vanilla.
Vanilla bean, cut small and
 bruised .... 3 ounces.
Sugar, granulated .... 6 ounces.
Alcohol .... ⎫ each sufficient to
Water .... ⎭ make 2 pints.
Mix alcohol and water in the proportion of two parts by weight of alcohol to one part by weight of water. Macerate the vanilla in one pint of this mixture for 12 hours; then drain off the liquid and set it aside. Transfer the vanilla to a mortar; beat it with the sugar into a uniform paste, then pack it into a percolator and pour upon it the reserved liquid; when this has disappeared from the surface, gradually pour on menstruum and continue the percolation until 2 pints of tincture are obtained.

2812. Tincture of Valerian Ethereal.
(Germ. Pharm.)
Valerian in powder .... 2½ ounces.
Spirit of ether........... q. s.
Mix the drug with 15 fluid ounces of spirit; macerate for 7 days, agitating occasionally, express, add enough spirit of ether to make 15 fluid ounces, and filter.

2813. Tincture of Veratri Viridis.
(Tincture of American Hellebore.)
American hellebore in 60
 powder .... 14½ ounces.
Alcohol, q. s. to make.... 2 pints.
Moisten the powder with 5 ounces of alcohol and macerate for 24 hours. Percolate with menstruum until 2 pints of tincture are obtained.

2814. Compound Tincture of Viburnum.
Cramp bark .... 2 ounces.
Cassia bark .... 1 ounce.
Skull cap................ ½ ounce.
Wild yam .... ½ ounce.
Cloves .... ¼ ounce.
Grind together to fine powder and percolate with a menstruum consisting of alcohol, 2 parts; water, 1 part, and glycerin, 1 part; first moistening, packing and macerating in the usual way. The product should measure 16 fluid ounces.

2815. Tincture of Wahoo.
(Brit. Form.)
Tincture of Euonymus.)
Wahoo bark, powdered.... 3¼ ounces.
Alcohol, 188 per cent...... q. s.
Extract the drug by percolation so as to obtain 16 fluid ounces of tincture.

2816. Warburg's Tincture—Modified.
Camphor .... 2 drams.
Rhubarb, coarse ground... 4 drams.
Aloes soc., powdered...... 4 drams.
Quinine sulphate .... 4 drams.
Cinchonidia sulphate ..... 4 drams.
Gum myrrh, powdered.... 8 drams.
Oil of angelica........... 10 drops.
Oil of caraway........... 10 drops.
Alcohol diluted, q. s. to
 make .... 4 pints.

2817. Tincture of Witch Hazel Bark.
(Brit. Form.)
Hamamelis bark, No. 20
 powder .... 1¾ ounces.
Diluted alcohol, enough to
 make .... 16 fl. ounces.
Extract the drug by percolation.

2818. Tincture of Wormwood.
(Ger. Phar.)
(Tincture of Absinthe.)
Wormwood .... 3 ounces.
Water .... 3½ fl. ounces.
Alcohol, 188 per cent...... 12½ fl. ounces.
Mix; macerate for 7 days, agitating occasionally, express, and filter.

2819. Tincture of Wormwood, Co.
(Bitter Stomach Drops.)
Wormwood .... 520 grains.
Blessed thistle .... 130 grains.
Galangal root .... 130 grains.
Orange berries .... 130 grains.
Diluted alcohol .... q. s.
Mix the drugs, reduce to powder, and extract by percolation with diluted alcohol so as to obtain 16 fluid ounces of tincture.

SOLUTIONS.

2820. Solution of Acid Phosphates. N. F.
(Co. Solution of Phosphoric Acid.)
Bone ash, in fine powder.. 17½ ounces.
Sulphuric acid (sp. gr.
  1.830).................... 13¼ ounces.
Water .... 64 ounces.

Mix the bone ash with 16 fluid ounces of water, add the sulphuric acid, diluted with 32 fluid ounces of water, and mix thoroughly with a porcelain or glass stirrer. Now add the remainder of the water and set the mixture aside for 24 hours, stirring occasionally. Then transfer the mixture to a strong muslin strainer, and subject this to a gradual pressure (avoiding contact with metals), so as to express as much of the liquid as possible. Lastly, filter this through paper.

2821. Solution of Aloes and Soda.
(Mettauer's Aperient.)
Aloes socotrine .... 5 drams.
Soda bicarb. .... 1½ ounces.
Tincture of lavender co.... ¾ ounce.
Water q. s. to make....... 16 ounces.

Macerate the drugs in the water for 2 weeks; filter and add the tincture of lavender co.

2822. Solution of Arsenious Acid.
(Solution Chloride of Arsenic.)
Arsenious acid in small
  pieces .... 74 grains.
Hydrochloric acid........ 135 minims.
Distilled water sufficient
  to make .... 1 pint.

Boil the arsenious acid with the hydrochloric acid, mixed with 4 fl. ounces of distilled water until it is dissolved. Filter the liquid and pass enough distilled water through the filter to make the solution measure one pint.

The medical properties of this solution are the same as Fowler's solution. The dose is from two to eight minims.

2823. Solution of Acetate of Ammonium.
(Spirit of mindererus.)
Diluted acetic acid .... 1 pint.
Carbonate of ammonia..... q. s.

Add a sufficient quantity of carbonate of ammonia to the diluted acetic acid, until it is neutralized. This preparation should be freshly made when required for use.

Solution of acetate of ammonium may also be prepared in the following manner:
Carbonate of ammonium.. 2 ounces.
Acetic acid .... 4¾ fl. ounces.
Distilled water .... 27 fl. ounces.

Dissolve the carbonate of ammonium in one pint of distilled water and filter the solution. To the acetic acid add enough distilled water to make one pint. Keep the solutions in separate well-stopped bottles, and when solution of acetate of ammonium is to be dispensed; measure equal quantites of each solution and mix them.

2824 Sol. of Acetate of Ammonium. Strong.
Carbonate ammonium . 5 ounces.
Acetic acid............q. s. or 13 fl. ounces.
Distilled water.......q. s.

Crush the carbonate of ammonium, and add it gradually to 12 ounces of the acetic acid; then add more of the acid until a neutral solution results. To this add sufficient water to make 16 fluid ounces.

2825. Solution of Citrate Bismuth and Ammonium.
(Br.)
Citrate bismuth .... 800 grains.
Solution of ammonia....... q. s.
Distilled water, ... q. s.

Rub the citrate of bismuth to a paste with a little distilled water; add the solution of ammonia gradually, and with stirring until the salt is just dissolved. Dilute with distilled water to form one pint.

2826. Solution of Magnesium Citrate. A
Carbonate of magnesium. 200 grains.
Citric acid .... 400 grains.
Syrup of citric acid....... 2 fl. ounces.
Bicarbonate of potassium in crystals........ 30 grains.
Water...................... q. s.

Dissolve the citric acid in 4 fluid ounces of water, and, having added the carbonate of magnesium, stir until it is dissolved. Filter the solution into a strong bottle of the capacity of 12 fluid ounces, containing the syrup of citric acid. Then add enough water, previously boiled and filtered, to nearly fill the bottle, drop in the bicarbonate of potassium, and immediately close the bottle with a cork, which must be secured with twine. Lastly, shake the mixture occasionally until the bicarbonate of potassium is dissolved.

2827. Solution of Citrate of Magnesia. B
Citric acid, crystals....... 60 grains.
Sulphate of magnesia...... ½ ounce.
Simple syrup .... 3 fl. ounces.
Extract of lemon.......... 10 drops.
Bicarbonate of potash
  (crystals) .... 2 scruples.
Water, q. s. to make...... 12 ounces.

Place the acid and epsom salts together in a 12-ounce citrate of magnesia bottle; add the simple syrup and extract of lemon; agitate for a moment and add the water; when dissolved add the bicarbonate of potash; cork the bottle and tie down with twine.

2828. Solution of Four Chlorides.
(Era.)

Alum	10 ounces.
Sal soda	10 ounces.
Sal ammoniac	2 ounces.
Common salt	2 ounces.
Chloride of zinc	1 ounce.
Muriatic acid, commercial	q. s.
Water, q. s. to make	1 gallon.

Dissolve the alum in ½ gallon of boiling water; then add the sal soda, which gives a precipitate of aluminum hydrate. Muriatic acid is then added in sufficient quantity to dissolve this precipitate, thereby forming aluminum chloride. The other salts are then dissolved in the remainder of the water and added to the first solution. The advantages claimed for this preparation are cheapness, ease of preparation, odorless, non-poisonous, and its adaptability for general use. Its freedom from iron in the disinfection of clothing is an important point, in so much that it will not injure the fabric in any way. It commends itself for the disinfection of rooms, by saturating a sheet with the diluted solution and hanging up in any convenient place.

This diluted solution may be made by mixing one pint of the concentrated solution with one gallon of water.

2829. Solution of Hydrastis—Colorless.
(Glycerite of Hydrastis.)

Hydrastis hydrochlorate	25 grains.
Aluminum chloride	50 grains.
Hydrochloric acid dil.	10 minims.
Water distilled	8 ounces.
Glycerine	8 ounces.

Dissolve the salts in the water by the aid of the diluted acid; filter; then add the glycerin.

2830. Solution of Iron Acetate.
(U. S.)

Solution of tersulphate of iron	14½ fl. ounces.
Glacial acetic acid	4¾ fl. ounces.
Water of ammonia	1 pint.
Water	
Distilled water, q. s. to make	1 pint.

To the water of ammonia diluted with 1½ pints of cold water add, constantly stirring, the solution of tersulphate of iron, previously diluted with 4 pints of cold water. Pour the whole on a wet muslin strainer, allow the precipitate to drain, then return it to the vessel and mix it intimately with 7 pints of cold water; again drain it on the strainer, and repeat the operation, until the washings cause but a slight cloudiness with test—solution of chloride of barium. Then allow the excess of water to drain off and press the precipitate, folded in the strainer, until its weight is reduced to fourteen ounces or less. Add the precipitate to the glacial acetic acid contained in a capacious porcelain capsule, and stir occasionally, until the oxide is entirely dissolved. Finally, add enough cold, distilled water to make the solution measure 1 pint, and filter if necessary. Solution of acetate of iron should be kept in well-stoppered bottles, protected from light.

2831. Solution of Iron Chloride.
(U. S.)

Iron, in the form of fine wire and cut into small pieces	3½ ounces.
Hydrochloric acid	16¾ fl. ounces.
Nitric acid	of each q. s.
Distilled water	to make 1 pint.

Put the iron wire into a flask capable of holding double the volume of the intended product. Pour upon it 10½ fluid ounces of hydrochloric acid previously diluted with 5¼ fluid ounces of distilled water, and let the mixture stand until effervescence ceases; then heat it to the boiling point, filter through paper, and, having rinsed the flask and iron wire with a little boiling distilled water, pass the washings through the filter. To the filtered liquid add 5¼ fluid ounces of hydrochloric acid, and pour the mixture, slowly and gradually, in a stream, in 1 fluid ounce and 3 fluid drams of nitric acid contained in a capacious porcelain vessel. After effervescence ceases, apply heat, by means of a sand bath, until the liquid is free from nitrous odor. Then test a small portion with freshly prepared test—solution of ferricyanide of potassium. Should this reagent produce a blue color, add a little more nitric acid and evaporate off the excess. Finally, add the remaining 1 fluid ounce of hydrochloric acid, and enough distilled water to make the solution measure 1 pint.

2832. Solution of Iron Citrate. (U. S.)

Solution of tersulphate of iron	10½ fl. ounces.
Citric acid	3 ounces.
Water of ammonia	8½ fl. ounces.
Water q. s. to make	10 ounces.

To the water of ammonia previously diluted with 20 fluid ounces of cold water, add, constantly stirring, the solution of tersulphate of iron previously diluted with 6 pints of cold water. Pour the whole on a wet muslin strainer, allow the precipitate to drain, then return it to the vessel and mix it intimately with 7½ pints of cold water. Again drain it on a strainer, and repeat the operation until the washings cause but a very slight cloudiness with test—solution of chloride of barium; then allow the excess of water to drain off. Transfer the moist precipitate to a porcelain dish, add the citric acid, and heat the mixture on a water-bath, to 60° C. (140° F.), stirring constantly until the precipitate is dissolved. Lastly, filter the liquid and evaporate it, at the above mentioned temperature, until it weighs 10 ounces.

2833. Solution of Iron Perchloride

| Strong solution of perchloride of iron | 5 fl. ounces. |
| Distilled water, q. s. to produce after admixture | 20 fl. ounces. |

Mix.

2834. Solution of Iodine Compound. (U. S.)

Iodine	½ ounce.
Iodide of potassium	1 ounce.
Distilled water 8 fluid ounces and 3 fluid drams, to make	9 fl. ounces.

Dissolve the iodine and iodide of potassium in the distilled water. Keep the solution in well-stoppered bottles.

2835. Solution of Lime. (Lime Water.)

Lime	one part ½ ounce.
Water	q. s.
Distilled water	q. s.

Slake the lime by the gradual addition of 3 fluid ounces of water; then add one pint of water and stir occasionally during half an hour. Allow the mixture to settle, decant the liquid and throw it away. Then add to the residue 8 pints of distilled water; stir well; wait a short time for the coarser articles to subside, and pour the liquid, holding the undissolved lime in suspension, into a glass stoppered bottle. Pour off the liquid when wanted for use.

2836. Solution of Lime.—Chlorinated. Br.

| Chlorinated lime | 1 pound. |
| Distilled water | 1 gallon. |

Mix well the water and the chlorinated lime by trituration in a large mortar, and having transferred the mixture to a stoppered bottle; let it be well shaken several times for the space of three hours. Pour out now the contents of the bottle on a calico filter, and let the solution which passes through be preserved in a stoppered bottle.

2837. Solution of Mercury and Arsenic Iodides. Donovan's Solution.

Iodide of arsenic	37 grains.
Red iodide of mercury	37 grains.
Distilled water, q. s. to make	½ pint.

Triturate the iodides with a fluid ounce of distilled water, until they are dissolved. Filter the liquid and pass enough distilled water through the filter to make the solution measure ½ pint.

2838. Solution of Morphine Acetate. (Br.)

Acetate of morphine	9 grains.
Diluted acetic acid	18 minims.
Rectified spirit	½ fl. ounce.
Distilled water	1½ fl. ounces.

Mix the acid, the spirit, and the water, and dissolve the acetate of morphine in the mixture.

2839. Sol. of Morphine Hydrochlorate. (Br.)

Hydrochlorate of morphine	9 grains.
Dil. hydrochloric acid	18 minims.
Rectified spirit	½ fl. ounce.
Distilled water	1½ fl. ounce.

Mix the hydrochloric acid, the spirit, and the water, and dissolve the hydrochlorate of morphine in the mixture.

2840. Solution of Pepsin. (U. S.)

Saccharated pepsin	400 grains.
Hydrochloric acid	110 minims.
Glycerin	7 fl. ounces.
Water	12 fl. ounces.

Dissolve the saccharated pepsin in the water, previously mixed with the hydrochloric acid, add the glycerin, let the mixture stand 24 hours, and filter.

2841. Solution of Lead Subacetate.
U. S.
Acetate of lead..... 4 ounces, 150 grains.
Oxide of lead ...... 3 ounces, 30 grains.
Distilled water, q. s. to
 make .... 20 fl. ounces.

Dissolve the acetate of lead in 20 fluid ounces of boiling distilled water, in a glass or porcelain vessel. Then add the oxide of lead and boil for half an hour, occasionally adding enough hot distilled water to make up the loss by evaporation. Remove the heat, allow the liquid to cool, and add enough distilled water, previously boiled and cooled, to make the product measure 20 fluid ounces. Finally, filter the liquid in a well-covered funnel. Solution of subacetate of lead should be kept in well-stoppered bottles.

2842. Solution of Potash.
Br.
Carbonate of potassium.... 1 pound.
Slaked lime, washed....... 12 ounces.
Distilled water............ 1 gallon.

Dissolve the carbonate of potassium in the water; and, having heated the solution to the boiling point, in a clean iron vessel, gradually mix with it the washed slaked lime and continue the boiling for ten minutes with constant stirring. Then remove the vessel from the fire; and, when by the subsidence of the insoluble matter the supernatant liquor has become perfectly clear, transfer it by means of a siphon to a green-glass bottle furnished with an air-tight stopper, and add distilled water, if necessary, to make it correspond with the tests of sp. gr. and neutralizing. The sp. gr. is 1.058.

2843. Solution of Potash.
U. S. P.
Potassium hydrate .... 1 ounce.
Water distilled .... 16 ounces.
Mix and dissolve.

2844. Solution of Potassium Arsenite.
Fowler's Solution, U. S.
Arsenious acid in small
 pieces .... 37 grains.
Bicarb. of potassium...... 37 grains.
Comp. tinct. lavender..... 130 minims.
Distilled water, q. s. to
 make .... ½ pint.

Boil the arsenious acid and bicarbonate of potassium in a glass vessel with six fluid drams of distilled water, until the acid is completely dissolved. Then add the compound tincture of lavender and enough distilled water to make the product measure half a pint. Lastly, set the mixture aside for eight days and then filter through paper.

2845. Solution of Soda.
U. S.
Soda hydrate .... 1 ounce.
Water distilled .... 16 ounces.
Mix and dissolve.

2846. Solution of Soda.—Chlorinated.
U. S.
Carbonate of sodium ...... 25 ounces.
Chlorinated lime.......... 20 ounces.
Water, q. s. to make....... 14 pints.

Mix the chlorinated lime intimately with 5½ pints of water in a tared vessel provided with a tightly fitting cover. Dissolve the carbonate of sodium in 5½ pints of boiling water, and immediately pour the latter solution into the former. Cover the vessel tightly, and when the contents are cold, add enough water to make them measure 14 pints. Lastly, strain the mixture through muslin, allow the precipitate to subside, and remove the clear solution by means of a siphon. Keep the product in well-stoppered bottles.

2847. Solution of Sodium Arseniate.
U. S.
Arseniate of sodium deprived of its water of crystallization by a heat not exceeding 149° (300° F.)............ 23 grains.
Distilled water .... 5 fl. ounces.

Dissolve the arseniate of sodium in the distilled water.

2848. Spiritus Acidi Formici.—N. F.
Spirit of Formic Acid.
Spiritus Formicarum (Germ. Pharm.). Spirit of Ants.
Formic acid.............. 250 minims.
Distilled water .... 3½ fl. ounces.
Alcohol enough to make.... 16 fl. ounces.

Mix the formic acid with the distilled water, and add enough alcohol to make sixteen (16) fluid ounces.

Note.—Formic acid is required by the Germ. Pharm. to have a specific gravity of 1.060 to 1.063.

2849. Spiritus Amygdalæ Amaræ.—N. F.
Spirit of Bitter Almond.
Essence of Bitter Almond.
Oil of bitter almond....... 160 minims.
Alcohol .... 14 fl. ounces.
Distilled water, enough
 to make .... 16 fl. ounces.

Dissolve the oil in the alcohol, and add enough distilled water to make sixteen (16) fluid ounces.

2850. Spiritus Aromaticus.—N. F.
Aromatic Spirit.

Comp. spirit of orange (N. F.)	8 fl. ounces.
Deodorized alcohol	7½ pints.

Mix them. Preserve the product, if it is to be kept in stock, in completely-filled and well-stoppered vials or bottles, and stored in a cool and dark place.

Aromatic spirit may also be prepared in the following manner:

Sweet orange peel, fresh, and deprived of the white, inner portion	16 tr. ounces.
Lemon peel, fresh	2 tr. ounces.
Coriander, bruised	2 tr. ounces.
Oil of star anise	16 minims.
Deodorized alcohol enough to make	1 gallon.

Macerate the solids during four days with 1 gallon of deodorized alcohol; then add the oil of star anise, filter, and pass enough deodorized alcohol through the filter to make the product measure one (1) gallon.

Note.—When good, fresh essential oils cannot be readily obtained for preparing the compound spirit of orange, the second formula may be used. But the product obtained by it should not be employed in mixtures containing iron, as the latter would cause a darkening of the mixture.

2851. Spiritus Aurantii Compositus.
N. F.
Compound Spirit of Orange.

Oil bitter orange peel	4 fl. ounces.
Oil of lemon	1 fl. ounce.
Oil of coriander	160 minims.
Oil of star anise	40 minims.
Deodorized alcohol enough to make	20 fl. ounces.

Mix them.

Note.—One fluid ounce of this spirit and 15 fluid ounces of deodorized alcohol make 1 pint of aromatic spirit. (See No. 2850.)

The essential oils used in this preparation, particularly those of orange and lemon, must be as fresh as possible, and absolutely free from any terebinthinate odor or taste. They should be diluted as soon as received, with a definite quantity of deodorized alcohol, which will retard deterioration. They should not be kept in stock, undiluted, for any length of time, or should at least be kept in bottles completely filled, and in a dark place. The alcoholic solution should be kept in the same manner. If oil of curacao orange of good quality can be obtained, it is advisable to use this, in place of ordinary oil of orange, as it imparts to the spirit a finer flavor than the latter.

2852. Spiritus Cardamomi Compositus.
N. F.
Compound Spirit of Cardamom.

Oil of cardamom,*	12 minims.
Oil of caraway	4 minims.
Oil of cinnamon, cassia	2 minims.
Alcohol	8 fl. ounces.
Glycerin	1 fl. ounce.
Water, enough to make	16 fl. ounces.

*The oil of cardamom may be replaced by 180 grains of freshly-bruised cardamom, and macerating for two days in the alcoholic solution of the oils.

Dissolve the oils in the alcohol, add the glycerin, and, lastly, enough water to make sixteen (16) fluid ounces.

Note.—This preparation is intended as a flavoring ingredient, being equivalent to the officinal tinctura cardamomi composita, without the coloring matter.

2853. Spiritus Curassao.
N. F.
Spirit of Curacao.

Oil of curacao orange	2 fl. ounces.
Oil of fennel	15 minims.
Oil of bitter almond	3 minims.
Deodorized alcohol	10 fl. ounces.

Mix the oils with the deodorized alcohol, and keep the spirit in completely-filled and well-corked bottles, and stored in a cool and dark place.

Note.—The essential oils used in this case must be as fresh as possible, and absolutely free from any terebinthinate odor or taste. Oil of curacao orange may be obtained without difficulty in the market, but it should be carefully examined as to its quality, immediately upon receipt, and should not be kept in stock for any length of time, without special precautions (see Note to No. 2851). A still finer quality of oil of orange is that derived from citrus nobilis, which is known in the market as oil of mandarin.

2854. Spiritus Glonoini.
Spirit of Glonoin.
Spirit of Nitroglycerin.   Solution of Nitroglycerin.

A solution of glonoin (or nitroglycerin) in officinal alcohol, containing one (1) per cent, by weight, of the former.

Note.—The specific gravity of this spirit, at 15° C. (59° F.) is 0.828. On mixing 10 C.c. of the solution with distilled water, in a test-tube having a diameter of ¾ inch, both liquids being at the temperature of 15° C. (59° F.), it will require about 16 C.c. of the water to render the liquid faintly turbid (when compared with the undiluted solution);

and about 4 C.c. more of water will be required to render it so opalescent that the eye cannot distinguish print placed behind the tube.

Glonoin (or nitroglycerin), for medical purposes, is usually procured by wholesale dealers in drugs directly from the factory where it is made, in form of a 10 per cent solution in alcohol. Such a solution is non-explosive, and may be diluted, as occasion requires, to the strength of 1 per cent. The specific gravity of the 10 per cent solution is 0.863 at 15° C. (59° F.). Ten C.c. of it require about 2.5 C.c. of distilled water to render it so opalescent that print cannot be distinguished through it under the conditions just described in the case of the 1 per cent solution.

Solutions of Glonoin, particularly the stronger (10 per cent), should always be transported or kept in tin cans, and never in glass or other fragile vessels. Should the container of a solution of glonoin be broken, and the contents be soaked up by wood, or packing material, the latter may become dangerously explosive when the alcohol has evaporated. Should the proportion of glonoin to porous material be not more than 70 parts of the former, and not less than 30 parts of the latter, the compound will be non-explosive (except by a detonator); and if the proportions are not more than 52 parts of the former, and not less than 48 parts of the latter, the compound cannot even be detonated. But, in presence of substances readily yielding oxygen, such as nitrates, chlorates, etc., so small a proportion as 5 per cent of glonoin will produce a dangerously explosive combination.

When handling an alcoholic solution of glonoin, care should be taken that it be not brought in prolonged or extended contact with the skin, as it is readily absorbed, and will then cause its characteristic physiological effects (distressing headache, nausea, etc.).

2855. Spiritus Olei Volatilis.
N. F.
Spirit of a Volatile Oil

Any spirit or alcoholic solution of a volatile oil, for which no formula is given by the U. S. Pharm. or by this Formulary, should be prepared in accordance with the following general formula:

Any volatile oil.............. 400 minims.
Deodorized alcohol, enough
  to make................. 16 fl. ounces.

Dissolve the volatile oil in the deodorized alcohol.

Note.—The strength of the spirit thus prepared is approximately 5 per cent by weight, provided the specific gravity of the oil is about 0.900.

2856. Spiritus Ophthalmicus.
N. F.
Ophthalmic Spirit
Alcoholic Eye-Wash.

Oil of lavender.............. 10 minims.
Oil of rosemary............. 30 minims.
Alcohol..................... 1 fl. ounce.

Mix them by agitation, and, if necessary, filter the liquid through paper.

2857. Spiritus Phosphori.
N. F.
Spirit of Phosphorus.
Tincture of Phosphorus

Phosphorus................. 10 grains.
Absolute alcohol, enough to
  make.................... 15 fl. ounces.

To the absolute alcohol, contained in a flask, add the phosphorus, cut into small pieces, and apply a moderate heat, by means of a water-bath, taking care to prevent, as much as possible, any loss of alcohol by evaporation, or making up any loss by adding, from time to time, a little more absolute alcohol. When the phosphorus is dissolved, allow the liquid to become cold, and add enough absolute alcohol, if necessary, to make fifteen (15) fluid ounces. Then transfer the spirit to small, dark amber-colored vials, stopper them securely, and keep them in a cool and dark place.

Each fluid dram contains 1/12 grain of phosphorus, or 14.4 minims contain 1/50 grain of phosphorus.

Note.—The phosphorus should be perfectly translucent, cut and weighed under water, and quickly dried with filtering paper before being dropped into the alcohol. The loss of alcohol, during the heating, may be avoided, and solution effected more expeditiously, by attaching to the flask a well-cooled upright condenser, which will cause the vapor of the alcohol to be condensed, and to flow back into the flask. In the absence of a condenser, a long glass tube, inserted through a tight-fitting cork into the neck of the flask, and maintained in an upright condition, will nearly answer the same purpose.

This preparation is intended for preparing the elixir of phosphorus (see No. 3072). It is unsuited for internal administration without corrigents. Care should be taken that it be not confounded with Thompson's solution of phosphorus.

2858. Spiritus Saponatus.
N. F.
Spirit of Soap

Castile soap, in shavings... 2½ tr. ounces.
Alcohol..................... 9 fl. ounces.
Water, enough to make... 16 fl. ounces.

Introduce the soap into a bottle, add the alcohol and three (3) fluid ounces of water, cork the bottle, and immerse it in hot water, frequently shaking. When the soap is dissolved, allow the bottle and contents to become cold, then add enough water to make sixteen (16) fluid ounces, and filter.

Note.—The spiritus saponatus of the Germ. Pharm. is prepared by saponifying olive oil with potassa, and then adding alcohol and water.

If time permits, the spirit ought to be set aside, in a moderately cold place, for about 12 hours, before it is filtered.

2859. Spiritus Sinapis.
N. F.
Spirit of Mustard
Volatile oil of mustard..... 190 minims.
Alcohol, enough to make.. 16 fl. ounces.
Mix them.

Note.—This preparation is officinal in the Germ. Pharm.

AROMATIC WATERS.

2860. Aqua Anethi.
Dill Water.
Oil of dill .... 15 minims.
Absorbent cotton .... 30 grains.
Distilled water q. s. to
make .... 1 pint.

Drop the oil on the cotton, pick and pack in a percolator or small glass funnel; run the distilled water through slowly until 1 pint is obtained.

2861. Aqua Anisi.
(Anise Water.)
Oil of anise star.......... 15 minims.
Absorbent cotton.......... 30 grains.
Distilled water q. s. to
make .... 1 pint.

Drop the oil on the cotton, pick and pack in a percolator or small glass funnel, run the distilled water through slowly until 1 pint is obtained.

2862. Aqua Aurantii Flor.
(Orange Flower Water.)
Oil of neroli petale....... 20 minims.
Absorbent cotton .... 30 grains.
Distilled water q. s. to
make .... 1 pint.

Drop the oil on the cotton, pick and pack in a percolator or small glass funnel; run the distilled water through slowly until 1 pint is obtained.

2863. Aqua Camphoræ.
(Camphor Water.)
Gum camphor.............. 1 dram.
Alcohol, 188 per cent...... 2 drams.
Absorbent cotton.......... 1 dram.
Distilled water q. s. to
make .... 1 pint.

Dissolve the camphor in the alcohol drop the solution on the cotton, pick and pack in a percolator or small glass funnel; run the water through slowly until 1 pint is obtained.

2864. Aqua Carui.
(Caraway Water.)
Oil of caraway .... 15 minims.
Absorbent cotton .... 30 grains.
Distilled water q. s. to
make .... 1 pint.
Proceed as directed for aqua aurantii.

2865. Aqua Chloroformi.
(Chloroform Water.)
Chloroform .... 1 fl. dram.
Distilled water .... 25 ounces.

Put them into a two-pint stoppered bottle and shake them together until the chloroform is entirely dissolved.

2866. Aqua Cinnamomi.
(Cinnamon Water.)
Oil of cinnamon........... 15 minims.
Absorbent cotton.......... 30 grains.
Distilled water q. s. to
make .... 1 pint.
Proceed as directed for aqua aurantii.

2867. Aqua Creasoti.
(Creasote Water.)
Creasote .... 72 minims.
Distilled water q. s. to
make .... 1 pint.
Proceed as directed for aqua chloroformi.

2868. Aqua Fœniculi.
(Fennel Water.)
Oil of fennel .... 15 minims.
Absorbent cotton.......... 30 grains.
Distilled water q. s. to
make .... 1 pint.
Proceed as directed for aqua cinnamomi.

2869. Aqua Lauro-Cerasi.
(Cherry Laurel Water.)
Oil of bitter almonds, essential .... 20 minims.
Alcohol .... 2 drams.
Absorbent cotton.......... 60 grains.
Distilled water q. s. to
make .... 1 pint
Proceed as directed for aqua camphora.

2870.   **Aqua Menthæ Pip.**
                (Peppermint Water.)
Oil of peppermint.......... 15 minims.
Absorbent cotton.......... 30 grains.
Distilled water q. s. to
   make .... 1 pint.
Proceed as directed for aqua aurantii.

2871.   **Aqua Menthæ Virid.**
                (Spearmint Water.)
Oil of spearmint........... 15 minims.
Absorbent cotton.......... 30 grains.
Distilled water q. s. to
   make .... 1 pint.
Proceed as directed for aqua aurantii.

2872.   **Aqua Pimentæ.**
                (Pimento Water.)
Oil of allspice............. 15 minims.
Absorbent cotton.......... 30 grains.
Distilled water q. s. to
   make .... 1 pint.
Proceed as directed for aqua aurantii.

2873.   **Aqua Rosæ.**
                (Rose Water.)
Oil of rose................ 5 drops.
Absorbent cotton.......... 15 grains.
Distilled water, warm, q. s.
   to make .... 1 pint.
Proceed as directed for aqua aurantii, and run through the warm water; the latter should have a temperature of about 120° F.

WINES—MEDICINAL.

2874.   **Wine of Aloes.**
                U. S. P.
Purified aloes............. 1 ounce.
Cardamom .... 75 grains.
Ginger .... 75 grains.
Alcohol .... q. s.
White wine................ q. s.

Mix the three drugs, reduce to coarse powder, add 2 fluid ounces of alcohol and 14 of wine; macerate for 7 days, agitating occasionally, and filter; add through the filter enough of a mixture of one part of alcohol to 7 of wine by volume to make the filtrate measure 16 fluid ounces.

2875.   **Wine of Beef and Iron.**
Extract of beef............ 256 grains.
Tincture of citro-chloride
   of iron .... 4¼ fl. drams.
Water, hot................ 1 fl. ounce.
Sherry wine, enough to
   make .... 16 fl. ounces.

Pour the hot water on the extract of beef contained in a mortar or other suitable vessel, and triturate until a smooth mixture results. Then gradually add, while stirring, 12 fluid ounces of sherry wine. Next add the tincture and the remainder of the wine. Transfer the mixture to a bottle, set this aside for a few days in a cold place, if convenient, filter, and pass enough sherry wine through the filter to restore the original volume.

2876. Wine of Beef, Iron and Cinchona.
Extract of beef............ 256 grains.
Tincture of citro-chloride
   of iron .... 4½ fl. drams.
Quinine sulphate .... 16 grains.
Cinchonidine sulphate...... 8 grains.
Citric acid .... 6 grains.
Water, hot................ 1 fl. ounce.
Angelica wine, enough to
   make .... 16 fl. ounces.

Dissolve the citric acid and the quinine and cinchonidine sulphates in the hot water, and pour the solution upon the extract of beef contained in a mortar or other suitable vessel. Triturate the liquid with the extract, until they form a smooth mixture, then gradually add, while stirring, 12 fluid ounces of angelica wine, and afterwards the tincture of citrochloride of iron. Transfer the mixture to a bottle, set this aside for a few days in a cold place; if convenient filter, and pass through the filter, the remainder of the angelica wine.

2877. Wine of Beef, Iron and Coca.
Extract of beef............ 256 grains.
Tincture of citro-chloride
   of iron .... 256 minims.
Water, hot................ 1 fl. ounce.
Simple syrup .... 1 fl. ounce.
Fluid extract of coca...... 10½ fl. drams.
Sherry wine, enough to
   make .... 16 fl. ounces.

Triturate the extract of beef with the water until dissolved, add 10 fluid ounces of wine, then the tincture, syrup, fluid extract, and the remainder of the wine, and filter.

Each ½ fluid ounce represents 8 grains of beef extract, 8 minims of tincture of iron, and 20 minims of coca.

2878.   **Wine of Cinchona.**
                Germ. Pharm.
Yellow cinchona, coarse
   powder .... ¾ ounce.
Port wine .... 16 fl. ounces.
Macerate for 8 days and filter.

2879. Wine of Cinchona Co.
Codex.

Yellow cinchona	1¾ ounces.
Bitter orange peel	75 grains.
Chamomile flowers	75 grains.
Alcohol, 188 per cent	4½ fl. ounces.
White wine	13 fl. ounces.

Bruise the drugs, macerate in the mixed alcohol and wine for 10 days, agitating occasionally, and filter.

2880. Wine of Cinchona and Cocoa.

Fluid extract of yellow cinchona	1 fl. ounce.
Tincture of cocoa	1 fl. ounce.
Simple syrup	2 fl. ounces.
Angelica wine	12 fl. ounces.

Mix and filter if necessary.

2881. Wine of Creasote.

Glycerite of creasote	4 fl. ounces.
Simple syrup	2½ fl. ounces.
Water	4 fl. ounces.
White wine	5½ fl. ounces.

This contains 2½ per cent of creasote.

2882. Wine of Creasote Co.

Creasote	2 fl. drams.
Alcohol	4 fl. drams.
Tincture of gentian	5 fl. ounces.
Sherry wine, enough to make	16 fl. ounces.

2883. Wine of Damiana.
Wine of Turnera.

Fluid extract of damiana	3 fl. ounces.
Simple elixir	3 fl. ounces.
Sherry wine	10 fl. ounces.

Mix and filter if necessary.

2884. Wine of Golden Seal Co.
Wine Bitters Eclectic.

Golden seal	20 grains.
Tulip tree bark	20 grains.
Bitter root (dogsbane)	20 grains.
Prickly ash berries	10 grains.
Sassafras bark	10 grains.
Capsicum	10 grains.
Sherry wine	q. s.

Extract the mixed drugs in coarse powder by percolation with the wine so as to obtain 16 fluid ounces.

2885. Wine of Iron.—Bitter.
U. S. P.

Iron and quinine citrate soluble	360 grains.
Tincture of sweet orange peel	2½ fl. ounces.
Simple syrup	5 ounces.
White wine, enough to make	16 fl. ounces.

Dissolve the iron and quinine citrate in 8 fluid ounces of wine, add to this the tincture, syrup, and remainder of the wine, set aside for several days, and filter.

2886. Wine of Iron.—Sweet.

Cinchona, powdered	60 grains.
Bitter orange peel, powdered	30 grains.
Citric acid	30 grains.
Citrate of iron soluble	120 grains.
Water	3½ fl. ounces.
Sherry wine	7 fl. ounces.
Tincture of sweet orange peel	3½ fl. ounces.
Simple syrup	14 fl. drams.

Mix the tincture with the water and with this percolate the mixed cinchona and orange peel, adding enough of the same menstruum to make 7 fluid ounces, add to this the citric acid and iron salt dissolved in the wine, then add the syrup and filter.

2887. Wine of Iron and Quinine Citrate.

Citrate of iron and quinine	48 grains.
Water, hot	2 fl. ounces.
Syrup of lemon	2 fl. ounces.
Sherry wine, enough to make	16 fl. ounces.

Dissolve the iron and quinine citrate in the water, add the other ingredients and filter if necessary.

2888. Wine of Iron and Potassium Tartrate.

Tartrate of iron and potassium	160 grains.
Water, hot	4 fl. drams.
Water of ammonia	q. s.
Angelica wine, enough to make	16 fl. ounces.

Dissolve the salt in the water, carefully neutralize the acid in the wine with ammonia water; mix the two liquids, and filter.

2889. Wine of Iron Citrate.
U. S. P.

Iron citrate, soluble	288 grains.
Tincture of sweet orange peel	2½ fl. ounces.

Simple syrup .... 13 fl. ounces.
White wine, enough to
 make .... 16 fl. ounces.

Dissolve the iron salt in 12 fluid ounces of wine, to this add the tincture, syrup, and remander of the wine, set the mixture aside for several days and filter.

2890. Wine of Orange.

Oil of orange.............. 5 minims.
Alcohol, 188 per cent..... 4 fl. drams
Magnesium carbonate..... 240 grains.
Simple syrup .... 2 fl. ounces.
Sherry wine............... 13½ fl. ounces.

Dissolve the oil in the alcohol, triturate with the magnesium carbonate, add the other ingredients and filter.

2891. Wine of Pancreatin.

Pancreatin, pure.......... 160 grains.
Simple elixir .... 5 fl. ounces.
Sherry wine............... 11 fl. ounces.

Macerate the pancreatin in the elixir for 24 hours, then add the wine and filter.

2892. Wine of Quinine.
Brit. Pharm.

Quinine sulphate .... 16 grains.
Citric acid .... 24 grains.
Orange wine .... 16 fl. ounces.

Mix, let stand for 3 days, agitating occasionally, and filter.

2893. Wine of Wormwood.—Codex.
Wine of Absinthium.

Wormwood, cut .... ½ ounce.
Alcohol, 188 per cent...... 1 fl. ounce.
Sherry wine............... 16 fl. ounces.

Mix, macerate for 7 days, agitating occasionally, and filter.

MISCELLANEOUS ELIXIRS.

2894. Elixir of Aletris.

Fluid extract of aletris
 farinosa .... 2 fl. ounces.
Simple elixir.............. 14 fl. ounces.

Mix, let stand for several days, and filter. Each fluid dram represents 7½ grains of aletris farinosa.

2895. Elixir of Ammonium Chloride.

Ammonium chloride....... 1280 grains.
Simple elixir, enough to
 make .... 16 fl. ounces.

Dissolve by agitation, and filter if necessary.

Each fluid dram contains 10 grains of ammonium chloride.

2896. Elixir of Ammonium Chloride and Licorice, Compound.

Ammonium chloride ...... 640 grains.
Compound elixir of licorice.
 enough to make .... 16 ounces.

Dissolve by agitation, and filter if necessary.

Each fluid dram contains 5 grains of ammonium chloride.

2897. Elixir of Ammonium, Quinine and Strychnine Valerianates.

Strychnine (alkaloid)....... 1¼ grains.
Valerianic acid .... q. s.
Quinine valerianate .... 64 grains.
Elixir of ammonium valerianate, N. F., enough to
 make .... 16 ounces.

Dissolve the strychnine in 2 fluid drams of the elixir of ammonium valerianate by the aid of a slight excess of valerianic acid. Triturate the quinine salt with this solution and add the remainder of the elixir of ammonium valerianate, agitate occasionally until dissolved, then filter.

In case the valerianic acid is in such excess that its odor is perceptible, the liquid must be cautiously neutralized by stirring it with a glass rod which is repeatedly moistened with very dilute ammonia water. Any excess of the latter must be avoided, as otherwise alkaloidal strychnine will be precipitated.

Each fluid dram contains 1-100 grain of strychnine valerianate, ¼ grain of quinine valerianate and 2 grains of ammonium valerianate.

2898. Elixir of Ammonium Valerianate with Sumbul.

(Elixir of Ammonium Valerianate with Musk Root.)

Fluid extract of sumbul... 2 ounces.
Elixir of ammonium valerianate.................. 14 ounces.

Mix, let stand for several hours and filter through purified talcum.

Each fluid dram contains nearly 2 grains of ammonium valerianate and represents 7½ grains of sumbul root.

2899. Elixir of Ammonium Valerianate with Strychnine.

Strychnine sulphate .... 1¼ grains.
Elixir of ammonium valerianate .... 16 fl. ounces.

Mix, dissolve by agitation, and filter.

2900. Elixir of Ammonium Valerianate with Cinchonidine, Iron Pyrophosphate and Quinine.

Iron pyrophosphate, soluble 64 grains.
Distilled water, hot........ 4 fl. drams.
Elixir of ammonium valerianate, with cinchonidine and quinine, enough to make .... 16 fl. ounces.

Dissolve the iron salt in the water and add the elixir.

Each fluid dram contains nearly 2 grains of ammonium valerianate, ½ grain of cinchonidine sulphate, and ¼ grain of quinine hydrochlorate, as well as ¼ grain of iron pyrophosphate.

2901. Elixir of Ammonium Valerianate with Cinchonidine, Iron Pyrophosphate Quinine and Strychnine.

Strychnine sulphate........ 1¼ grains.
Distilled water............. 2 drams.
Elixir of ammonium valerianate, cinchonidine, iron pyrophosphate, and quinine, enough to make.... 16 ounces.

Dissolve the strychnine salt in the water and add the elixir.

2902. Elixir of Ammonium Valerianate with Cinchonidine and Quinine.

Quinine hydrochlorate...... 32 grains.
Cinchonidine sulphate...... 64 grains.
Elixir of ammonium valerianate, N. F., enough to make .... 16 ounces.

Mix, dissolve by agitation and filter.

Each fluid dram contains 2 grains of ammonium valerianate, ½ grain of cinchonidine sulphate and ¼ grain of quinine hydrochlorate.

2903. Elixir of Ammonium Valerianate with Cinchonidine, Quinine and Strychnine.

Strychnine sulphate .... 1¼ grains.
Distilled water .... 2 drams.
Elixir of ammonium valerianate with cinchonidine and quinine, enough to make .... 16 ounces.

Dissolve the strychnine in the water and add the elixir.

2904. Elixir of Ammonium Valerianate with Cinchonidine and Strychnine.

Strychnine sulphate........ 1¼ grains.
Distilled water .... 2 drams.
Elixir of ammonium valerianate with cinchonidine, enough to make.......... 16 ounces.

Dissolve the strychnine sulphate in the water, add the elixir and filter if necessary.

Each fluid dram contains 1-100 grain of strychnine sulphate, ½ grain of cinchonidine sulphate and 2 grains of ammonium valerianate.

2905. Elixir of Ammonium Valerianate and Iron.

Iron pyrophosphate, soluble 128 grains.
Distilled water, hot........ 1 ounce.
Elixir of ammonium valerianate, N. F................ 15 ounces.

2906. Elixir of Ammonium Valerianate with Iron, Quinine and Strychnine.

Strychnine sulphate........ 1¼ grains.
Distilled water .... 2 drams.
Elixir of ammonium valerianate with iron and quinine, enough to make.... 16 ounces.

Dissolve the strychnine sulphate in the water and add the elixir.

2907. Elixir of Antifebrin.

Acetanilid .... 128 grains.
Simple elixir .... 16 ounces.

Dissolve by agitation. Each fluid dram contains one grain of antifebrin.

2908. Elixir of Antipyrin.

Antipyrin .... 640 grains.
Simple elixir .... 16 ounces.

Dissolve by agitation.

Each fluid dram contains 5 grains of antipyrin.

2909. Elixir of Arsenic and Quinine.

Solution of arsenious acid.. 10½ drams.
Quinine sulphate........... 128 grains.
Simple elixir, enough to make .... 16 ounces.

Dissolve by agitation and filter if necessary.

Each fluid dram contains 1-20 grain of arsenious acid, and 2 grains of quinine sulphate.

2910. Elixir of Arsenic and Strychnine.

Solution of arsenious acid.. 10½ fl. drams.
Strychnine sulphate........ 1¼ grains.
Simple elixir, enough to make .... 16 fl. ounces.

Dissolve by agitation and filter.

Each fluid dram contains 1-20 grain of arsenious acid, and 1-100 grain of strychnine sulphate.

2911.   Elixir of Beef.

    Extract of beef............ 256 grains.
    Distilled water............ 1 fl. ounce.
    Simple elixir, enough to
      make .... 16 fl. ounces.

Dissolve the extract in the water, add the elixir, let stand for several days if possible, and filter.

Each fluid dram contains 2 grains of extract of beef.

The extract of beef suitable for this and similar preparations is that which is prepared by Liebig's method.

2912.   Elixir Aurantii.
           U. S. P.

    Oil of orange peel......... 2½ fl. drams.
    Cotton .... ½ ounce.
    Sugar, in coarse powder.... 25 ounces.
    Alcohol ....
    Water q. s. to make........ 4 pints.

Mix alcohol and water in the proportion of 1 pint of alcohol to 2½ pints of water. Add the oil of orange to the cotton, in small portions at a time; distributing it thoroughly by picking the cotton apart after each addition; then pack tightly in a conical percolator, and gradually pour on the mixture of alcohol and water, until 3¼ pints of filtered liquid are obtained. In this liquid dissolve the sugar by agitation, without heat, and strain.

2913.   Elixir of Beef and Iron.

    Citrate of iron and am-
      monium .... 128 grains.
    Distilled water, warm...... 1 fl. ounce.
    Elixir of beef, enough to
      make .... 16 fl. ounces.

Dissolve the iron salt in the water and add the elixir.

Each fluid dram contains 1 grain of iron salt and 1¾ grains of extract of beef.

2914. Elixir of Beef, Iron and Malt.

    Extract of beef............ 256 grains.
    Extract of malt (thick).... 4 av. ounces.
    Citrate of iron and am-
      monium .... 128 grains.
    Spirit of orange........... 1 fl. dram.
    Alcohol .... 2 fl. ounces.
    Sherry wine................ 9 fl. ounces.
    Water...................... } of each
    Ferric hydrate............. } sufficient.

Dissolve the extract of beef in one fluid ounce of hot water, and add the alcohol containing the spirit of orange, then the wine with which the malt extract has previously been mixed; shake frequently during 2 or 3 days, filter, and wash the filter with a mixture of alcohol and water in the proportion of 1 of the former to 4 of the latter by measure, so as to obtain a filtrate of 15 fluid ounces. Dissolve the iron salt in 6 fluid drams of water, add to the filtrate, and then add enough water to make 16 fluid ounces.

The ferric hydrate may be prepared as described under the heading of elixir of gentian; the amount to be used must be sufficient to detannate the mixture, and if an insufficient amount has been used, more must be added, allowing to stand for several days more. The test to be applied is the usual one—filtering a small amount of liquid and testing the filtrate with solution of iron chloride to note if any discoloration occur.

2915.   Elixir of Berberine.

    Berberine phosphate....... 32 grains.
    Distilled water, hot...... 1 fl. ounce.
    Simple elixir .... 15 fl. ounces.

Dissolve the berberine in the water and add the elixir.

Each fluid dram contains ¼ grain of berberine phosphate.

2916.   Elixir of Berberine and Iron.

    Iron pyrophosphate, soluble 128 grains.
    Distilled water, hot....... 1 fl. ounce.
    Elixir of berberine, enough
      to make .... 16 fl. ounces.

Dissolve the iron salt in the water, add the elixir, and filter if necessary.

Each fluid dram contains 1 grain of iron pyrophosphate and nearly ¼ grain of berberine phosphate.

2917.   Elixir of Bismuth.

    Bismuth subnitrate........ 180 grains.
    Nitric acid, C. P......... 3 fl. drams.
    Tartaric acid............. ⎫
    Sodium bicarbonate, C. P.. ⎬ of each
    Distilled water........... ⎭ sufficient.
    Simple elixir, enough to
      make .... 16 fl. ounces

Mix 3 fluid drams of nitric acid with an equal measure of distilled water, and to this add the bismuth subnitrate, stirring until solution is effected; add enough distilled water to make 3 fluid ounces. Now dissolve 135 grains of tartaric acid in 12 fluid drams of distilled water, and pour this into the bismuth solution, stirring constantly during mixing. To this mixture gradually add 150 grains of sodium bicarbonate, stirring constantly during mixing. Dilute the magma thus obtained with 5 fluid ounces of distilled water, and after the lapse of several hours, pour the whole upon a plain filter; allow the liquid to drain, and wash the precipitate with distilled water until the washings pass tasteless.

Now mix 150 grains of sodium bicarbonate with 1 fluid ounce of distilled water, and add 135 grains of tartaric acid gradually, with constant stirring. When reaction has ceased, and a clear solution has formed, add the washed precipitate of bismuth tartrate and stir until it is dissolved. Now add enough distilled water to make 3 fluid ounces and then the elixir. Allow to stand for 24 hours and filter.

The 3 fluid ounces of solution to which elixir is added is a solution of tartrate of bismuth and sodium, and may be used to advantage, instead of citrate of bismuth and ammonium, in all preparations containing a soluble compound of bismuth.

Each of the elixirs of bismuth contains about 2 grains of the respective bismuth salt.

2918. Elixir of Bismuth and Cinchona.

Citrate of bismuth and ammonium .... 128 grains.
Distilled water, hot........ 4 fl. drams.
Ammonia water .... sufficient.
Detannated elixir of cinchona, N. F., enough to make .... 16 fl. ounces.

Mix the bismuth salt with the hot water, allow the solution to stand to permit any undissolved matter to subside; decant the clear liquid and add to the residue just enough ammonia water to dissolve. Mix this solution with the decanted liquid, and if alkaline, neutralize the mixture with dilute solution of citric acid gradually added. To the whole add the elixir of cinchona, let stand 24 hours, and filter if necessary.

Each fluid dram contains 1 grain of bismuth salt and represents 1½ grains of calisaya.

2919. Elixir of Bismuth, Cinchona, Iron and Pepsin.

Citrate of bismuth and ammonium .... 128 grains.
Detannated tincture of cinchona .... 2½ fl. ounces
Iron pyrophosphate, soluble 256 grains.
Pepsin, pure................ 128 grains.
Distilled water, hot........ 1½ fl. ounces.
Aromatic spirit............ 1 fl. ounce.
Simple syrup .... 5 fl. ounces.
Simple elixir, enough to make .... 16 fl. ounces.
Water of ammonia......... sufficient.

Add the bismuth salt to 4 fluid drams of the water, triturate well for a moment, allow to stand until the insoluble portion subsides, decant the clear liquid, carefully add to the residue just sufficient ammonia water to dissolve it, carefully avoiding any excess, and mix this solution with the decanted portion.

Add the pepsin to 5 fluid ounces of simple elixir and agitate occasionally until dissolved; also dissolve the iron salt in the remainder of the water.

Now mix the three liquids, add the tincture, the spirit, syrup, and the remainder of the elixir, allow to stand for 24 hours, and filter.

Each fluid dram represents 1 grain each of citrate of bismuth and ammonium and of pepsin, nearly 2 grains of cinchona, and 2 grains of iron pyrophosphate.

2920. Elixir of Bismuth, Cinchona, Iron Pepsin and Strychnine.

Strychnine sulphate........ 1¼ grains.
Distilled water............. 4 fl. drams.
Elixir of bismuth, cinchona, iron and pepsin... 15½ fl. ounces.

Dissolve the strychnine sulphate in the water, add the elixir, and filter.

2921. Elixir of Bismuth, Cinchona and Pepsin.

Detannated tincture of cinchona .... 2½ fl. ounces
Citrate of bismuth and ammonium .... 128 grains.
Pepsin, pure .... 128 grains.
Distilled water, hot........ 4 fl. drams.
Water of ammonia ..... sufficient.
Aromatic spirit .... 1 fl. ounce.
Simple syrup .... 4 fl. ounces.
Simple elixir, enough to make .... 16 fl. ounces.

Triturate the citrate of bismuth and ammonium with the water, allow to stand until the insoluble matter subsides, to the residue add ammonia water until solution takes place, carefully avoiding any excess, and mix the two liquids. Add the pepsin to 7 fluid ounces of elixir, agitate occasionally until dissolved; mix this with the preceding liquid, add the tincture, spirit, syrup and remainder of the elixir, allow to stand for 24 hours, and filter.

Each fluid dram represents nearly 2 grains of cinchona, and contains 1 grain each of pepsin, and of citrate of bismuth and ammonium.

2922. Elixir of Bismuth and Gentian.

Citrate of bismuth and ammonium	128 grains.
Distilled water, hot	4 fl. drams
Ammonia water	sufficient.
Elixir of gentian, N. F., enough to make	16 fl. ounces.

Treat the bismuth salt as described under elixir of bismuth and cinchona, add the elixir of gentian, allow to stand for 24 hours, and filter if necessary.

Each fluid dram contains 1 grain of bismuth salt and represents about 2 grains of gentian.

2923. Elixir of Bismuth, Gentian and Iron.

Citrate of bismuth and ammonium	128 grains.
Distilled water, hot	4 fl. drams.
Ammonia water	sufficient
Elixir of gentian and iron phosphate, enough to make	16 fl. ounces.

Treat the bismuth salt as in the preceding elixir, add the elixir of gentian and iron, let stand 24 hours, and filter if necessary.

Each fluid dram contains 1 grain of bismuth salt and nearly 1 grain of iron phosphate, and represents about 1½ grains of gentian.

2924. Elixir of Bismuth, Gentian, Iron and Strychnine.

Strychnine sulphate	1¼ grains.
Distilled water	4 fl. drams.
Elixir of bismuth, gentian and iron, enough to make	16 fl. ounces.

Dissolve the strychnine in the water, add the elixir, let stand a few hours and filter.

Each fluid dram contains 1-100 grain of strychnine sulphate, nearly 1 grain bismuth salt and nearly 1 grain of iron phosphate, and represents about 1½ grains of gentian.

2925. Elixir of Bismuth, Gentian and Strychnine.

Strychnine sulphate	1¼ grains.
Distilled water	4 fl. drams.
Elixir of bismuth and gentian, enough to make	16 fl. ounces.

Dissolve the strychnine in the water, add the elixir, let stand a few hours, and filter.

Each fluid dram contains 1-100 grain of strychnine sulphate, and nearly 1 grain of bismuth salt and represents about 1½ grains of gentian.

2926. Elixir of Bismuth, Golden Seal and Iron.

Iron pyrophosphate, soluble	128 grains.
Glycerite of hydrastis	1 fl. ounce.
Distilled water, hot	4 fl. drams.
Elixir of bismuth, enough to make	16 fl. ounces.

Dissolve the iron salt in the water, and the glycerite and elixir, let stand for a day or two, and filter. The elixir must be perfectly neutral.

Each fluid dram contains 1 grain of iron pyrophosphate, and nearly 2 grains of bismuth salt and represents 3¾ grains of hydrastis.

2927. Elixir of Bismuth and Golden Seal.

(Elixir of Bismuth and Hydrastis.)

| Glycerite of hydrastis | 1 fl. ounce. |
| Elixir of bismuth | 15 fl. ounces. |

Mix, let stand for several days if possible, and filter. The elixir of bismuth must be exactly neutral before adding the glycerite.

Each fluid dram represents 3¾ grains of hydrastis and contains nearly 2 grains of citrate of bismuth and ammonium.

2928. Elixir Bismuth and Iron.

Iron pyrophosphate, soluble	128 grains.
Distilled water, hot	4 fl. drams.
Elixir of bismuth	8 fl. ounces.
Simple elixir, enough to make	16 fl. ounces.

Dissolve the iron salt in water and add the elixirs.

Each fluid dram contains 1 grain each of iron pyrophosphate and bismuth salt.

2929. Elixir of Bismuth, Iron and Pepsin.

Citrate of bismuth and ammonium	128 grains.
Iron pyrophosphate	128 grains.
Pepsin, pure	128 grains.
Distilled water, hot	1 fl. ounce.
Water of ammonia	sufficient.
Simple elixir, enough to make	16 fl. ounces.

Triturate the bismuth with 4 fluid drams of water, allow the insoluble matter to subside, decant the clear liquid, to the residue add gradually ammonia water until solution occurs, carefully avoiding any excess, and mix this with the decanted portion. Dissolve the iron pyrophosphate in the remainder of the water; also dissolve the pepsin in 12 fluid ounces of elixir by frequent agitation. Mix the three liquids, add the remainder of the elixir, and filter.

Each fluid dram contains 1 grain each of iron pyrophosphate, pepsin, and citrate of bismuth and ammonium.

2930. Elixir of Bismuth, Iron, Pepsin and Quinine.

Quinine hydrochlorate ... 32 grains.
Elixir of bismuth, iron and
  pepsin .... 16 fl. ounces.

Mix, dissolve by agitation, and filter, if necessary.

Each fluid dram contains 1 grain each of pepsin, iron pyrophosphate and citrate of bismuth and ammonium and ¼ grain of quinine hydrochlorate.

2931. Elixir of Bismuth, Iron and Strychnine.

Iron pyrophosphate, soluble 128 grains.
Strychnine sulphate ...... 1¼ grains.
Distilled water............ 1 fl. ounce.
Elixir of bismuth......... 8 fl. ounces.
Simple elixir, enough to
  make .... 16 fl. ounces.

Dissolve the iron salt and strychnine salt separately in 4 fluid drams of the water; add the two elixirs, and filter if necessary. The elixir of bismuth must be perfectly neutral.

Each fluid dram contains 1-100 grain of strychnine sulphate and 1 grain each of iron pyrophosphate and bismuth salt.

2932. Elixir of Bismuth, Nux Vomica and Pepsin.

Tincture of nux vomica... 5½ fl. drams.
Elixir of pepsin and bismuth, N. F., enough to
  make .... 16 fl. ounces.

Each fluid dram contains 1 grain each of pepsin and 2 grains of citrate of bismuth and ammonium and represents about ½ grain of nux vomica.

2933. Elixir of Bismuth and Pancreatin.

Citrate of bismuth and ammonium .... 128 grains.
Pancreatin, pure .... 128 grains.
Distilled water............ 1 fl. ounce.
Water of ammonia ....sufficient.
Tincture of cudbear....... 2 fl. drams.
Simple elixir, enough to
  make .... 16 fl. ounces.

Triturate the bismuth salt with the water, allow the insoluble portion to subside, decant the clear liquid, add sufficient ammonia water to dissolve the residue, add this solution and the decanted portion to 12 fluid ounces of elixir mixed with the tincture, then add the pancreatin, agitate occasionally until the latter is apparently dissolved, filter in a well-covered funnel, and add enough elixir through the filter to make the filtrate measure 16 fluid ounces.

Each fluid dram contains 1 grain each of pancreatin and citrate of bismuth and ammonium.

2934. Elixir of Bismuth, Pepsin and Quinine.

Quinine hydrochlorate..... 32 grains.
Elixir of pepsin and bismuth, N. F............. 16 fl. ounces.

Mix and dissolve by agitation.

Each fluid dram contains ¼ grain of quinine, hydrochlorate of pepsin, and 2 grains of citrate of bismuth and ammonium.

2935. Elixir of Bismuth and Quinine.

Quinine hydrochlorate..... 32 grains.
Elixir of bismuth, enough
  to make .... 16 fl. ounces.

Dissolve the quinine salt in the elixir (which should be neutral) by agitation and filter, if necessary.

Each fluid dram contains 1 grain of quinine hydrochlorate and 2 grains of bismuth salt.

2936. Elixir of Bismuth and Strychnine.

Strychnine sulphate....... 1¼ grains.
Distilled water .... 4 fl. drams.
Elixir of bismuth......... 15½ fl. ounces.

Dissolve the alkaloidal salt in the water and add to the elixir, which latter should be neutral.

Each fluid dram contains 1-100 grain of strychnine sulphate and nearly 2 grains of bismuth salt.

2937. Elixir, Bitter.

(Elixir Amarum.)
Germ. Pharm.

Extract of wormwood..... 3¼ av. ounces
Oleosaccharate of peppermint .... 1¾ av. ounces
Aromatic tincture, N. F. 1¾ fl. ounces.
Bitter tincture, N. F...... 1¾ fl. ounces.
Water................... 8½ fl. ounces.

Triturate the extract and oleosaccharate with the water to a smooth condition and add the other ingredients. This preparation should be cloudy and of a dark brown color.

NON-SECRET FORMULAS.

2938. Elixir of Blackberry.
Fluid extract of rubus.... 2 fl. ounces.
Tincture of vanilla .... 4 fl. drams.
Compound elixir of taraxa-
 cum .... 4 fl. ounces.
Simple elixir, enough to
 make .... 16 fl. ounces.
Each fluid dram represents 7½ grains of blackberry root bark.

2939. Elixir of Black Haw.
(Elixir of Viburnum Prunifolium.)
Fluid extract of black haw 2 fl. ounces.
Compound tincture of car-
 damom.................. 9½ fl. drams.
Aromatic elixir, enough to
 make .... 16 fl. ounces.
Mix, allow the mixture to stand a few days, if convenient, and filter.

2940. Elixir of Black Cohosh.
(Elixir of Cimicifuga.)
Fluid extract of black
 cohosh .... 4 fl. ounces.
Alcohol .... 1 fl. ounce.
Simple elixir .... 11 fl. ounces.
Mix, let stand 24 hours, and filter through purified talcum.
Each fluid dram represents 7½ grains of cimicifuga.

2941. Elixir of Black Haw, Compound.
(Compound Elixir of Viburnum Prunifolium.)
Fluid extract of black haw 2 fl. ounces.
Fluid extract of hydrastis. 2 fl. ounces.
Fluid extract of Jamaica
 dogwood .... 1 fl. ounce.
Simple elixir .... 11 fl. ounces.
Mix, allow to stand for 24 hours and filter.
Each fluid dram represents 7½ grains each of black haw and golden seal and 3¾ grains of Jamaica dogwood.

2942. Elixir of Blue Flag.
Fluid extract of blue flag. 4 fl. ounces.
Alcohol .... 1 fl. ounce.
Simple elixir .... 11 fl. ounces.
Mix, allow to stand for 24 hours, and filter.
Each fluid dram represents 15 grains of blue flag.

2943. Elixir of Blue Flag and Wahoo.
Fluid extract of blue flag. 2¾ fl. ounces.
Fluid extract of wahoo.... 2¾ fl. ounces.
Alcohol .... ½ fl. ounce.
Simple elixir .... 10 fl. ounces.
Mix, allow to stand for 24 hours and filter through talcum.
Each fluid dram represents about 10 grains each of blue flag and wahoo.

2944. Elixir of Three (or Triple) Bromides.
Potassium bromide .... 128 grains.
Sodium bromide .... 128 grains.
Elixir of caffeine, enough
 to make .... 16 fl. ounces.
Mix, dissolve by agitation, and filter, if necessary.
Each fluid dram contains 8 grains of each of the bromides of potassium, sodium, and caffeine.

2945. Elixir of Six Bromides.
Potassium bromide......... 640 grains.
Sodium bromide .... 640 grains.
Ammonium bromide ...... 384 grains.
Calcium bromide .... 192 grains.
Lithium bromide .... 64 grains.
Iron bromide .... 64 grains.
Compound tincture of car-
 bear .... 2 fl. drams.
Simple elixir, enough to
 make .... 16 fl. ounces.
Dissolve by agitation and filter, if necessary.
Each fluid dram contains 5 grains each of potassium and sodium bromides, 3 grains of ammonium bromide, 1½ grains of calcium bromide, and 1 grain each of lithium and iron bromides.

2946. Elixir of Bromide of Zinc.
Zinc bromide .... 128 grains.
Citric acid .... 3 grains.
Simple elixir .... 16 fl. ounces.
Dissolve by agitation and filter, if necessary.
Each fluid dram contains 1 grain of zinc bromide.

2947. Elixir of Buchu and Juniper, Compound.
(Rheumatic Elixir.)
Fluid extract of buchu .... 6½ fl. drams.
Fluid extract of barberry
 bark .... 3¼ fl. drams.
Fluid extract of juniper
 berries.................. 3¼ fl. drams.
Sodium salicylate .... 160 grains.
Simple syrup .... 1 fl. ounce.
Alcohol .... 1 fl. ounce.
Simple elixir enough to
 make .... 16 fl. ounces.
Mix all, let stand for 24 hours, and filter through purified talcum.
Each fluid dram contains 1¼ grains of sodium salicylate, and represents 3 grains of buchu, and 1½ grains each of barberry bark and juniper berries.

2948. Elixir of Buchu, Juniper and Potassium Acetate.

Fluid extract of buchu	12 fl. drams.
Fluid extract of juniper berries	4 fl. drams.
Potassium acetate	192 grains.
Alcohol	1 fl. ounce.
Simple syrup	1 fl. ounce.
Simple elixir	12 fl. ounces.

Mix, allow to stand for 24 hours and filter through talcum.

Each fluid dram contains 1½ grains of potassium acetate, and represents about 5½ grains of buchu, and 2 grains of juniper berries.

2949. Elixir of Buchu, Juniper, Uva Ursi and Potassium Acetate.

Fluid extract of buchu	2 fl. ounces.
Fluid extract of uva ursi	11 fl. drams.
Fluid extract of juniper berries	5½ fl. drams.
Potassium acetate	1½ av ounces.
Alcohol	1 fl. ounce.
Simple syrup	1 fl. ounce.
Simple elixir, enough to make	16 fl. ounces.

Mix, allow to stand for 24 hours, and filter through purified talcum.

Each fluid dram contains 5 grains of potassium acetate, and represents 7½ grains of buchu, 5 grains of uva ursi, and 2½ of juniper berries.

2950. Elixir of Buchu and Pareira.

Fluid extract of buchu	2 fl. ounces.
Fluid extract of pareira brava	2 fl. ounces.
Alcohol	1 fl. ounce.
Simple syrup	1 fl. ounce.
Simple elixir	10 fl. ounces.

Mix, allow to stand for 24 hours, and filter through purified talcum.

Each fluid dram represents 7½ grains each of buchu and pareira brava.

2951. Elixir of Buchu and Pareira, Compound.

Fluid extract of buchu	8 fl. drams.
Fluid extract of juniper berries	4 fl. drams.
Fluid extract of pareira brava	2 fl. drams.
Fluid extract of stone-root	2 fl. drams.
Alcohol	1 fl. ounce.
Simple syrup	1 fl. ounce.
Simple elixir	12 fl. ounces.

Mix, allow to stand for 24 hours, and filter through purified talcum.

Each fluid dram represents about 4 grains of buchu, 2 grains of juniper berries, and 1 grain each of pareira brava and collinsonia.

2952. Elixir of Buckthorn and Senna.

Fluid extract of frangula	2 fl. ounces.
Elixir of senna	14 fl. ounces.

Each fluid dram represents 7½ grains of buckthorn bark, and 26 grains of senna.

2953. Elixir of Calcium and Sodium Hypophosphites with Malt.

Calcium hypophosphite	128 grains.
Sodium hypophosphite	128 grains.
Adjuvant elixir	8 fl. ounces.
Fluid extract of malt, N. F.	8 fl. ounces.

Dissolve the salts in the elixir by trituration, filter, and add the malt extract.

Each fluid dram contains 1 grain each of the hypophosphites of calcium and sodium.

2954. Elixir of Calcium and Sodium Hypophosphites with Tar.

Calcium hypophosphite	128 grains.
Sodium hypophosphite	128 grains.
Distilled water, hot	2 fl. ounces.
Elixir of tar, enough to make	16 fl. ounces.

Dissolve the salts in the water, add the elixir, and filter.

Each fluid dram contains 1 grain each of the hypophosphites.

2955. Elixir of Calcium Iodide.

Calcium iodide	1½ ounces av.
Simple elixir, enough to make	16 fl. ounces.

Dissolve by agitation, and filter.

Inasmuch as calcium iodide is an unstable compound, it should be prepared as needed, and the following formula should therefore receive preference:

Solution of iron iodide, N. F., prepared without hypophosphorous acid	13½ fl. drams.
Calcium oxide, C. P.	2 ounces av.
Distilled water	sufficient.
Sugar	3½ ounces av.
Compound spirit of orange	2 fl. drams.
Alcohol	4 fl. ounces.

Hydrate the calcium oxide with 6 fluid ounces of water, add the solution of iron oxide, heat to boiling, allow to stand a few minutes, decant the clear liquid, add to the residue a fresh portion of distilled water, heat again to boiling, decant as before, and repeat the process again until the mixed decantates measure 10 fluid ounces; add the alcohol containing the spirit, let stand for an hour or more, filter, in the filtrate dissolve the sugar by agitation, and strain if necessary.

Each fluid dram contains 5 grains of calcium iodide.

2956. Elixir of Iodo-Bromide of Calcium, Compound.

(Compound Elixir of Calcium Bromide with Iodides.)

Calcium bromide	256 grains.
Sodium iodide	256 grains.
Potassium iodide	256 grains.
Magnesium chloride	256 grains.
Compound fluid extract of sarsaparilla	2 fl. ounces.
Compound fluid extract of stillingia	2 fl. ounces.
Aromatic elixir	4 fl. ounces.
Sugar	4½ ounces.
Water, enough to make	16 fl. ounces.

Dissolve the salts in the water, add the sugar, and to this syrup add the fluid extracts previously mixed with the aromatic elixir; after standing for 2 days, filter, and add the remainder of the water.

2957. Elixir of Calcium Lactophosphate and Cinchona.

Detannated elixir of cinchona	8 fl. ounces.
Elixir of calcium lactophosphate	8 fl. ounces.

2958. Elixir of Calcium Phosphate.

Calcium phosphate	640 grains.
Hydrochloric acid, concentrated	5 fl. drams.
Water	1 fl. ounce.
Tincture of cudbear	2 fl. drams.
Simple elixir, enough to make	16 fl. ounces.

Mix the calcium phosphate with the water, add the acid, dissolve, add the elixir, and then the tincture.

Each fluid dram contains 5 grains of calcium phosphate.

2959. Elixir of Cascara Sagrada with Sodium Salicylate.

Elixir of cascara sagrada	5 fl. ounces.
Sodium salicylate	2½ ounces av.
Simple elixir, enough to make	16 fl. ounces.

Mix, dissolve by shaking, and filter if necessary.

Each fluid dram represents approximately 2 grains cascara sagrada, and contains very nearly 1 grain of sodium salicylate.

2960. Elixir, Castillon's.

Cinchona, coarsely powd.	160 grains.
Gentian, coarsely powd.	160 grains.
Ipecac, coarsely powd.	80 grains.
Columbo, coarsely powd.	80 grains.
Cinnamon, coarsely powd.	20 grains.
Aqueous extract of opium	20 grains.
Diluted alcohol	sufficient.

Macerate the drugs with 16 fluid ounces of diluted alcohol for 7 days, and filter, adding enough menstruum through the filter to make up 16 fluid ounces of filtrate.

2961. Elixir of Celery and Guarana.

Fluid extract of celery seed	2 fl. ounces.
Fluid extract of guarana	2 fl. ounces.
Aromatic elixir	12 fl. ounces.

Mix, allow to stand for 24 hours, and filter through talcum.

Each fluid dram represents 7½ grains each of celery and guarana.

2962. Elixir of Cherries.

(Elixir Cerasorum.)

Ripe, sour cherries, free from stems	8 ounces av.
Alcohol	2 fl. ounces.
Glycerin	1 fl. ounce.
Simple syrup	sufficient.

Crush the cherries and stones to a pulp, add the alcohol and glycerine, macerate for 7 days, press and filter, and to the filtrate add simple syrup enough to make 16 fluid ounces.

2963. Elixir of Cherries with Calcium and Sodium Hypophosphites.

Calcium hypophosphite	128 grains.
Sodium hypophosphite	128 grains.
Elixir of cherries, enough to make	16 fl. ounces.

Triturate the two salts to fine powder, add to the elixir, dissolve by agitation, and filter.

Each fluid dram contains 1 grain each of sodium and calcium hypophosphites.

2964. Elixir of Chloral Hydrate.

Chloral hydrate, crystal	640 grains.
Simple elixir, enough to make	16 fl. ounces.

Mix, dissolve by agitation, and filter, if necessary.

Each fluid dram contains 5 grains of chloral hydrate.

2965. Elixir of Chirata.

Tincture of chirata	4 fl. ounces.
Simple elixir	12 fl. ounces.

Each fluid dram represents 1½ grains of chirata.

2966. Elixir of Chloral Hydrate and Ammonium Valerianate.

Refer to "Elixir of Ammonium Valerianate" and its combinations.

2967. Elixir of Chlorides of Arsenic and Iron.

(Elixir of Two Chlorides.)

Solution of arsenious acid.	10½ fl. drams.
Tincture of citrochloride of iron	5¼ fl. drams.
Simple elixir	14 fl. ounces.

Each fluid dram contains 1-20 grain of arsenious acid (as so-called "chloride of arsenic") and about ¼ grain of iron chloride.

2968. Elixir of Chlorides of Arsenic, Iron and Mercury.

(Elixir of Three Chlorides.)

Solution of protochloride of iron, N. F.	48 minims.
Mercuric chloride	1 grain.
Solution of arsenious acid	50 minims.
Compound elixir of quinine, N. F., enough to make	16 fl. ounces.

Mix, dissolve, and filter.

Each fluid dram contains ⅛ grain of iron protochloride, 1-128 grain of mercuric chloride and 1-256 grain of arsenious acid (as so-called "chloride of arsenic").

2969. Elixir of Four Chlorides.

(Four Chlorides.)

Mercuric chloride	2 grains.
Solution of arsenic	5½ fl. drams.
Tincture of ferric chloride	2 fl. ounces.
Hydrochloric acid, diluted	11 fl. drams.
Syrup of ginger	4 fl. ounces.
Water, enough to make	16 fl. ounces.

Mix, dissolve, and filter, if necessary.

Each fluid dram contains about 1-40 grain of arsenious acid (as so-called "chloride of arsenic"), 1-64 grain of mercuric chloride, about ¾ grain of ferric chloride, and about 5 minims of diluted hydrochloric acid.

2970. Elixir of Chloroform.

Chloroform	4 fl. drams.
Alcohol	2 fl. ounces.
Simple elixir, enough to make	16 fl. ounces.

Mix the alcohol and chloroform, and add the elixir.

Each fluid dram contains very nearly 2 minims of chloroform.

2971. Elixir of Cinchona Detannated.

Yellow cinchona	480 grains.
Saigon cassia	80 grains.
Coriander	80 grains.
Nutmeg	20 grains.
Star anise	20 grains.
Sugar	10 av. ounces.
Alcohol	} of each
Water	} sufficient.
Spirit of orange	2 fl. drams.
Purified talcum	120 grains.

Reduce the cinchona, cassia, coriander, nutmeg and anise to a moderately fine powder, and extract by percolation with a mixture of alcohol and water, in the proportion of 1 by measure of the former to 3 of the latter, until 22 fluid ounces of percolate are obtained. Now beat the white of 1 egg with a portion of the percolate, add the remainder of the percolate, and set aside for 24 hours, agitating occasionally. Test at the end of the specified period of time with solution of ferric chloride and if discoloration occurs, the white of another egg may be added as before, allowing to stand 24 hours, then filtering. Wash the filter with a liquid similar to the menstruum used until 25 fluid ounces of filtrate are obtained. To this add the spirit of orange and purified talcum, filter; to the filtrate add the sugar, dissolve by agitation, and strain, or filter, if necessary.

Each fluid dram represents about 1¾ grains of cinchona.

2972. Elixir of Cinchona, Compound.

(Elixir of Cinchona and Coca.)

Fluid extract of cinchona	10 fl. drams.
Fluid extract of coca	10 fl. drams.
Tincture of cacao	2½ fl. ounces.
Simple elixir	11 fl. ounces.

Mix, and filter, if necessary.

Each fluid dram represents about 4½ grains each of cinchona and coca.

2973. Elixir of Cinchona, Gentian and Iron Malate.

Malate of iron ("scales")	128 grains.
Extract of gentian	35 grains.
Simple syrup	4 fl. ounces.
Elixir of cinchona	6 fl. ounces.
Tincture of vanilla	2 fl. drams.
Oil of cinnamon	1 drop.
Water, hot	1 fl. ounce.
Aromatic elixir, enough to make	16 fl. ounces.

Dissolve the iron salt and extract in the water, add the other ingredients and filter.

Each fluid dram represents about 1 grain of gentian and ½ grain of cinchona, and contains 1 grain of iron malate.

The malate of iron to be used should not be the ferrated extract of apples, but the pure malate of iron which appears in the scale form.

2974. Elixir of Cinchona and "Protoxide" of Iron.

Solution of "protoxide" of
  iron .... 1½ fl. ounces.
Glycerin .... 1½ fl. ounces.
Elixir of cinchona, N. F.... 13 fl. ounces.

Mix the solution and the glycerin and add the elixir.

2975. Elixir of Cinchona, Iron and Phosphorous.

Spirit of phosphorus....... 7½ fl. drams.
Elixir of cinchona and iron,
  enough to make.......... 16 fl. ounces.

Each fluid dram contains 1-200 grain of phosphorus, 2 grains of iron phosphate, and represents nearly 2 grains of cinchona.

2976. Elixir of Cinchona and Pepsin. A

Quinine sulphate .... 16 grains.
Cinchonine sulphate....... 8 grains.
Elixir of pepsin .... 16 fl. ounces.

Dissolve the alkaloidal salts in the elixir and filter if necessary.

2977. Elixir of Cinchona and Pepsin. B

Pure pepsin .... 128 grains.
Hydrochloric acid .... ½ fl. dram.
Detannated elixir of cin-
  chona, enough to make... 16 fl. ounces.

Dissolve by agitation and filter, using purified talcum, if necessary.

2978. Elixir of Cinchona with Phosphates. A

Syrup of calcium lacto-
  phosphate, U. S. P....... 4 fl. ounces.
Syrup of iron lactophos-
  phate .... 2 fl. ounces.
Diluted phosphoric acid.... 1 fl. ounce.
Quinine sulphate .... 32 grains.
Alcohol .... 4 fl. ounces.
Spirit of orange........... 4 fl. drams.
Water .... 4½ fl. ounces.

Dissolve the quinine salt in the alcohol previously mixed with the acid and spirit, pour this solution into the syrups previously mixed with the water, allow to stand for 2 days, and filter.

2979. Elixir of Cinchona with Phosphates. B

Elixir of cinchona......... 8 fl. ounces.
Compound syrup of phos-
  phates................... 8 fl. ounces.

The elixir of cinchona, iron and calcium lactophosphate, N. F., may be dispensed under the above title.

2980. Elixir of Cinchona and Strychnine.

Strychnine sulphate .... 1¼ grains.
Detannated elixir of cin-
  chona .... 16 fl. ounces.

Dissolve by agitation.

Each fluid dram contains 1-100 grain of strychnine sulphate, and represents nearly 2 grains of cinchona.

2981. Elixir of Cinchonidine.

Cinchonidine sulphate ..... 128 grains.
Simple elixir .... 16 fl. ounces.

Dissolve by agitation, and filter, if necessary.

Each fluid dram contains 1 grain of cinchonidine sulphate.

2982. Elixir of Cinchonidine and Iron.

Iron pyrophosphate, soluble 256 grains.
Cinchonidine sulphate ..... 128 grains.
Distilled water, hot ...... 6 fl. drams.
Simple elixir .... 15 fl. ounces.

Dissolve the iron pyrophosphate in the water, and the cinchonidine in the elixir; mix the two solutions and filter if necessary.

Each fluid dram contains 1 grain of cinchonidine sulphate and 2 grains of iron pyrophosphate.

2983. Elixir of Cinchonidine, Iron and Strychnine.

Make this either by adding 1¼ grains of strychnine sulphate to the preceding, or the elixir of iron phosphate, cinchonidine and strychnine may be employed.

2984. Elixir of Coca and Phosphorus.

Spirit of phosphorus....... 15 fl. drams.
Elixir of coca, enough to
  make .... 16 fl. ounces.

Mix and filter if necessary.

Each fluid dram contains 1-100 grain of phosphorus and represents 6½ grains of coca.

2985. Elixir of Codeine.
Codeine sulphate .... 16 grains.
Simple elixir .... 16 fl. ounces.
Dissolve by agitation.

Each fluid dram contains ⅛ grain of codeine sulphate.

2986. Elixir of Corydalis, Compound.
(Alterative Elixir.)
Fluid extract of corydalis.. 1 fl. ounce.
Fluid extract of stillingia.. 1 fl. ounce.
Fl. ext. of prickly ash bark. 4 fl. drams.
Fluid extract of blue flag.. 1½ fl. ounces.
Alcohol .... 2 fl. ounces.
Potassium iodide .... 384 grains.
Aromatic elixir, enough to
make .... 16 fl. ounces.

Mix the alcohol with the fluid extracts, dissolve the potassium iodide in the mixture, and add the aromatic elixir. Let the mixture stand a few days, if convenient, and filter.

Each fluid dram contains 3 grains of potassium iodide, and small quantities of the several fluid extracts.

2987. Elixir of Codeine and Terpin Hydrate.
Codeine sulphate .... 16 grains.
Terpin hydrate............ 256 grains.
Simple elixir, enough to
make .... 16 fl. ounces.

Dissolve by agitation and filter if necessary.

Each fluid dram contains ⅛ grain of codeine sulphate, and 2 grains of terpin hydrate.

2988. Elixir of Crampbark, Compound.
(Compound Elixir of Viburnum Opulus.)
Fluid extract of crampbark 10 fl. drams.
Fluid extract of trillium... 2½ fl. ounces.
Fluid extract of aletris..... 10 fl. drams.
Comp. elixir of taraxacum. 11 fl. ounces.

Mix, allow to stand a few days, if convenient, and filter.—N. F.

2989. Elixir of Croton Chloral Hydrate.
(Elixir of Butyl Chloral Hydrate.)
Croton chloral hydrate..... 256 grains.
Alcohol .... 1 fl. ounce.
Tincture of cacao .... 2 fl. ounces.
Simple elixir, enough to
make .... 16 fl. ounces.

Dissolve the croton chloral in the alcohol, add the tincture and elixir, and filter, if necessary.

Each fluid dram contains 2 grains of croton chloral hydrate.

2990. Elixir of Croton Chloral Hydrate and Quinine.
Quinine sulphate .... 128 grains.
Elixir of croton chloral
hydrate .... 16 fl. ounces.

Reduce the quinine salt to fine powder, add the elixir, dissolve by agitation, and filter, if necessary.

Each fluid dram contains 1 grain of quinine sulphate and 2 grains of croton chloral hydrate.

2991. Elixir of Damiana, Iron, Nux Vomica and Phosphorus.
Fluid extract of damiana.. 2 fl. ounces.
Tincture of nux vomica... 10½ fl. drams.
Iron pyrophosphate, soluble 128 grains.
Elixir of phosphorus....... 4 fl. ounces.
Alcohol .... 2 fl. ounces.
Distilled water, hot .... 4 fl. drams.
Simple elixir, enough to
make .... 16 fl. ounces.

Mix the fluid extract, tincture, elixir of phosphorus, alcohol, and 6 fluid ounces of simple elixir, also dissolve the iron salt in the water, mix the two liquids, add the remainder of the simple elixir, and filter, if necessary, in a well-covered funnel.

Each fluid dram represents 7½ grains of damiana and about 1 grain of nux vomica, and contains 1-200 grain of phosphorus and 1 grain of iron pyrophosphate.

2992. Elixir of Damiana, Iron and Phosphorus.
Fluid extract of damiana.. 2 fl. ounces.
Elixir of phosphorus....... 4 fl. ounces.
Iron pyrophosphate, soluble 128 grains.
Alcohol .... 1 fl. ounce.
Distilled water, hot........ 4 fl. drams.
Simple elixir, enough to
make .... 16 fl. ounces.

Mix the fluid extract, elixir of phosphorus, alcohol, and 8 fluid ounces of simple elixir, dissolve the iron pyrophosphate in the water, mix the two liquids, add the remainder of the elixir, and filter, if necessary, in a well-covered funnel.

Each fluid dram contains 1-200 grain of phosphorus and 1 grain of iron pyrophosphate and represents 7½ grains of damiana.

2993. Elixir of Damiana, Nux Vomica and Phosphorus.
Fluid extract of damiana.. 2 fl. ounces.
Tincture of nux vomica.... 10½ fl. drams.
Elixir of phosphorus....... 2 fl. ounces.

Alcohol .... 2 fl. ounces.
Simple elixir, enough to
 make .... 16 fl. ounces.
Mix the above ingredients in the order given and filter, if necessary, in a well-covered funnel.

Each fluid dram represents 1-200 grain of phosphorus, about 1 grain of nux vomica, and 7½ grains of damiana.

2994. Elixir of Damiana and Phosphorus.
Elixir of phosphorus...... 8 fl. ounces.
Fluid extract of damiana. 2 fl. ounces.
Alcohol .... 2 fl. ounces.
Simple elixir .... 4 fl ounces.
Mix the elixir of phosphorus, alcohol, and fluid extract and add the simple elixir.

Each fluid dram represents 1-100 grain of phosphorus and 7½ grains of damiana.

2995. Elixir of Damiana, Phosphorus and Strychnine.
Elixir of phosphorus ...... 8 fl. ounces.
Fluid extract of damiana... 2 fl. ounces.
Alcohol .... 2 fl. ounces.
Strychnine sulphate .... 1¼ grains.
Simple elixir .... 4 fl. ounces.
Mix the elixir of phosphorus, alcohol, and fluid extract and add the simple elixir, having first dissolved the alkaloidal salt in the latter.

Each fluid dram represents 7½ grains of damiana and contains 1-100 grain each of phosphorus and strychnine sulphate.

2996. Elixir of Dewberry Root, Compound.
Dewberry root, in coarse
 powder .... 2¼ av. ounces
Galls, powdered........... 120 grains.
Kino, powdered........... 120 grains.
Cinnamon, powdered ...... 60 grains
Cloves, powdered .... 30 grains.
Capsicum, powdered ...... 5 grains.
Tincture of opium .... 4 fl. drams.
Spirit of peppermint....... 45 minims.
Brandy .... 16 fl. ounces.
Sugar .... 7½ av. ounces.
Macerate all of the above, sugar, excepted, for 14 days, shaking occasionally; express, filter, and in the filtrate dissolve the sugar.

2997. Elixir of Dandelion.
Fluid extract of dandelion. 6 fl. ounces.
Simple elixir, enough to
 make .... 16 fl. ounces.
Each fluid dram represents 22½ grains of dandelion.

2998. Elixir of Dandelion, Compound. A
Compound Elixir of Taraxacum.
Fluid extract of dandelion. 4 fl. drams.
Fluid extract of sweet
 orange peel............ 2½ fl. drams.
Fluid extract of wild cherry 2½ fl. drams.
Fluid extract of licorice
 root .... 1 fl. ounce.
Tincture of cinnamon...... 4 fl. drams.
Compound tincture of car-
 damom .... 4 fl. drams.
Aromatic elixir, enough to
 make .... 16 fl. ounces.
Mix, let stand a few days, and filter.—N. F. (last edition).

2999. Elixir of Dandelion, Compound. B
Dandelion................. 320 grains.
Wild cherry............... 320 grains.
Sweet orange peel, recently
 dried .... 320 grains.
Licorice, Russian, peeled... 2¼ av. ounces.
Cinnamon, Saigon......... 80 grains.
Cardamom .... 80 grains.
Canada snake root........ 80 grains.
Caraway .... 80 grains.
Cloves .... 27 grains.
Simple syrup............. 21 fl. ounces.
Alcohol .... } of each
Water................... } sufficient.

3000. Elixir of Dandelion, Compound. C
A formula for a preparation of the same name, which is also much in use and which is much different in some respects from either of the preceding, is the following:
Fluid extract of dandelion. 5 fl. drams.
Fluid extract of wild cherry 3 fl. drams.
Fluid extract of gentian.. 1 fl. dram.
Fluid extract of licorice
 root .... 1 fl. dram.
Simple elixir, enough to
 make .... 16 fl. ounces.
Mix and filter.

3001. Elixir, Emmenagogue.
Rue .... 96 grains.
Spanish saffron........... 96 grains.
Savin .... 96 grains.
Socotrine aloes........... 192 grains.
Adjuvant elixir, enough to
 make .... 16 fl. ounces.
Reduce the drugs to moderately fine powder, mix with 12 fluid ounces of adjuvant elixir, macerate for 7 days, agitating occasionally, filter, and through the filter add the remainder of the elixir.

Each fluid dram represents ¾ grain each of rue, saffron and savin, and 1½ grains of aloes.

3002. Elixir, Flavoring.

Oil of orange sweet	1½ drams.
Oil of lemon	½ dram.
Oil of cardamom	10 minims.
Oil of coriander	5 minims.
Tincture of vanillin	2 ounces.
Made from vanillin	1 ounce.
Cologne spirits, 188%	1 gallon.

The above amount is for one gallon of simple elixir. For mode of manufacture see Elixir Simple, No. 3093.

3003. Elixir of Galls, Aromatic.

Galls	1 av. ounce.
Nutmegs	½ av. ounce.
Cinnamon	½ av. ounce.
Brandy	sufficient.
Elixir of orange	10 fl. ounces.

Reduce the drugs to moderately coarse powder, moisten with brandy, pack in a percolator and percolate until 6 fluid ounces of liquid are obtained, to which add the elixir.

3004. Elixir de Garus. A
(Elixir Gari.)

Cinnamon	30 grains.
Canella	30 grains.
Cloves	30 grains.
Nutmeg	30 grains.
Myrrh	110 grains.
Aloes	220 grains.
Spanish saffron	8 grains.
Orange flower water	1 fl. ounce.
Water	8 fl. ounces.
Simple syrup	16 fl. ounces.
Alcohol	16 fl. ounces.

Reduce the drugs, except the saffron, to a moderately coarse powder, macerate for 24 hours in a small still with 8 fluid ounces of alcohol and the water, then distil off 8 fluid ounces; to this distillate add the saffron, the remainder of the alcohol and the orange flower water, macerate for 2 days, agitating occasionally; add the syrup, and filter.

3005. Elixir de Garus. B

Oil of cassia	8 drops.
Oil of cloves	8 drops.
Oil of mace	8 drops.
Saffron	20 grains.
Tincture of vanilla	½ fl. dram.
Alcohol	5 fl. ounces.
Orange flower water	6½ fl. ounces.
Sugar	7 av. ounces.

Mix the oil, saffron, tincture and alcohol, macerate for 2 days, agitating occasionally; strain to remove the saffron, add the orange flower water and sugar, agitate until the latter is dissolved, and filter.—H. modified.

3006. Elixir of Gentian.

Fluid extract of gentian	5½ fl. drams.
Compound spirit of cardamom	4 fl. drams.
Solution of tersulphate of iron	4 fl. drams.
Water of ammonia	4½ fl. drams.
Alcohol	of each
Distilled water	sufficient.
Aromatic elixir	

Dilute the solution of tersulphate of iron with 4 fluid ounces of cold water, and add it, constantly stirring, to the water of ammonia, previously diluted with an equal volume of cold water. Collect the precipitate on a well-wetted muslin strainer, allow it to drain completely, return it to the vessel, mix it intimately with 4 fluid ounces of water, and again drain. Repeat this operation once more with the same quantity of water. When the precipitate has been completely drained for the third time, fold the strainer, and press it gently so as to remove the water as completely as possible without loss of magma; then remove the magma into a tared bottle, and ascertain its weight. Now add to the magma one-fifth of its weight of alcohol, the fluid extract, compound tincture and 12 fluid ounces of aromatic elixir, and shake the mixture occasionally during 24 hours: Filter through paper, and pass enough aromatic elixir through the filter to make the product measure 16 fluid ounces.

Each fluid dram represents about 2 grains of gentian.—N. F. (last edition).

3007. Elixir of Gentian, Compound. A

Stronger compound infusion of gentian, N. F.	4½ fl. ounces.
Aromatic elixir	11¾ fl. ounces.

3008. Elixir of Gentian, Compound. B

Gentian	256 grains.
Coriander	64 grains.
Bitter orange peel	64 grains.
Alcohol	of each
Water	sufficient.
Sugar	5 av. ounces.
Aromatic spirit	1 fl. ounce.
Egg albumen	120 grains.
Citric acid	5 grains.

Mix alcohol and water in the proportion of 1 of the former to 2 of the latter by measure, and with this mixture percolate the drugs, previously ground to moderately fine powder, until 12 fluid ounces of percolate are obtained. To this percolate add the albumen and citric acid, agitate until the latter is dissolved, add the aromatic spirit and filter. In the absence of dried egg albumen, the white of 1 egg may be employed.

3009. Elixir of Gentian, Compound. C
Compound tincture of gentian .... 5¼ fl. ounces.
Simple elixir............. 10¾ fl. ounces.
Each fluid dram represents 2 grains of gentian.

3010. Elixir of Gentian and Iron Pyrophosphate.
Iron pyrophosphate, soluble 128 grains.
Distilled water, hot....... 4 fl. drams.
Elixir of gentian, enough to make................. 16 fl. ounces.
Dissolve the iron salt in the water, add the elixir, and filter, if necessary.
Each fluid dram contains 1 grain of iron salt and represents nearly 2 grains of gentian.

3011. Elixir of Gentian, Iron Phosphate, Nux Vomica and Quassia.
Tincture of nux vomica... 256 minims.
Iron phosphate........... 128 grains.
Distilled water, hot....... 4 fl. drams.
Fluid extract of quassia... 4 fl. drams.
Compound fluid extract of gentian .... 4 fl. drams.
Simple elixir, enough to make .... 16 fl. ounces.
Dissolve the iron phosphate in the water, add the other ingredients and filter.
Each fluid dram contains 1 grain of iron phosphate, and represents 2/3 grains of nux vomica, nearly 2 grains of quassia, and 1¼ grains of gentian.

3012. Elixir of Gentian and Phosphorous.
Fluid extract of gentian... 10 fl. drams.
Elixir of phosphorus...... 8 fl. ounces.
Compound elixir of taraxacum .... 5 fl. ounces.
Aromatic elixir, enough to make .... 16 fl. ounces.
Each fluid dram represents 1/100 grains of phosphorus and 5 grains of gentian.

3013. Elixir of Guaiac.
Tincture of guaiac......... 4 fl. ounces.
Potassium carbonate.......20 grains.
Water .... 2 fl. drams.
Glycerin .... 4 fl. ounces.
Compound elixir of taraxacum .... 4 fl. ounces.
Simple syrup .... 4 fl. ounces.
Dissolve the potassium carbonate in the water, add to the tincture of guaiac and to this mixture add the remaining ingredients in the order given above.

3014. Elixir of Golden Seal.
(Elixir of Hydrastis.)
Glycerite of hydrastis..... 10½ fl. drams.
Simple elixir, enough to make .... 16 fl. ounces.
Each fluid dram represents 5 grains of golden seal.

3015. Elixir of Guarana.
Br.
Guarana, powdered........ 3¼ av. ounces.
Light magnesia........... 175 grains.
Oil of cinnamon........... 5 drops.
Simple syrup............. 13 fl. drams.
Diluted alcohol........... sufficient.
Sand, clean and coarse.... 6½ av. ounces.
Mix the guarana and magnesia, moisten with 2½ fluid ounces of diluted alcohol, set aside for 24 hours, then mix with the sand, pack in a percolator, percolate until 13 fluid ounces of liquid are obtained, then remove the mass from the percolator, inclose it in a cloth and express in a tincture press; to the percolate add the oil and syrup, and make up to 16 fluid ounces by addition of the expressed liquid, previously concentrating the latter, if necessary, by evaporation.
Each fluid dram represents about 11 grains of guarana.

3016. Elixir of Helonias.
Fluid extract of helonias.. 4 fl. ounces.
Simple elixir............. 12 fl. ounces.
Mix, allow to stand for 24 hours and filter.
Each fluid dram represents 15 grains of helonias.

3017. Elixir of Helonias, Compound.
(Compound Elixir of Squaw-vine.—Compound Elixir of Mitchella.)
Fluid extract of false unicorn (helonias dioica).... 2 fl. ounces.
Fluid extract of mitchella. 4 fl. ounces.
Fluid extract of blue cohosh 2 fl. ounces.
Fluid extract of crampbark 2 fl. ounces.
Purified talcum........... ½ av. ounce.
Aromatic elixir, enough to make .... 16 fl. ounces.
Mix and filter.
Each fluid dram represents nearly 14 grains of mitchella, and 7 grains each of helonias, blue cohosh and crampbark.

3018. Elixir of Hypophosphites of Iron and Quinine. A
Iron hypophosphite........ 128 grains.
Potassium citrate......... 128 grains.
Quinine sulphate.......... 128 grains.
Calcium hypophosphite.... 30 grains.

Spirit of orange	2 fl. drams.
Orange flower water	1 fl. ounce.
Sugar	5 av. ounces.
Alcohol	of each
Distilled water	sufficient.

Dissolve the iron hypophosphite with the aid of the potassium citrate in the orange flower water, and enough water to make the solution measure 6½ fluid ounces, and in this dissolve the sugar. Triturate the quinine sulphate with 5 fluid ounces of alcohol, add a solution of the calcium hypophosphite in 4 fluid drams of water, and shake the mixture occasionally during 1 hour; filter, and wash the filter with enough alcohol to make 6½ fluid ounces. Add this solution to the spirit of orange, mix this with the iron solution and sugar solution previously prepared, and filter the whole.

Each fluid dram contains 1 grain each of the hypophosphites of iron and quinine.

3019. Elixir of Hypophosphites of Iron and Quinine. B

Solution of Iron hypophosphite, N. F.	12¾ fl. drams.
Quinine hypophosphite	128 grains.
Hypophosphorous acid	sufficient.
Simple elixir, enough to make	16 fl. ounces

Mix the quinine hypophosphite with 8 fluid ounces of elixir, add enough of the acid to dissolve the quinine, add the solution of iron hypophosphite, and then enough elixir to make 16 fluid ounces, and filter.

This is of the same strength as the preceding.

3020. Elixir of Hypophosphites of Iron, Quinine and Strychnine.

This may be prepared by dissolving 1¼ grains of strychnine sulphate in 4 fluid drams of distilled water, and adding enough of the preceding elixir to make 16 fluid ounces.

3021. Elixir of Hypophosphites with Malt.

Refer for above to Elixir of Calcium Hypophosphite and its combinations.

3022. Elixir of Six Iodides.

Arsenic iodide	1 grain.
Mercuric iodide	1 grain.
Manganese iodide	13 grains.
Sodium iodide	128 grains.
Potassium iodide	128 grains.
Solution of Iron Iodide, N. F.	15 minims.
Sodium hypophosphite	sufficient.
Simple elixir, enough to make	16 fl. ounces.

Add the six iodides to the elixir, dissolve by agitation, add a few grains of sodium hypophosphite, or sufficient to decolorize the liquid, and filter.

Each fluid dram contains 1/128 grains each of arsenic and mercury iodides, 1/12 grain of ferrous iodide, 1/10 grain of manganese iodide, and 1 grain each of sodium and potassium iodides.

3023. Elixir of Iodide of Potassium, Compound.
(Alterative Elixir.)

Potassium iodide	640 grains.
Tincture of citrochloride of iron	10½ fl. drams.
Spirit of orange	4 fl. drams.
Fluid extract of saxifrage	12 fl. drams.
Fluid extract of stillingia	12 fl. drams.
Fluid extract of menispermum	12 fl. drams.
Fluid extract of helonias	12 fl. drams.
Sugar	4½ av. ounces.
Water, enough to make	16 fl. ounces.

Dissolve the potassium iodide in the water, add the tincture or iron, and in this mixture dissolve the sugar by agitation. Mix the fluid extracts, add the spirit, then the syrup, allow the whole to stand for two days, and filter.

Each fluid dram contains 5 grains of potassium iodide, and represents about ½ grain of ferric chloride, and about 5½ grains each of saxifraga, stillingia, menispermum and helonias.

3024. Elixir of Iodide of Potassium.

Potassium iodide	640 grains.
Aromatic elixir of licorice, enough to make	16 fl. ounces.

Dissolve by agitation.

Each fluid dram contains 5 grains of potassium iodide.

3025. Elixir of Iron, Pepsin and Quinine.

Iron pyrophosphate, soluble	256 grains.
Quinine hydrochlorate	32 grains.
Distilled water, hot	1 fl. ounce.
Elixir of pepsin, N. F., enough to make	16 fl. ounces.

Dissolve the iron salt in the water, add the elixir and the quinine salt, agitate occasionally until dissolved, and filter. Each fluid dram contains 2 grains of iron pyrophosphate, ¼ grain of quinine hydrochlorate, and nearly 1 grain of pepsin.

3026. Elixir of Iron, Quinine and Arsenic.

Iron pyrophosphate	128 grains.
Quinine hydrochlorate	64 grains.
Solution of arsenious acid	400 minims.
Distilled water, hot	4 fl. drams.
Simple elixir, enough to make	16 fl. ounces.

Dissolve the iron pyrophosphate in the water, dissolve the quinine in about 12 fluid ounces of elixir by agitation, mix the solutions, add the acid solution and the remainder of the elixir, then neutralize exactly with ammonia water, carefully added, and filter.

Each fluid dram contains 1 grain of iron pyrophosphate, ½ grain of quinine hydrochlorate, and 1/32 grain of arsenious acid.

3027. Elixir of Iron and Wild Cherry.
(Ferrated Elixir of Wild Cherry.)

Iron pyrophosphate	128 grains.
Distilled water, hot	4 fl. drams.
Fluid extract of wild cherry	2 fl. ounces.
Alcohol	2 fl. ounces.
Simple elixir, enough to make	16 fl. ounces.

Mix the alcohol and fluid extract, add the elixir, and then the iron salt previously dissolved in the water, and filter through purified talcum.

Each fluid dram contains 1 grain of iron pyrophosphate, and represents 7½ grains of wild cherry.

3028. Elixir of Iron and Quinine Citrate.
(Elixir of Iron and Quinine.)

Citrate of iron and quinine	256 grains.
Water	1 fl. ounce.
Aromatic elixir, enough to make	16 fl. ounces.

Dissolve the citrate in the water, add the elixir, and filter. Each fluid dram contains 2 grains of iron and quinine citrate.

3029. Elixir of Iron Peptonate. A

Dried egg albumen	75 grains.
(Or fresh egg albumen	560 grains.)
Distilled water	sufficient.
Hydrochloric acid	2 fl. drams.
Pepsin, pure	4 grains.
Solution of iron oxychloride	15 fl. dr.
Solution of soda	sufficient.
Brandy	14 fl. dr.

Dissolve the albumen in 16 fluid ounces of distilled water, add the hydrochloric acid and pepsin, digest the mixture at a temperature of 40 degrees C., until it produces only a faint turbidity with nitric acid; allow to cool, neutralize with solution of soda, strain, mix the colature with the solution of iron oxychloride, to which has been added 16 fluid ounces of distilled water. The mixture is again neutralized with solution of soda, the precipitate is washed by decantation with distilled water, until the washings are no longer affected by silver nitrate. The precipitate is now drained on a well-wetted muslin strainer, transferred to a porcelain capsule, 10 minims of hydrochloric acid are added, and the mixture heated on a water bath and stirred until solution occurs. To this solution is now added distilled water to make 14¼ fluid ounces, and lastly, the brandy is added.—D.

Iron peptonate may be obtained by spreading the solution in the porcelain capsule upon glass plates and allowing to dry.

3030. Elixir of Iron Peptonate. B

Pepsin, pure	4 grains.
Dried egg albumen	30 grains.
Simple syrup	4 fl. drams.
Solution of dialized iron or ironoxychloride	12½ fl. drams.
Aromatic elixir	12½ fl. drams.
Distilled water, enough to make	16 fl. ounces.

Dissolve the albumen in 3¼ fluid ounces of water, add the pepsin and digest for four hours at 50 degrees C. Mix the syrup and solution of iron with 9 fluid ounces of the water, then add to the pepsin solution and heat to 90 degrees C. Cool, add the elixir and the remainder of the water. Set aside for 8 days and then decant the clear solution.

3031. Elixir of Iron Phosphate, Quinine and Strychnine. A

Strychnine (alkaloid)	1¼ grains.
Quinine sulphate	64 grains.
Citric acid	5 grains.
Iron phosphate, soluble	256 grains.
Alcohol	3 fl. ounces.
Simple syrup	6 fl. ounces.
Distilled water, hot	4 fl. ounces.
Orange flower water	3 fl. ounces.
Sodium bicarbonate	sufficient.

Triturate the strychnine and quinine sulphate with the acid until well mixed, and rub this mixture with the alcohol gradually added. Heat the syrup to about 65 degrees C., add to it the alcoholic liquid, and stir until clear. Dissolve the iron salt in the water, add the orange flower water, mix this with the preceding liquid, and allow to cool. Then add sodium bicarbonate in very small amounts, stirring thoroughly after each addition, until the elixir remains but slightly acid. Allow to stand for a few hours, then filter through white filter paper. Any excess of soda must be avoided.

3032. Elixir of Iron Phosphate, Quinine and Strychnine. B

Strychnine sulphate	1¼ grains.
Quinine hydrochlorate	128 grains.
Iron phosphate, soluble	256 grains.
Potassium citrate	32 grains.
Alcohol	1½ fl. ounces.
Distilled water, hot	1 fl. ounce.
Glycerin	18 fl. drams.
Aromatic elixir, enough to make	16 fl. ounces.

Dissolve the quinine salt in 10 fluid ounces of elixir, mixed with the alcohol, by agitation, and mix this solution with the strychnine sulphate previously dissolved in 2 fluid drams of the water.

Dissolve the iron phosphate in 6 fluid drams of the water, add 2 fluid ounces of glycerin and mix this solution with the preceding liquid. Now to this mixture add the potassium citrate dissolved in 1½ fluid ounces of aromatic elixir mixed with 2 fluid drams of glycerin. Allow the whole to stand for several hours, then filter.

3033. Elixir of Iron Phosphate, Quinine and Strychnine. C

Quinine sulphate	128 grains.
Iron phosphate, soluble	256 grains.
Strychnine sulphate	1¼ grains.
Alcohol	2 fl. ounces.
Glycerin	2 fl. ounces.
Simple syrup	2 fl. ounces.
Distilled water, hot	1 fl. ounce.
Aromatic elixir, enough to make	16 fl. ounces.

Dissolve the strychnine salt in the alcohol, and add the quinine; mix the glycerin and syrup, and heat, and when warm add to the alkaloidal solution; continue heating carefully, until quinine is dissolved, and add enough elixir to make 15 fluid ounces. Dissolve the iron salt in the water, add this to previous liquid, let stand three or four hours, and filter.

3034. Elixir of Iron Phosphate, Quinine and Strychnine. D

Iron phosphate, soluble	256 grains.
Quinine sulphate	128 grains.
Strychnine sulphate	1¼ grains.
Alcohol	1 fl. ounce.
Simple syrup	8 fl. ounces.
Aromatic elixir, enough to make	16 fl. ounces.

Dissolve the iron phosphate in the syrup by the aid of heat, and raise the temperature to near the boiling point. Dissolve the alkaloidal salts in 6 fluid ounces of aromatic elixir, contained in a flask, by the aid of heat, and while still hot add this solution all at once to the iron solution, shaking immediately. Allow to stand 24 hours, then filter.

3035. Elixir of Iron, Quinine and Strychnine Phosphates.
(Elixir of Three Phosphates.)

Nearly all of the preparations dispensed under this name contain the iron as phosphate or pyrophosphate, and the quinine and strychnine in some other form than as phosphate. If it be desired to dispense such a preparation as "elixir of three phosphates," then any of the preparations made according to formulas given in this formulary under elixir of iron phosphate, or pyrophosphate, quinine and strychnine may be dispensed.

The following formula does actually contain the three bases in the form of phosphates, which are maintained in solution by the excess of hydrochloric acid:

Solution of iron chloride, U. S. P.	7½ fl. drams.
Quinine (alkaloid)	110 grains.
Strychnine (alkaloid)	1 grain.
Phosphoric acid, U. S. P.	2½ fl. drams.
Distilled water	2 fl. drams.
Alcohol	1 fl. ounce.
Simple elixir	10 fl. ounces.
Simple syrup, enough to make	16 fl. ounces.

Mix the iron solution, phosphoric acid and water, and in this mixture dissolve the alkaloids; to this solution add the syrup, and then elixir and alcohol previously mixed.

However, any elixir containing iron in the form of phosphate or pyrophosphate will inevitably darken upon exposure to light, and therefore some manufacturers place upon the market a so-called "permanent elixir of three phosphates," which contains the iron as citro-chloride; a preparation of this character would be well represented by the elixir of iron, quinine and strychnine of the National Formulary.

3036. Elixir of Iron "Protoxide."

Solution of "protoxide" of iron	2 fl. ounces.
Simple elixir	14 fl. ounces.

3037. Elixir of Iron Pyrophosphate, Quinine and Strychnine. A

Iron pyrophosphate, soluble	256 grains.
Quinine sulphate	64 grains.
Strychnine	1¼ grains.
Citric acid	5 grains.
Alcohol	3 fl. ounces.
Spirit of orange	1½ fl. drams.
Distilled water	7 fl. ounces.

Simple syrup.............. 6 fl. ounces.
Ammonia water........... sufficient.

Triturate the quinine sulphate, strychnine and acid together, until minutely divided, and add the alcohol and spirit of orange; warm the syrup to about 65 degrees C., and add to the alcoholic mixture, stirring until clear. To this add the iron salt previously dissolved in the water; to the mixture add ammonia water, drop by drop, until the mixture is clear, and finally filter.

3038. Elixir of Iron Pyrophosphate, Quinine and Strychnine. B

Strychnine (alkaloid)....... 1¼ grains.
Quinine (alkaloid).......... 64 grains.
Iron pyrophosphate........ 128 grains.
Alcohol .... 2 fl. ounces.
Distilled water, hot........ 3 fl. ounces.
Simple syrup.............. 3 fl. ounces.
Aromatic elixir............ 8 fl. ounces.

Dissolve the strychnine and quinine in the alcohol, also the iron salt in the water, mix the two solutions, add the syrup and then the elixir, and filter, if necessary.

3039. Elixir of Iron Pyrophosphate, Quinine and Strychnine. C

Strychnine (alkaloid)....... 1¼ grains.
Quinine sulphate.......... 64 grains.
Citric acid................. 5 grains.
Alcohol .... 3 fl. ounces.
Simple syrup.............. 6 fl. ounces.
Distilled water, hot........ 4 fl. ounces.
Orange flower water...... 3 fl. ounces.
Iron pyrophosphate, soluble 256 grains.
Sodium bicarbonate........ sufficient.

Triturate together the alkaloids and the acids until thoroughly mixed; rub this with the alcohol gradually added. Heat the syrup to about 65 degrees C., add it to the alcoholic mixture, and stir until clear. Dissolve the iron salt in the water, and add the orange flower water; mix the two solutions, and when cold, add carefully bicarbonate of sodium in small portions until the elixir remains but slightly acid. Allow to stand for a few hours, then filter through white filter paper. Excess of soda must be carefully avoided.

3040. Elixir of Iron Pyrophosphate and Strychnine.

Iron pyrophosphate........ 256 grains.
Strychnine sulphate....... 1¼ grains.
Distilled water, hot........ 2 fl. ounces.
Simple elixir, enough to
 make .... 16 fl. ounces.

Dissolve the iron salt and strychnine sulphate in the hot water, add the elixir, and filter.

Each fluid dram contains 2 grains of iron pyrophosphate and 1/100 grains of strychnine sulphate.

3041. Elixir of Iron Salicylate.

Iron salicylate............. 640 grains.
Distilled water, hot........ 2¼ fl. ounces.
Glycerin .... 2¼ fl. ounces.
Simple elixir, enough to
 make .... 16 fl. ounces.

Dissolve the iron salt in the hot water and glycerin, add the elixir, allow to stand for a few days and filter.

Each fluid dram contains 5 grains of iron salicylate.

3042. Elixir of Iron Salicylate, Compound.

Iron salicylate............. 640 grains.
Distilled water, hot........ 2¼ fl. ounces.
Glycerin .... 2¼ fl. ounces.
Fluid extract of colchicum
 root .... 9 fl. drams.
Deodorized tincture of
 opium .... 4½ fl. drams.
Simple elixir, enough to
 make .... 16 fl. ounces.

Dissolve the iron salt in the hot water and glycerin, add the other ingredients, allow to stand a few days, and filter.

Each fluid dram contains 5 grains of iron salicylate and represents about 4¼ grains of colchicum root and 2 minims of deodorized tincture of opium.

3043. Elixir of Iron Valerianate.

Iron valerianate............ 128 grains.
Alcohol .... 1 fl. ounce.
Simple elixir.............. 15 fl. ounces.

Dissolve the iron salt in the alcohol, add the elixir, and filter.

Each fluid dram contains 1 grain of iron valerianate.

3044. Elixir of Kola.

Fluid extract of kola...... 2 fl. ounces.
Ammoniated glycyrrhizin.. 60 grains.
Saccharin .... 60 grains.
Oil of orange.............. 5 drops.
Water .... 7 fl. ounces.
Alcohol .... 3½ fl. ounces.
Simple syrup.............. 3½ fl. ounces.
Simple elixir, enough to
 make .... 16 fl. ounces.

Dissolve the ammoniated glycyrrhizin in the water and in this dissolve the saccharin; add the syrup and alcohol, followed by the fluid extract of kola, to which has been added the oil of orange; set aside for 5 or 6 hours, agitating occasionally; filter, and add the simple elixir.

Each fluid dram represents 7½ grains of kola.

3045. Elixir of Licorice Aromatic. A

Cardamom (seed without capsule)	16 grains.
Cinnamon	16 grains.
Staranise	16 grains.
Coriander	8 grains.
Caraway	8 grains.
Canella	4 grains.
Nutmeg	4 grains.
Cloves	4 grains.
Vanilla	24 grains.
Ammoniated glycyrrhizin	110 grains.
Diluted alcohol	6½ fl. ounces.
Water, hot	1 fl. ounce.
Simple syrup, enough to make	16 fl. ounces

Reduce the drugs to moderately coarse powder, macerate for 7 days in the diluted alcohol, and filter, adding, if necessary, enough diluted alcohol through the filter to make the filtrate measure 6½ fluid ounces. Dissolve the glycyrrhizin in the water, mix this solution with the filtrate, and add the syrup.

3046. Elixir of Licorice-Aromatic. B

Select licorice root, cut and slightly bruised	2¼ av. ounces.
Water of ammonia	4 fl. drams.
Glycerin	1 fl. ounce.
Water	16 fl. ounces.

Macerate for 24 hours, strain, boil for 10 minutes, filter, and evaporate at gentle heat until reduced to 6 fluid ounces.

Now add to this evaporated infusion.

Simple syrup	6 fl. ounces.
Alcohol	4 fl. ounces.
Spirit of orange	2 fl. drams.
Oil of cinnamon (Ceylon)	2 drops.

This elixir is employed for disguising the taste of bitter medicines, particularly quinine. No acid should be used because it dissolves the quinine and makes its bitter taste more perceptible, and at the same time liberates the glycyrrhizin from its combination with ammonia and renders it insoluble, and therefore valueless for the purpose of disguising or modifying taste.

3047. Elixir of Licorice Compound.

Pure extract of licorice, (U. S. P.)	½ av. ounce.
Wine of antimony	1 fl. ounce.
Paregoric	2 fl. ounces.
Spirit of nitrous ether	4 fl. drams.
Elixir of cherries, enough to make	16 fl. ounces.

Dissolve the extract in a portion of the elixir and add the remaining ingredients.

The above replaces "brown mixture" in the form of an elixir.

3048. Elixir of Long Life.

("Elixir ad Longam Vitam."—"Elixir of Life."—Compound Tincture of Aloes. (Germ. Pharm.) ("Swedish Bitters.")

Aloes	200 grains.
Rhubarb	35 grains.
Gentian	35 grains.
Zedoary	35 grains.
Spanish saffron	35 grains.
Water	4 fl. ounces.
Alcohol	12 fl. ounces.

Mix the drugs in coarse powder with the two liquids, macerate for 3 days, agitating frequently; express and filter. Sometimes 35 grains of agaric is added to the other drugs, and the menstruum generally employed is diluted alcohol.

The following is a simple formula which may be used for the preparation of this ancient and complicated remedy.

Tincture of aloes and myrrh	8 fl. ounces.
Tincture of rhubarb	2 fl. ounces.
Compound tincture of gentian	1 fl. ounce.
Water	1 fl. ounce.
Alcohol	4 fl. ounces.

3049. Elixir of Lupulin.

Fluid extract of lupulin	1 fl. ounce.
Magnesium carbonate	1 av. ounce.
Simple elixir, enough to make	16 fl. ounces.

Triturate the fluid extract with the talcum, add the elixir, transfer to a bottle, set aside for several hours, and filter.

The above is of the strength usually furnished by manufacturers; Diehl's formula, which is largely used, directs the use of 2 fluid ounces of the fluid extract to the pint of finished elixir.

3050. Elixir of Lupulin and Sodium Bromide.

Fluid extract of lupulin	10½ fl. drams.
Purified talcum	120 grains.
Sodium bromide	640 grains.
Aromatic elixir of licorice, enough to make	16 fl. ounces.

Triturate the fluid extract with the talcum, add some of the elixir, transfer to a bottle, add the sodium salt and the remainder of the elixir, dissolve by agitation, and filter after several hours.

Each fluid dram represents 5 grains of lupulin and contains 5 grains of sodium bromide.

3051. Elixir of Malt.

Extract of malt............ 4 fl. ounces.
Simple elixir.............. 12 fl. ounces.

3052. Elixir of Malt and Pepsin.

Elixir of malt............ 8 fl. ounces.
Elixir of pepsin, N. F..... 8 fl. ounces.

Mix and filter.

Each fluid dram represents ½ grain of pepsin and 15 minims of extract of malt.

3053. Elixir of Manaca and Salicylates.

Fluid extract of manaca... 2½ fl. ounces.
Sodium salicylate......... 1¾ av. ounces
Potassium salicylate...... 384 grains.
Lithium salicylate........ 96 grains.
Simple elixir, enough to
 make .... 16 fl. ounces.

Dissolve the salicylates in some of the elixir add the fluid extract and the remainder of the elixir, allow to stand for a few hours, and filter through talcum.

Each fluid dram contains 6 grains of sodium salicylate, 3 grains of potassium salicylate, and ¾ grain of lithium salicylate, and represents nearly 10 grains of manaca.

3054. Elixir of Matico, Compound.

Fluid extract of matico.... 3 fl. ounces.
Fluid extract of buchu..... 1½ fl. ounces.
Fluid extract of cubeb..... 1½ fl. ounces.
Alcohol .... 2 fl. ounces.
Simple elixir.............. 4 fl. ounces.
Compound elixir of taraxacum .... 4 fl. ounces.

Mix, set aside for 3 days, and filter through talcum.

Each fluid dram represents 11 grains of matico and nearly 4 grains each of buchu and cubeb.

3055. Elixir of Morphine Valerianate.

Morphine valerianate...... 16 grains.
Simple elixir............. 16 fl. ounces.

Dissolve by agitation and filter.

Each fluid dram contains ⅛ grain of morphine valerianate.

3056. Elixir of Orange.

Oil of orange............. 4½ fl. drams.
Alcohol .... 14 fl. ounces.
Water .... 22 fl. ounces.
Simple syrup.............. 28 fl. ounces.
Purified talcum........... ½ av. ounce.

Mix the oil and alcohol, add the talcum, shake well, and then add the other ingredients in small portions at a time, agitating well after each addition.—U. S. P. 1880 modified.

The oil used should be a perfectly fresh sweet oil of orange peel.

3057. Elixir of Orange, Compound.

(Compound Wine of Orange.—Vinum Amarum, Bitter Wine.—Elixir Stomachicum, Stomachic Elixir.—Elixir Viscerale Hoffmani.)

Bitter orange peel, cut.... 1600 grains.
Cinnamon, bruised......... 320 grains.
Potassium carbonate....... 80 grains.
Extract of gentian........ 160 grains.
Extract of wormwood...... 160 grains.
Extract of buckbean....... 160 grains.
Extract of cascarilla...... 160 grains.
Sherry wine, enough to
 make .... 16 fl. ounces.

Macerate the orange peel, cinnamon and potassium carbonate with 16 fluid ounces of sherry wine for 8 days, agitating occasionally; express the liquid portion, in the latter dissolve the extracts, filter, and add enough sherry wine through the filter to make the filtrate measure 16 fluid ounces.—Germ. Pharm.

The National Formulary also recognizes what is identically the same preparation under the title of "compound wine of orange;" in the latter no extracts are used, but the drugs themselves are mixed with the orange peel, cinnamon, and potassium carbonate, the whole being extracted by percolation.

3058. Elixir of Pancreas.

Take 1 pig pancreas, chop into pieces, and macerate in a cool place for 3 days in a mixture of

Water .... 32 fl. ounces.
Glycerin .... 6½ fl. ounces.
Hydrochloric acid......... 5 fl. ounces.

Strain, add ½ fluid dram of oil of orange and enough glycerin to make 48 fluid ounces, and filter.

3059. Elixir of Pancreatin.

Pancreatin, pure.......... 128 grains.
Sodium bicarbonate........ 16 grains.
Water .... 2 fl. ounces.
Simple elixir enough to
 make .... 16 fl. ounces.

Macerate the pancreatin in the water for 24 hours, add the sodium bicarbonate, triturate until dissolved, gradually add the elixir and filter.

Each fluid dram represents 1 grain of pancreatin.

The elixir of pancreas may be substituted for the above, if deemed desirable.

3060. Elixir of Pancreatin, Bismuth and Pepsin.

Citrate of bismuth and ammonium	128 grains.
Pancreatin, pure	64 grains.
Pepsin, pure	64 grains.
Distilled water, hot	1 fl. ounce.
Water of ammonia	sufficient.
Glycerin	2 fl. ounces.
Water	2 fl. ounces.
Tincture of cudbear	2 fl. drams.
Simple elixir, enough to make	16 fl. ounces.

Triturate the bismuth salt with the water, allow the insoluble portion to subside, decant the clear portion, to the residue add ammonia water very gradually, until the solution occurs, carefully avoiding any excess, and mix this liquid with the decanted portion.

Macerate the pepsin and pancreatin with the glycerin and water for 24 hours, agitating occasionally; add the tincture, the bismuth solution, and the elixir, and filter through purified talcum.

Each fluid dram contains 1 grain each of pepsin and of citrate of bismuth and ammonium, and ½ grain of pancreatin.

3061. Elixir of Pancreatin and Pepsin.

Pancreatin, pure	64 grains.
Pepsin, pure	128 grains.
Glycerin	2 fl. ounces.
Water	2 fl. ounces.
Tincture of cudbear	2 fl. drams.
Simple elixir, enough to make	16 fl. ounces.

Macerate the pepsin and pancreatin with the glycerin and water for 24 hours, agitating occasionally; add the tincture and elixir, and filter through talcum.

Each fluid dram contains 1 grain of pepsin and ½ grain of pancreatin.

3062. Elixir of Papain.

Papain	256 grains.
Glycerin	3¼ fl. ounces.
Sherry wine	8 fl. ounces.
Saccharin	10 grains.
Chloroform water	4¾ fl. ounces.

Mix, let stand for 7 days, agitating occasionally, and filter.

Each fluid dram contains 2 grains of papain.

3063. Elixir of Paraldehyde.

Paraldehyde	4 fl. ounces.
Glycerin	2 fl. ounces.
Alcohol	5 fl. ounces.
Tincture of cardamom	2½ fl. drams.
Oil of orange	15 minims.
Oil of cinnamon	15 minims.
Compound tincture of cudbear	2 fl. drams.
Aromatic elixir, enough to make	16 fl. ounces.

Mix the ingredients in the order given, and filter, if necessary.—N. F.

Each fluid dram contains 15 minims of paraldehyde.

Elixir of paraldehyde varies in strength from 10 to 25 per cent, as prescribed in different localities. The formula here given produces a 25 per cent elixir, and from this the weaker preparations may readily be made by the addition of aromatic elixir colored with compound tincture of cudbear in the proportion used in the above formula.

To make a 20 per cent elixir of paraldehyde, for instance, 4 fluid ounces of the 25 per cent elixir are mixed with 1 fluid ounce of colored aromatic elixir. To make 5 fluid ounces of 15 per cent elixir, 3 fluid ounces of the 25 per cent elixir are required, and to make the same quantity of 10 per cent elixir, 2 fluid ounces of the above elixir are required.

3064. Elixir of Pareira Brava.

Fluid extract of pareira	2 fl. ounces.
Simple elixir	14 fl. ounces.

Mix, allow to stand for 24 hours and filter through talcum.

Each fluid dram represents 7½ grains of pareira brava.

3065. Elixir of Pepsin.

Pepsin, pure	128 grains.
Hydrochloric acid	½ fl. dram.
Glycerin	2 fl. ounces.
Compound elixir of taraxacum	1 fl. ounce.
Alcohol	3 fl. ounces.
Purified talcum	120 grains.
Sugar	4½ av. ounces.
Water, enough to make	16 fl. ounces

Mix the pepsin with 6 fluid ounces of water, add the glycerin and acid, and agitate until solution has been effected. Then add the compound elixir of taraxacum, alcohol, and the talcum, and mix thoroughly. Set the mixture aside for a few hours, occasionally agitating. Then filter it through a wetted filter, dissolve the sugar in the filtrate, and pass the remainder of the water through the filter.

Each fluid dram represents 1 grain of pepsin.—N. F.

3066. Elixir of Pepsin, Compound. A
(Elixir of Lactated or Lactinated Pepsin.—Compound Digestive Elixir.)

Pepsin, soluble scales......	75 grains.
Pancreatin, pure...........	8 grains.
Diastase	8 grains.
Lactic acid................	20 minims.
Hydrochloric acid..........	40 minims.
Glycerin	4 fl. ounces.
Water	2 fl. ounces.
Tincture of cudbear, N. F..	2 fl. drams.
Talcum, purified...........	120 grains.
Aromatic elixir, enough to make	16 fl. ounces.

Add the acid to the water and glycerin, and to this mixture add the pepsin, pancreatin, and diastase, and macerate until apparently dissolved; then add the tincture and aromatic elixir; thoroughly incorporate the purified talcum and filter.

3067. Elixir of Pepsin, Compound. B

Pepsin, pure...............	80 grains.
Pancreatin	40 grains.
Diastase of ptyolin........	10 grains.
Cudbear, powdered.........	180 grains.
Diluted hydrochloric acid..	20 minims.
Lactic acid................	3 drops.
Alcohol	3 fl. ounces.
Water	7 fl. ounces.
Simple syrup..............	6 fl. ounces.

Mix all the above except the syrup, macerate for 3 days, agitating frequently; filter, to the filtrate add the syrup, and then through the filter add enough of a mixture of alcohol and water, in the proportion of 5 to 7 by measure, to make the liquid measure 16 fluid ounces.

3068. Elixir of Pepsin and Quinine.

Quinine sulphate...........	32 grains.
Elixir of pepsin............	16 fl. ounces.

Agitate until dissolved and filter.

Each fluid dram contains 1 grain of pepsin and ¼ grain of quinine sulphate.

3069. Elixir of Pepsin, Quinine and Strychnine.

Strychnine sulphate........	1¼ grains.
Distilled water.............	4 fl. drams.
Elixir of pepsin and quinine	15½ fl. ounces.

Dissolve the alkaloidal salt in the water and add the elixir.

Each fluid dram contains 1/100 grain of strychnine sulphate, nearly ¼ grain of quinine sulphate, and nearly 1 grain of pepsin.

3070. Elixir of Pepsin and Strychnine.

Strychnine sulphate.......	1¼ grains.
Distilled water............	4 fl. drams.
Elixir of pepsin............	15½ fl. ounces.

Dissolve the alkaloidal salt in the water and add the elixir.

Each fluid dram contains 1/100 grain of strychnine sulphate and nearly 1 grain of pepsin.

3071. Elixir of Pepsin and Wafer Ash.
(Elixir Pepsin and Ptelea.)

Pepsin, pure...............	128 grains.
Simple elixir...............	14 fl. ounces.
Fluid extract of wafer ash.	2 fl. ounces.
Purified talcum............	120 grains.

Add the pepsin to the simple elixir, agitate until dissolved, add the remaining ingredients, set aside for 24 hours, and filter.

Each fluid dram contains 1 grain of pepsin and represents 7½ grains of wafer ash.

3072. Elixir of Phosphorus. A

Spirit of phosphorus.......	3¾ fl. ounces.
Oil of anise................	16 minims.
Glycerin	9 fl. ounces.
Aromatic elixir, enough to make	16 fl. ounces.

To the spirit contained in a bottle, add the oil and glycerin, and mix by repeatedly inverting bottle until a clear liquid is obtained. Then add the elixir in several portions, gently agitating after each addition, until all is added.—U. S. P.

3073. Elixir of Phosphorus. B

Phosphorus	2½ grains.
Chloroform	4 fl. drams.
Alcohol	2¾ fl. ounces.
Glycerin, enough to make.	16 fl. ounces.

Dissolve the phosphorus in the chloroform, add the alcohol, and then the glycerin.—Brit. Form.

Each fluid dram contains 1/50 grain of phosphorus.

3074. Elixir of Phosphorus, Compound.

Strychnine sulphate........	1¼ grains.
Quinine sulphate..........	64 grains.
Iron pyrophosphate........	128 grains.
Distilled water, hot........	1 fl. ounce.
Alcohol	1 fl. ounce.

Elixir of phosphorus...... 8 fl. ounces.
Simple elixir, enough to
make .... 16 fl. ounces.

Dissolve the strychnine salt in 4 fluid drams of the water, and the iron salt in the remainder of the water.

Mix the alcohol and elixir of phosphorus, add the two solutions already prepared, then the quinine salt and the simple elixir, agitate until dissolved, and filter in a well-covered funnel.

Each fluid dram contains 1/100 grain of strychnine sulphate, 1 grain of iron pyrophosphate, ½ grain of quinine sulphate and 1/100 grain of phosphorus.

3075. Elixir of Phosphorus, Quinine and Strychnine.

Elixir of phosphorus...... 8 fl. ounces.
Quinine hydrochlorate..... 32 grains.
Strychnine sulphate....... 1¼ grains.
Distilled water........... 4 fl. drams.
Tincture of cudbear....... 2 fl. drams.
Simple elixir, enough to
make .... 16 fl. ounces.

Dissolve the quinine salt in 7 fluid ounces of simple elixir, and the strychnine salt in the water, mix the two solutions, and then add the other ingredients.

Each fluid dram contains 1/100 grain of strychnine sulphate, ¼ grain of quinine sulphate, and 1/100 grain of phosphorus.

3076. Elixir of Phosphorus and Strychnine.

Strychnine sulphate....... 1¼ grains.
Distilled water........... 4 fl. drams.
Elixir of phosphorus...... 8 fl. ounces.
Tincture of cudbear....... 2 fl. drams.
Simple elixir, enough to
make .... 16 fl. ounces.

Dissolve the quinine salt in the water and add the remaining ingredients.

Each fluid dram contains 1/100 grain of of phosphorus and strychnine sulphate.

3077. Elixir Pulmonic.
(Pectoral Elixir.)

Pure extract of licorice, U.
S. P.................... 300 grains.
Fluid extract of squill..... 128 minims.
Fluid extract of senega.... 128 minims.
Fluid extract of henbane
leaves .... 128 minims.
Fluid extract of ipecac.... 64 minims.
Morphine sulphate......... 8 grains.
Distilled water........... 4 fl. drams.
Tincture of cacao......... 1 fl. ounce.
Elixir of cherries, enough
to make............... 16 fl. ounces.

Dissolve the morphine salt in the water, add the licorice extract, mix well, add the remaining ingredients, and filter.

Each fluid dram contains 1/16 grain of morphine sulphate.

3078. Elixir of Quinine Bisulphate.

Quinine bisulphate......... 128 grains.
Simple elixir.............. 16 fl. ounces.

Dissolve by agitation and filter, if necessary.

Each fluid dram contains 1 grain of quinine bisulphate.

Elixir of Quinine, Phosphorus and Strychnine.

Refer to Elixir of Phosphorus and its combinations.

3079. Elixir of Quinine and Strychnine.

Quinine sulphate........... 64 grains.
Strychnine sulphate........ 1¼ grains.
Simple elixir.............. 16 fl. ounces.

Dissolve the alkaloidal salts in the elixir by agitation, and filter.

Each fluid dram contains ½ grain of quinine sulphate and 1/100 grain of strychnine sulphate.

3080. Elixir of Quinine Valerianate.

Quinine valerianate........ 128 grains.
Tincture of cudbear....... 2 fl. drams.
Simple elixir, enough to
make .... 16 fl. ounces.

Triturate the quinine valerianate with a little of the elixir to a smooth paste. Add about 8 fluid ounces more of elixir, triturate until dissolved, add the tincture and the remainder of the elixir.

Each fluid dram contains 1 grain of quinine valerianate.

3081. Elixir of Quinine and Strychnine Valerianates.

Strychnine (alkaloid)...... 1¼ grains.
Valerianic acid............ sufficient.
Quinine valerianate........ 128 grains.
Tincture of cudbear....... 2 fl. drams.
Simple elixir, enough to
make .... 16 fl. ounces.

Triturate the strychnine and quinine sulphate with a little elixir to a smooth paste, add 4 fluid ounces of elixir and just enough valerianic acid to dissolve the alkaloids; then add the tincture and the remainder of the elixir, neutralize any excess of valerianic acid as described in the formula preceding, and filter.

Each fluid dram contains 1 grain of quinine valerianate and 1/100 grain of strychnine valerianate.

3082. Elixir of Rhubarb-Aromatic.

Aromatic fluid extract of rhubarb	1 fl. ounce.
Simple elixir	15 fl. ounces.

This is of the same strength as the aromatic syrup of rhubarb of the United States pharmacopoeia.

3083. Elixir of Rhubarb and Potassium with Pancreatin.

Rhubarb	320 grains.
Golden seal	160 grains.
Cinnamon	160 grains.
Potassium bicarbonate	320 grains.
Pancreatin	320 grains.
Spirit of peppermint	1 fl. dram.
Simple syrup	2 fl. ounces.
Diluted alcohol	} of each
Simple elixir	} sufficient.

Moisten the rhubarb, golden seal and cinnamon (first reduced to a suitable powder) with diluted alcohol, and pack moderately in a percolator; allow to macerate 48 hours and then percolate with diluted alcohol until 6 ounces have been obtained; in the percolate dissolve the potassium bicarbonate and add the pancreatin previously dissolved in the syrup, and about 4 fluid ounces of elixir; mix thoroughly, add the spirit and enough elixir to make the whole measure 16 fluid ounces, and filter.

This is similar to the preceding, containing only pancreatin in addition. Like the preceding, also, it may be prepared with fluid extracts.

3084. Elixir of Rhubarb and Potassium.
(Neutralizing Elixir.)

Rhubarb	320 grains.
Golden seal	160 grains.
Cinnamon	160 grains.
Potassium bicarbonate	320 grains.
Spirit of peppermint	1 fl. dram.
Simple syrup	2 fl. ounces.
Diluted alcohol	} of each
Simple elixir	} sufficient.

Reduce the three drugs to moderately coarse powder, extract them in the usual way by percolation with diluted alcohol until 6 fluid ounces of percolate are obtained. In this percolate dissolve the potassium bicarbonate, add the spirit of peppermint, syrup, and enough elixir to make 16 fluid ounces of product, and filter.

This preparation represents the well-known syrup of rhubarb and potassium in the elixir form.

3085. Elixir of Rhubarb, Magnesia and Senna.

Magnesia, calcined	144 grains.
Acetic acid	sufficient.
Fluid extract of rhubarb	8½ fl. drams.
Fluid extract of senna	8½ fl. drams.
Simple elixir, enough to make	16 fl. ounces.

Dissolve the magnesia in 2½ fluid ounces of acetic acid with the aid of a gentle heat, adding, if necessary, a little more acetic acid, drop by drop, until the solution is neutral to test paper; then add the fluid extracts and elixir, and filter.

Each fluid dram contains 4 grains of magnesium acetate and represents 4 grains each of rhubarb and senna.

3086. Elixir of Rhubarb and Senna.

Fluid extract of rhubarb	2 fl. ounces.
Fluid extract of senna	2 fl. ounces.
Tincture of cacao	2 fl. ounces.
Simple elixir	10 fl. ounces.

Mix and filter, if necessary.

Each fluid dram represents 7½ grains each of senna and rhubarb.

3087. Elixir of Salicylic Acid-Compound.

Salicylic acid	640 grains.
Sodium bicarbonate	480 grains.
Potassium iodide	192 grains.
Fluid extract of black cohosh	4 fl. drams.
Fluid extract of gelsemium	2 fl. drams.
Compound spirit of orange	1 fl. dram.
Glycerin	4 fl. ounces.
Water	4 fl. ounces.
Alcohol	4 fl. ounces.
Simple syrup, enough to make	16 fl. ounces.

Mix the acid, sodium bicarbonate and water in a capacious mortar, stir occasionally until reaction is completed, add the potassium iodide, stir until dissolved, then add the alcohol, glycerin, fluid extracts, spirit and syrup, and filter.

3088. Elixir of Senna. A

Deodorized fluid extract of senna	8 fl. ounces.
Compound tincture of cardamom	½ fl. ounce.
Simple elixir	7½ fl. ounces.

3089. Elixir of Senna. B

Alexandria senna	11 av. ounces.
Sugar	8 av. ounces.
Water	⎫
Alcohol	⎬ of each sufficient.
Diluted alcohol	⎭
Chloroform	16 minims.
Oil of coriander	2 drops.
Tincture of capsicum	20 minims.

Mix 2¾ fluid ounces of alcohol with 8¼ fluid ounces of water, and with it evenly moisten the senna; pack tightly in a closed vessel, macerate for 3 days, express forcibly, break up the marc, macerate it with enough more of the same kind of menstruum to furnish, in all, 11 fluid ounces of liquid, express in 24 hours, mix the two liquids, add the sugar, heat in a closed vessel by means of a waterbath to 94 degrees C., maintain at this temperature 10 minutes, allow to cool, strain, add the chloroform, tincture of capsicum, and oil of coriander, first mixed with 2 fluid drams of alcohol, and finally add, if necessary, enough diluted alcohol to make 16 fluid ounces.—Brit. Form.

3090. Elixir of Senna-Compound.

Fluid extract of senna	2 fl. ounces.
Purified tamarind pulp	4 av. ounces.
Oil of coriander	12 drops.
Alcohol	2 fl. drams.
Simple elixir, enough to make	16 fl. ounces.

Dissolve the oil in the alcohol, add to the fluid extract and pulp, then add the elixir.

3091. Elixir of Saw Palmetto and Pichi.

Fluid extract of saw palmetto	2 ounces.
Fluid extract pichi	1 ounce.
Oil of sandalwood	¼ ounce.
Potassium iodide	512 grains.
Ammonium chloride	512 grains.
Simple elixir enough to make	16 fl. ounces.

3092. Elixir of Saw Palmetto and Sandalwood-Compound.

Fluid extract of saw palmetto	2 ounces.
Oil of sandalwood	¼ ounce.
Alcohol	1¾ fl. ounces.
Simple elixir, enough to make	16 fl. ounces.

3093. Elixir Simple. A

Oil of orange	1½ drams.
Oil of lemon	¼ dram.
Oil of cardamom	10 minims.
Oil of coriander	5 minims.
Tincture of vanilla, made from vanillin	2 ounces.
Cologne spirits, 188 per cent	2 pints.
Simple syrup	3 pints.
Rose water	1 pint.
Water, distilled	2 pints.
Magnesia carbonate	1 ounce.

Dissolve the oils in 4 ounces of the cologne spirits; place the magnesia in a large mortar; pour on the solution of oils and triturate well.

Take 12 ounces of the spirits, mix with the 32 ounces of water, and slowly add to the contents of the mortar, stirring constantly and uniformly for 10 minutes to ensure its solubility; filter and set aside. Mix the syrup and rose water, and to this mixture add the remaining pint of spirits, then add the 2 ounces of vanillin extract, and shake well. To this add the soluble flavoring and mix thoroughly. If the syrup is clear (as it should be) no further filtration is needed—if red elixir is desired, color with carmine and caramel, q. s. This elixir has a very fine flavor, is easily made and can be used with iron salts.

3094. Elixir Simple. B

Oil of orange	½ fl. dram.
Oil of cinnamon	5 drops.
Oil of anise	2 drops.
Oil of bitter almond	1 drop.
Tincture of cardamom	5 fl. drams.
Alcohol	16¾ fl. ounces.
Water	36 fl. ounces.
Sugar	20 ounces.
Cacao (Baker's)	240 grains.
Magnesium carbonate	480 grains.

Mix the oils, tincture and alcohol, and triturate with the cacao and magnesium carbonate, having first mixed the latter intimately; transfer the mixture to a bottle, add the water gradually, agitate occasionally for several hours, filter, express the filter between muslin, filter the expressed liquid, mix the two filtrates, in the liquid dissolve the sugar by agitation, and filter or strain as may be necessary.

3095. Elixir Simple. C

Oil of orange	70 minims.
Alcohol	27½ fl. ounces.
Purified talcum	120 grains.
Orange flower water	18¼ fl. ounces.
Simple syrup	18¼ fl. ounces.

Mix the oil and alcohol, add the talcum, shake well, add the other ingredients, shake again, and filter.

3096. Elixir Simple. D

Tincture of fresh orange peel	12 fl. ounces.
Tincture of fresh lemon peel	4 fl. ounces.
Alcohol	8 fl. ounces.
Orange flower water	8 fl. ounces.
Purified talcum	2 av. ounces.
Simple syrup	32 fl. ounces.

Mix the whole well and filter.

This and the preceding have been known as elixir of orange.

3097. Elixir Simple. E

Oil of sweet orange	1½ fl. ounces.
Oil of caraway	20 drops.
Alcohol	14½ fl. ounces.
Spirit of cinnamon	32 drops.
Simple syrup	36 fl. ounces.
Glycerin	8 fl. ounces.
Distilled water	4 fl. ounces.
Calcium phosphate	1½ ounces.

Mix the oils and alcohol, add the calcium phosphate, shake well, add the other ingredients, shake again, and filter.

3098. Elixir Simple. F

Oil of orange	2¼ fl. drams.
Oil of Ceylon cinnamon	3 drops.
Oil of anise	3 drops.
Oil of caraway	6 drops.
Tincture of vanilla	9 fl. drams.
Simple syrup	26 fl. ounces.
Sherry wine	3 fl. ounces.
Alcohol	12½ fl. ounces.
Water	23 fl. ounces.
Purified talcum	1 av. ounce.

Mix the oils with the talcum; mix the alcohol, wine and water, add to the mixture of talcum and oils, then add the vanilla and the syrup; let stand one hour, shaking often, and filter.

3099. Elixir Simple. G

Saccharin solution	24 grains.
Oil of anise	160 minims.
Alcohol	16 fl. ounces.
Distilled water, enough to make	64 fl. ounces.

Dissolve the saccharin in 40 fluid ounces of water, add the oil of anise, previously dissolved in 16 fluid ounces of alcohol, and the remainder of the water. Add 1 av. ounce of purified talcum; let stand 24 hours, occasionally shaking, and filter.

3100. Elixir Simple. H

Cinnamon water	24 fl. ounces.
Simple syrup	24 fl. ounces.
Alcohol	16 fl. ounces.
Spirit of orange	2 fl. ounces.

This may be clarified by shaking with paper pulp or purified talcum, and filtering. The pulp can be made by beating ½ av. ounce filter paper in a mortar with sufficient water just to moisten it.

3101. Elixir Simple. I

Ceylon cinnamon	90 grains.
Star anise	60 grains.
Coriander	90 grains.
Nutmeg	30 grains.
Caraway	90 grains.
Oil of sweet orange	½ fl. dram.
Diluted alcohol	sufficient.
Simple syrup	32 fl. ounces.

Percolate the aromatics, previously reduced to coarse powder, with diluted alcohol previously mixed with the oil of orange, continuing the percolation until 32 fluid ounces of aromatic tincture are obtained, and mix with the syrup, filtering through talcum, if necessary.

3102. Elixir Simple. J

Orange flower water	32 fl. ounces.
Bitter almond water	8 fl. ounces.
Simple syrup	8 fl. ounces.
Glycerin	8 fl. ounces.
Alcohol	8 fl. ounces.

Mix all and filter through purified talcum.

3103. Elixir of Stillingia. A

Fluid extract of stillingia	2 fl. ounces.
Alcohol	4 fl. drams.
Simple elixir, enough to make	16 fl. ounces.

Mix the fluid extract and alcohol, add the elixir, and filter through purified talcum.

Each fluid dram represents 7½ grains of stillingia.

3104. Elixir of Stillingia. B

Compound fluid extract of stillingia	2 fl. ounces.
Alcohol	2 fl. ounces.
Compound elixir of taraxacum	2 fl. ounces.
Simple elixir	10 fl. ounces.

Mix the fluid extract and alcohol, add the elixirs, and filter through talcum.

3105. Elixir of Sumbul.
(Elixir of Musk Root.)

Fluid extract of sumbul...	2½ fl. ounces.
Alcohol	1 fl. ounce.
Elixir simple	12½ fl. ounces.
Purified talcum	½ av. ounce.

Triturate the fluid extract with the talcum, add the alcohol and elixir, and filter.

Each fluid dram represents about 10 grains of sumbul.

3106. Elixir of Sumbul, Compound.

Fluid extract of sumbul...	2 fl. ounces.
Fluid extract of skullcap..	4 fl. drams.
Fluid extract of valerian..	1 fl. dram.
Alcohol	1 fl. ounce.
Adjuvant elixir, enough to make	16 fl. ounces.
Purified talcum	½ av. ounce.

Mix the fluid extracts and alcohol, add the talcum, shake well, then add the elixir, shake again, and filter.

Each fluid dram represents 7½ grains of sumbul, about 2 grains of skullcap, and about ½ grain of valerian.

3107. Elixir of Tar, Compound.
N. F.

Syrup of wild cherry	3¼ fl. ounces.
Syrup of tolu	3¼ fl. ounces.
Morphine sulphate	2½ grains.
Methylic alcohol	6 fl. drams.
Distilled water, hot	1 fl. dram.
Wine of tar, enough to make	16 fl. ounces.

Dissolve the morphine sulphate in the water, add the solution to the two syrups previously mixed, then add the methylic alcohol and the wine of tar.

Each fluid dram contains 1-50 grain of morphine sulphate.

3108. Elixir of Terpin Hydrate.

Terpin hydrate	128 grains.
Glycerin	1 fl. ounce.
Alcohol	2 fl. ounces.
Simple elixir, enough to make	16 fl. ounces.

Each fluid dram contains 1 grain of terpin hydrate.

3109. Elixir of Triple Valerianates.

Iron valerianate	64 grains.
Quinine valerianate	64 grains.
Zinc valerianate	64 grains.
Tincture of cudbear	2 fl. drams.
Valerianic acid	sufficient.
Simple elixir enough to make	16 fl. ounces.

Triturate the 3 valerianates with 8 fluid ounces of elixir to a smooth paste, add, if necessary, a very small amount of the acid, just enough to dissolve the salts, then add the tincture and the remainder of the elixir, and filter.

If too much valerianic acid has been added so that it is betrayed by its odor, it should be exactly neutralized by stirring with a glass rod repeatedly dipped in dilute ammonia water.

Each fluid dram contains ½ grain each of the valerianates of iron, quinine and zinc.

3110. Elixir of Wafer Ash.
(Elixir of Ptelea.)

Fluid extract of wafer ash.	2¾ fl. ounces.
Simple elixir, enough to make	16 fl. ounces.

Mix, and allow to stand for about 24 hours, then filter through purified talcum.

Each fluid dram represents 10 grains of wafer ash.

3111. Elixir of Wahoo.
N. F.
(Elixir of Euonymus.)

Fluid extract of wahoo	2½ fl. ounces.
Water	2 fl. ounces.
Syrup of coffee	2 fl. ounces.
Compound elixir of taraxacum	9½ fl. ounces.

Mix them, let the mixture stand 48 hours, and filter.

Each fluid dram represents about 9½ grains of wahoo.

3112. Elixir of White Pine, Compound.

Fluid extract of white pine bark	1 fl. ounce.
Fluid extract of balsam Gilead buds	64 minims.
Fluid extract of spikenard.	64 minims.
Fluid extract of wild cherry bark	1 fl. ounce.
Sanguinarine nitrate	2 grains.
Morphine acetate	3 grains.
Chloroform	64 minims.
Alcohol	4 fl. ounces.
Water	7 fl. ounces.
Simple syrup	3 fl. ounces.

Mix the fluid extracts with the alcohol, water and syrup previously mixed, and filter through purified talcum until clear; add the chloroform and dissolve the sanguinarine and morphine salts in the mixture.

The above represents the now well-known "white pine cough syrup" in the elixir form.

3113. Elixir of Wild Cherry.

Fluid extract of wild cherry	4 fl. ounces.
Alcohol	1 fl. ounce.
Simple elixir	11 fl. ounces.

Mix, allow to stand for 24 hours, and filter through purified talcum.

Each fluid dram represents 15 grains of wild cherry.

3114. Elixir of Yerba Santa. A
(Elixir of Eriodictyon.)

Fluid extract of yerba santa	2 fl. ounces.
Pumice stone, powdered	1 av. ounce.
Alcohol	1 fl. ounce.
Simple elixir, enough to make	16 fl. ounces.

Triturate the fluid extract with the pumice stone until well mixed, add the alcohol, mix again, then add 13 fluid ounces of elixir, mix once more, let the whole stand for several hours, stirring occasionally, then filter, returning the first portions of filtrate to the filter until the liquid is clear, and finally adding enough simple elixir through the filter until the filtrate measures the requisite amount.

Each fluid dram represents 7½ grains of yerba santa.

3115. Elixir of Yerba Santa, Aromatic. B
(Elixir Corrigens.)
N. F.

Fl. ext. of yerba santa	1 fl. ounce.
Simple syrup	8 fl. ounces.
Pumice, fine powder	240 grains.
Magnesium carbonate	80 grains.
Compound elixir of taraxacum, enough to make	16 fl. ounces.

Mix 7 fluid ounces of compound elixir of taraxacum with the syrup and pumice, then add the fluid extract, and mix the whole thoroughly by agitation. Shake the mixture occasionally during 2 hours, then allow it to settle, and carefully decant the liquid into a funnel, the neck of which contains a small pellet of absorbent cotton. Afterwards add the dregs and allow them to drain. To the filtrate add the magnesium carbonate, and shake occasionally during several hours. Let the mixture stand at rest during 12 hours. If convenient, then decant the liquid and filter it through paper. To the filtrate add enough compound elixir of taraxacum, if necessary, to make 16 fluid ounces.

3116. Elixir of Yerba Santa, Aromatic. C

Yerba santa, coarse powder	360 grains.
Sweet orange peel, recently dried and in coarse powder	120 grains.
Liquor potassa	1 fl. dram.
Oil of cloves	4 drops.
Oil of cinnamon	4 drops.
Oil of caraway	2 drops.
Oil of coriander	1 drop.
Comp. tinct. of cardamom	1 fl. dram.
Sugar	7 av. ounces.
Glycerin	} of each sufficient.
Water	
Alcohol	

Mix the oils and tincture with the drugs and extract by percolation in the usual way, employing as a menstruum a mixture of 1 part of alcohol, 1 of glycerin, and 3 of water, all by measure, with 1 per cent of liquor potassa; 10 fluid ounces of percolate are to be obtained, which is to be returned to the percolator. If not clear; to this add the remainder of the liquor potassa and 2 fluid ounces of alcohol, and in the whole dissolve the sugar by agitation.

3117. Elixir of Yerba Santa, Aromatic. D

Yerba santa	1 av. ounce.
Sweet orange peel	144 grains.
Cardamom (without capsule)	28 grains.
Cloves	28 grains.
Cinnamon	28 grains.
Anise	20 grains.
Coriander	20 grains.
Caraway	20 grains.
Red saunders	10 grains.
Sugar	7 av. ounces.
Alcohol	} of each sufficient.
Glycerin	
Distilled water	

Mix the drugs, reduce to moderately coarse powder, extract by percolation with a menstruum composed of 1 part of alcohol, 1 of glycerin, and 3 of water, all by measure, until 12 fluid ounces of percolate are obtained; in the latter dissolve the sugar by agitation, and filter.

3118. Elixir of Yerba Santa, Compound.

Fluid extract of yerba santa	1 fl. ounce.
Fluid extract of grindelia	1 fl. ounce.
Alcohol	1 fl. ounce.
Pumice stone, powdered	1 av. ounce.
Simple elixir enough to make	16 fl. ounces.

Mix the fluid extracts, triturate with pumice stone, add 13 fluid ounces of simple elixir, mix again, allow the whole to stand for several hours, stirring occasionally, and filter.

Each fluid dram represents nearly 4 grains each of yerba santa and grindelia.

ELIXIRS OF THE NATIONAL FORMULARY.

3119.   Elixir of Acidi Salicylic.
(N. F.)
Salicylic acid.............. 640 grains.
Citrate of potassium....... 2 tr. ounces.
Glycerin .... 8 fl. ounces.
Aromatic elixir enough to
  make .... 16 fl. ounces.

Dissolve the citrate of potassium in the glycerin, with the aid of a gentle heat; add the salicylic acid, and continue the heat until it is dissolved. Then add enough aromatic elixir to make sixteen fluid ounces.

This elixir should be freshly made when wanted for use.

Each fluid dram contains 5 grains of salicylic acid.

3120.   Elixir Adjuvants.
(N. F. Adjuvant Elixir.)
Sweet orange peel, recently
  dried .... 2 tr. ounces.
Wild cherry................ 4 tr. ounces.
Glycyrrhiza, Russian,
  peeled .... 8 tr. ounces.
Coriander .... 1 tr. ounce.
Caraway .... 1 tr. ounce.
Alcohol .... ⎫
Water .... ⎬ of each sufficient
Syrup .... ⎭
quantity, enough to make 1 gallon.

Grind the wild cherry to a moderately coarse (No. 40) powder, moisten it with four (4) fluid ounces of water and set it aside for twelve hours. Reduce the other solids also to a moderately coarse (No. 40) powder, mix this intimately with the wild cherry, and having mixed one (1) volume of alcohol with two (2) volumes of water, moisten the powder with four (4) fluid ounces of the mixture, and pack tightly in a percolator. Then gradually pour menstruum on top until ninety-six (96) fluid ounces of percolate are obtained. Mix this with thirty-two (32) fluid ounces of syrup, and filter.

NOTE.—This preparation is chiefly intended as a vehicle, particularly for acrid or saline remedies.

3121.   Elixir Ammonii Bromidi.
(Elixir of Bromide of Ammonium.)
Bromide of ammonium..... 640 grains.
Citric acid................. 30 grains.
Adjuvant elixir, enough to
  make .... 16 fl. ounces.

Dissolve the bromide of ammonium and the citric acid in about eight (8) fluid ounces of adjuvant elixir, by agitation. Then add enough adjuvant elixir to make sixteen (16) fluid ounces, and filter, if necessary.

Each fluid dram contains 5 grains of bromide of ammonium.

3122.   Elixir Ammonii Valerianatis.
(Elixir of Valerianate of Ammonium.)
Valerianate of ammonium.. 256 grains.
Water of ammonia......... sufficient.
Chloroform .... 6 minims.
Tincture of vanilla........ 120 minims.
Compound tincture of cudbear .... 120 minims.
Aromatic elixir, enough to
  make .... 16 fl. ounces.

Dissolve the valerianate of ammonium in about twelve (12) fluid ounces of aromatic elixir, in a graduated vessel, and add enough water of ammonia, in drops, until a faint excess of it is perceptible in the liquid. Then add the chloroform, tincture of vanilla, and compound tincture of cudbear, and, finally, enough aromatic elixir to make sixteen (16) fluid ounces. Filter, if necessary.

Each fluid dram contains 2 grains of valerianate of ammonium.

Note.—Should the odor of valerianic acid become perceptible after the elixir has been kept for some time, it may be overcome by slightly supersaturating with water of ammonia.

3123.   Elixir Ammonii Valerianatis et Quininæ.
(Elixir of Valerianate of Ammonium and of Quinine.)
Hydrochlorate of quinine.. 32 grains.
Elixir of valerianate of ammonium .... 16 fl. ounces.

Dissolve the hydrochlorate of quinine in the elixir by agitation, and, if necessary, by occasionally immersing the bottle containing the ingredients in hot water, until solution has been effected. Finally, filter.

Each fluid dram contains ¼ grain of hydrochlorate of quinine and 2 grains of valerianate of ammonium.

3124.   Elixir Anisi.
(N. F.)
(Elixir of Anise. Aniseed Cordial.)
Anethol .... 25 minims.
Oil of fennel.............. 5 minims.
Oil of bitter almond....... 1 drop.
Deodorized alcohol........ 4 fl. ounces.

Syrup .... 10 fl. ounces.
Water .... 2 fl. ounces.
Purified talcum........... 120 grains.

Mix the anethol and the oils with the deodorized alcohol, add the syrup and water, and set the mixture aside for twelve hours. Then mix it intimately with the purified talcum, and filter it through a wetted filter, returning the first portions of the filtrate until it runs through clear.

Note.—This elixir is liable to become cloudy from separation of essential oils, when it is exposed to a temperature lower than that at which it has been filtered. In general, it is recommended that it be cooled to, and filtered at, a temperature of about 15° C. (59° F.). In the northern sections of this country, or in winter time, it should be cooled to a proportionately lower temperature previous to filtration.

Anethol is the stearopten of oil of anise, and possesses a finer and purer aroma and taste than any commercial variety of oil of anise. If it cannot be readily obtained, the so-called Saxon oil of anise may be substituted for it. Oil of star-anise, which is usually supplied by dealers when "oil of anise" without specification is ordered, does not answer well for this purpose. The oil of fennel should be that from the seed ("sweet"), and not that from the chaff.

3125. Elixir Apii Graveolentis Compositum
(N. F.)

(Compound Elixir of Celery.)

Fluid extract of celery root 1 fl. ounce.
Fluid extract of erythroxylon .... 1 fl. ounce.
Fluid extract of kola........ 1 fl. ounce.
Fluid extract of viburnum prunifolium .... 1 fl. ounce.
Alcohol .... 2 fl. ounces.
Aromatic elixir, enough to make .... 16 fl. ounces.

Mix the alcohol with four (4) fluid ounces of aromatic elixir. To this add the fluid extract of celery root in several portions, shaking after each addition, and afterwards the other fluid extracts. Finally, add enough aromatic elixir to make sixteen (16) fluid ounces; allow the mixture to stand twenty-four hours, and filter.

Note.—If this preparation is prescribed or quoted under its Latin title, it is recommended that the full title be given, so that the word "Apii" may not be mistaken for "Opii."

3126. Elixir Aromaticum.
(N. F.)
(Aromatic Elixir.)

Aromatic spirit........... 16 fl. ounces.
Syrup .... 24 fl. ounces.
Water .... 24 fl. ounces.
Purified talcum........... 1 tr. ounce.

Mix the aromatic spirit with twelve (12) fluid ounces of syrup, and add the water. Incorporate the purified talcum thoroughly with the mixture; set the latter aside during a few days, if possible, occasionally agitating, then stir it well, and filter it through a wetted filter, returning the first portions of the filtrate until it runs through clear. Finally, mix the filtrate with the remainder of the syrup.

Note.—When this elixir is to be used in preparations containing iron, the aromatic spirit to be used in its preparation should be that made from the essential oils. (See Spiritus Aromaticus.)

If it is desired to color this elixir, this may be effected by the addition of two (2) fluid drams of compound tincture of cudbear to each pint.

3127. Elixir Bismuthi.
N. F.
(Elixir of Bismuth.)

Citrate of bismuth and ammonium .... 256 grains.
Water, hot................. 1 fl. ounce.
Water of ammonia......... sufficient.
Aromatic elixir, enough to make .... 16 fl. ounces.

Dissolve the citrate of bismuth and ammonium in the hot water, allow the solution to stand until any undissolved matter has subsided; then decant the clear liquid, and add to the residue just enough water of ammonia to dissolve it. Then mix it with the decanted portion and add enough aromatic elixir to make sixteen (16) fluid ounces. Filter, if necessary.

Each fluid dram represents 2 grains of citrate of bismuth and ammonium.

3128. Elixir Buchu.
N. F.
(Elixir of Buchu.)

Fluid extract of buchu.... 2 fl. ounces.
Alcohol .... 1 fl. ounce.
Syrup .... 1 fl. ounce.
Purified talcum........... 120 grains.
Adjuvant elixir, enough to make .... 16 fl. ounces.

Mix the fluid extract of buchu with the alcohol, then add twelve (12) fluid ounces of adjuvant elixir, and the syrup. Incorporate with it the purified talcum, and filter. Finally, pass enough adjuvant elixir through the filter to make sixteen (16) fluid ounces.

Each fluid dram represents about 7½ grains of buchu.

3129. Elixir Buchu Compositum.
N. F.
(Compound Elixir of Buchu.)
Compound fluid extract of
  buchu .... 4 fl. ounces.
Alcohol .... 1 fl. ounce.
Syrup .... 1 fl. ounce.
Purified talcum............. 120 grains.
Adjuvant elixir, enough to
  make .... 16 fl. ounces.

Mix the compound fluid extract of buchu with the alcohol, then add eight (8) fluid ounces of adjuvant elixir, and the syrup. Incorporate with it the purified talcum, and filter. Finally, pass enough adjuvant elixir through the filter to make sixteen (16) fluid ounces.

Each fluid dram represents 15 minims of compound fluid extract of buchu.

Note.—It is advisable to allow the mixture of liquids with the purified talcum to remain at rest for several days before filtering.

3130. Elixir Buchu et Potassii Acetatis.
N. F.
(Elixir of Buchu and Acetate of Potassium.)
Acetate of potassium...... 640 grains.
Elixir of buchu, enough to
  make .... 16 fl. ounces.

Dissolve the acetate of potassium in about twelve (12) fluid ounces of elixir of buchu, filter, if necessary, and add enough elixir of buchu to make sixteen (16) fluid ounces.

Each fluid dram represents 5 grains of acetate of potassium and about 7 grains of buchu.

3131. Elixir Caffeinæ.
N. F.
(Elixir of Caffeine.)
Caffeine .... 128 grains.
Diluted hydrobromic acid
  (U. S. P.)............... 32 grains.
Syrup of coffee........... 4 fl. ounces.
Aromatic elixir, enough to
  make .... 16 fl. ounces.

Rub the caffeine in a mortar, with the diluted hydrobromic acid and about two (2) fluid ounces of aromatic elixir, until solution is effected. Then add the syrup of coffee, and, lastly, enough aromatic elixir to make sixteen (16) fluid ounces. Filter, if necessary.

Each fluid dram contains 1 grain of caffeine.

3132. Elixir Calcii Bromidi.
(Elixir of Bromide of Calcium.)
Bromide of calcium........ 640 grains.
Citric acid................ 30 grains.
Adjuvant elixir, enough to
  make .... 16 fl. ounces.

Dissolve the bromide of calcium and the citric acid in about twelve (12) fluid ounces of adjuvant elixir by agitation. Then add enough adjuvant elixir to make sixteen (16) fluid ounces, and filter, if necessary.

Each fluid dram contains 5 grains of bromide of calcium.

3133. Elixir Calcii Hypophosphitis.
(Elixir of Hypophosphite of Calcium.)
Hypophosphite of calcium. 256 grains.
Citric acid................ 30 grains.
Aromatic elixir, enough to
  make .... 16 fl. ounces.

Dissolve the hypophosphite of calcium in fourteen (14) fluid ounces of aromatic elixir, and filter. Dissolve the citric acid in the filtrate and pass enough aromatic elixir through the filter to make sixteen (16) fluid ounces.

Each fluid dram contains 2 grains of hypophosphite of calcium.

3134. Elixir Calcii Lactophosphatis.
(Elixir of Lactophosphate of Calcium.)
Lactate of calcium........ 128 grains.
Phosphoric acid (U. S. P.)
  50 per cent)............ 128 minims.
Water .... 1 fl. ounce.
Syrup .... 1 fl. ounce.
Aromatic elixir, enough to
  make .... 16 fl. ounces.

Triturate the lactate of calcium with the phosphoric acid, the water, and the syrup, until the salt is dissolved. Then add enough aromatic elixir to make sixteen (16) fluid ounces, and filter.

Each fluid dram represents 1 grain of lactate of calcium, or about 1½ grains of so-called lactophosphate of calcium.

3135. Elixir Catharticum Compositum.
(N. F.)
(Compound Cathartic Elixir.)
Fluid extract of senna..... 2 fl. ounces.
Fluid extract of podophyllum
  .... 1 fl. ounce.
Fluid extract of leptandra. 360 minims.
Fluid extract of jalap..... 360 minims.
Tartrate of potassium and
  sodium .... 2 tr. ounces.
Bicarbonate of sodium..... 120 grains.

Compound elixir of taraxa-
   cum .... 4 fl. ounces.
Elixir of glycyrrhiza,
   enough to make.......... 16 fl. ounces.

Mix the liquids, add the salts, and dissolve them by agitation.

The product should not be filtered, and should be shaken up whenever any of it is dispensed.

The average dose for an adult is 2 fluid drams.

3136. Elixir Chloroformi Compositum.
(N. F.)
Compound Elixir of Chloroform.
Chloroform .... 3 fl. ounces.
Tincture of opium......... 3 fl. ounces.
Spirit of camphor.......... 3 fl. ounces.
Aromatic spirit of ammonia 3 fl. ounces.
Alcohol .... 3 fl. ounces.
Oil of cinnamon (cassia)... 40 minims.
Water, enough to make.... 16 fl. ounces.

Mix the chloroform with the alcohol, then add the oil of cinnamon, aromatic spirit of ammonia, spirit of camphor, tincture of opium, and lastly, enough water to make sixteen (16) fluid ounces. Allow the mixture to stand a few hours, and filter in a well-covered funnel.

Each fluid dram represents about 1 grain of opium and 11 minims of chloroform.

Note.—This preparation is called chloroform paregoric in some sections of the country. It is recommended that this title be abandoned, to prevent confusion with the official paregoric or tincture opii camphorata.

3137.   Elixir Cinchonæ.
(N. F.)
(Elixir of Cinchona. Elixir of Calisaya.)
Tincture of cinchona (U. S.
   P. 1880)................. 2½ fl. ounces.
Aromatic spirit........... 2 fl. ounces.
Syrup .... 6 fl. ounces
Purified talcum........... 120 grains.
Water, enough to make.... 16 fl. ounces.

Mix the liquids, allow the mixture to stand for twenty-four hours or longer, if convenient, then incorporate the purified talcum, and filter through a wetted filter, returning the first portions of the filtrate, until it runs through clear.

Each fluid ounce represents about 14 grains of yellow cinchona.

Note.—When elixir of cinchona is directed in combination with preparations of iron, the elixir cinchonae detannatum should be used in place of the above preparation.

3138. Elixir Cinchonæ et Hypophosphitum.
(Elixir of Cinchona with Hypophosphites.)
(Elixir of Calisaya and Hypophosphites.)
Hypophosphite of calcium.. 128 grains.
Hyphosphite of sodium.... 128 grains.
Citric acid................ 30 grains.
Water .... 2 fl. ounces.
Elixir of cinchona, enough
   to make .... 16 fl. ounces.

Dissolve the hypophosphites and the citric acid in the water, add enough elixir of cinchona to make sixteen (16) fluid ounces, and filter.

Each fluid dram contains 1 grain each of the hypophosphites of calcium and sodium.

3139. Elixir Cinchonæ Detannatum.
(N. F.)
(Detannated Elixir of Cinchona.)
(Detannated Elixir of Calisaya.)
Detannated tincture of cin-
   chona .... 2½ fl. ounces.
Aromatic spirit............ 2 fl. ounces.
Syrup .... 6 fl. ounces.
Purified talcum............ 120 grains.
Water, enough to make.... 16 fl. ounces.

Mix the liquids, allow the mixture to stand twenty-four hours or longer, if convenient, then incorporate the purified talcum, and filter through a wetted filter, returning the first portions of the filtrate, until it runs through clear.

Each fluid ounce represents about 14 grains of yellow cinchona.

Note.—This preparation is to be used when elixir cinchonae is directed in combination with preparations of iron.

When detannated elixir of cinchona is not available, and the preparation, of which it forms a constituent, is required at once, an equivalent quantity of compound elixir of quinine, colored by the addition of 120 minims of compound tincture of cudbear to each pint, may be substituted for it.

3140. Elixir of Cinchonæ et Ferri.
N. F.
Elixir of Cinchona and Iron.
Elixir of Calisaya and Iron. Ferrated Elixir of Calisaya.
Phosphate of Iron (U. S. P.
   1880) .... 256 grains.
Water, boiling .... 1 fl. ounce.
Detannated elixir of cin-
   chona, enough to make... 16 fl. ounces.

Dissolve the phosphate of iron in the boiling water, then add enough detannated elixir of cinchona, to make sixteen (16) fluid ounces, and filter.

Each fluid dram contains 2 grains of phosphate of iron.

3141. Elixir Cinchonæ, Ferri, Bismuthi, et Strychninæ.
N. F.
Elixir of Cinchona, Iron, Bismuth, and Strychnine.
Elixir of Calisaya, Iron, Bismuth, and Strychnine.

Citrate of bismuth and ammonium .... 128 grains.
Sulphate of strychnine..... 1¼ grains.
Water, hot .... q. s.
Elixir of cinchona and iron,
    enough to make.......... 16 fl. ounces.

Dissolve the citrate of bismuth and ammonium in one-half (½) fluid ounce of hot water; allow the solution to stand until any undissolved matter has subsided; then decant the clear liquid, and add to the residue enough water of ammonia to dissolve it, carefully avoiding an excess. Dissolve the sulphate of strychnine in one (1) fluid dram of hot water, and having mixed the two solutions, add enough elixir of cinchona and iron to make sixteen (16) fluid ounces. Let the mixture stand twenty-four hours, if convenient, and filter.

Each fluid dram contains 1 grain of citrate of bismuth and ammonium, 1-100 grain of sulphate of strychnine, and nearly 2 grains of phosphate of iron.

3142. Elixir Cinchonæ, Ferri, et Bismuthi.
N. F.
Elixir of Cinchona, Iron, and Bismuth.
Elixir of Calisaya, Iron, and Bismuth.

Citrate of bismuth and ammonium .... 128 grains.
Water, hot................. ½ fl. ounce.
Elixir of cinchona and iron,
    enough to make .... 16 fl. ounces.

Dissolve the citrate of bismuth and ammonium in the hot water, allow the solution to stand until any undissolved matter has subsided; then decant the clear liquid, and add to the residue enough water of ammonia to dissolve it, carefully avoiding an excess. Then mix the solution with enough elixir of cinchona and iron to make sixteen (16) fluid ounces. Let the mixture stand twenty-four hours, if convenient, and filter.

Each fluid dram contains 1 grain of citrate of bismuth and ammonium and nearly 2 grains of phosphate of iron.

3143. Elixir Cinchonæ, Ferri, et Calcii Lactophosphatis.
N. F.
Elixir of Cinchona, Iron, and Lactophosphate of Calcium.
Elixir of Calisaya, Iron and Lactophosphate of Lime.

Lactate of calcium......... 64 grains.
Phosphoric acid (50 per cent) .... 64 minims.
Water of ammonia .... ½ fl. ounce.
Citric acid.................120 grains.
Elixir of cinchona and iron,
    enough to make.......... 16 fl. ounces.

Dissolve the lactate of calcium in seven (7) fluid ounces of elixir of cinchona and iron, with the aid of the phosphoric acid. Then add the citric acid, and when this is dissolved, the water of ammonia. Finally, add enough elixir of cinchona and iron to make sixteen (16) fluid ounces, and filter.

Each fluid dram contains ½ grain of lactate of calcium (or about ¾ grain of so-called lactophosphate of calcium) and nearly 2 grains of phosphate of iron.

3144. Elixir Cinchonæ, Ferri et Pepsini.
N. F.
Elixir of Cinchona, Iron and Pepsin.
Elixir of Calisaya, Iron and Pepsin.

Pepsin (N. F.)..............128 grains.
Hydrochloric acid .... 30 minims.
Water .... 3 fl. ounces.
Elixir of cinchona and iron,
    enough to make.......... 16 fl. ounces.

Dissolve the pepsin in the water mixed with the hydrochloric acid; then add enough elixir of cinchona and iron to make sixteen (16) fluid ounces. Let the mixture stand a few days, if convenient, and filter.

Each fluid dram represents 1 grain of pepsin (N. F.) and about 1½ grains of phosphate of iron.

3145. Elixir Cinchonæ, Ferri, et Strychninæ.
N. F.
Elixir of Cinchona, Iron and Strychnine.
Elixir of Calisaya, Iron and Strychnine.

Sulphate of strychnine...... 1¼ grains.
Water..................... 120 minims.
Elixir of Cinchona and Iron
    enough to make.......... 16 fl. ounces.

Dissolve the sulphate of strychnine in the water, and add enough elixir of cinchona and iron to make sixteen (16) fluid ounces.

Each fluid dram contains 1-100 grain of sulphate of strychnine and about 2 grains of phosphate of iron.

3146. Elixir Cinchonæ, Pepsini, et Strychninæ.
N. F.
Elixir of Cinchona, Pepsin, and Strychnine.
Elixir of Calisaya, Pepsin, and Strychnine.

Sulphate of quinine........ 16 grains.
Sulphate of cinchonine .... 8 grains.

Sulphate of strychnine..... 1¼ grains.
Elixir of pepsin .... 16 fl. ounces.

Dissolve the alkaloidal salts in the elixir, and filter, if necessary.

Each fluid dram represents small quantities of cinchona alkaloids, 1-100 grain of sulphate of strychnine, and 1 grain of pepsin (N. F.).

3147. Elixir Corydalis Compositum.
N. F.
Compound Elixir of Corydalis.

Fluid extract of corydalis.. 1 fl. ounce.
Fluid extract of stillingia.. 1 fl. ounce.
Fl. ext. of xanthoxylum.... ½ fl. ounce.
Fluid extract of iris........ 1½ fl. ounces
Alcohol .... 2 fl. ounces
Iodide of potassium .... 384 grains.
Aromatic elixir, enough to
  make .... 16 fl. ounces

Mix the alcohol with the fluid extracts, dissolve the iodide of potassium in the mixture, and add enough aromatic elixir to make sixteen (16) fluid ounces. Let the mixture stand a few days, if convenient, and filter.

Each fluid dram contains 3 grains of iodide of potassium and small quantities of the several fluid extracts.

3148. Elixir Curassao.
N. F.
Elixir of Curacao.
Curacao Cordial.

Spirit of curacao........... 120 minims.
Orris root, in fine powder.. 30 grains.
Deodorized alcohol .... 4 fl. ounces.
Citric acid .... 50 grains.
Syrup .... 8 fl. ounces.
Purified talcum .... 120 grains.
Water, enough to make.... 16 fl. ounces.

Mix the spirit of curacao with the alcohol, add the orris root, the purified talcum, and three (3) fluid ounces of water. Allow the mixture to stand twelve hours, occasionally agitating; then pour it on a wetted filter, returning the first portions of the filtrate until it runs through clear, and pass enough water through the filter to make the filtrate measure eight (8) fluid ounces. In this dissolve the citric acid, and finally add the syrup.

3149. Elixir Eriodictyi Aromaticum.
N. F.
Aromatic Elixir of Eriodictyon.
Aromatic Elixir of Yerba Santa; Elixir Corrigens.

Fluid extract of eriodictyon 1 fl. ounce.
Syrup .... 8 fl. ounces.
Pumice, in fine powder..... ½ tr. ounce.
Carbonate of magnesium... 80 grains.
Compound elixir of taraxa-
  cum, enough to make..... 16 fl. ounces.

Mix seven (7) fluid ounces of compound elixir of taraxacum with the syrup and pumice, then add the fluid extract, and mix the whole thoroughly by agitation. Shake the mixture occasionally during two hours, then allow it to settle, and carefully decant the liquid into a funnel, the neck of which contains a small pellet of absorbent cotton. Afterwards add the dregs and allow them to drain. To the filtrate add the carbonate of magnesium and shake occasionally during several hours. Let the mixture stand at rest during twelve hours, if convenient, then decant the liquid and filter it through paper. To the filtrate add enough compound elixir of taraxacum, if necessary, to make sixteen (16) fluid ounces.

Note.—This preparation is chiefly intended as a vehicle for quinine and other bitter remedies.

3150. Elixir Erythroxyli.
N. F.
Elixir of Erythroxylon.
Elixir of Coca.

Fluid ext. of erythroxylon.... 2 fl. ounces.
Alcohol .... 1 fl. ounce.
Syrup .... 2 fl. ounces.
Tincture of vanilla .... 120 minims.
Purified talcum .... 120 grains.
Aromatic elixir, enough to
  make .... 16 fl. ounces.

Mix the fluid extract with the alcohol, the syrup, and ten (10) fluid ounces of aromatic elixir, add the purified talcum and incorporate the latter thoroughly. Let the mixture stand during forty-eight hours, if convenient, shaking occasionally; then filter, add the tincture of vanilla to the filtrate, and pass enough aromatic elixir through the filter to make the product measure sixteen (16) fluid ounces.

Each fluid dram represents 7½ grains of erythroxylon (coca).

3151. Elixir Erythroxyli et Guaranae.
N. F.
Elixir of Erythroxylon and Guarana.
Elixir of Coca and Guarana.

Fl. ext. of erythroxylon.... 2 fl. ounces
Fluid extract of guarana... 2 fl. ounces.
Purified talcum .... 120 grains.
Comp. elixir of taraxacum. 12 fl. ounces.

Mix the liquids, and thoroughly incorporate the purified talcum with the mixture. Let it stand during forty-eight hours, if convenient, occasionally agitating, then filter.

Each fluid dram represents 7½ grains each of erythroxylon (coca) and guarana.

3152. Elixir Eucalypti.
N. F.
Elixir of Eucalyptus.

Fluid extract of eucalyptus   2 fl. ounces.
Alcohol   2 fl. ounces.
Carbonate of magnesium   120 grains.
Syrup of coffee   6 fl. ounces.
Comp. elixir of taraxacum   6 fl. ounces.

Mix the fluid extract with the alcohol, then add the other ingredients, shake the mixture occasionally during forty-eight hours, and filter.

Each fluid dram represents 7½ grains of eucalyptus.

3153. Elixir Euonymi.
N. F.
Elixir of Euonymus.
Elixir of Wahoo.

Fluid extract of euonymus   2½ fl. ounces.
Water   2 fl. ounces.
Syrup of coffee   2 fl. ounces.
Comp. elixir of taraxacum   9½ fl. ounces.

Mix them, let the mixture stand forty-eight hours, and filter.

Each fluid dram represents about 9½ grains of euonymus.

3154. Elixir Ferri Hypophosphitis.
N. F.
Elixir of Hypophosphite of Iron.

Solution of hypophosphite of iron   768 minims.
Aromatic elixir, enough to make   16 fl. ounces.

Mix the solution of hypophosphite of iron with enough aromatic elixir to make sixteen (16) fluid ounces. Allow the mixture to stand a few days in a cool place, and filter if necessary.

Each fluid dram contains 1 grain of hypophosphite of iron (ferric).

3155. Elixir Ferri Lactatis.
N. F.
Elixir of Lactate of Iron.

Lactate of iron, in crusts   128 grains.
Citrate of potassium   384 grains.
Aromatic elixir, enough to make   16 fl. ounces.

Triturate the lactate of iron with the citrate of potassium and about four (4) fluid ounces of aromatic elixir, gradually added, until solution has been effected. Then add enough aromatic elixir to make sixteen (16) fluid ounces, and filter.

Each fluid dram contains 1 grain of lactate of iron.

3156. Elixir Ferri Phosphatis.
N. F.
Elixir of Phosphate of Iron.

Phosphate of iron (U. S. P. 1880)   256 grains.
Water   1 fl. ounce.
Aromatic elixir, enough to make   16 fl. ounces.

Dissolve the phosphate of iron in the water with the aid of heat; then mix this solution with a sufficient quantity of aromatic elixir to make sixteen (16) fluid ounces. Filter, if necessary.

Each fluid dram contains 2 grains of phosphate of iron.

3157. Elixir Ferri Phosphatis, Cinchonidinæ, et Strychninæ.
N. F.
Elixir of Phosphate of Iron, Cinchonidine, and Strychnine.

Phosphate of iron (U. S. P. 1880)   256 grains.
Citrate of potassium   32 grains.
Sulphate of cinchonidine   128 grains.
Sulphate of strychnine   1¼ grains.
Alcohol   1 fl. ounce.
Water   360 minims.
Aromatic elixir enough to make   16 fl. ounces.

Dissolve the phosphate of iron and citrate of potassium in the water, using heat, if necessary. To twelve (12) fluid ounces of aromatic elixir, contained in a bottle, add the alcohol, and afterwards the alkaloidal salts, and agitate until the latter are dissolved, or nearly so. Then mix the two solutions, and, having shaken the mixture, add enough aromatic elixir to make sixteen (16) fluid ounces. Finally filter.

Each fluid dram contains 2 grains of phosphate of iron, 1 grain of sulphate of cinchonidine, and 1-100 grain of sulphate of strychnine.

Note.—When this elixir is mixed with water, it will become cloudy or opaque through the separation of some of its constituents.

3158. Elixir Ferri Phosphatis, Quininæ, et Strychninæ.
N. F.
Elixir of Phosphate of Iron, Quinine, and Strychnine.

Phosphate of iron (U. S. P. 1880)   256 grains.
Citrate of potassium   32 grains.
Hydrochlorate of quinine   128 grains.
Sulphate of strychnine   1¼ grains.

Alcohol .... 1 fl. ounce.
Water .... 360 minims.
Aromatic elixir, enough to
 make .... 16 fl. ounces.

Dissolve the phosphate of iron and citrate of potassium in the water, using heat, if necessary. To twelve (12) fluid ounces of aromatic elixir, contained in a bottle, add the alcohol, and afterwards the alkaloidal salts, and agitate until the latter are dissolved, or nearly so. Then mix the two solutions, and, having shaken the mixture, add enough aromatic elixir to make sixteen (16) fluid ounces. Finally filter.

Each fluid dram contains 2 grains of phosphate of iron, 1 grain of hydrochlorate of quinine, and 1-100 grain of sulphate of strychnine.

Note.—When this elixir is mixed with water, it will become cloudy or opaque through the separation of some of its constituents.

3159. Elixir Ferri Pyrophosphatis.
N. F.

Elixir of Pyrophosphate of Iron.

Pyrophosphate of iron (U.
 S. P. 1880) .... 256 grains.
Water .... 1 fl. ounce.
Aromatic elixir, enough to
 make .... 16 fl. ounces.

Dissolve the pyrophosphate of iron in the water, and add enough aromatic elixir to make sixteen (16) fluid ounces. Filter, if necessary.

Each fluid dram contains 2 grains of pyrophosphate of iron.

3160. Elixir Ferri, Quininæ, et Strychninæ.
N. F.

Elixir of Iron, Quinine, and Strychnine.

Tincture of citro-chloride
 of iron .... 2 fl. ounces.
Sulphate of quinine .... 128 grains.
Sulphate of strychnine ..... 1¼ grains.
Alcohol .... ½ fl. ounce.
Aromatic elixir, enough to
 make .... 16 fl. ounces.

Dissolve the alkaloidal salts in about twelve (12) fluid ounces of aromatic elixir, then add the tincture and the alcohol, and, finally, enough aromatic elixir to make sixteen (16) fluid ounces. Filter, if necessary.

Each fluid dram represents about 1 grain of ferric chloride, 1 grain of sulphate of quinine, and 1-100 grain of sulphate of strychnine.

3161. Elixir Frangulæ.
N. F.

Elixir of Frangula.
Elixir of Buckthorn.

Fl. ext. of frangula (U. S.
 P.) .... 4 fl. ounces.
Alcohol .... 1 fl. ounce.
Comp. elixir of taraxacum. 4 fl. ounces.
Aromatic elixir .... 7 fl. ounces.

Mix them, allow the mixture to stand during forty-eight hours, if convenient, and filter.

Each fluid dram represents 15 grains of frangula.

3162. Elixir Gentianæ.
N. F.

Elixir of Gentian.

Extract of Gentian (U. S.
 P.) .... 70 grains.
Aromatic spirit .... 180 minims.
Tincture of vanilla .... 120 minims.
Syrup .... 1 fl. ounce.
Aromatic elixir, enough to
 make .... 16 fl. ounces.

Dissolve the extract of gentian in about two (2) fluid ounces of aromatic elixir, next add the syrup, aromatic spirit, and tincture of vanilla, and, lastly, enough aromatic elixir to make sixteen (16) fluid ounces. Filter, if necessary.

Each fluid dram represents about 2 grains of gentian.

Note.—This elixir will be more likely to remain clear if, after the liquids are mixed together, 360 grains of purified talcum are added, the whole allowed to stand a few days, and then filtered.

3163. Elixir Gentianæ et Ferri Phosphatis.
N. F.

Elixir of Gentian and Phosphate of Iron.

Elixir Gentianae Ferratum. Ferrated Elixir of Gentian. Ferrophosphated Elixir of Gentian.

Phosphate of iron (U. S. P.
 1880) .... 128 grains.
Water .... ½ fl. ounce.
Elixir of gentian, enough to
 make .... 16 fl. ounces

Dissolve the phosphate of iron in the water with the aid of heat, and add enough elixir of gentian to make sixteen (16) fluid ounces. Filter, if necessary.

Each fluid dram represents 1 grain of phosphate of iron and nearly 2 grains of gentian.

3164. Elixir Gentianae cum Tinctura Ferri Chloridi.
N. F.
Elixir of Gentian with Tincture of Chloride of Iron.

Tincture of citro-chloride
of iron .... 640 minims.
Elixir of gentian, enough to
make .... 16 fl. ounces.

Mix the tincture of citro-chloride of iron with enough elixir of gentian to make sixteen (16) fluid ounces, and filter, if necessary.

Each fluid dram represents about 2-3 grain of ferric chloride and nearly 2 grains of gentian.

3165. Elixir Glycyrrhizae.
N. F.
Elixir of Glycyrrhiza.
Elixir of Licorice.

Purified ext. of glycyrrhiza 1 tr. ounce.
Water of ammonia......... q. s.
Aromatic elixir, enough to
make .... 16 fl. ounces.

Triturate the purified extract of glycyrrhiza with twelve (12) fluid ounces of aromatic elixir gradually added. To ten (10) fluid ounces of this mixture add water of ammonia in drops, until it is in slight excess. Mix this with the reserved portion, and, finally, add enough aromatic elixir to make sixteen (16) fluid ounces. Filter, if necessary.

3166. Elixir Glycyrrhizae Aromaticum.
N. F.
Aromatic Elixir of Glycyrrhiza.
Aromatic Elixir of Licorice.

Fl. ext. of glycyrrhiza..... 2 fl. ounces.
Oil of cloves .... 6 minims.
Oil of cinnamon (Ceylon).. 6 minims.
Oil of nutmeg............. 4 minims.
Oil of fennel .... 12 minims.
Purified talcum .... 360 grains.
Aromatic elixir, enough to
make .... 16 fl. ounces.

Triturate the oils with the purified talcum and the fluid extract, then add fourteen (14) fluid ounces of aromatic elixir, filter, and pass enough aromatic elixir through the filter to make sixteen (16) fluid ounces.

3167. Elixir Grindeliae.
N. F.
Elixir of Grindelia.

Fluid extract of grindelia.. 1 fl. ounce.
Aromatic spirit .... 2 fl. ounces.
Comp. elixir of taraxacum. 13 fl. ounces.

Mix them, allow the mixture to stand a few days, if convenient, then filter.

Each fluid ounce represents 30 grains of grindelia.

3168. Elixir Guaranae.
N. F.
Elixir of guarana.

Fluid extract of guarana
(U. S. P.)................ 3 fl. ounces.
Aromatic elixir .... 3 fl. ounces.
Comp. elixir of taraxacum. 10 fl. ounces.

Mix them, allow the mixture to stand during forty-eight hours, if convenient, and filter.

Each fluid dram represents about 11 grains of guarana.

3169. Elixir Humuli.
N. F.
Elixir of Humulus.
Elixir of Hops.

Fl. ext. of hops (N. F.)..... 2 fl. ounces.
Carbonate of magnesium... 120 grains.
Tincture of vanilla .... 240 minims.
Comp. elixir of taraxacum. 2 fl. ounces.
Aromatic elixir, enough to
make .... 16 fl. ounces.

Triturate the fluid extract of hops with the carbonate of magnesium, then gradually add the compound elixir of taraxacum, tincture of vanilla, and enough aromatic elixir to make sixteen (16) fluid ounces. Allow the mixture to stand several days, if convenient, occasionally agitating, then filter.

Each fluid dram represents 7½ grains of humulus (hops).

3170. Elixir Hypophosphitum.
N. F.
Elixir of Hypophosphites.

Hypophosphite of calcium...384 grains.
Hypophosphite of sodium...128 grains.
Hypophosphite of potassium .... 128 grains.
Citric acid .... 30 grains.
Water .... 4 fl. ounces.
Glycerin .... ½ fl. ounce.
Comp. spirit of cardamom.. ½ fl. ounce.
Aromatic elixir, enough to
make .... 16 fl. ounces.

Dissolve the hypophosphites and the citric acid in the water; then add the glycerin, compound spirit of cardamom, and enough aromatic elixir to make sixteen (16) fluid ounces. Filter, if necessary.

Each fluid dram contains 3 grains of hypophosphite of calcium and 1 grain, each, of the hypophosphites of sodium and potassium.

3171. Elixir Hypophosphitum cum Ferro.
N. F.
Elixir of Hypophosphites with Iron.

Hypophosphite of calcium	188 grains.
Hypophosphite of sodium	128 grains.
Hypophosphite of potassium	64 grains.
Sulphate of iron, in clear crystals	96 grains.
Citric acid	30 grains.
Water	4 fl. ounces.
Syrup	4 fl. ounces.
Aromatic elixir, enough to make	16 fl. ounces.

Dissolve the hypophosphites in three (3) fluid ounces of water, and add the syrup. Dissolve the sulphate of iron in the remainder of the water, and mix this with the other solution. Then add six (6) fluid ounces of aromatic elixir, set the mixture aside, in a cold place, for twelve hours, and filter from the deposited sulphate of calcium. Finally, dissolve the citric acid in the filtrate, and pass enough aromatic elixir through the filter to make sixteen (16) fluid ounces.

Each fluid dram contains about ½ grain of hypophosphite of iron (ferrous), about 1 grain each of the hypophosphites of calcium and sodium, and ½ grain of hypophosphite of potassium.

3172. Elixir Lithii Bromidi.
N. F.
Elixir of Bromide of Lithium.

Bromide of lithium	640 grains.
Citric acid	30 grains.
Adjuvant elixir, enough to make	16 fl. ounces.

Dissolve the bromide of lithium and the citric acid in about twelve (12) fluid ounces of adjuvant elixir, by agitation. Then add enough adjuvant elixir to make sixteen (16) fluid ounces, and filter.

Each fluid dram contains 5 grains of bromide of lithium.

3173. Elixir Lithii Citratis.
N. F.
Elixir of Citrate of Lithium.

Citrate of lithium	640 grains.
Adjuvant elixir, enough to make	16 fl. ounces.

Dissolve the citrate of lithium in about twelve (12) fluid ounces of adjuvant elixir, by agitation. Then add enough adjuvant elixir to make sixteen (16) fluid ounces, and filter.

Each fluid dram contains 5 grains of citrate of lithium.

3174. Elixir Lithii Salicylatis.
N. F.
Elixir of Salicylate of Lithium.

Salicylate of lithium	640 grains.
Adjuvant elixir, enough to make	16 fl. ounces.

Dissolve the salicylate of lithium in about twelve (12) fluid ounces of adjuvant elixir, by agitation. Then add enough adjuvant elixir to make sixteen (16) fluid ounces, and filter.

Each fluid dram contains 5 grains of salicylate of lithium.

3175. Elixir Malti et Ferri.
N. F.
Elixir of Malt and Iron.

Extract of malt	4 fl. ounces.
Phosphate of iron, (U. S. P. 1880)	128 grains.
Water	½ fl. ounce.
Aromatic elixir, enough to make	16 fl. ounces.

Dissolve the phosphate of iron in the water by the aid of heat, mix the solution with the extract of malt previously introduced into a graduated bottle, and add enough aromatic elixir to make sixteen (16) fluid ounces. Set the mixture aside for twenty-four hours, and filter.

Each fluid dram represents 1 grain of phosphate of iron and 15 grains of extract of malt.

Note.—Extract of malt, most suitable for this preparation, should have about the consistence of balsam of peru, at a temperature of about 15° C. (59° F.) The filtration of this preparation will be greatly facilitated by allowing the mixture to stand a few days before pouring it on the filter.

6176. Elixir Pepsini.
N. F.
Elixir of Pepsin.

Pepsin (N. F.)	128 grains.
Hydrochloric acid	30 minims.
Glycerin	2 fl. ounces.
Comp. elixir of taraxacum	1 fl. ounce.
Alcohol	3 fl. ounces.
Purified talcum	120 grains.
Sugar	4 tr. ounces.
Water, enough to make	16 fl. ounces.

Mix the pepsin with six (6) fluid ounces of water, add the glycerin and acid, and agitate until solution has been effected. Then add the compound elixir of taraxacum, alcohol, and the purified talcum, and mix thoroughly. Set the mixture aside for a few hours, occasionally agitating. Then filter it through a wetted filter, dissolve the sugar in the filtrate, and pass enough water through the filter to make the whole product measure sixteen (16) fluid ounces.

Each fluid dram represents 1 grain of pepsin (N. F.).

Note.—The filtration of this preparation will be greatly facilitated by allowing the mixture to stand a few days before pouring it on the filter

3177. Elixir Pepsini, Bismuthi, et Strychninæ.
N. F.
Elixir of Pepsin, Bismuth, and Strychnine.

Sulphate of strychnine	1¼ grains.
Elixir of pepsin and bismuth	16 fl. ounces.

Dissolve the sulphate of strychnine in the elixir.

Each fluid dram represents 1-100 grain of sulphate of strychnine, 1 grain of pepsin (N. F.), and 2 grains of citrate of bismuth and ammonium.

3178. Elixir Pepsini et Bismuthi.
N. F.
Elixir of Pepsin and Bismuth.

Pepsin (N. F.)	128 grains.
Citrate of bismuth and ammonium	256 grains.
Water of ammonia	q. s.
Glycerin	2 fl. ounces.
Alcohol	3 fl. ounces.
Syrup	3 fl. ounces.
Comp. elixir of taraxacum	1 fl. ounce.
Purified talcum	120 grains.
Water, enough to make	16 fl. ounces.

Dissolve the pepsin in four (4) fluid ounces of water. Dissolve the citrate of bismuth and ammonium in one (1) fluid ounce of warm water, allow the solution to stand until clear, if necessary; then decant the clear liquid, and add to the residue just enough water of ammonia to dissolve it, carefully avoiding an excess. Then mix the two solutions, and add the glycerin, compound elixir of taraxacum, and alcohol. Thoroughly incorporate the purified talcum with the mixture, filter it through a wetted filter, and pass enough water through the filter to make the filtrate measure thirteen (13) fluid ounces. To this add the syrup.

Each fluid dram represents 1 grain of pepsin (N. F.) and 2 grains of citrate of bismuth and ammonium.

3179. Elixir Pepsini et Ferri.
N. F.
Elixir of Pepsin and Iron.

Tincture of citro-chloride of iron	512 minims.
Elixir of pepsin, enough to make	16 fl. ounces.

Mix the tincture of citro-chloride of iron with a sufficient quantity of elixir of pepsin to make sixteen (16) fluid ounces, and filter, if necessary.

Each fluid dram represents about ½ grain of chloride of iron (ferric) and nearly 1 grain of pepsin (N. F.).

3180. Elixir Phosphori.
N. F.
Elixir of Phosphorus.

Spirit of phosphorus	3¾ fl. ounces.
Oil of star-anise	16 minims.
Glycerin	9 fl. ounces.
Aromatic elixir, enough to make	16 fl. ounces.

To the spirit of phosphorus add the oil of star-anise and glycerin, and shake gently until they form a clear liquid. Then add the aromatic elixir, in small portions at a time, gently agitating after each addition, until a clear mixture results.

Keep the product in dark amber-colored vials, in a cool and dark place. It should not be prepared in quantities larger than will be consumed within a few months.

Each fluid dram contains 1-50 grain of phosphorus.

3181. Elixir Phosphori et Nucis Vomicæ.
N. F.
Elixir of Phosphorus and Nux Vomica.

Tincture of nux vomica	256 minims.
Elix. of phosphorus, enough to make	16 fl. ounces.

Mix them. This preparation should be freshly made, when wanted for use.

Each fluid dram represents 2 minims of tincture of nux vomica and nearly 1-50 grain of phosphorus.

3182. Elixir Picis Compositum.
N. F.
Compound Elixir of Tar.

Syrup of wild cherry	3 fl. ounces.
Syrup of tolu	3 fl. ounces.
Sulphate of morphine	2½ grains.
Methylic alcohol	360 minims.
Water	q. s.
Wine of tar, enough to make	16 fl. ounces.

Dissolve the sulphate of morphine in about one (1) fluid dram of hot water, and add the solution to the two syrups previously mixed. Then add the methylic alcohol and enough wine of tar to make sixteen (16) fluid ounces.

Each fluid dram contains about 1-50 grain of sulphate of morphine.

Note.—Much of the commercial "wood spirit" or "wood naphtha" is unfit for medicinal purposes. Refined wood naphtha or methylic alcohol should be colorless and freely miscible to a clear liquid with water, alcohol, and ether. Its odor, which is characteristic, should be free from empyreuma. It should contain at least 90 per cent of absolute methylic alcohol, which corresponds to a specific gravity of 0.846 at 15° C. (59° F.) On mixing methylic alcohol cautiously with one-fourth its volume of sulphuric acid, the liquid should remain colorless or acquire not more than a very pale yellowish-red tint; and on gently heating methylic alcohol with an equal volume of a 10 per cent solution of potassa, the mixture should not acquire a brown color.

3183. Elixir Pilocarpi.
N. F.
Elixir of Pilocarpus.
Elixir of Jaborandi.
Fluid extract of pilocarpus.. 1 fl. ounce.
Syrup of coffee............ 3 fl. ounces.
Tincture of vanilla......... ½ fl. ounce.
Comp. elixir of taraxacum,
  enough to make.......... 16 fl. ounces.

Mix them, allow the mixture to stand during four days, if convenient, and filter.

Each fluid dram represents 3¾ grains of pilocarpus.

3184. Elixir Potassii Acetatis.
N. F.
Elixir of Acetate of Potassium.
Acetate of potassium....... 640 grains.
Aromatic elixir, enough to
  make .... 16 fl. ounces.

Dissolve the acetate of potassium in twelve (12) fluid ounces of aromatic elixir, then add enough of the latter to make sixteen (16) fluid ounces. Filter, if necessary.

Each fluid dram contains 5 grains of acetate of potassium.

3185. Elixir Potassii Acetatis et Juniperi.
N. F.
Elixir of Acetate of Potassium and Juniper.
Acetate of potassium....... 640 grains.
Fluid extract of juniper ... 2 fl. ounces.
Carbonate of magnesium.. 120 grains.
Aromatic elixir, enough to
  make .... 16 fl. ounces.

Triturate the fluid extract of juniper with the carbonate of magnesium, then add twelve (12) fluid ounces of aromatic elixir in which the acetate of potassium had previously been dissolved. Filter, and add enough aromatic elixir through the filter to make sixteen (16) fluid ounces.

Each fluid dram represents 5 grains of acetate of potassium and 7½ grains of juniper.

3186. Elixir Potassii Bromidi.
N. F.
Elixir of bromide of potassium.
Bromide of potassium .....1280 grains.
Citric acid................. 30 grains.
Adjuvant elixir, enough to
  make .... 16 fl. ounces.

Dissolve the bromide of potassium and the citric acid in about twelve (12) fluid ounces of adjuvant elixir, by agitation. Then add enough adjuvant elixir to make sixteen (16) fluid ounces, and filter.

Each fluid dram contains 10 grains of bromide of potassium.

3187. Elixir Quininæ Compositum.
N. F.
Compound Elixir of Quinine.
Sulphate of quinine .... 16 grains.
Sulphate of cinchonidine .. 8 grains.
Sulphate of cinchonine .... 8 grains.
Aromatic elixir............ 16 fl. ounces.

Add the alkaloidal salts to the aromatic elixir, and dissolve them by agitation. Finally, filter.

Each fluid ounce contains 1 grain of sulphate of quinine and ½ grain each of the sulphates of cinchonidine and cinchonine.

Note.—This preparation is chiefly intended as a substitute for elixir of cinchona in certain cases, when the presence of other constituents of cinchona is deemed unnecessary, or where the elixir is intended rather as a vehicle than a medicine.

If it is desired to impart a color to this elixir, this may be effected by the addition of 120 minims of compound tincture of cudbear to each pint.

3188. Elixir Quininæ et Phosphatum Compositum.
N. F.
Compound Elixir of Quinine and Phosphates.
Sulphate of quinine........ 32 grains.
Phosphate of iron (U. S. P.
  1880) .... 128 grains.
Citrate of potassium ...... 128 grains.
Syrup of lactophosphate of
  calcium .... 4 fl ounces.
Water .... ½ fl. ounce.
Aromatic elixir, enough to
  make .... 16 fl. ounces.

Dissolve the sulphate of quinine in ten (10) fluid ounces of aromatic elixir, if necessary with the aid of a gentle heat. Dissolve the phosphate of iron and the citrate of potassium in the water, and add the solution to that first prepared. Then add the syrup of lactophosphate of calcium, and, lastly, enough aromatic elixir to make sixteen (16) fluid ounces. Filter, if necessary.

Each fluid dram contains ¼ grain of sulphate of quinine, 1 grain of phosphate of iron, and about ¾ grain of so-called lactophosphate of calcium.

3189. Elixir Quininæ Valerianatis et Strychninæ.
N. F.

Elixir of Valerianate of Quinine and Strychnine.

Valerianate of quinine	128 grains.
Sulphate of strychnine	1¼ grains.
Comp. tinct. of cudbear	120 minims.
Aromatic elixir, enough to make	16 fl. ounces.

Triturate the valerianate of quinine and the sulphate of strychnine with about eight (8) fluid ounces of aromatic elixir, until they are dissolved. Then add the compound tincture of cudbear, and, lastly, enough aromatic elixir to make sixteen (16) fluid ounces. Filter, if necessary.

Each fluid dram contains 1 grain of valerianate of quinine and 1-100 grain of sulphate of strychnine.

3190. Elixir Rhamni Purshianæ.
N. F.

Elixir of Rhamnus Purshiana. Elixir of Cascara Sagrada.

Fl. ext. of rhamnus purshiana	4 fl. ounces.
Elixir of glycyrrhiza	4 fl. ounces.
Comp. elixir of taraxacum	8 fl. ounces.

Mix them. Allow the mixture to stand a few days, if convenient, and filter.

Each fluid dram represents 15 grains of rhamnus purshiana.

3191. Elixir Rhamni Purshianæ Compositum.
N. F.

Compound Elixir of Rhamnus Purshiana. Compound Elixir of Cascara Sagrada. Elixir Laxativum; Elixir Purgans; Laxative Elixir.

Fl. ext. of rhamnus purshiana	2 fl. ounces.
Fluid extract of senna	1¼ fl. ounces.
Fluid extract of juglans	1 fl. ounce.
Fluid extract of glycyrrhiza	½ fl. ounce.
Comp. tinct. of cardamom	½ fl. ounce.
Aromatic spirit	2 fl. ounces.
Syrup	6 fl. ounces.
Purified talcum	120 grains.
Water, enough to make	16 fl. ounces.

Mix the fluid extracts with the compound tincture of cardamom and the aromatic spirit; then add the syrup, and, lastly, enough water to make sixteen (16) fluid ounces. Incorporate the purified talcum thoroughly with the mixture, and filter.

The average dose for an adult of this preparation is 1 to 2 teaspoonfuls.

3192. Elixir Rhei.
N. F.

Elixir of Rhubarb.

Sweet tincture of rhubarb (U. S. P.)	8 fl. ounces.
Deodorized alcohol	1 fl. ounce.
Water	3 fl. ounces.
Glycerin	2 fl. ounces.
Syrup	2 fl. ounces.

Mix them, and filter.

Each fluid dram represents about 2¼ grains of rhubarb.

3193. Elixir Rhei et Magnesii Acetatis.
N. F.

Elixir of Rhubarb and Acetate of Magnesium. Elixir Rhei et Magnesiae. Elixir of Rhubarb and Magnesia.

Magnesia, calcined	144 grains
Acetic acid (U. S. P.)	q. s.
Fl. ext. of rhubarb	2 fl. ounces.
Aromatic elixir, enough to make	16 fl. ounces.

Dissolve the magnesia in two and one-half (2½) fluid ounces of acetic acid, with the aid of a gentle heat, adding, if necessary, a little more acetic acid, drop by drop, until the solution is neutral to test-paper. Then add the fluid extract and enough aromatic elixir to make sixteen (16) fluid ounces, and filter.

Each fluid dram represents about 4 grains of acetate of magnesium and 7½ grains of rhubarb.

3194. Elixir Rubi Compositum.
N. F.

Compound Elixir of Blackberry.

Blackberry root	2 tr. ounces.
Galls	2 tr. ounces.
Cinnamon, saigon	2 tr. ounces.
Cloves	½ tr. ounce.
Mace	¼ tr. ounce.
Ginger	¼ tr. ounce.

Diluted alcohol .... q. s.
Blackberry juice, recently
  expressed .... 3 pints.
Syrup .... 3 pints.

Reduce the solids to a moderately coarse (No. 40) powder, moisten it with diluted alcohol, and percolate it with this menstruum in the usual manner, until two (2) pints of percolate are obtained. To this add the blackberry juice and syrup, and mix thoroughly.

3195.   Elixir Sodii Bromidi.
            N. F.
      Elixir of Bromide of Sodium.

Bromide of sodium......... 1280 grains.
Citric acid .... 30 grains.
Adjuvant elixir, enough to
  make .... 16 fl. ounces.

Dissolve the bromide of sodium and the citric acid in about twelve (12) fluid ounces of adjuvant elixir by agitation. Then add enough adjuvant elixir to make sixteen (16) fluid ounces, and filter, if necessary.

Each fluid dram contains 10 grains of bromide of sodium.

3196.   Elixir Sodii Hypophosphitis.
            N. F.
     Elixir of Hypophosphite of Sodium.

Hypophosphite of sodium... 256 grains.
Citric acid................. 30 grains.
Aromatic elixir, enough to
  make .... 16 fl. ounces.

Dissolve the hypophosphite of sodium and the citric acid in about twelve (12) fluid ounces of aromatic elixir, by agitation. Then add enough aromatic elixir to make sixteen (16) fluid ounces, and filter, if necessary.

Each fluid dram contains 2 grains of hypophosphite of sodium.

3197.   Elixir Sodii Salicylatis.
            N. F.
      Elixir of Salicylate of Sodium.

Salicylate of sodium .... 640 grains.
Aromatic elixir, enough to
  make .... 16 fl. ounces.

Dissolve the salicylate of sodium in about twelve (12) fluid ounces of aromatic elixir, by agitation. Then add enough aromatic elixir to make sixteen (16) fluid ounces, and filter if necessary.

This preparation should be freshly prepared when required for use.

Each fluid dram contains 5 grains of salicylate of sodium.

3198.   Elixir Stillingiæ Compositum.
            N. F.
      Compound Elixir of Stillingia.

Comp. fl. ext. of stillingia.. 4 fl. ounces.
Aromatic elixir............ 12 fl. ounces.

Mix them, allow the mixture to stand a few days, or longer, if convenient, and filter.

Each fluid dram represents 15 minims of compound fluid extract of stillingia.

3199.   Elixir Strychninæ Valerianatis.
            N. F.
      Elixir of Valerianate of Strychnine.

Valerianate of strychnine.. 1¼ grains.
Acetic acid .... q. s.
Tincture of vanilla .... 120 minims.
Comp. tinct. of cudbear.... 120 minims.
Aromatic elixir, enough to
  make .... 16 fl. ounces.

Triturate the valerianate of strychnine with about one (1) fluid ounce of aromatic elixir, gradually added, and effect complete solution by the addition of one or more drops of acetic acid, avoiding an excess. Then add the tinctures, and, lastly, enough aromatic elixir to make sixteen (16) fluid ounces. Filter, if necessary.

Each fluid dram contains 1-100 grain of valerianate of strychnine.

3200.   Elixir Taraxaci Compositum.
            N. F.
      Compound Elixir of Taraxacum.

Taraxacum .... 1 tr. ounce.
Wild cherry .... 1 tr. ounce.
Sweet orange peel, recently
  dried .... 1 tr. ounce.
Glycyrrhiza, Russian, peel.. 3 tr. ounces.
Cinnamon, saigon ....120 grains.
Cardamom ....120 grains.
Canada snake root.........120 grains.
Caraway .... 120 grains.
Cloves .... 40 grains.
Alcohol ....
Water, each............... q. s.
Syrup .... 32 fl. ounces.

Reduce the solid substances to a moderately coarse (No. 40) powder, and percolate, in the usual manner, with a mixture of one (1) volume of alcohol and two (2) volumes of water, until sixteen (16) fluid ounces of percolate are obtained. Lastly, add the syrup, let the mixture stand a few days, if possible, and filter.

Note.—If a precipitate should make its appearance in this preparation on standing, it ought to be removed by filtration. This elixir is chiefly intended as a vehicle or corrigent, to cover the bitter taste of quinine and similar substances.

3201. Elixir Turneræ.
N. F.
Elixir of Turnera.
Elixir of Damiana.

Fluid extract of turnera....	2½ fl. ounces.
Carbonate of magnesium...	240 grains.
Alcohol	4 fl. ounces.
Glycerin	1 fl. ounce.
Aromatic elixir, enough to make	16 fl. ounces.

Mix the fluid extract with the alcohol, glycerin, and eight (8) fluid ounces of aromatic elixir. Incorporate the carbonate of magnesium thoroughly with the mixture by trituration. Then filter through a wetted filter, and pass enough aromatic elixir through the filter to make sixteen (16) fluid ounces.

Each fluid dram represents about 9½ grains of turnera.

3202. Elixir Viburni Opuli Compositum.
N. F.
Compound Elixir of Viburnum Opulus.
Compound Elixir of Crampbark.

Fl. ext. of viburnum opuli	1¼ fl. ounces.
Fluid extract of trillium...	2½ fl. ounces.
Fluid extract of aletris.....	1¼ fl. ounces.
Comp. elixir of taraxacum..	11 fl. ounces.

Mix them, allow the mixture to stand a few days, and filter.

3203. Elixir Viburnum Prunifolium.
N. F.
Elixir of Black Haw.

Fl. ext. of viburnum prunifolium	2 fl. ounces.
Comp. tinct. of cardamom..	1 fl. ounce.
Aromatic elixir	13 fl. ounces.

Mix them, allow the mixture to stand a few days, and filter.

Each fluid dram represents about 7½ grains of viburnum prunifolium.

3204. Elixir Zinci Valerianatis.
N. F.

Valerianate of zinc.........	128 grains.
Stronger solution of citrate of ammonium	1½ fl. ounces.
Alcohol	2 fl. ounces.
Oil of bitter almond........	1 drop.
Comp. tinct. of cudbear.....	120 minims.
Aromatic elixir, enough to make	16 fl. ounces.

Mix the stronger solution of citrate of ammonium with 4 fluid ounces of aromatic elixir and the alcohol, and triturate the valerianate of zinc with this mixture, added gradually and in portions, until solution has been effected. Then add the oil of bitter almond, the comp. tincture of cudbear, and, finally, enough aromatic elixir to make 16 fluid ounces. Allow the mixture to stand a few days, and filter.

Each fluid dram contains 1 grain of valerianate of zinc.

GLYCERITES.

3205. Glycerite of Alum.
Brit. Pharm.

Alum, powder	3 av. ounces
Glycerin	14½ fl. ounces.

Stir together in a porcelain dish, apply a gentle heat until solution is effected, set aside and decant the clear fluid from any deposited matter.

3206. Glycerite of Bismuth.
N. F.
Liquor Bismuthi Concentratus. Concentrated Solution of Bismuth.

Subnitrate of bismuth......	1480 grains.
Nitric acid	4 tr. ounces
Citric acid	1200 grains.
Water of ammonia.........	q. s.
Glycerin	8 fl. ounces.
Water, enough to make.....	16 fl. ounces.

Dissolve the subnitrate of bismuth in the nitric acid mixed with an equal volume of water. Add the citric acid previously dissolved in four (4) fluid ounces of water. Divide the solution into two equal portions. To one portion add water of ammonia until the precipitate first formed is redissolved, and then dilute with water to eight (8) pints. To this add the reserved portion, stirring constantly. Let the mixture stand about six hours, then transfer it to a paper filter, inside of a muslin strainer, both being folded together. Wash the precipitate with water, until it is free from nitric acid, and by gentle pressure remove as much of the water as possible. Dissolve the precipitate in a sufficient quantity of water of ammonia, evaporate the solution on the water-bath, in a tared capsule, to eight (8) troy ounces, then transfer it to a graduate, allow it to cool, and wash the capsule with a little water so as to make the whole volume of liquid measure eight (8) fluid ounces. Finally, add the glycerin, and filter, if necessary.

Glycerite of bismuth, when required for immediate use, may also be prepared as follows:

Citrate of bismuth and am-
    monium .... 2048 grains.
Stronger water of ammonia   q. s.
Glycerin .... 8 fl. ounces.
Water, enough to make..... 16 fl. ounces.

Triturate the citrate of bismuth and ammonium with six (6) fluid ounces of water and four (4) fluid ounces of glycerin, and add to it gradually just enough stronger water of ammonia to dissolve the salt, and to produce a neutral solution. Then add the remainder of the glycerin and enough water to make sixteen (16) fluid ounces, and filter.

Each fluid dram contains 16 grains of citrate of bismuth and ammonium.

Note.—When this preparation is directed as an ingredient in other preparations, which are required to be filtered when completed, it may be added to them without previous filtration.

If glycerite of bismuth should at any time deposit a precipitate, this may be redissolved by the addition of just sufficient stronger water of ammonia.

3207.   Glycerite of Borax.
U. S. P.

Borax, powdered.......... 4 av. ounces.
Glycerin .... 14½ fl. ounces.

Triturate together until dissolved, or else warm gently, stirring constantly until dissolved.

3208. Glycerite of Boric and Tannic Acids.

Boric acid .... 1 av. ounce.
Tannic acid .... 1¾ av. ounces.
Glycerin .... 13 fl. ounces.

Mix the acids with the glycerin, heat on a water bath until dissolved, and strain.

3209.   Glycerite of Boroglycerin.
N. F.

Glycerite of Glyceryl Borate. Solution of Boroglyceride.

Boric acid, in powder....... 62 parts.
Glycerin, enough to make...200 parts.

Heat ninety-two (92) parts of glycerin in a tared porcelain capsule to a temperature not exceeding 150° C. (302° F.), and add the boric acid in portions, constantly stirring. When all is added and dissolved, continue the heat at the same temperature, frequently stirring, and breaking up the film which forms on the surface. When the mixture has been reduced to the weight of one hundred (100) parts, add to it one hundred (100) parts of glycerin, mix thoroughly, and transfer it to suitable vessels.

Two parts, by weight, of this preparation represent 1 part of solid boroglycerin.

Note.—The product, which is a clear, viscid liquid, is more readily soluble in, and miscible with, other liquids than the solid boroglycerin. (See boroglycerinum.)

It may be found more convenient, if the glycerite is needed immediately, to place one ounce (av.) of boroglyceride in a dish and add one ounce (av.) of glycerin, heating gently and stirring until it is dissolved.

3210.   Glycerite of Carbolic Acid.
U. S. P.

Carbolic acid, crystals...... 3½ av. ounces.
Glycerin .... 12¾ fl. ounces.

Warm the acid, add the glycerin, and stir until mixed.

3211.   Glycerite of Creasote.

Creasote .... 1¾ fl. ounces.
Alcohol .... 2 fl. ounces.
Glycerin .... 5½ fl. ounces.
Water .... 6¾ fl. ounces.
Magnesium carbonate ...... 1 av. ounce.

Triturate the magnesium carbonate, alcohol and creasote together in a mortar, add the water and the glycerin, put the whole in a bottle, let stand for several days and filter. The product represents about 10 per cent by weight of creasote, and may be used for making other preparations of this agent.

3212.   Glycerite of Chloroform.

Chloroform .... 1¼ fl. ounces.
Alcohol .... 4½ fl. ounces.
Glycerin .... 10¼ fl. ounces.

Dissolve the chloroform in the alcohol, add the glycerin, and shake well.

The product represents 10 per cent by weight of chloroform.—D.

3213.   Glycerite of Guaiac.
N. F.

Resin of guaiac, powder... 640 grains.
Solution of potassa........ 1 fl. ounce.
Glycerin .... 9½ fl. ounces.
Water, enough to make.... 16 fl. ounces.

Mix the solution of potassa with 5 fluid ounces of water, and in this liquid macerate the resin for 24 hours. Then filter, and pass enough water through the filter to make the filtrate measure 6½ fluid ounces, and mix this with the glycerin.

3214. Glycerite of Gallic Acid.
Br.

Gallic acid	3½ av. ounces.
Glycerin	12¾ fl. ounces.

Mix well, heat on a water bath until the acid is dissolved, and strain.

3215. Glycerite of Lead Subacetate.
Br.

Lead acetate	3½ av. ounces.
Lead oxide, powd.	2 av. oz. 20 grains.
Glycerin	15 fl. ounces.
Distilled water	9 fl. ounces.

Mix all, boil together for 15 minutes, then filter, and heat again until all the water has evaporated.

This is of the same strength as the solution of lead subacetate U. S. P., and may be employed in making the diluted solution of lead subacetate.

3216. Glycerite of Pepsin.
N. F.

Pepsin (N. F.)	640 grains.
Hydrochloric acid	80 minims.
Purified talcum	120 grains.
Glycerin	8 fl. ounces.
Water, enough to make	16 fl. ounces.

Mix the pepsin with 7 fluid ounces of water and the hydrochloric acid, and agitate until solution has been effected. Then incorporate the purified talcum with the liquid, filter, returning the first portions of the filtrate until it runs through clear, and pass enough water through the filter to make the filtrate measure eight fluid ounces. To this add the glycerin, and mix.

Each fluid dram represents 5 grains of pepsin.

3217. Glycerite of Starch.

Starch	1 av. ounce.
Water	1 fl. ounce.
Glycerin	6½ fl. oz., or 8 av. ounces.

To the starch, contained in a porcelain capsule, add the water and glycerin, and stir until a homogeneous mixture results. Then apply heat, gradually raising the temperature to a point between 140 and 144 degrees C., stirring constantly until a transparent jelly is formed.

3218. Glycerite of Tannin.
U. S. P.

Tannic acid	2 tr. ounces.
Glycerin	8 fl. ounces.

Dissolve the tannin in the glycerin with the aid of a gentle heat.

3219. Glycerite of Tar.
N. F.

Tar	1 tr. ounce.
Carbonate of magnesium	2 tr. ounces.
Glycerin	4 fl. ounces.
Alcohol	2 fl. ounces.
Water, enough to make	16 fl. ounces.

Upon the tar, contained in a mortar, pour 3 fluid ounces of cold water, stir them thoroughly together, and pour off the water. Repeat this once or twice, until the water only feebly reddens blue litmus-paper. Now triturate the washed tar with the alcohol, gradually incorporate the carbonate of magnesium and glycerin, and, lastly, 10 fluid ounces of water. Pour the mixture upon a filter of loose texture spread over a piece of straining muslin, and, after the liquid portion has passed through, wash the residue on the filter with water, until the whole filtrate measures 16 fluid ounces.

3220. Glycerite of Tragacanth.
N. F.

Tragacanth, in fine powder	2 tr. ounces.
Glycerin	12½ fl. ounces.
Water	3 fl. ounces.

Triturate the tragacanth with the glycerin in a mortar, add the water, and continue the trituration, until a homogenous, thick paste results.

MEDICATED HONEY.

3221. Honey of Borax.
U. S. P.

Borax powder	2 av. ounces.
Clarified honey	16 av. ounces.

Mix and dissolve by the aid of a gentle heat.

3222. Honey of Borax.
Br.

Borax	2 av. ounces.
Glycerin	1 fl. ounce.
Honey	14½ av. ounces

Prepare like the preceding.

3223. Honey of Rose with Borax.

Honey of rose, U. S. P.	10 av. ounces.
Borax	1 av. ounce.

Mix and dissolve borax by aid of a gentle heat.

NON-SECRET FORMULAS.

3224.   **Honey of Rose.**
                U. S. P.

Red rose leaves in No. 40 powder............ 2 av. ounces.
Honey clarified .... 23 av. ounces.
Alcohol diluted q. s. to make the product measure .... 22 fl. ounces.

Moisten the powder, with half a fluid ounce of diluted alcohol, pack it firmly in a conical glass percolator and gradually pour diluted alcohol upon it until eight fluid ounces of percolate are obtained. Reserve six fluid drams of the percolate, evaporate the remainder by means of a water bath to ten fluid drams, add the reserved portion, and mix the whole with the clarified honey.

3225. Honey of Rose with Salicylic Acid.
Honey of rose.............. 16 av. ounces.
Salicylic acid ....140 grains.

Triturate the acid intimately with a small portion of the honey of rose, then add the remainder of the honey.

3226. Honey of Rose with Tannic Acid.
Honey of rose.............. 16 av. ounces.
Tannic acid ....370 grains.

Triturate the acid intimately with a small portion of the honey of rose, then add the remainder of the rose honey.

3227.   **Hydromel.**
Honey .... 1 fl. ounce.
Water .... 9 fl. ounces.

TREATMENT OF INEBRIETY OR NARCOMANIA.

BY NORMAN KERR, M. D., F. L. S.

Reparation of Damaged Tissue and Function.

In the essential work of reparation of tissue by the construction of new healthy structure, good sound food suited to the digestive and assimilative capacities of the patient is a leading factor.

Good Sound Food.

Healthful nutriment alone will aid in the reproduction of healthy material. By no other process can sound blood, flesh, sinew, bone, and nerve be renovated, and the diet must be such as the stomach and duodenum can thoroughly digest. Unless completely broken up and dissolved so as to be readily absorbed by the lacteals, the best and most judiciously chosen articles of food will be inadequate.

Vegetarian Claim as Best Renovator of Tissue and Function Unfounded.

It has been claimed on behalf of certain restricted dietaries that they afford the fittest pabulum for the renewal of strength. No such claim can justly be conceded.

Different Diet Needed by Different Individuals.

No one limited course of feeding can suit every constitution. It is physiologically true that a rigid dietary cannot be universal. A purely vegetarian diet excluding fish, flesh, and fowl suits many very well, provided due care be bestowed on the selection of the different edibles and on their cooking. It is imperative to exercise this caution, as owing to improperly chosen substances and the defective preparation of wisely chosen vegetarian products, I have seen dyspepsia so depressing and prostration so extreme as to have driven the sufferer to the beer, wine, and spirit bottle for relief from his sufferings, with the unfortunate result of fully developed inebriety. The adoption of a vegetarian mode of life involves in these islands often greater care than does the use of a mixed animal and vegetable diet. For example, in Scotland, Ireland, and North of England, most persons can digest and thrive on that excellent national diet of my native land, of which I am not ashamed to own, that a day begun without it always seems wanting in something good.

I refer to oatmeal porridge.

Yet in the southern portion of England, including the Metropolis, I have had under my care many persons, young and old, who have been quite unable to assimilate it, a perseverance in taking it daily for a week, never failing to set up most aggravated and well-nigh unendurable symptoms of indigestion. There are, too, not a few constitutions in which oatmeal acts as an irritant, and gives rise to a sense of intolerable heat, with skin trouble. Again, I have seen persons leading sedentary lives, who rushed from animal food at least twice a day to as frequent meals composed mainly of peas, beans and other legumes. The issue here was indeed disastrous.

Diet must be Judiciously Selected.

I am, therefore, especially desirous to warn inebriates who hope to find, as they are sometimes told they will find, in vegetarian diet a cure for their inebriety, of the need for great circumspection in the practice of that system. No one can have any excuse for imputing this warning to any prejudice against vegetarian habits. I have none, being of opinion that we English eat far too much meat; that excessive flesh eating tends to the production of narcotic intemperance, and that a judicious dietary, excluding fish, flesh and fowl, is ample for the physical and mental requirements of the great majority of mankind.

Inebriates and embryo—inebriates who are flesh eaters, also stand in need of admonition.

Excess in Animal Food Injurious.

Though I have no sympathy with those who teach that the moderate consumption of animal food creates a thirst for alcoholic liquors, no unprejudiced physician, with much experience in the treatment of inebriety, can have failed to discern the mischievous influence of a gluttonous indulgence in this variety of food. Persons who are the greater part of their time in the open air can assimilate a very much greater quantity of animal food than those who follow a sedentary occupation. Yet it is not uncommon for the latter to be inordinate consumers of strong meat, eating it largely and eating it often. In such cases, though the meat eater may be thin and pale-faced, a physically gross habit of body is apt to be engendered; the blood is surcharged with effete products, the circulation is impeded, and the infatuated kreophagist, instead of lessening the oppression, by eating less of the oppressor, resorts to the British alcoholic panacea for all the ills to which flesh is heir, and ere long may be an inebriate indeed. In these cases the patient is easily tired; has a feeling of general weariness; sometimes gets thinner and is altogether miserable. The urine has usually a high specific gravity. Alcohol relieves the discomfort for the moment and inebriety gradually sets in.

Food should be Slowly and Moderately Partaken of.

As a general rule the subjects of congenital and acquired inebriety will derive most bodily vigor and nervous tone from a plain, mixed diet of fish, flesh, and vegetables, with fruits, roots and grain. Probably fatty foods should have a prominent place in the dietary. As another general rule, animal food at one daily meal is enough. Above and beyond all else, whatever the food, it should be eaten slowly. The German proverb, "Food well masticated is half digested," is physiologically true. Deliberate eating would save no inconsiderable number of human beings from falling into inebriate courses. The bottle has a potent ally in the bolting of food. The hasty despatch of a meal leaves masses of food, not properly broken up and dissolved, in the mouth for the stomach to encounter, a task never intended to be thrown on that organ. The result is that digestion is attended with considerable difficulty, followed frequently by flatulence, severe pain and depression of spirits. This diseased condition craves for relief, and an alcoholic soother is employed—in too many cases the introduction to a course of periodic or constant inebriety.

Selection of Drinks.

In the restoration of physical and mental strength an important question is, "What should the inebriate drink?"

Intoxicants must be Excluded.

I am aware that the moderate use of certain intoxicating beers and wines has been recommended. To this recommendation I cannot assent, and I feel assured that it is a vital error. It is fatal to multitudes who are beguiled by the treacherous and false alcoholic promiser of strength into limited drinking, drunkenness and death. It is all a delusion. Neither alcohol, nor chloral, nor chloroform, nor opium, nor any narcotic, is a strength giver. "Wine is a mocker," physically as well as morally. All the alcohol in the world will not contribute a drop of blood, a filament of nerve, a fibrilla of muscle, a spiculum of bone, to the human economy. On the contrary, there is death in the cup; waste of strength, decay of substance, destruction of tissue, degradation of function, material death. In the most unequivocal terms I denounce alcoholic and other intoxicants as useless, unsafe, perilous remedies in the treatment of inebriety, bearers to the convalescent from this disease of physical feebleness, mental unstableness, moral perversion, volitional disablement.

Medicated Wines to be Avoided.

Some who are alive to the danger involved in the prescription of alcoholic intoxicant beverages to inebriates, have, in pure innocence, recommended medicated wines of various kinds, under the mistaken impression that these pharmaceutic articles contain only a minute proportion of alcohol for preservative purposes. These alcoholized medicaments, though they have some amount of nutriment, are all unsafe for narcomaniacs, the proportion of proof spirit sometimes being as high as 32 per cent. All such intoxicating alcoholic alleged "nutrient" and "restorative" preparations should be resolutely withheld in the therapeutic treatment of inebriety.

Water is Best.

There is a host of drinks at once restorative, refreshing and safe. Of water, the best of all beverages, the veritable "water of life," body-life, brain-life, it is impossible to speak in too high terms. Even in the height of inebriate madness, the thirsting dipsomaniac craves for water. None need be afraid of it. If, as is the case with some, it is not acceptable or comforting when drank cold, it can be taken hot. When desired, it can be flavored to suit any variety of palate by the addition of some non-intoxicating preparation of lime-juice or other similar fruit syrup. Sweet milk stands next—at once nourishing and thirst-quenching to most. There are some with whom it does not agree, taken cold and neat, but the addition of lime or soda or apollinaris water will probably render it grateful. Sometimes it suits better iced, sometimes when swallowed hot. There are, however, a few individuals who cannot assimilate milk in any form. Buttermilk is a delicious and reviving drink when the ordinary sweet milk does not agree. Whey is useful to some. Separated milk is often retained and assimilated when the heavier sweet milk would give rise to troublesome digestive disturbance.

Tea, Cocoa and Coffee.

Tea should be partaken of weak, rapidly infused and in moderate quantity. Cocoa and chocolate are delightful forms of combined food and drink. Coffee, genuine coffee properly prepared, is the most stimulating and enlivening of all artificial potables, with an aroma and a charm of its own.

Port with Bark.

Port (unfermented and unintoxicating) with bark, is an elegant and valuable aid to nerve and muscle rehabiliment.

Ærated Drinks.

Zoedone, and other non-intoxicating drinks, are sometimes of service, but special caution must be exercised to use these with moderation, as many of them contain iron, and their gaseous form is apt to cause cardiac distension.

Still Lemonade and Ginger Beer.

Oxygenated water, charged with oxygen from the atmosphere by Brin's process, made pleasant to the taste by lemon or other flavoring, is a new and palatable non-intoxicant. I have found no drink more useful than two very common and venerable favorites, viz.: For a still drink, home-made lemonade or lemon water; for an effervescent, ginger beer.

Only Intoxicants to be Absolutely Excluded.

To sum up, no hard and fast line of feeding or drinking can be laid down for every inebriate. The peculiarities of each case must be taken into account, as what would suit one admirably would be most unsuitable for another. Only one article should be absolutely excluded. That article is intoxicating liquor of every kind and strength.

Abstinence must be Unconditional.

The abstinence should be unconditional, with no exception in favor of birthday or other celebrations.

No Exception on Religious or Medical Grounds.

Such exceptions have been the rule of not a few, as has also the exception for religious purposes at the communion. Every intelligent and honest physician when asked, as I have frequently been, if it is safe for the reformed inebriate to partake of intoxicating liquor in such circumstances, should at once reply. "No, it is not safe." A high medical authority once publicly asserted that there was no probable danger, and that if there were, there would be greater risk in calling the special attention of the reformed inebriate to his weakness by any provision to meet it. Such an opinion could only have been delivered in utter ignorance of what inebriety really is. This is a physical disease, a paroxysm of which is provoked by the application of an exciting cause. Alcohol is such an excitant, probably the most potent of all, and the purely physical effect of the sip of a sacramental intoxicant is sufficient, in many cases, to arouse to activity the latent disease. Most reformed inebriates know this and avoid the risk. The great temperance orator, John B. Gough, during his reformation period of some forty years of abstinence, never would run this risk. Cases of excitation to paroxysmal drunkenness on this solemn occasion, after long terms of absolute sobriety, have not been unknown.

Unintoxicating Wine should be used at the Communion.

There need be no difficulty on the part of the clergy. In the Roman Catholic community the cup is withheld from the laity. For the Protestants, a variety of genuine unintoxicating wines (much more entitled to be considered pure and fit for sacred purposes than most of the fortified commercial so-called "pure sacramental wines" in general use at present) are now available.

Intoxicants should not be Prescribed as Medicine.

Nor should there be an exception in medicinal treatment. Other stimulant remedies can be applied, and if alcohol be in a rare case deemed necessary, it can be given in accurate doses, a precision impossible when intoxicating drinks are prescribed. It can be ordered either in the form of proof spirit, diluted, or, as I prefer, in the form of tr. cardamomi co., spirit ammoniae aromat., or spirit chloroform. In opium, morphine, chloral, and other forms of inebriety, this condition of abstention from alcoholic intoxicants should be insisted on. The danger in alcoholic inebriety is greater than in any of the other kinds, because the inherited tendency is more intense with alcohol, and this narcotic sets up organic and structural pathological lesions which are rarely, if ever, met with in opiism, morphinomania, chloralism, or any non-alcoholic narcomania. The physician should be wary in ordinary alcoholic intoxicants, even as therapeutic remedies, for in the subjects of inherited alcoholism (or tendency to alcoholism) medical prescription has been known to re-awaken the old irresistible crave or impulse. He should also administer opium, chloral, and narcotics generally with never-failing caution. In no case, with an inebriate diathesis, should he continue the use of opium or any sedative without a break. Especially should the self-administration of morphine hypodermically, be prohibited. The absolute discontinuance of all narcotics is of the highest importance; and the medical practitioner should never resort to them if any other remedy will answer the purpose. When required, these potent and dangerous drugs should be given in accurately defined doses for the occasion only.

For the remaining articles of food and drink, common sense and medical skill must be brought to bear upon the diet problem. The peculiarities, the likes and dislikes, the tastes and distastes, of each inebriate should be carefully considered, while due weight should be given to considerations as to the idiosyncrasies of digestion, and to the nutritious and other properties of the various articles of diet. Eating and drinking should be a pleasure not a task—a welcome interlude, not a serious and forbidding duty.

Correction of Prior Morbid Condition.

The correction of the pre-inebriate morbid condition is most essential. In many cases, if the pathological physical antecedent can be transformed into a physiological physical antecedent, a cure will be effected. If the unhealthy state of organ or of function, which has originated the inebriate impulse or crave, can be converted into organic and functional good health, the work is accomplished. The attention of the physician, therefore, ought to be chiefly directed, for the removal of internal exciting causes as well as for the correction of the diseased antecedent cause of the drink impulse or crave, to the bodily and mental soundness of the patient; to the rectification of abnormal departures from health. If, for example, an inebriate female dates her initiation into inebriety to, or is suffering from some ovarian or uterine affection, that trouble must be at once attacked.

Importance of Sound Hygienic Conditions.

The convalescent from inebriety, who so urgently needs restoration of the healthy nutrition of the brain, should live, as far as is practicable, under sound hygienic conditions.

Air, Exercise, Cleanliness, Activity.

Fresh air and exercise are almost as important as diet. Personal cleanliness is of the highest value. No one can over-estimate the influence of a life of vigor and activity, physical and intellectual exertion being withal kept within due bounds, in preserving and elevating the healthy tone of the human constitution. After a few weeks of abstention from inebriates, there is an extraordinary access of bodily strength and nerve force. This new and superabundant supply of vigor must find an outlet, and the great point is to have a healthy outlet in energetic work of some kind. A word of caution as to moderation will not be amiss. If the amount of exercise be immoderate, a feeling of cardiac exhaustion and general weariness may be induced, which may reawake the crave for a neurotic but temporary dissipator of lassitude. If the brain work be excessive a pathological state of neurasthenia (or nerve exhaustion) may ensue, which may prove but the prelude to a fresh inebriate paroxysm. I have witnessed this in several painful cases of relapse.

Amusement and Recreation.

Recreation and wholesome amusement are powerful allies. "All work and no play makes Jack a dull boy" is as true of the inebriate as of the teetotaler. The lack of diversion has driven many a sober man to drink; has brought on a melancholia which has transformed an abstainer into a sot. Music and the fine arts have saved many a young man and woman from being confirmed inebriates.

The Exhibitory Power must be Strengthened.

Not less essential is the strengthening of the inhibitory power. No matter how strong and active a man may be, if he have the strength of a Samson or the agility of a harlequin, no matter what his intellectual prowess, if he have the intellect of a Newton, or the logic of a Locke, if the faculty of inhibition be not cultivated, he may lapse into as abject servitude to inebriety as the most clownish and unlettered rustic. Education is no safeguard against drunkenness. The most learned man I ever knew was a habitual inebriate for years before he died. He was drunk regularly every evening, and I have known him occasionally attend meetings of important bodies, of which he was a member, in a state of intoxication during the earlier part of the day. His learning was profound and his memory phenomenal. Simple in his taste, unostentatious in his mode of life, and so warm-hearted withal, that no more touching and generous bequests were ever made by man. The ranks of opium, chloral, chloroform, and chlorodyne inebriates have been conspicuous by the presence of men and women of towering intellect, close reasoning, brilliant genius, perfect culture, and manifold accomplishments. All else that man can desire on earth may be his; all else that woman can wish for may be hers, but if moral control be allowed to lie fallow, none more likely to become a victim to inebriety, if temptation, or any other exciting cause present itself.

By Exercise.

Exercise is as essential to the health of each organ as it is to the general health. If a fractured arm is kept in splints too long the muscles are atrophied and weakened, and are unable to fulfil their office till exercise has restored their pristine vigor. If the brain be not kept at work, the power of thought is lessened. In the same way, if the moral control is not actively employed, it, too, will sustain loss. Each time mere impulse is obeyed without an effort at restraint the moral government loses strength. Therefore it is that resistance to the beginning of evil is so plainly enforced in the Scriptures. "My son, if sinners entice thee, consent thou not." The moral governance can be strong only when its efficiency is preserved by use. Its idleness is its death. On the other hand, each occasion on which control is wisely enforced, it is invigorated and strengthened. Each renewed judicious effort contributes to its stability and its mastery.

By Moral Influences.

It is of the highest importance, therefore, that firmness and perseverance in the paths of rectitude be sedulously cultivated. Every influence tending to aid in this consummation is a remedial agent urgently called for.

By Healthful Influences.

The physical tone is affected by pathological states of bodily organs, and also by the slightest physical disturbance of the nervous organization. That is to say, the integrity of the higher nerve centres, to a great extent, depends on the normal state of the nerve tissue and nerve function. Every derangement of the human economy wields a certain influence on mental tonicity. Therefore it is that the remedying of all morbid exciting causes is so vital a necessity in the cure of inebriety. By this rational and strictly scientific procedure, the controlling power is protected from a very common source of weakness.

Difference between Narcomania and Mere Moral Evils.

Something more is indispensable. Besides the enfeebling of inhibition by neglect of its exercise, alcohol and other narcotics exert a directly debilitating and enervating influence on the inhibitory power. For this latter reason it is imperative to call in every auxiliary to the bracing up of the control. This immediate and serious enervation by the anaesthetic paralyzing action of the narcotic, over and above the psychical disturbance by the functional commotion aroused by the poison, renders narcomania a more difficult disease to cope with than mischiefs free from a material narcotising factor. Herein, too, is a radical distinction between intoxication and other evils, such as lying or swearing, which are non-material actions. The operation of a destructive and deceptive chemical agent is peculiar to acts of inebriety, no one becoming inebriated without either drinking, smoking, inhaling, or having introduced into the body in some manner, the inebriating substance.

By Reasoning and Sound Instruction on Alcohol and other Narcotics.

To aid in the buttressing of the central inhibitory power many allies can be summoned. The reason ought to be appealed to by sound instruction on the nature and effects of narcotics and anaesthetics. By the exposition of the uselessness of these substances in a state of health, of the delusiveness of the plea that they are food for either body or brain, and of the hidden perils, all the more dangerous because they are concealed under the disguise of healthfulness, from which their use is never wholly free. The mind should be further enlightened as to the physical effects of the physical poison on body and brain, on organ and function, and as to the physical aspect of the narcotic bondage in which the inebriate is held fast. Inebriates should be shown that they labor under a physical disease, which is frequently curable, especially in its early stages, when exciting causes can be ascertained and removed, before the volition has been seriously weakened and moral control seriously diminished. It should emphatically be made clear to them, when cured, that their brain and nervous system will still remain peculiarly susceptible to the anaesthetic and paralyzing influence of narcotics and that, to their dying day, their only safe course is to be abstainers in all circumstances from all such drinks and drugs.

"No Good to Fight against my Fate."

It has been objected that to tell inebriates that they are diseased, is to dishearten them, and to set a seal on their fate. They will say, "What is the good of my fighting against my inclination to drink? I can never be cured." Or, "I have an inherited drinking tendency. What is the use of my struggling to keep sober?" The contrary ought to be the effect on the inebriate. If told judiciously, he will understand that to find a cure for any disease, it is important first to recognize the disease and then to comprehend its immediate and remote causes. With this knowledge, a hope of cure is as good as in rheumatism or neuralgia or almost any other disease. The fact of having any special abnormal heredity is no reason why we should necessarily yield to it. We all have heredity of some kind. When this is unhealthful, if we know its form, we can avoid the causes and occasions of it—we can strengthen our body and invigorate our brain—we can add to our inhibitory power. By these means we can, if we have an inebriate diathesis, hand down to our children a weaker inebriate inheritance, with a greatly increased power of resistance and moral control.

By Religious Influences.

Conscience should be approached by the inculcation of the duties owed by the inebriate to his family and to the community, and the value of the hallowed and strength-giving power of true religion should be plainly laid down "not by might nor by power, but by my spirit, saith the Lord." I have seen many a wasted waif, many a despairing drunkard, many a forlorn inebriate, who had failed again and again when trusting in his own strength to resist the impulse to excess, succeeding at last when invoking help from on High. Not spiritual hysteria, not theological dogma, but true and unsullied religion, is a grand support to the feeble, fitful, and unstable will of the diseased inebriate. It is a strengthener of the volition as well as a purifier of the affections, a mental tonic as well as a moral alterative. In opium inebriety religion has wrought marvels. Men will submit to being locked up in uncomfortable quarters for a month to rehabilitate the system that they may be able to do with a small allowance of the drug, they having applied for restraint because they needed a quantity greater than they could afford to procure. Their hearts have been touched when their brain was freed from the opium and its effects, and they have continued steadfast after their discharge. On the other hand, many who have left determining to abstain, have broken down after a longer or shorter interval. With opium users religion has been the faithful and helpful ally of medicine in strengthening resolution and supporting firmness.

"In the invigoration of the control the resources of pharmacy play a secondary part. It is a common belief that there can be no medical treatment without the profuse prescription of pharmaceutical preparations; that the advice of the physician is valueless, unless he orders drugs with a lavish hand. For this reason, unfortunately, the inebriate and his friends usually regard the consulting of a medical man as altogether useless. There can be no more grievous and mischievous error. Medicines are but one stone in the aesculapian sling; one resource of the art of healing. The intelligent medical practitioner knows that physic is a good stick but a bad crutch. He uses it, but does not lean on it. He employs drugs as one means of combating ill-health but these are not the only weapons with which he essays to slay disease. Scientific medical treatment includes attention to hygiene, to diet, to the body, brain, mind and morale. Everything which can contribute to the improvement of the soul and spirit, as well as to the reparation of tissue, has its place in the medical armamentarium.

Sometimes a Placebo is Demanded.

Yet there are many who do not believe that they are properly cared for unless they are directed to swallow or otherwise apply unmistakable medicaments. This is a natural feeling. When laid aside by illness we can with difficulty realize that we are making progress, unless we are using special means to assist us on our way. The act of swallowing, especially if the medicine has a taste of physic, is palpable to our senses, and each time we take a dose we feel that we are doing our part to promote recovery. I have myself experienced this feeling, and have never failed to feel benefited by the medicine ordered by a professional colleague, even when I knew that rest and fair play to the Vis medicatrix naturae were the only real needs. The mere fact of taking a medicine which has been prescribed, is of itself a remedy not to be slighted. For such inebriates of strong will and dogged perseverance, even if no medicine is indicated, it is useful to prescribe some course of gentle tonic physic, or at least some placebo. In such cases (they are few in number) a daily pill of half a grain each of ferrous sulphate and pil. asafoetid. co. will generally be found of advantage. Or this might be tried:

3228. A Gentle Tonic.

　　Tr. gentian co............ ½ fl. dram.
　　Acid. nitro-muriatic, dilut. ½ fl. dram.
　　Tr. cardamom co......... 1 fl. dram.
　　Aq. destillat, ad.......... 6 fl. ounces.
　　Sig: A sixth part twice daily.

In many cases of this kind any other simple and harmless, though slightly alterative, and tonic prescription, will answer. I have generally found that if the medicine be ordered to be taken for from ten to twenty days, every useful purpose will be served.

In a few cases I have found that nothing but something like this nauseous compound seemed to make the patient realize that he was actually taking the medicine which he felt he wanted:

3229. Mild Tonic Anti-Spasmodic.

　　Tr. valerian............... ½ fl. dram.
　　Tr. calumbae.............. ½ fl. dram.
　　Aq. destillat. ad.......... 6 fl. ounces.
　　Sig.: A sixth part twice daily.

There are, however, no inconsiderable numbers of convalescent inebriates, whose general tone and whose recovery of moral control are decidedly aided by medicinal remedies.

Medicines Sometimes Needed in Larger Doses.

For alcoholic and other narcomaniacs, Beckett's syrup of orange and quinine diluted with water, which forms an elegant and palatable substitute for the bitter beer of the drinker, has often answered well as has also, at times, the following:

3230. Bark with Acid.

　　Tr. cinchon. co............ 1 fl. dram.
　　Acid nitro—muriatic dilut. ½ fl. dram.
　　Aq. destillat. ad.......... 6 fl. ounces.
　　Sig: A sixth part twice daily.

Strychnine.

Strychnine is in some cases useful. It may be given in the form of pill, prepared by trituration with sugar of milk and glycerine of tragacanth in one daily dose of 1-30 grain, or still better, two daily doses of 1-50 grain each. This remedy may also be administered in liquid form which I, on the whole, prefer.

3231.

　　Liquor, strychnin. hydro-
　　　chlorat .... 12 fl. minims.
　　Aq. chloroform............ 1 fl. ounces.
　　Aq. destillat. ad.......... 6 fl. ounces.
　　Sig.: A sixth part twice daily.

Nitrate of strychnine, in pill or solution, in doses of 1-50 grain twice daily, is sometimes efficacious when other preparations have failed. Other occasionally useful preparations are the hydrobromate of strychnine, 1-50 grain, and arseniate of strychnine, 1-100 grain, once daily.

Iron and Strychnine.

Citrate of iron and strychnine and the triple citrate of iron, quinine and strychnine in two grain doses, three times daily, are in many cases of undoubted value.

Nux Vomica.

Of the various therapeutic remedies which I have found serviceable in the treatment of narcomania, none has been more satisfactory than nux vomica. The following has been a frequent prescription:

3232.

　　Ex. nucis vomicae......... ¼ grain.
　　Ex. belladonnae .... ¼ grain.
　　Sig.: One pill to be taken twice daily.

Nux vomica with phosphoric acid is of unmistakable service to many in the restoration of healthy tissue and tone, as thus:

3233. Nux Vomica with Phosphoric Acid.

　　Tr. nucis vomicae........ ½ fl. dram.
　　Acid phosphoric dilute ... 1 fl. dram.
　　Aq. chloroform............ 1 fl. ounce.
　　Aq. destillat. ad.......... 6 fl. ounces.
　　Sig.: A sixth part three times daily.

With Nitric Acid and Taraxacum.

Generally speaking, in all the forms of narcomania when the liver is affected, as evidenced by coating of the tongue, slight jaundice, languor, depression (more frequent in opiate than in alcoholic inebriety) mix with dilute nitric acid and taraxacum is invaluable.

Blue Pill.

An occasional four-grain dose of blue pill, followed by a saline aperient draught (such as epsom salts, hunyadijanos, rubinat or condal mineral water), will unload the oppressed viscera, relieve the malaise, and infuse a healthy glow of cheerfulness and hope.

Gold.

Especially in the United States chloride of gold and sodium is held to be efficacious by some physicians. I have no experience of this medicine, but if I were to prescribe any preparation of gold, I would prefer the bromide, which is in the proportion of four parts to one of the metal. Others lay stress on sulphate of manganese.

Cod Liver Oil and Hypophosphites Malt with Phosphates.

In some cases cod-liver oil with hypophosphites is a genuine heightener of nerve tone. Maltine or other non-intoxicating malted preparations, with phosphates, is also good. A well-known reformed drunkard, Mr. John Vine Hall, found the following, which he took regularly for seven months, a valuable remedy:

3234.

Ferri sulphate............ 5 grains.
Magnesiae sulphate....... 4 grains.
Sp. myristicae............ 1 fl. dram.
Aq. menth. pip. ad....... 1½ fl. ounces.
Sig.: The draught to be taken twice daily.

Antifebrin and Antipyrin.

Antifebrin, in tabloids, or suspended in an aqueous vehicle by mucilage, and antipyrine, in tabloids or in a watery solution, may sometimes be given in 3 to 6-grain doses twice daily with advantage, especially when neuralgic or obscure pain are present.

Objection to Hypodermic Injection.

With reference to the mode of administration of drugs, I have a strong aversion from hypodermic injection, and never resort to it where the medicine ordered can be administered by the mouth. The latter method I have found as effective though not quite so immediate in action. I have seen so many troubles, generally local, though sometimes followed by constitutional complications, that I cannot recommend, under ordinary conditions, the introduction of physic under the skin. There is also, too, the risk of the celerity and fascination of the needle operation proving irresistible for self-administration by the patient.

From the foregoing directions and prescriptions it will be apparent that I have indicated only general lines of treatment.

Special Pathological State of Inebriate must be Treated.

No two patients will be found alike. Each case is a study in itself. Where, as is frequently the fact, there are diseased conditions other than inebriety present, these must be met. If there is a syphilitic taint, combinations of iodine and mercury will probably be found necessary; if there is a history of malarial trouble, quinine, bebeerine, or arsenic may be indicated. No pains should be spared to trace and to cope with every morbid disturbance or tendency.

Tobacco in Treatment.

In most homes for the treatment of male inebriates the majority of the patients are allowed to smoke. I apprehend, not because this habit is considered an aid to cure, but because most male inebriates have used tobacco and it would be difficult to prohibit both intoxicating drink and tobacco in all such cases. In a few instances I have known a pipe or cigar prove the most efficacious means of tiding over the involuntary impulse or crave for intoxication. But these cases have been rare. With these exceptions tobacco has no legitimate place in the therapeutic treatment of inebriety. In the renovation of sound brain tissue, it is not a help, but a hindrance. Were I in charge of a home for the treatment of inebriates, the consumption of tobacco would be restricted within very narrow limits in exceptional cases, if allowed at all.

Treatment of Complications.

Various alcoholic disorders, which may effect the inebriate call for special treatment. Such a complication is delirium tremens. This is most successfully combated by the careful sustenance of the strength by frequent supplies of light nutriment readily assimilated. For medicines a brisk hepatic purge at the outset is often useful. I used to rely thereafter on the administration of the bromides with chloral and henbane. Whenever a hot, wet pack could be applied it seemed to do excellent service.

Delirium Tremens.

What is delirium tremens? Is it a morbid condition produced by nervous exhaustion, or a malady developed as an effect of alcoholic poisoning? I believe it to be the latter, and that the disease arises from the cumulative specific action of the poison on the cerebral tissues, through the alcoholization of the blood. Acting on this belief for some time past, I have aimed at eliminating the brain poison as speedily as possible, leaving as a rule, the healing power of nature to do the rest. So far as I know this plan was first suggested by Dr. Alexander Peddie in 1854, who generally prescribed antimony. The most serviceable drug in my hands has, however, been liq. amm. acet. The main point is to avoid the administration of alcoholic liquors, opiates, chloral, bromide of potassium, and the like. These potent drugs tend only to aggravate the symptoms. The best hope of cure lies in natural exhaustion, inducing sound refreshing sleep.

Treatment by Liq. Amm. Acetat.

The differing results of narcotic and non-narcotic treatment were strikingly exemplified in the case of a publican, who, at 48, was treated, during his second attack, by opium, and pot. bromid., and in his third attack, two years later, by liq. amm. acet. In the former seizure, the patient, though the narcotic draught at bedtime induced some sleep after the second night, invariably awoke feeling confused and heavy, stuperose, and with no relish for even the lightest food. The only crave was for spirits, and the delirium steadily became more intense, until it took four strong men to control him. The patient persisting in refusing food, dashing the cup with great force against the wall whenever he had a chance and becoming more and more maniacal, to save his life, as a favor, I procured him admission into the workhouse. He was there put into a padded room and left to rave and storm at his pleasure. Strong coffee was given to him which he at first angrily refused, but latterly craved for, no medicine at all being administered. Though, at first, he was hardly expected to survive, he made a good recovery in a week, but felt very weak and languid for some weeks afterwards. His succeeding attack was characterized by even graver symptoms, he having a fit (apparently epileptic) in the early stage of the delirium. As it was extremely undesirable, for various reasons, that he should be taken to the workhouse again, I treated him at home. From first to last I gave him no narcotic nor anaesthetic. The only medicine given was liq. amm. acet., beginning with a dram every hour till he perspired freely, and after that gradually diminishing the dose down to 15 minims and extending the intervals to 4 hours. In about 70 hours he had a short sleep of four hours, and in four hours more a quiet, sound sleep extending over 20 hours. Thereafter, except when aroused to take nourishment, he slept naturally. All delusions and hallucinations disappeared on the fourth day of the attack. In 7 days he was at his usual work again behind the bar.

Contrasted with Previous Attacks.

The contrast between the effects of the treatment during the two illnesses was most marked. During the first, when awake, he was constantly delirious, heavily stuperose or violent, continually trying to get in and out of bed. During the second he always awoke with head clearer, less confused, and with a readiness to take food. During both attacks, milk and soda, beef tea, meat juice, and chicken broth were relied on to sustain the strength. No alcohol was prescribed on either occasion. These were both typical examples of the graver form of delirium tremens.

In incipient cases, whenever I can, I rely upon its proper administration (or indeed during the height of the attack) I would prefer a cold or hot wet pack, frequently repeated, if necessary, to induce sleep. But in the absence of a skilled bath attendant, I have found the liq. amm. acet., by far the most effective, acceptable and reliable remedy which I have tried. By this method of wooing natural sleep, the first step in the cure, we leave the patient's brain and nervous system undisturbed by any narcotic or anaesthetic, and the vis medicatrix, which, after all is the most powerful factor in recovery from disease, has "a fair field and no favor." The delirious patient must be closely and unceasingly watched.

Other Complications to be Discriminated.

In all cases of inebriety a careful out-look should be kept for complications. Frequently only convalescence from a paroxysm gradually reveals epileptic neuritic or other symptoms masked during the intensity of an outbreak. Care, too, must be taken to discriminate these complicatory morbid affections. Obscure pains and aches, commonly credited to gout or especially rheumatism, are really symptoms of alcoholic neuritis, the treatment being different. It is in these obscure post-drunken pains that antipyrin is so valuable. But all such painful, as well as other unhealthful symptoms, call still more loudly for remedial measures to restore the general health. Probably the greatest relief will be found from Turkish and other hot baths, which promote the elimination of the unduly retained waste products and thoroughly cleanse the body.

Importance of Detecting Original Causes.

Let me once more call attention to the importance, after the patient has recovered to a considerable extent from acute symptoms of alcoholization, of discovering the preceding body or brain degenerations or functional perversions which, in so many cases, have originated a morbid inebriate impulse or crave. Adequate treatment must be applied, adapted to the special degenerative or physically depraved disorder. If, for example, syphilitic brain affections have been the predisposing cause, some preparation of mercury or iodine with tonics must be administered. A favorite prescription of mine has been Donovan's triple solution of mercury, iodine and arsenic.

If scrofula or some anaemic lowering of vitality has been the source of the mischief, recourse must be had to some such drug as ol. morrhuae, or arsenic with iron. If the intoxication craze has arisen from brain-fag, rest is a vital part of the treatment. If the exciting cause has been locality, a change of residence is indicated.

After combating the pre-inebriate or the past-inebriate degeneration, comes the physical regeneration of brain structure and nerve tissue, following on, though with unequal pace and occupying a greatly longer period, the physical reconstruction of muscle texture. In all stages of the therapeusis, after the first or acute stages, in the repairment of the physical structural degradation, as in the renovation of healthy tissue, active muscular exercise, fresh air, appropriate bathing, the adoption of hygienic measures, suitable bodily nutriment, cheerful society, and above all, occupation, are essential to successful treatment. All through, the ennobling and elevating influences of intellect, morals, and religion are of the highest value."

DRUNKENNESS CURES. MISCELLANEOUS.

To Allay the Craving for Alcohol.

The Practitioner.

3235.

Tinct. capsici	2 drams.
Tinct. nucis vomicae	1 dram.
Acid. nitrohydrochlor. dil.	1 dram.
Infus. gentian	ad 12 ounces.

M.

Two tablespoonfuls as required.

ALCOHOLISM.

C. & D.

Alcohol, taken to excess, destroys, hardens, and renders useless every organ of the body.

Intemperance is most pronounced in persons of an active excitable temperament, and obtains on them a greater hold. Idleness, great trouble or grief, an irritable brain, the thoughtless recommendation by a doctor of wine to a susceptible patient, are common starting-points of excess. It is generally agreed that alcohol in any form is bad for children.

TREATMENT.

Entire abstinence from all intoxicants is the only real cure for those who, possessing an unstable brain, drink to excess. If combined with a stay in an inebriate-home until the craving has ceased, permanent good may be done.

The Swedish Cure consists in isolating the patient and saturating all his food with alcohol until he absolutely loathes the sight and smell of the poison. Cures are often permanent. The ordeal is much dreaded by would-be drunkards who have once tried it.

Vinegar.—A wineglassful taken neat will steady a drunken person. Liq. ammon. acetatis, a full dose, is more pleasant and equally efficacious.

Diet-cures.—Many articles of food have been recommended from time to time. Copious water-drinking allays thirst and washes out the alcohol from the blood. If sufferers can be induced to drink skimmed milk or buttermilk they will continue taking it and avoid the spirit. Milk repairs alcohol-damaged organs, and is a wholesome nutritious substitute. Eating apples or fruit of any kind in large quantities is asserted to destroy craving for drink. Almonds, raisins, lump sugar, or pure sweets—even chocolate—are not merely nutriment, but in a measure quench thirst and diminish desire. Such articles can be carried in the pocket and eaten to escape temptation.

Chamomile-tea.—The soothing effect of inf. anthemidis on the digestive organs is well known. Put about a dozen heads in a teacup, pour on them boiling water, and let the hot infusion be taken habitually. It is a pleasant drink, and many people like it.

Liq. Ammoniae is a very old remedy for alcoholism and a very good one—7 to 8 drops in half a wineglassful of water. It modifies the sensibility of the stomach and so acts on the nervous system.

Potassium Bromide ½ dram doses combined, if desirable, with chloral and Indian hemp. Given alone in full doses it is one of the best remedies for dypsomania. It soothes the nervous system, and is especially valuable if patients are idle or sleepless.

Cocaine Hydrochlorate 1-10 grain to ½ grain internally restores appetite, soothes the brain, and induces a feeling of contentment and calmness. A useful form for administration, if patient requires a stimulant, is coca-wine.

Capsicum.—Ten minims of the tincture, combined with other hot camphoraceous drugs, is useful to allay sinking feeling and the morning nausea and sickness. Capsicum enters into the composition of many reputed cures:

Iron has been recommended. A good formula is:

3236.

Ferri sulph.	5 grains.
Magnesiae	10 grains.
Spt. myrist.	1 dram.
Aq. menth. pip.	1½ ounces.

One dram t. d. s. in water.

Ext. Cannab. Ind., ½ grain in pill t. d. s. arrests craving for drink by substituting another sedative for the alcohol.

Morphia.—Liq. morph. hydrochlor. ½ dram, combined with Inf. gent. co. 1 ounce or other tonics, allays the pain of alcoholic diseases. As a rule morphia should be avoided in treating dypsomaniacs, as they are very apt to continue it and become morphiomaniacs.

DRUNKENNESS CURES.
Ph. Era.

The following formulas have been going the rounds for nearly two years past, and secured by Dr. C. F. Chapman in one of the "Institoots." They are again published here in answer to several requests.

"No. 1.—Tonic, known as the 'dope.'

3237.

Aurii et sodii chlorid.	12 grains.
Strych. nit.	1 grain.
Atropiae sulph.	¼ grain.
Ammonii muriat.	6 grains.
Aloin	1 grain.
Hydrastin.	2 grains.
Glycerinae	1 ounce.
F. E. cinch. co.	3 ounces.
F. E. coca erythrox.	1 dram.
Aquae	1 dram.

M. Sig.: 1 dram every two hours.

"No. 2.—Injection, known as the 'shot.'

3238.

Strychniae nit.	0 1-10 grains.
Aq. dest.	4 ounces.
Potas. permangan.	q. s. to color.

M. Sig.: Begin with five drops, which equals 1-40 of a grain of strychnine, and increase one drop at each injection until the physiological effect is produced. Four hypodermic injections to be given daily at 8 A. M., 12 M., 4 and 8 P. M.

"No. 3.—Used with No. 2.

3239.

| Aurii et sodii chlorid. | 2½ grains. |
| Aq. dest. | 1 ounce. |

M. Sig.: Three drops every four hours in combination with the strychnine solution for the first four days.

"This last prescription is used only for the moral effect, which is produced in the following manner: Five drops of the strychnine solution are drawn into the syringe, then three drops of the gold solution are drawn in and mixed. This produces a golden yellow color, to which attention is called, and the patient is further assured as to the reality of the presence of the gold by the stain left on the skin after the hypodermic needle has been removed. A positive disgust is, in almost if not in every instance, produced in the following manner: The patient is given a drink of whisky, then the so-called bichloride of gold solution (really a solution of strychnine) is injected in his arm, but at the same time, and without his knowledge, he receives one-tenth of a grain of apomorphine. It takes but a comparatively short time for the emetic to produce its effect. Now the patient acknowledges the wonderful power of the hypothetical gold compound and surrenders unconditionally. From an unbelieving scoffer, he is changed into a disciple and supporter of the prophet."

HOT MILK AND VICHY.

"There are a great many men who are overworked and under-fed," said an up-town physician; "they think they are too busy to eat lunch at midday, and resort to stimulants as a substitute for food. It only takes a minute to step into a barroom and take a drink. This makes them feel better for a time, but the effect soon passes away and another is taken to get rid of the empty feeling. The habit grows until it takes eight, ten, or more drinks a day to keep them going. Alcoholic stimulants are the worst thing in the world for an empty stomach, finally causing catarrh of the stomach, interfering with the secretions of the liver, and destroying the ability to assimilate food. When a man comes to me in this condition the first thing I do is to cut off his whisky or whatever form of stimulant he is addicted to, and substitute food for it. I can't substitute solid food, because his stomach won't retain it. I must get him to take something that it will. This is where hot milk and vichy come in. Cold milk is too harsh. It shocks his weakened stomach. Hence I give it to him hot. Vichy lightens and livens it; makes it more easily digested. I tell him to take a glass, two-thirds milk, one third vichy, twice a day; to order it over a bar, anywhere he can get it, and to let whisky and all stimulants severely alone. If he obeys the orders I will cure him and save his life. A great many men among my own patients fast growing prematurely old, and bringing upon themselves a multitude of ills by the steady and excessive use of alcoholic stimulants instead of the nutritious food which they should take, have been reclaimed by the use of hot milk and vichy. If you find you are losing your appetite for food and correspondingly gaining that for alcoholic stimulants, try it. It will do you good."—American Carbonator.

KEELEY CURE.—HOME TREATMENT.

3240. Tincture of Willow Bark.
Tincture of gentian......... 4 ounces.
Tincture of calumba........ 4 ounces.
Tincture of cinchona....... 4 ounces.
Salicin .... 4 ounces.

Dissolve the salicin in the tinctures.

Dose: One teaspoonful every two hours.

This is given as a specific for the drink habit and will effect a cure in every instance where the patient desires to lead a sober life. The remedy will antagonize and eliminate the poison of alcohol—restore the brain cells to a natural condition, so that there will be no desire for alcoholic stimulants. The medicine should be put up in two eight ounce bottles labeled No. 1 and No. 2, and to ensure its being taken with regularity ought to be placed in charge of some member of the family or nurse, who will see that eight doses of 1 teaspoonful each are taken every day and two hours apart. When bottle number 1 is exhausted, begin with number 2 and take the same as number 1.

This remedy is for the Home Treatment of patients who cannot spare the time to take Institute treatment. Its bitter taste cannot be disguised and it should not be given without the full consent of the patient, as experience has proven that the one who does not feel the necessity for a cure will not appreciate the remedy.

Dissolve the Salicin in four ounces of boiling water before adding to the tinctures. This makes up the 16 ounces required by the formula

HOW TO DO THE PHOTOGRAPHIC TRADE.

From the Chemists' and Druggists' Diary, London.

When a chemist, finding he has the necessary space and that there is apparently an opening for a dealer in photographic goods in his neighborhood, decides to add this department to his business, he is frequently at a loss to know how to do it. The purpose of this article is to make the matter clear. It will be a distinct advantage to a chemist taking up this branch if he is himself a practical amateur—in fact, without some such knowledge, the business can only be conducted with difficulty. Therefore, every would-be dealer should master the elements of this art-science before embarking in it.

The amount of stock to be carried depends on the amount of capital it is wished to invest. It is, perhaps, best to commence with a small, well-assorted stock, buying in larger quantity those goods which experience shows to be most in request. It is as well to state here the standard sizes of plates, by which sizes, cameras, &c., to take them, are also known:

Lantern-plates .... 3¼ by 3¼ inches.
Quarter-plate .... 4¼ by 3¼ inches.
(On which carte de visites are taken.)
Half-plate .... 6½ by 4¾ inches.
(Used also for cabinet portraits.)
Whole-plate .... 8½ by 6½ inches.

Other sizes are:—5 by 4, 6½ by 3¼, 6½ by 4¼, 7 by 5, 7½ by 5, 10 by 8, and 15 by 12 inches.

Most of these find advocates for special purposes. It is best, however, to avoid recommending unusual sizes, as they cause a lot of trouble in obtaining the necessary plates, as many dealers do not stock any but well-known sizes. The quarter-plate camera is the most popular with beginners, but they invariably, as soon as proficient, obtain either the half-plate or whole-plate size.

The next thing to consider is the

DARK-ROOM.

If a good-sized room can be set apart for photographic uses so much the better; if not, a stock room can be found, which, with very little difficulty, may be converted into a dark-room, whilst still used for storage purposes. Temporary erections of laths and twill should be avoided, as they are eminently unsatisfactory and no saving of expense. The room selected must be made perfectly light-tight. If the window is large get a carpenter to make a well-fitting shutter to cover it. In the shutter a hole should be cut, about 8 by 12 inches, and glazed with a piece of the deepest ruby glass procurable. Should the door not be quite light-tight it must be made so by nailing cloth-edging round it or by hanging a curtain outside. Provide a catch on the inside of the door, so that it cannot be accidently opened from the outside when in use. The ventilation of the room must not be neglected, as the door and window, which are frequently the only sources of air, will have been made airtight as well as light-tight. In addition to the ruby window a dark lamp will be required for night use. A lamp burning gas is best; but where gas is not available a large paraffin lamp, with an ample oil-reservoir, should be provided. A water-supply and sink are very desirable in the dark-room. A table will be required, or, better, a bench projecting from the wall about 18 or 24 inches, 3 feet from the ground. Some shelving can be placed over for the bottles of developer, etc. A width of 5 inches admits of bottles with a capacity of 30 ounces. A perforated-zinc shelf over the sink should be arranged for draining-measures. A few dishes—say, three of each quarter-plate, half-plate, and whole-plate—will be conveniently stored in spaces beneath the bench. A distinctive dish for "hypo" is desirable. For measures, one each of 2-drams, 1-ounce, 4-ounce and 20-ounce size will be needed; these are not required stamped. Some stoppered bottles for solutions are wanted—say, of 30-ounce capacity and some of 10-ounce size. Developers to be kept ready will depend on the demand. At the end of this article will be found some useful formulae for them. Alum-solution (strength 2 ounces in a pint of water) had better be kept in a Winchester quart, as it is required rather freely. A similar-sized bottle of concentrated "hypo" (1 pound in 20 ounces) will form a stock solution, to be diluted when required for use. Intensifying-solution, oxalate-of-potash solution (1 pound in 54 ounces of water) for platinotypes, solution of ferrocyanide of potassium for reducing, and sulphocyanide of ammonia in solution are some of the other chemicals required to be ready for use. All these bottles should be plainly labelled in black or blue ink, so as to be readily seen in the dim light of the ruby lamp. A notice that a dark-room is available should be placed in a prominent place in the pharmacy, and notice sent round to the various photographic papers. The charges for use of dark-room depend on circumstances. It is policy to let customers use it for nothing for plate-changing. For developing it is usual to charge 1s. an hour (with 1s. as a minimum) or terms for a week might be, say, 5s. for changing and developing.

Of the apparatus to be stocked the first in importance will be the

CAMERA.

There are two kinds of cameras—one with a sliding wooden centre, the other with the centre in the form of a bellows. The use of the latter kind is now almost universal. There are two types of bellows, square and kinnear (tapering). The kinnear bellows are more used than the square kind, as they reduce the weight of the camera somewhat, although square bellows are indispensable when much architectural work is attempted. The fittings of cameras vary very much, the number of movements and quality of workmanship combining to make the large differences in price which will be noticed. When a worker who has been using a cheap camera purchases a good one, he will more appreciate the difference in use than can be conveyed by a page of letter-press. Cameras may be roughly divided into two classes—"stand" and "hand"—the former requiring a tripod stand for use, whilst the latter are intended to be used by holding in the hand either against the body or some convenient resting place. In hand-cameras there are three general types—those with an automatic changing arrangement, those with a changing box, and those in which dark slides are used.

THE LENS

will demand careful attention, as a defective lens is an effectual bar to good negatives. There are commercially but three main types of lenses, each type with many varieties. The types are (1) the single or landscape lens, the most suitable for taking views, but on account of the distortion they produce not suitable for architectural subjects; (2) the portrait lens, for portraits only, obviously of limited application to most amateurs; (3) the doublet, or rapid rectilinear lens, suitable for architectural subjects, landscapes, groups, and portraits, which convenient combination of properties makes this lens the most suitable for amateurs. The names for lenses used by the various makers are often as fanciful as they are numerous. The focus of a lens is the measure of the distance between the ground glass of the camera and the lens when a distant view is sharply defined on the ground glass. Makers of lenses generally aim at including certain proportions of a view on the ground glass, an angle of 45° being the most usual. Thus, a quarter-plate lens should have a focus of 4 to 5 inches; a half-plate 8 to 9 inches; a whole-plate 10 to 11 inches. The amount of light passing through the lens is variously limited by means of "diaphragms," or "stops," with the object of obtaining sharp definition over the whole of the plate. The marked values of the stops are obtained by dividing the focus of the lens by the diameter of the stop. It is useful to know how to find the focus of a lens. One of the simplest methods, but requiring a long-extension camera, is to focus a given object (such as a foot rule, or part of it) the same size, on the ground glass; then measure the distance between the object and the ground glass, which, divided by four, gives the focal length or focus of the lens. Extra rapid rectilinear lenses are so called on account of a claimed extra clearness in the glass used in their construction. A wide-angle lens, is one in which the focus is relatively short in proportion to the diagonal of the plate. The telephotographic lens is a lens which gives a much-enlarged image. It is used for taking distant objects on a larger scale than they are rendered by an ordinary lens.

THE STAND

which the chemist dealer will be most interested in is the tripod kind. Stands made of various woods and designs, the different designs claiming some advantage either as regards lightness, rigidity, or durability. As may be expected a stand combining these qualities would reach the ideal. The top of the stand should be as large as possible, as this contributes to rigidity in a great degree. The points of the legs are shod with more or less substantial spikes, to prevent slipping when in use. Some stands possess distinct advantages in regard to the ease in which they are folded up. Absence of loose parts is a point which saves a deal of discomfort from their tendency to get mislaid at critical moments.

MISCELLANEOUS APPARATUS.

The following are a few other requisites required: Instantaneous shutters of various makes, camera and lens cases, exposure-meters for gauging correct exposure, backgrounds (of which only plain ones are in demand), focussing-glasses, flash-lamps for evening portraiture, dark-lamps to take candles or oil, developing and other dishes in porcelain, glass or celluloid measures and graduated glass jugs, scales and weights, washers for plates and prints, drying-racks of wood or metal, grooved boxes for storing plates, printing frames, masks and discs; vignetting glasses, retouching desks and pencils, cutting shapes and knives, squeegees (both roller and flat), ground glass and ferrotype plates, blotting-paper and boards, albums of different designs, and, lastly,

MOUNTS.

A good selection of these must be stocked. "A good mount improves a good photograph, and to some extent a bad photograph." Mounts for portraits are supplied in a variety of sizes. It will only be necessary to stock carte de visite, quarter-plate, cabinet, half-plate, and whole-plate sizes at the commencement. Sizes like promenade, victoria, boudoir, imperial, panel, and stereoscopic can always be obtained in a day or two, unless a local demand justifies carrying a stock. The surface of a mount is either enamelled or plain, whilst they are obtainable in all manner of tints, such as cream, lemon, buff, salmon, pale-blue, pink, black, chocolate, brown, slate, cerise, mauve, crimson, and various shades of green and grey.

The edges may be either bevelled or plain. If bevelled, they are either left plain or gilded, silvered or colored. The corners are either square or rounded. Some cards, again, have lines or rands on the front. In mounts for views the same range of tints holds good, but here it is enlarged by combining various tints. The impression of a plate is marked on some kinds to convey the idea of an engraving to bromide or platinum prints. Just now a very popular mount for gelatine-chloride prints which have been squeegeed, is the push-in variety. These do away with the use of a mountant, as the photograph is merely pushed through a slit in the end, which may or may not be afterwards secured by an adhesive.

The best way of storing mounts is to have a box made for each kind, and plainly mark the variety and prices on the end. If these are again classed into different sizes in a cupboard they will readily be accessible. For convenience in retailing mounts, a sample of each kind should be kept together, each plainly marked with the price per dozen, hundred, and thousand, and, if thought necessary, a private mark of the cost may be added.

The next thing to consider is

DRY PLATES AND FILMS.

In stocking these it is well to bear in mind that all plates are good, although an amateur will always swear by the ones he has been accustomed to using. Local demand will quickly show what kinds to stock.

There is a great range of developers for all these plates; for instance, in the case of pyro-developer it runs from 1 grain to 5½ grains to the ounce. With each kind of plate full developing directions are given, and it is only fair to the makers to use solutions of the strength which experience has shown them is most suited for their particular plates.

The various

SENSITIVE PAPERS

are not less numerous than the varieties of plates. The sensitive salts were formerly held on the surface of the paper by means of albumen; this has now nearly given way to gelatin. The demand for albumen-paper is so slight that it may be disregarded in keeping stock. The gelatino-chloride, or printing-out, paper, as it is called, is made by several makers. The Eastman Company call theirs "Solio;" the Britannia Works Company's make is known as as the "Ilford P. O. P." Then there is the "Paget P. O. P.," the "Imperial Kloro," and Wellington & Ward's "Sylvio." A variety of surface is offered, such as shiny or matt, and various tints like pink and mauve.

Other kinds of papers are bromide-paper for printing and enlarging, of which there are numerous makers, each paper, with slight differences in composition and working, giving a variety of results; platinum-paper, issued with very complete instructions for producing platinotypes; carbon-paper, depending on the action of light on bichromated gelatine; and ferro-prussiate paper, much used for copying large plans and architect's drawings. These last three papers do not keep well, and are best procured as wanted, until such time as the demand would justify a stock being kept. Sepiatype, mezzotype, collodio-chloride, and citrate-of-silver papers are kinds occasionally asked for.

A few labels will be required for photographic chemicals and for such specialties as it is decided to put up. The formulae at the end of this article will give an idea of what are usually in demand. It is also necessary to make arrangements with a firm of printers and enlargers, so as to be able to get work of that kind done promptly for such customers as require it. If it is desirable to issue a price-list, most big firms will lend their blocks, if it is wished to include a few illustrations.

NON-SECRET FORMULAS.

3241.   **Flash Light Powder.**   A
    Chlorate of potash....... 16 parts.
    Aluminum powder....... 5.46 parts.
    Black antimony.......... 3.4 parts.

3242.   **Flash Light Powder.**   B
    Chlorate potash.......... 6 parts.
    Magnesium powder....... 3 parts.
    Black antimony.......... 1 part.

In either formula the black antimony must be an absolutely pure article—the commercial being too variable and doubtful as to purity.

MISCELLANEOUS FORMULAE

for such preparations as are likely to be in demand from photographic dealers. These are all well-tried formulae, many having previously appeared in the pages of The Chemist and Druggist:

3243.   **Concentrated Pyro Developer.**   A
    Pyrogallol .... 146 grains.
    Nitric acid............... 3 drops.
    Water to................. 10 ounces.

3244.   **Concentrated Pyro Developer.**   B
    Sodium carbonate........ 2 ounces.
    Sodium sulphite.......... 2 ounces.
    Potass. bromide.......... 20 grains.
    Water to................. 10 ounces.

For use, to develop a quarter-plate, mix 2 drams of each, and dilute with an equal quantity of water.

3245.   **Concentrated Hydroquinone Developer.**   A
    Hydroquinone .... ½ ounce.
    Sodium sulphite.......... 1 ounce.
    Water to................. 10 ounces.

3246.   **Concentrated Hydroquinone Developer.**   B
    Caustic soda............. ¼ ounce.
    Potass. bromide.......... ⅛ ounce.
    Water to................. 10 ounces.

For use for a quarter-plate, mix 80 minims of each, and dilute to 1 ounce with water.

3247.   **Metol Developer.**   A
    Metol .... 50 grains.
    Sodium sulphite.......... 1 ounce.
    Potass. bromide.......... 6 grains.
    Water to................. 10 ounces.

3248.   **Metol Developer.**   B
    Potass. carbonate........ 1 ounce.
    Water to................. 10 ounces.

For use, mix 3 parts of A with 1 part of B.

3249.   **Metol-Quinol Developer.**   A
    Metol .... 40 grains.
    Quinol .... 50 grains.
    Sodium sulphite.......... 1¼ ounces.
    Water to................. 10 ounces.

3250.   **Metol-Quinol Developer.**   B
    Sodium carbonate........ 300 grains.
    Water to................. 10 ounces.

For use, mix equal parts of A and B.

3251.   **Mercurial Intensifier.**   A
    Mercuric chloride......... ½ ounce.
    Hydrochloric acid......... 45 minims.
    Water .... 10 ounces.

3252.   **Mercurial Intensifier.**   B
    Liq. ammonia............. 1 ounce.
    Water to................. 10 ounces.

Immerse the negative in A till bleached, well wash, and tone in B till black throughout.

3253.   **Uranium Intensifier.**
    Potass. ferricyanide...... ½ ounce.
    Uranium nitrate.......... ¼ ounce.
    Glacial acetic acid........ ½ ounce.
    Water to................. 20 ounces.

Dissolve the salts separately, mix; after twenty-four hours filter and add the glacial acetic acid.

3254.   **Mountants.**   A
    Powdered starch.......... 2 ounces.
    Gelatine .... ½ ounce.
    Spirit .... 2 ounces.
    Carbolic acid............. ½ ounce.
    Water .... 12 ounces.

Heat the starch with 10 ounces of water until the granules are completely tumified and a translucent jelly is formed; then add the gelatine, previously dissolved, in the remaining 2 ounces of water; and lastly, the spirit and carbolic acid.

3255. Mountants.

Gelatine	4 ounces.
Glycerine	1 ounce.
Spirit	5 ounces.
Water	25 ounces.

Mix.

3256. Backing Preparation.

Mucilage	1 ounce.
Caramel	1 ounce.
Burnt sienna (ground in water)	2 ounces.

Mix well and add

Spirit	2 ounces.

3257. Backing Fluid.

Hard soap (in fine shavings)	½ ounce.
Spirit	10 ounces.

Digest at a temperature not exceeding 70° F., agitating occasionally for seven days; filter, and dissolve in the filtrate

Erythrosin	50 grains.
Aurin	50 grains.

3258. Concentrated Toning Bath.

Gold chloride	15 grains.
Ammon. sulphocyanide	225 grains.
Water to	3 ounces 6 drams.

Dissolve the gold chloride in 15 drams of water, neutralize with a little chalk, and filter. Dissolve the ammon. sulphocyanide in 1½ ounces of water and add to the gold solution, and make up to 3 ounces 6 drams. Label "Shake the bottle." To make a toning-bath add 4 drams to 15½ ounces water.

3259. Combined Toning and Fixing Bath.

Sodium hyposulphite	1¼ pound.
Acid citric	½ ounce.
Lead acetate	¼ ounce.
Ammon. sulphocyanide	2 ounces.
Water	80 ounces.

Dissolve in the water (warm), in above order, filter bright, and add

Gold chloride	12 grains.

3260. Platinum Toning Bath.

Potass. chloroplatinite	15 to 30 grains.
Acid lactic	3 drams.
Water to	35 ounces.

Mix.

3261. Negative Varnish.

Sandarac	½ pound.
Venice turpentine	2 ounces.
Oil of turpentine	4 ounces.
Spirit	½ gallon.

Mix.

3262. Matt Varnish.

Sandarac	1 ounce.
Mastic	90 grains.
Ether	10 ounces.

Dissolve and add

Toluol	4 ounces.

3263. Black Varnish.

Asphaltum	3 ounces.
Guttapercha	20 grains.
Lampblack	½ ounce.
Benzine	10 ounces.

Macerate the asphalt and guttapercha in the benzine till dissolved, then mix in the lampblack.

PHOTOGRAPHY.

From the Scientific American Cyclopedia.

The subject of photography has received much attention in compiling this book. Only those formulas were selected that came from undoubted authorities. The recipes do not form merely a collection of old recipes of the collodion process, but are the very latest that could be obtained, and the subject of photography has been thoroughly revised as the book passed through the press and it is hoped the result will prove a valuable acquisition to the art science. Special attention has been given to the Elkonoger developer which is considered the best. Look for the main subjects, as Developers, Toning Baths, etc.

3264. Aphorisms, Photographic.

1. When focusing, remember that the nearer the camera is to the subject the further away must the ground glass be from the lens, and vice versa.

2. Always endeavor to shade the lens as much as possible, and the resulting picture will have its brilliancy proportionately augmented. Many landscape artists use a large cone-shaped hood on the lens for this purpose.

3. On a hot summer day the atmosphere is often hazy and highly charged with non actinic light, while after, or even during a shower of rain the atmosphere is clear and bright.

4. Give your plants full exposure; over exposure is more easily corrected in the developer than is under exposure.

5. Clouds, being eight or ten times more actinic than the rest of the picture, will be proportionately over exposed, and unless they receive much less exposure than the foreground, which may be attained by the use of a drop shutter, they will appear in the finished picture as a blank space. They may, however, be afterward printed in from a separate negative by what is termed combination printing.

6. The color of the object is a great factor in the exposure required; whites and blues are rapid; red, brown, yellow, etc., are slow, according to their actinism.

7. Buildings taken full front elevation never look well; the camera should be placed in a position to include the front and one side, showing the building in perspective.

8. When the two sides of a picture are very similar, as in a street scene, for example, symmetry should generally be avoided. By placing the camera a little to one side, and pointing the lens at the other, the facsimile of the sides may be subdued.

9. Aim at the quality rather than the quantity of the views taken.

10. Remember that photography, being a witness, needs to be treated with much judgment, lest it tell lies. Also that those who use the most art betray the least. And lastly, never go forth without a large reserve of patience, as it is sure to be needed. See also Negative, Failures, Photographing.

3265. Autotypes, Flexible Supports for.

Yellow resin	6 drams.
Yellow beeswax	2 drams.
Rectified spirits of turpentine	20 ounces.

3266. Backgrounds, Photographic.

Purchase close-grained packing canvas cloth. Tack on frame and pull out projecting fibres. The cloth does not need to be stretched too tight, as it shrinks when painted. Coat it two or three times with the following mixture:

Low grade of gelatine	¼ pound.
Water	1 gallon.
Molasses	2 ounces.
Whiting	¼ pound.

Sandpaper after drying to make it smooth, then paint with one coat of ordinary oil paint. The white lead ground in oil is thinned with turpentine and mixed with lampblack, part of which has been ground in oil, and part in powder. The color should be a dark brown. One coat of flatting is next put on, usually by two persons, one to paint and the other to dab with a soft brush. A drab colored cloth, merino or woolen, answers very well.

3267. Backing Prints, to Prevent Halation.
See Halation.

3268. Baths, Silver, to Clear.
Agitate with China clay or kaolin.

3269. Baths, Silver, to Renovate.

1. Dilute with 3 volumes of distilled water, expose to sunlight, filter, add sodium carbonate till slightly turbid. Expose to sunlight six hours more, filter, add sodium carbonate till the silver is all thrown down. Wash precipitate by decantation, then dissolve in nitric acid. Filter again, make up to 35 grams; neutralize, expose to the sun a week, and the bath is ready for use.

2. Neutralize with ammonia till just alkaline; boil till black; let it cool, filter, acidify with pure nitric acid and evaporate to crystallization, then fuse. When cool add distilled water, shake and let stand exposed to light. Filter and add drained crystals; dissolve and make solution acid with pure nitric acid. Expose again to sunlight, filter, and the bath is ready for use.

3. Add potassium permanganate, expose to sunlight, filter, acidify, put in clean bottles four-fifths full, cork and freeze in a tray; thaw gradually till a ball of ice ⅛ size of the bottle remains. Remove this and use the rest. [This recipe should be used with caution, if at all; if the freezing is carried too far the bottle will inevitably be broken. —Ed.]

3270. To Blacken Cameras.

A good dead black is made as follows: Mix drop black, ground in turps, with gold size and turps—enough gold size to keep the black from rubbing off when dry.

3271. Blistering of Albumen Paper.

1. Have the room warm, but do not dry the paper by excessive heat.

2. Avoid acidity in solutions. Test with litmus paper. Moisten the print before washing with a sponge saturated in alcohol.

3. Add a slight trace of ammonia to the hypo.

4. Soak the print before fixing in a weak alum bath.

3272. Blisters, to Prevent.

After toning, immerse in a mixture of 8 parts methylated spirit and 2 parts of water.

3273. Blue Prints.

Float the paper for one minute in a solution of

| Ferricyanide of potash | 1 ounce. |
| Water | 5 ounces. |

Dry it in a dark room and then expose beneath negative until the dark shades have assumed a deep blue color; then immerse the print in a solution of

| Water | 2 ounces. |
| Bichloride mercury | 1 grain. |

Wash the print and then immerse it in a hot solution of

| Oxalic acid | 4 drams. |
| Water | 4 ounces. |

Wash again and dry.

For other prints in red, etc., see Printing Processes below.

3274. Blue Print Process.

1. Cover a flat board, the size of the drawing to be copied, with two or three thicknesses of common blanket or its equivalent.

2. Upon this place the prepared paper, sensitive side uppermost.

3. Press the tracing firmly and smoothly upon this paper by means of a plate of clear glass laid over both and clamped to the board.

4. Expose the whole in a clear sunlight from four to six minutes. In a winter's sun from six to ten minutes. In a clear sky from twenty to thirty minutes.

5. Remove the prepared paper and pour clear water on it for one or two minutes, saturating it thoroughly, and hang up to dry.

The sensitive paper may be readily prepared, the only requisite quality in the paper itself being its ability to stand washing.

Cover the surface evenly with the following solution, using such a brush as is generally employed for the letter press: One part soluble citrate of iron (or citrate of iron and ammonia), 1 part red prussiate of potash and dissolve in 10 parts of water.

The solution must be kept carefully protected from light, and better results are obtained by not mixing the ingredients until immediately required. After being coated with the solution the paper must be laid away to dry in a dark place, and must be shielded entirely from light until used. When dry, the paper is of a yellow and bronze color. After exposure the surface becomes darker, with the lines of the tracing still darker. Upon washing the characteristic blue tint appears, with the lines of the tracing in vivid contrast. Excellent results have been obtained from glass negatives by this process.— R. W. Jones, Proc. Eng. Club, Phila.

Use two separate solutions of

| Iron and ammonium citrate | 1 ounce. |
| Water | 4 ounces. |

and

| Potassium ferricyanide | 1 ounce. |
| Water | 4 ounces. |

For use, mix equal quantities and float paper for two minutes.

3275. Blue Prints, to Change to Brown.

| Borax | 2½ ounces. |
| Hot water | 38 ounces. |

When cool add sulphuric acid in small quantities until blue litmus paper turns slightly red, then add a few drops of ammonia until the alkaline reaction appears and red litmus paper turns blue. Then add to the solution 154 grains of red crude gum catechu. Allow it to dissolve with occasional stirring. The solution will keep indefinitely. After the print has been washed out in the usual way, immerse it in the above bath a minute or so longer than it appears when the desired tone is reached. An olive brown or a blackish brown is the result.

3276. To Make Blue Prints Green.

Make four solutions as follows:

Solution A.—Water 8 ounces and a crystal of nitrate of silver as big as a pea.

Solution B.—Hydrochloric acid 1 ounce and water 8 ounces.

Solution C.—Pour a solution of iodide of potassium (iodide of potassium 1 ounce and water 8 ounces) into a saturated solution of bichloride of mercury until the red precipitate is just dissolved, and then add four times as much water as the resulting solution.

Solution D.—Water 16 ounces, and iodide of potassium 1 dram.

Then take the blue print and bleach it with solution A, when the image will become pale slate color or sometimes a pale yellow.

Then wash thoroughly and immerse the print in solution B., when the image will again become blue.

Then, without washing, immerse the print in solution C., when the image will become green but the "whites" will be of a yellow tint.

Then put the print in solution B again, without washing.

Then wash and pour solution D over the print to purify the whites and to give the green image a bluer tint; but do not leave print in this solution too long, as it has a tendency to make the print blue again.

3277. Converting Blue Prints into Brown Prints.

Immerse the blue print after it is dried in a solution of aqua ammonia containing 22 per cent. am. gas, 2 parts; distilled water, 18 parts. Leave the print in this solution from two to four minutes, or until the blue color entirely disappears, then rinse in clear water, and plunge in a filtered solution of tannic acid, 2 parts; distilled water, 100 parts. Keep in this solution about twelve hours. If not as dark as desired, intensify by adding to the bath a few drops of ammonia water. Take out after a few minutes and wash thoroughly. The prints resemble sepia drawings. A greenish tone may be given blue prints by immersing after washing in a 1 per cent solution of sulphuric acid.

3278. Obtaining Warm Brown Tones on Bromide Paper or Lantern Slides.

Two formulae given by Mr. Robert Talbot in the Photographische Neuheiten, the author states, have proved to be very successful in his hands:

1. With uranium nitrate. This method is very well suited for Eastman positive paper, as well as for transferrotype paper. After the prints have been fixed, washed, and eventually transferred, the following two solutions are prepared:

Solution A.
Ferricyanide of potassium.. 5 grams.
Water. .... 500 c. c.

Solution B.
Uranium nitrate. .... 5 grams.
Water. .... 500 c. c.

Just before use, equal parts of solutions A and B are mixed. The print is immersed in the solution until the desired tone has been obtained, then washed thoroughly, and placed once more in the fixing bath.

Water. .... 100 c. c.
Hyposulphite of soda...... 20 grams.

After five minutes it is removed and well washed. The above gives warm red tones. Warm brown tones are obtained if the print is allowed to remain in the above bath until it begins to acquire a brown color; it is then immersed in a weak alum solution, when it is rinsed, fixed as above, and again thoroughly washed.

2. With potassium chloride. Three solutions are prepared:

Solution A.
Water. .... 1,000 c. c.
Potassium oxalate. .... 330 grams.

Solution B.
Water. .... 1,000 c. c.
Potassium chloride........ 130 grams.

Solution C.
Water. .... 500 c. c.
Sulphate of iron. .... 24 grams.
Citric acid. .... 2 grams.
Potassium bromide. .... 2 grams.

The paper should be fully exposed, and then soaked in clean water. Then mix.
Solution A. .... 20 c. c.
Solution B. .... 5 c. c.
Solution C. .... 5 c. c.

The more of B, if taken, the browner will be the tone. The print is cleared, fixed, and washed as usual.—Photo News.

3279. Silver Bromide Emulsions.

Over exposed gelatino bromide prints may be cleared by treating them with a very dilute solution of potassium cyanide, to which a small quantity of iodine has been added. Fog at the edges of the paper may be removed by applying a somewhat stronger solution with a brush, care being taken not to touch the image.—C. T. F. Phot. A., 31.

Bromide prints on paper or opal may be toned with the Oberpetter toning solution for gelatino-chloride paper, viz.: (A) Gold chloride, 15 grains; sodium acetate, 1 ounce; water, 39 ounces. (B) Gold chloride, 15 grains; ammonium sulphocyanide, 300 grains; water, 39 ounces. Mix 10 parts of A with 3 parts of B. Wash thoroughly after toning.—F. Golby, Y. B. Photo., 1891.

Another toning formula, designed especially for Eastman's paper, is ammonium sulphocyanide, 120 grains (120 parts); gold chloride, 4 grains (4 parts); water, 16 ounces (7,000 parts). The prints must not be left in after they become blue gray, or they will be deep blue when dried. This last color is suitable for moonlight effects.—H. W. B. Bruno.

Developing formulae: (D) Hydrochinon, 80 grains; sodium sulphite, 240 grains; water, 10 ounces. (A) Sodium carbonate solution, saturated at 60° F. Mix in equal volumes, and dilute the mixture with its own volume of water.—Pringle, A. Phot., 11.

(D) Hydrochinon, 80 grains; potassium bromide, 15 grains; sodium sulphite, 1 ounce; water, 20 ounces; citric acid, 60 grains. (A) Potassium carbonate, 2 ounces; sodium carbonate, 2 ounces; water, 20 ounces. Mix in equal proportions; gives warm tones.—B. Alfieri, A. Phot., 11.

(D) Eikonogen, 15 parts; sodium sulphite, 60 parts; water, 600 parts. (A) Potassium carbonate, 24 parts; water, 600 parts; mix in equal proportions, and add few drops 10 per cent potassium bromide solution.—Carbutt, Phot. T.

Eikonogen, 4 grains; sodium sulphite, 32 grains; lithium carbonate, 2 grains; water to 1 ounce.—Cowan, Phot. N., 34.

Quinol, 2 grains; sodium sulphite, 8 grains; potassium carbonate, 10 grains; water to 1 ounce.—Cowan, ibid.—[Quinol—Hydrochinon.—Ed.]

3280. Bromide Prints, to Secure Pure Whites in.

If the whites of bromide prints are found on completion to be yellowed, the stain can be completely removed by immersing the print after fixing, and thorough washing in a strong solution of tartaric acid, keeping it in the solution for an hour or more, if necessary, and finally washing in clean water.

3281. Burnishing, Lubricator for.

A.
Paraffine. . . . . 8 drams.
Benzine. . . . . 10 ounces.

B.
Gum ammoniacum. . . . . 30 grains

Alcohol, quantity sufficient to prevent the gum from sticking to the pestle while grinding the gum in a mortar. Add A and B together, and shake well and apply with a flannel or rag. The above give a fine polish.

3282. Lubricator for Hot Burnishing.

Cetaceum. . . . . 1 part.
Castile soap. . . . . 1 part.
Alcohol. . . . . 100 parts.

3283. Glacè Lubricator.

If a greater polish is desired than can be produced by the ordinary soap and alcohol lubricator, the following may be employed: Alcohol, absolute, 4 fl. ounces; castile soap (white), 25 grains; spermaceti, 25 grains. Dissolve by heat; add 1 fl. ounce chloroform. Apply in the usual manner. Dry thoroughly, and remove all traces of the lubricator with a piece of Canton flannel. Burnish; have the burnisher quite hot. (Swain.)

3284. Burnishing Solution.

Castile soap. . . . . 4 grains.
Alcohol (90 per cent). . . . . . 1 ounce.

Rub on the surface of the print, allow to dry, then burnish.

3285. Carbon Tissue, Sensitizing Solution for.

Potassic bichromate, 1½ ounce; water, 30 ounces; ammonia, at least 1½ drams. No more ammonia should be used than will change the reddish color of the bichromate solution to yellow.

Catechol. See Developers.

3286. To Cleanse the Hands from Silver and Iron Stains.

Dilute hydrochloric acid to half its strength; or, better still, chloride of lime in strong solution; pour ¼ ounce of this on the hands, and rub well in till the stains disappear. Next rinse the hands and apply a little dilute solution of potassium oxalate.

3287. To Clean Negatives Stained by Silver.

Make a weak solution of cyanide potassium. Rub the negative gently all over with a plug of cotton wool well wet in this solution, rubbing a little harder on the stained parts. Wash the negative well, and dry on blotting paper. If desired to revarnish, the plate may be flooded once or twice with methylated spirit. After drying it may be varnished in the ordinary way.

3288. Clearing Solution.
Edwards.

Alum. . . . . 1 ounce.
Citric acid. . . . . 1 ounce.
Sulphate of iron. . . . . 3 ounces.
Water . . . . 20 ounces.

Soak for a minute or two, when clearing should be complete.

3289. Clearing Solution for Pyro-Negatives.
J. Hay Taylor.

Alum. . . . . 2 ounces.
Hydrochloric acid. . . . . 2 fl. ounces.
Boracic acid. . . . . 1 ounce.
Water. 32 fl. ounces.

The solution can be used over and over again. It will do its work in ½ minute. The negative should be well washed.

3290. Clearing Solution for Gelatine Bromide Plates.

Alum.	2 ounces.
Citric acid.	2 ounces.
Sulphate Iron.	6 ounces.
Water.	40 ounces.

3291.

Sometimes by prolonged development negatives become stained, and usually clearing solutions are employed after the negative is fixed.

Mr. T. Bedding, in the British Journal of Photography, advises the use of an alum and citric acid bath, one part of citric acid to thirty of alum, before fixing. When the developer has been poured off the negative, the latter has been washed in a couple of changes of water, and the clearing solution applied for a few minutes, after which it may be returned to the bottle for future use. It is then important that the negative be carefully washed prior to immersion in the fixing bath.

3292.

Saturated solution of alum, 10 fluid ounces; hydrochloric acid (commercial), ½ ounce. After fixing and washing the negative, immerse in the above solution. Wash well.

3293.

Negatives which, after development by ferrous oxalate, are opalescent from oxalate of lime, are immersed in the following solution:

Water.	100 parts.
Oxalate of iron.	2 parts.
Alum.	8 parts

By which the opalescence will be completely cleared, and the whites of the negative will remain transparent.

3294. Clearing Solution.
Cowel's.

Alum.	2 ounces.
Citric acid.	1 ounce.
Water.	10 ounces.

Wash moderately after fixing, and immerse the negative in the above.

3295.

Saturated solution of alum.	20 ounces.
Hydrochloric acid (commercial).	1 ounce.

Immerse the negative after fixing, having previously washed it for two or three minutes under the tap; wash well after removal from the alum and acid.

3296. Chautauqua Clearing Solution.

Alum.	2 ounces.
Water.	30 fl. ounces.
Citric acid.	½ ounce.

3297. Clouds, Photographing of.

The best time to photograph clouds is in the spring, say March or April, when, after a storm, the heavy cloud banks assume fantastic forms. To successfully photograph clouds, the photographer must take up a position where his view will be unobstructed, by trees, houses, telegraph posts, chimneys, or other high objects. Then focusing upon the extreme distance, and including but a small portion of the landscape in his picture, let him, if he has not fixed upon the cloud, wait until the effect is most striking, then with a rapid shutter and a medium stop, say f/22, and a slow plate, let him make his exposure. Development should not be too heavy and should be stopped when all detail is fully out and sufficiently dense not to disappear in the fixing. With a suitably selected and properly developed negative of cloudland, landscape pictures can very frequently be considerably improved by the operation of printing in from the cloud negatives.

Clouds, Printing in.

Many pictures are improved by the addition of clouds. A bare expanse of white sky is very rarely attractive. To do this, special cloud negatives must be made or purchased. It is essential, to secure a satisfactory and pleasing effect, that the cloud should be lit from the same direction as the negative. Having made a suitable selection, of two negatives, a print is first taken of the landscape. If the negative is very dense in the sky, it will print out quite white. Two prints should be taken, one to make the final picture, the other to serve as a mask. This must be carefully cut through along the line dividing the blank sky from the objects in the picture. Fine branches of trees and such like projections need not be troubled with. Having carefully fitted this mask over the printed portion of the picture, it is placed in contact with the cloud negative and printed in the usual way, the mask protecting the lower portion of the printed picture from further action of the light. If the sky portion of the original negative is thin and it would in the ordinary course of printing print out more or less tinted, the sky must be blocked out. This can be done by running a brush filled with vermilion along the face of the negative for an eighth of an inch above the sky line, and then cutting a rough mask of paper and pasting on to meet this and cover up the rest of the sky. This will enable the sky portion to print perfectly white, when it is ready for the reception of the cloud impressions in the manner just described.

3298. Collodio Bromide Emulsion.

Ether, s. g. 0:720.	4 fl. ounces.
Alcohol, s. g. 0:820.	2½ fl. ounces.
Pyroxyline.	40 grains.
Castile soap dissolved in alcohol.	30 grains.
Bromide of ammonium and cadmium.	56 grains.

Dissolve 125 grains nitrate of silver in 1 ounce boiling alcohol and sensitize the emulsion by adding 1 dram of the silver solution at a time thoroughly stirring with a glass rod until the silver is well incorporated. After the whole has stood for twelve hours, add 30 grains more of the double bromide of ammonium and cadmium dissolved in ½ ounce alcohol. After standing for a few hours longer the emulsion is poured into a flat dish and allowed to evaporate and dry. It is then washed with distilled water by repeated soakings until all the soluble salts are removed. After drying it is again re-dissolved in equal parts of alcohol, at the rate of from 20 to 24 grains to the ounce of solvents. Then it is ready for use, and plates may be used wet or dry.

Collodion Formula.—Mix 6 ounces sulphuric acid, 4 ounces nitric acid at 1.450 sp. gr. and 2 ounces water. The temperature will rise to about 170° F., 77° C. When it is cooled down to about 100° F., 38° C., immerse perfectly dry cotton wool, best carded and of long fibre, pull it in under the acid with a piece of glass rod, and let each piece be well saturated before adding another. Cover the vessel and leave it for twelve to twenty hours in a situation where any fumes generated may escape into the outer air. Next lift the cotton out and plunge it quickly into a large quantity of water, separating the tufts with pieces of glass; wash in changes of water till no acid is left. Wring the cotton in a coarse towel as dry as possible, and then pull out the tufts and place them in the air to dry. Collodion made with this cotton will be very soluble and leave no sediment. 5 to 6 grains will dissolve in 1 ounce mixed ether and alcohol and still the collodion will be very fluid.

To prepare one pint of collodion with above—

3299.

Alcohol	10 ounces.
Sulphuric ether	5 ounces.
Cotton as above	100 grains.

3300. To Iodize.

Alcohol	5 ounces.
Ammonium iodide	60 grains.
Cadmium iodide	30 grains.
Cadmium bromide	20 grains.

Shake till dissolved and then pour into 1. Another plan, better for small quantities: Dissolve the iodides, as above, in 10 ounces alcohol, then put in 100 grains cotton and shake well. Lastly, add 10 ounces ether and shake till cotton is dissolved. This collodion will be ready for use in a few hours, but will improve with age.

3301.

For Washed Emulsion (for Transparencies)—

Ether, s. g. 720.	5 fl. ounces.
Alcohol, s. g. 0.820.	3 fl. ounces.
Pyroxiline or papyroxyline.	60 grains.
Bromide of cadmium and ammonium	100 grains.

Or—

3302.

Bromide of zinc	96 grains.
Hydrochloric acid, s. g. 1.2	8 minims.

Sensitize with 20 grains of nitrate of silver to each ounce dissolved in a minimum of water with two drams of boiling alcohol. Allow to stand for two or three days.

N. B.—In the last three formulae, the emulsion, after being allowed to ripen for the time stated, should be poured into a dish and allowed to become thoroughly dry. The mass of dry emulsion is then washed, to remove all the soluble salts, and is then again dried and redissolved in equal parts of ether and alcohol at the rate of from 20 to 24 grains to the ounce of solvents.

3303. Organifiers for Unwashed Emulsions.

For Landscape Work.

Tannin	½ ounce.
Gallic acid	60 grains.
Water	20 fl. ounces.

3304.

Tannin	300 grains.
Water	20 fl. ounces.

3305.
For Landscapes or Transparencies (warm, brown tone).
Freshly ground coffee..... 1 ounce.
Boiling water............ 1 pint.

3306.
For Transparencies (brownish black tone).
Tannin................... 30 grains.
Pyrogallic acid........... 60 grains.
Water.................... 20 fl. ounces.

3307. Developing Solutions for Collodion Emulsion.
A
Pyrogallic acid........... 96 grains.
Alcohol.................. 1 fl. ounce.

3308.
B
Bromide of potassium..... 10 grains.
Water................... 1 fl. ounce.

3309.
C
Liquor ammonia, s. g. 0.880 1 fl. dram.
Water................... 15 fl. drams.

3310.
D
Carbonate of ammonia..... 2 grains.
Water.................... 1 fl. ounce.

For each dram of developer take, for a normal exposure, 5 minims of A, 1 or 2 minims of B, and 1 or 2 minims of C; or if D be used, add the above quantities of A, B and C to 1 dram of D. When the details of the image are out, add double the quantities of B and C.

3311. Intensifying Solutions for Collodion Emulsion.
Nitrate of silver.......... 60 grains.
Citric acid............... 80 grains.
Nitric acid............... 30 minims.
Water.................... 2 ounces.

To each dram of a 3-grain solution of pyrogallic acid add 2 or 3 minims of the above, and apply until sufficient density is attained.

3312. Collodion Bottles, to Clean.
Collodion Bottles, to Clean.—Leave the stopper out until all the ether and alcohol have evaporated; when dry, remove the film with water and a bottle brush. Rinse with alcohol.

Dry Collodion Processes.—Pyroxyline.—For Collodio-Bromide or Unwashed Emulsion.

3313.
Nitric acid, sp. gr. 1.45.... 2 fl. ounces.
Sulphuric acid, sp. gr. 1.845 4 fl. ounces.
Water.................... 1 fl. ounce.
Cotton (cleaned and carded) 100 grains.
Temperature.............. 150° F.
Time of immersion, ten minutes.

3314.
For Washed Emulsion.
Nitric acid, sp. gr. 1.45.... 2 fl. ounces.
Sulphuric acid, sp. gr. 1.845 6 fl. ounces.
Water.................... 1 fl. ounce.
Cotton (cleaned and carded) 100 grains.
Temperature.............. 140° F.
Time of immersion, ten minutes.

3315.
Nitric acid, sp. gr. 1.45.... 2 fl. ounces.
Sulphuric acid, sp. gr. 1.845 3 fl. ounces.
White blotting paper...... 145 grains.
Temperature.............. 100° F.
Time of immersion, thirty minutes.

3316.
Collodio-Bromide Emulsion.
Ether, sp. gr. 0.720....... 5 fl. ounces.
Alcohol, sp. gr. 0.820..... 3 fl. ounces.
Pyroxyline............... 50 grains.
Bromide of cadmium and ammonium............ 80 grains.
or Bromide of zinc........ 76 grains.

Sensitize by adding to each ounce 15 grains of nitrate of silver, dissolved in a few drops of water and one dram of boiling alcohol. This is suitable for slow landscape work or for transparencies.

3317.
Washed Emulsion (for Landscapes).
Ether, sp. gr. 0.720....... 4 fl. ounces.
Alcohol, sp. gr. 0.820..... 2¾ fl. ounces.
Pyroxyline............... 40 grains.
Castile soap (dissolved in alcohol)................ 30 grains.
Bromide of ammonium and cadmium............... 84 grains.

Sensitize with 100 grains nitrate of silver dissolved in 1 ounce boiling alcohol; and after standing ten days, add a further 20 grains silver dissolved as before in 2 drams alcohol.

3318.
Rapid.
Ether, sp. gr. 0.720....... 4 fl. ounces.
Alcohol, sp. gr. 0.820..... 2½ fl. ounces.
Pyroxyline............... 40 grains.
Castile soap.............. 30 grains.
Bromide of ammonium and cadmium................ 56 grains.

3319. The Wet Collodion Process.
Iodized Collodion (for Negatives).

Ether, sp. gr., 0.725	10 fl. ounces.
Alcohol, sp. gr., 0.805	8 fl. ounces.
Pyroxyline	120 grains.
Iodide of ammonium	12 grains.
Iodide of cadmium	20 grains.

3320.
Bromo-Iodized Collodion.
(For Negatives.)

Ether, sp. gr., 0.725	10 fl. ounces.
Alcohol, sp. gr., 0.805	10 fl. ounces.
Pyroxyline	120 grains.
Iodide of ammonium	40 grains.
Iodide of cadmium	40 grains.
Bromide of cadmium	20 grains.

3321.
Bromo-Iodized Collodion.
(For Positives or Ferrotypes.)

Ether, sp. gr., 0.725	10 fl. ounces.
Alcohol, sp. gr., 0.805	10 fl. ounces.
Pyroxyline	100 grains.
Iodide of cadmium	50 grains.
Bromide of ammonium	20 grains.

3322.
The Nitrate Bath.
(For Negatives.)

Nitrate of silver (recrystallized)	6 ounces.
Distilled water	80 fl. ounces.
Nitric acid (pure)	10 minims.

Saturate with iodide of silver and filter.

3323.
For Positives or Ferrotypes.—

Nitrate of silver (recrystallized)	5 ounces.
Distilled water	80 fl. ounces.
Nitric acid (pure)	12 minims.

Saturate with iodide of silver and filter.

3324.
Developer.
For Negatives.

Protosulphate of iron	¼ ounce.
Glacial acetic acid	¼ ounce.
Alcohol	½ ounce.
Water	8 ounces.

3325.

Protosulphate of iron	15 grains.
Acetate of soda	15 grains.
Glacial acetic acid	30 minims.
Alcohol	30 minims.
Water	1 ounce.

3326.

Protosulphate of iron	1 ounce.
Glacial acetic acid	1 ounce.
Citric acid	½ dram.
Water	1 pint.

3327.

Ammonio-sulphate of iron	75 grains.
Glacial acetic acid	75 grains.
Sulphate of copper	7 grains.
Water	3 ounces.

3328.

Protosulphate of iron	7 drams.
Water	20 ounces.
Collocine	2 drops.
Alcohol	q. s.

This developer can also be used for glass positives and ferrotypes.

3329.
For Collodion Positives or Ferrotypes.

Protosulphate of iron	1½ ounces.
Nitrate of baryta	1 ounce.
Water	1 pint.
Alcohol	1 ounce.
Nitric acid	40 drops.

3330.
For Collodion Transfers.

Pyrogallic acid	5 grains.
Citric acid	3 grains.
Acetic acid	45 minims.
Water	1 ounce.
Alcohol	q. s.

3331.
Intensifying Solution.
A.

Pyrogallic acid	3 grains.
Water	1 ounce.

3332.
B.

Nitrate of silver	10 grains.
Citric acid	20 grains.
Acetic acid	1 dram.
Water	1 ounce.

For use, mix in a few drops of B with enough of A to cover the surface of the plate.

3333. Curling, to Prevent Prints from.
Try a very little glycerine in the toning and fixing baths.

3334.

A more correct heading of this receipt would perhaps be to flatten prints after they are curled. Lay the photograph face down upon a pad composed of several sheets of paper and place upon it at the left-hand margin a straight and rather sharp edge of a smooth ivory or boxwood rule. Move the rule slowly to the right, and with the left hand raise up the margin of the print nearest to that hand, pulling up rather strongly, yet so as not to allow the print to drag over the pad upon which it is laid. This will flatten the print and remove any further tendency to curl.

3335.

Immerse the finished prints in the following solution for a few minutes:

Water	1 part.
Alcohol	4 parts.
Glycerine	3 parts.

3336. Gelatine Paper Prints, to Prevent the Curling of.

After the print has been fixed and washed, it is immersed for a few minutes in a 5 per cent solution of glycerine and water, then removed, and directly squeegeed on a sheet of smooth hard rubber, then left to dry. When pulled off, it will lie as flat as a sheet of glass.

3337. Daguerreotypes, to Restore.

Daguerreotypes do not fade, but become stained if much exposed to air and dampness, and need cleaning. To clean daguerreotypes according to P. C. Duchochois, take hold of the daguerreotype with pinchers by one corner, and, keeping the plate level, cover it with a solution of potassium cyanide (1 part to 25 of water), and if the picture be much stained, heat it moderately with an alcohol lamp for fifteen or twenty seconds, when the solution is thrown off and the plate rinsed. This done, flow the plate with clear water, heat it as before, and holding it then almost vertically, dry it; in commencing, heat it at one of the upper corners and dry the water by blowing upon it toward the opposite corner. The whole operation should be quickly done, and the plate not too strongly heated, especially when covered with cyanide: otherwise the image might be obliterated. The daguerreotypes may be dusted with a fine camel's hair brush, but not touched with the fingers nor rubbed with any hard material. They are very easily scratched.

To Clean a Tarnished Daguerreotype.

Wash the plate gently, pour on carefully a 3 per cent solution of cyanide of potassium. Keep the plate in motion. Keep the solution only a short time on the plate, pour off, and wash well. If the tarnish remains, pour on more solution, repeat until the plate is clean. Wash with distilled water, and dry over a flame. Blow on the plate constantly, so that the water may be driven off evenly.

3338. Negatives, Density of, Reducing.

Solution for Reducing Over-Density.

A.

Hyposulphite of soda	2 ounces.
Water	1 pint.

B.

Ferrocyanide of potassium	2 drams.
Water	5 ounces.

Mix ½ ounce of B with 5 ounces of A just before use.

3339.

According to the Beacon, the following formula of L. Belizki is said to possess several advantages over Farmer's well-known potassium ferricyanide and hypo. It must be mixed in the order given.

Water	200 parts.
Potassium ferric oxalate	10 parts.
Sodium sulphite (neutral)	8 parts.
Oxalic acid	3 parts.
Sodium hyposulphite	50 parts.

It will retain its working strength if kept in the dark, and may be used over and over so long as it has a green color.

3340.

Red prussiate of potash	30 grammes.
Water	500 c. c.

Hypo. Solution.

Hypo	30 grains.
Water	500 c. c.

In cases of error in development the negative is too intense. The high lights may be safely reduced by the method of Mr. Howard Farmer, viz.: Ferricyanide of potassium (red prussiate of potash), 1 ounce; water, 16 ounces; hyposulphite of soda, 1 ounce; water, 16 ounces; immerse the negative in sufficient hypo solution to cover it, to which have been added a few drops to each ounce of the above ferricyanide solution; the speed of reduction depends on the quantity of ferricyanide present. When sufficiently reduced, wash thoroughly. To reduce locally, apply the mixed solution to the wet negative with a camel's hair brush to the parts requiring reducing.

3341.

There are three principal methods of reducing density:

a. The image may be changed in color, so as to be more transparent to actinic light. b. It can be partly converted into some compound, which can be dissolved out in hypo. or other solvent. c. The gelatine film can be reduced in thickness by solution or mechanical means.

Mr. W. E. Debenham's Method with Ozone Bleach.

Two solutions are required:

No. 1.

Chrome alum	1 ounce.
Water	1 pint.

No. 2.

The plate is immersed in a solution composed of ½ ounce of each of these in 5 ounces of water, and then in the hypo. bath. To reduce locally a stronger solution is poured in a stream on the part desired, the operation being repeated, if necessary.

3342.

Method with Chloride of Lime or with Eau de Javelle.

Hypochlorite of Potash.

For the first a saturated solution of chloride of lime is prepared, and for the second:

Chloride of lime	2 ounces.
Carbonate of potash	4 ounces.
Water	40 ounces.

The lime is mixed with 30 ounces of the water, and the carbonate dissolved in the other 10 ounces. The solutions are mixed, boiled and filtered. Either of these are diluted and the plate immersed until the required reduction is produced; it is then passed through the fixing bath and washed. In these cases a double action occurs; part of film being dissolved off and a portion of the silver being converted into chloride, which is removed in the fixing bath.

3343.

Method with Ferric Chloride.

A solution is prepared with—

Ferric chloride	1 dram.
Water	4 ounces.

The plate is immersed in this, which converts the silver into silver chloride, and on washing and immersing in the hypo. bath this is dissolved out.

3344.

Other Methods.—There are various other methods extant for reducing density. One or two, requiring only a single solution, have been found to answer very well.

No. 1.

Copper sulphate	½ ounce.
Ammonia	q. s.
Water	1 pint.

The quantity of ammonia is such as to redissolve the precipitate first formed on adding it to the copper sulphate and water.

No. 2.

Potassium ferricyanide (red prussiate of potash)	1 ounce.
Water	1 pint.

A few drops of ether should be added to 1 ounce of the hypo. bath diluted with 4 ounces of water, and the plate immersed until the requisite reduction is obtained and washed. In the first case silver sulphate, and in the second silver ferrocyanide, are formed, and immediately dissolved out by the hypo.—Br. Jour. of Photo.

3345.

(Seed).—Saturated solution chloride of lime, 2 fluid ounces; water, 8 fluid ounces. This solution should be poured over the negative in a tray. Soak for two or three minutes. Rub gently with the finger the spot to be reduced, until the desired intensity is obtained. Wash five minutes and dry.

3346.

The Hypochlorite Method.

It is often advisable to harden the film by immersion for some minutes in a solution made by dissolving 80 to 100 grains of chrome alum in a pint of water, after which it is immersed in the following hyposulphite of potash solution until nearly sufficient reduction is effected. Finally immerse in the hyposulphite fixing bath, and thoroughly wash.

3347.

The Hyposulphite of Potash Solution.

Agitate 3 ounces of good chloride of lime (bleaching powder) with 30 ounces of water, then add 5 ounces of carbonate of potassium dissolved in 10 ounces of water, agitate well, and filter through calico.

3348.

Reducing Over Printed Proofs (Salomon's).

Immerse for a short time in the following solution: Cyanide of potassium, 10 grains; liquid ammonia, 10 drops; water, 1 quart. Watch the prints carefully, and wash well.

Developers.—The following large collection of developers comprises all that are of any value, and the very latest formulas are published. The elkonogen developer is perhaps the best, and the developers using elkonogen and hydrochinon are also recommended.

3349.
Catechol.

Catechol (pyrocatechin) gives clear good printing negatives with less density and no greater detail for a given exposure than pyro or quinol, but has the advantage that it works well in dilute solutions. The following formula is given: (A.) Caustic potash, 10 parts; water, 1,000 parts. (D.) Catechol, 2 parts; sodium sulphite, 10 parts; water, 100 parts. Mix 5 parts of both with 100 parts of water, and, if necessary, add potassium bromide. The two solutions may be kept ready mixed.—L. Backelandt, A. Phot. B., xxi., 77-79.

3350.
Elkonogen.

The elkonogen developer allows of much shorter exposure than with pyro, does not deteriorate, and is not poisonous, and gives a fine deposit on the negative. The solutions can be used until exhausted, and over-exposure can be remedied by its use. Elkonogen is frequently contracted to elko, aspyro, hydro, etc.

No. 1.
Distilled water............ 20 ounces.
Sulphite of soda crystals.. 2 ounces.
Elkonogen crystals........ ½ av. ounce.

No. 2.
Distilled water............ 20 ounces.
Carbonate of potash....... ¾ ounce.

Mix Nos. 1 and 2 in equal parts, and to each ounce add 2 to 4 drops 10 per cent solution bromide of sodium. A few drops of a 10 per cent solution caustic soda will give additional energy for instantaneous exposures. The after treatment is same as with any other developer.

Although the above developer will keep if made up in one solution, we recommend making up stock in separate solutions, and mixing as wanted. The mixed developer can be kept in separate bottles for future use.

A mixture of equal parts elkonogen and hydrochinon developer yields lantern slides of great beauty, and we strongly recommend it also for negatives.

3351.
Elkonogen Developer for Short Exposures.

Distilled water, 100 parts; sulphate of soda, 40 parts. Dissolve and add crystallized elkonogen, 10 parts; caustic potash, 10 parts. For use dilute with three to ten times its value of water.

An elkonogen developer, said to be very simple, and to work good for lantern slide plates, is advised by T. A. Sinclair.

No. 1.
Elkonogen................. ½ ounce.
Sulphite soda............. 2 ounces.
Water .... 20 ounces.

No. 2.
Washing soda.............. 2 ounces.
Carbonate of potash....... 2 ounces.
Water .... 20 ounces.

Take one ounce of No. 1, half an ounce of No. 2, and add half an ounce of water. This will develop eight or ten plates in succession.

3352.
Elkonogen and Soda Developer.
A.
Sodium sulphite (crystals C. P.) .... 4 ounces.
Distilled water............ 60 ounces.
Elkonogen................. 2 ounces.

B.
Sodium carbonate (crystals) .... 3 ounces.
Distilled water............ 20 ounces.

Dissolve in order named. A developer is made by adding to 3 ounces of A, 1 ounce of B.

Single Solution, Elkonogen and Soda Developer.
Sodium sulphite (crystals C. P.)................... 4 ounces.
Sodium carbonate......... 3 ounces.
Distilled water............ 80 ounces.
Elkonogen .... 1 ounce.

Dissolve in the order named. Add a few drops of the hypo. solution during development. All of the formulas are based on 437½ grains to the ounce.

The usual alum and fixing baths may be employed.

3353.

With any developer that may be devised it is impossible to produce an image if the light has had no effect on the sensitive film, as is the case when a plate is described as being rather under exposed. Generally such exposures only develop on the surface, as the light has not had time to affect the underlying particles of silver. We advise the use of the eikonogen and potash developer. If this fails to produce an effect, no other developer is likely to. Make the eikonogen as follows:

No. 1.
Warm water.............. 40 ounces.
Sulphite sodium........... 2 ounces.
Eikonogen................ 1 ounce.

No. 2.
Water .... 3 ounces.
Carbonate of potash...... 1 ounce.

Take 2 ounces of No. 1, and add from 1 to 2 drams of No. 2, or 3 drams if necessary, to bring out the details; allow from half to three-quarters of an hour's time for the development of one plate, should it be greatly under exposed, and see that the temperature of the solutions is 70° Fah. Density is only obtained by a strong eikonogen solution and length of time of development.

3354.

6. The developing and fixing baths must be kept separate. An energetic developer is made by dissolving in warm
Water .... 40 ounces.
Sulphite sodium, c. p..... 2 ounces.
Eikonogen .... 1 ounce.

To 2 ounces of the above add 1 dram of following solution:
Water .... 3 ounces
Carbonate of potash...... 1 ounce.

Begin by soaking the plate in the first solution a few minutes; then, should the plate refuse to develop, add the second. A fixing bath is made by dissolving 1 ounce of hyposulphite of soda in 6 ounces of water.

3355.

Himly's Eikonogen Developer.
Captain Himly recommends the following:
Water .... 1000 parts.
Glycerine .... 100 parts.
Metabisulphite of potassium .... 2 parts.
Bisulphite of sodium...... 75 parts.
Eikonogen .... 12 parts.
Carbonate of potassium... 60 parts.
Yellow prussiate of potassium .... 40 parts.

3356.

Hubert's Eikonogen Developer.
Rain water................ 300 parts.
Sulphite of soda.......... 50 parts.
Eikonogen .... 10 parts.

The water should be warm and the salts dissolved in the order given in the formula; then add
Carbonate of soda........ 30 parts.

For extremely rapid exposures the undiluted developer is to be used. For shutter exposures of medium rapidity a sufficient quantity of the developer is diluted with half its bulk of water. For time exposures take equal parts of developer and water.—Le Progres Photographique.

	Eikonogen.	Sodium Sulphite.	Potassium Carbonate.	Sodium Carbonate.	Potassium Bromide.	Distilled Water.	Glycerine.	Potassium Ferrocyanide.	Sodium Sulphide, grn. to the oz. of solution.	Potassium Carbonate, grn. to the oz. of solution.
	oz.	oz.	oz.	oz.	oz.	oz.	oz.	oz.		
Formula of manufacturers of eikonogen......	1	2	15	16	....	1 16	45	......	17 1/2	9 1/7
Seed Dry Plate Co	1	6	1 1/2	....	....	60	......	......	43 2/3	10 1/2
Cramer Dry Plate Works....................	1	2 1/2	1 1/2	....	....	53	......	......	22	11
Eagle Dry Plate Works, for time exposures....	1	2	6	....	....	128	......	......	7	20 31/36
Eagle Dry Plate Works, instantaneous exposures............................	1	2	1	....	....	30	......	......	29	14 1/2
Harvard Dry Plate Works....................	1	2	2	....	....	80	......	......	11	11
Allen & Rowell Co.........................	1	4	2	....	....	80	......	......	22	11
Allen & Rowell Co., for instantaneous exposures....................................	1	4	2	....	....	40	......	......	43 7/10	22
Allen & Rowell Co., for bromide paper........	1	3	2	....	....	128	1	......	10 1/4	6 53/64
Allen & Rowell Co., for lantern slides........	1	5	1	1	....	128	1	1/2	17	3 1/2
Allen & Rowell Co., average for plates, bromide paper and lantern slides.............	1	3 1/2	2 1/2	....	....	74 2/3	......	......	......	......

3357.
Development with Separate Solutions.

A. Sulphite of soda, 1½ ounces, 30 grains; elkonogen, 180 grains; water, 26½ ounces. B. Carbonate of soda, 1 ounce, 1 dram, 40 grains; water, 8 ounces, 6 drams, 50 minims.

Note.—Dissolve the sulphite of soda in the water, and then add the elkonogen. For use employ three parts of No. 1 and 1 part of No. 2. N. B.—Be sure the sulphite is dissolved before adding the elkonogen.

3358.
Development with Single Solution.

Sulphite of soda, 1½ ounces, 30 grains; carbonate of soda, 1 ounce, 1 dram, 40 grains; elkonogen, 180 grains; water, 35 ounces, 1½ drams.

Note.—Dissolve the sodas in the water, and afterward add the elkonogen. This solution is used direct for developing without the addition of water. The sulphite of soda must be pure and fresh.

3359.

For very short instantaneous exposures (1-1000 of a second), and for increasing the power of the developers Nos. 20 and 21, in cases where the plate has not been sufficiently exposed:

Sulphite soda...............	5 parts.
Carbonate of potassium....	2 parts.
Elkonogen	1 part.
Water	30 parts.

Allowed to cool and preserved in a tightly closed stoppered bottle. To prepare this developer, place the chemicals in an earthenware jar, and add the water; stand the jar in a saucepan of boiling water, and bring about dissolution by boiling and stirring.

Preliminary Bath for No. 22.—

Hyposulphite soda..........	15 grains.
Chloride of mercury solution (1 in 100)............	15 minims.
Water	55 ounces.

Place the plate in this bath for one minute, and develop without rinsing.

3360.
Messrs. Fradelle and Young's Formula for Portraiture.

A. For normal exposures in the studio: Sulphite of soda, 4 ounces; elkonogen, 1 ounce; distilled water, hot, 100 ounces. B. Carbonate of soda, 1 ounce; distilled water, 100 ounces.

Notes.—For normal exposures take equal quantities of each, but varied at discretion. For instantaneous work and certain effects of lighting the face, use a stronger solution by reducing the water to 50 ounces in both A and B. Solutions of bromide of potassium and carbonate of soda, 1 in 10, may be kept in reserve for correcting over and under exposure. These are called 10 per cent solutions.

3361.
Dr. Mitchell's (Photo. Soc. of Philadelphia) Formula.
For lantern slides and transparencies.

A. Sulphite of soda, 1 ounce; elkonogen, ¼ ounce; water, 1 pint. B. Carbonate of soda, ¼ ounce; water, 1 pint. (N. B.—The American pint is 16 ounces.)

Notes.—For normal exposure take equal parts of A and B and add 2 parts water. For warm tones use half of No. 2 only and give a longer exposure.

3362.
Formula by Dr. H. G. Piffard (New York Camera Club).
With Ammonia Addition.

Sulphite of soda, 2 ounces avoirdupois; elkonogen, 1 ounce avoirdupois; bromide of potassium, 8 grains; boiling distilled water, 1 quart.

Notes.—Dr. Andresen forbids ammonia with elkonogen; but Dr. Piffard says it can be used as the alkali,' and works beautifully; time alone will show. Dr. Piffard's directions are—To 1 ounce of above solution add from 1 to 2 drops of liquid ammonia; but this should be used only in cases of decidedly under exposure. 1 to 1½ drops will do for a properly exposed plate. Instead of ammonia, add, if preferred, from ½ to 1 dram of an 8 per cent solution of carbonate of potassium, which gives more density than ammonia.

3363.
Warnerke's Formula.
For Copying Line Drawings and Engravings.

Sulphite of soda............	40 parts.
Elkonogen..................	20 parts.
Caustic potassium..........	20 parts.
Distilled boiling water......	100 parts.

Use 1 part of developer to 3 of water. Restrain with bromide if necessary. Dissolve the sulphite, then the elkonogen, and lastly the alkali. Filter while still hot, and store away for use. This developer has been used by M. Marey, in Paris, who is working on physiological subjects requiring extreme rapidity of exposure. He had previously been using hydrokinone, but he found a marked increase in the amount of detail obtained when using elkonogen instead.

3364.
Formula by Herr Eugen Von Gothard, Hérenz Observatory.
For Stellar Photography.

A. Sulphite of soda, 200 grammes; elkonogen, 50 grammes; water, 3 liters. B. Carbonate of soda, 150 grammes; water, 1 liter.

For use.—Take 3 parts solution A and 1 part solution B.

3365.
Combined Hydrokinone and Elkonogen Developer.

Sulphite of soda	300 grains
Carbonate of soda	200 grains
Hydrate of soda	30 grains
Bromide of soda	5 grains
Hydrokinone	20 grains
Elkonogen	30 grains
Water	10 ounces

This developer possesses the rapid action of the elkonogen combined with the sustaining energy of the hydrokinone, and keeps indefinitely. This is the latest phase of a single solution developer, presumably for instantaneous subjects, but I have not yet tried its powers.

3366.
Dr. Andresen's Fixing Bath.

Plates which have been developed with elkonogen should be well washed, and will greatly benefit by being fixed in the following bath:

Hyposulphite of soda	4 parts
Bisulphite of soda	1 part
Water	20 parts

The advantages of fixing in this bath are that—

a. The negatives have a perfect tone, which enables very fast printing.

b. This new fixing bath remains, even after frequent usage, clear, and water white.

3367.
Elkonogen, 10; potassium caustic, 10; sodium sulphite, 20; water, 100; dilute with 3 to 10 vols. water, according to result required, adding potassium bromide in case of over exposure.—Warnerke, Phot. J., xiv., 57.

3368.
(D.) Elkonogen, 25; sodium sulphite, 50; water, 1,000. (A.) Potassium carbonate, 100; water, 100. (R.) Potassium bromide, 10; water, 100. Mix (D) 3 parts, (A) 1 part, and add small quantity (R) if developer is new.—Cramer, Phot. T., xx., 208-210.

3369.
(D.) Elkonogen, 1; sodium sulphite, 2; water, to 32. (A.) Potassium carbonate, 1; sodium sulphite, 0.5; water to 64. Mix in equal volumes.—C. A. Dundore, Phot. T., xx., 233, 234.

3370.
(D.) Elkonogen, 25; sodium sulphite, 50; sodium carbonate crystal, 50; potassium bromide, 0.5; water, 1,000.—C. Jones, B. J., Phot. A., 1891, 560, 561.

3371.
(A.) Potassium carbonate, 9; sodium carbonate, 18; sodium sulphite, 120; water, 950. Dilute 100 parts with an equal volume of water, and add elkonogen, 5 parts.—Phot. A., xxxi., 35, 36, from Amer. A. Phot.

3372.
Elkonogen, 50; sodium sulphite, 250; boiled distilled water, 400. (A.) Potassium carbonate, 1; sodium carbonate cryst., 1; boiled distilled water, 10. To 100 parts (D) add 4 parts (A), or more as required.—A. Phot. B., xxi., 60.

3373.
(D.) Elkonogen, 1 ounce; sodium sulphite, 2 ounces; water, 40 ounces; potassium bromide, 8 grains. To 1 fluid ounce add not more than 2 drops strong ammonia solution; to get density add 30 to 60 drops of a solution of potassium carbonate (1.8).—H. Piffard.

3374.
(D.) Elkonogen, 5 to 6; sodium sulphite, 25; water, 500. When dissolved add 20 parts of a mixture of 500 parts of a saturated solution of sodium sulphite with 40 parts hydrochloric acid. (A.) Sodium carbonate, 20; potassium carbonate, 5; water, 500. Mix 3 parts (A) with 10 parts (D).—T. H. Veight, Phot. A., xxxi., 144.

3375.

Eikonogen Developer for Bromide Paper, by M. V. Portman.

The following is the process I advise for Eastman's bromide paper. (Workers may, of course, try the ferrous oxalate developer recommended in the instruction with this paper, but I admit that after a considerable experience with it, I have a strong objection to it).

Developer A.

Eikonogen	2 drams.
Sulphite of soda	4 drams.
Water	8 ounces.

To be mixed according to the instructions sent with the eikonogen.

Developer B.

Carbonate of soda	4 drams.
Water	1½ ounces.

Mix just before use. This amount will develop a 15"x12" print. Use fresh developer for each print, and take care, by experiment, that your exposure is correct. Always do your contact printing by a standard artificial light.

After development and washing in water (not under a tap), place the print in a fixing bath of—

Hyposulphite of soda	10 ounces.
Sulphite of soda	2 ounces.
Water	45 ounces.
Sulphuric acid	110 minims.

Leave the print in this bath for half an hour; then wash, not under tap, but in a print washer (I always use the Godstone print washer, which answers very well) for half an hour. Then immerse the print for one minute in a tanning bath.

Sulphite of soda	2½ drams.
Water	7½ ounces.

Dissolve and add—

Tannin	15 grains.
Hydrochloric acid	1½ drams.

Wash in a Godstone washer for three hours. If after washing the print is muddy in the high lights, immerse it for a short time (sufficient to clear it only) in—

Cyanide of potassium	½ ounce.
Water	40 ounces.
Iodine	1 grain.

Then wash it again thoroughly.

3376. Formaldehyde.

Formaldehyde, which, with some of its compounds, has been recommended as a constituent of developers, has been further investigated by W. Eschweiler and G. Grossman (Annalen, cclviii., 95-110). Formaldehyde sodium bisulphite (sodium oxymethyl sulphonate) is obtained by mixing a strong solution of sodium bisulphite with crude formaldehyde, and adding ethyl alcohol. It forms transparent crystals, easily soluble in water or in methyl alcohol, but only slightly soluble in ethyl alcohol. The crystals have the composition, $CH2O, NaHSO3, H2O$, but effloresce and lose water slowly when exposed to dry air. The salt can also be obtained in long, needle shaped crystals containing only half as much water $(CH2O, NaHSO3)2, H2O$. Formaldehyde-potassium bisulphite is obtained in a similar manner, and forms large tabular crystals, which contain no water of crystallization, and have the composition $CH2O, KHSO3$.

Formaldehyde sodium bisulphite, when added to a pyrogallol developer produces variable effects, though in some cases greater detail is obtained with less fog. When used in dilute solution (1 : 1000 or 1 : 2000) as a preliminary bath before ferrous oxalate development, it reduces the time of development, and gives stronger images, with more detail. The plate should be washed, after immersion in the bath, before being placed in the ferrous oxalate, or fog may result.—Eder, Phot. C., xxvii., 105-107.

P. Richter (Phot. Mitt., xxvi., 352) was unable to recognize any advantages arising from the addition of formaldehyde sodium bisulphite to the developer.

3377. Hydrochinon Developers.

These are excellent developers and are excelled only by the eikonogen developer. The word is spelled hydrochinon, hydrochinone, hydrokinone, hydroquinone, quinol, hydro, etc.

Water	10 ounces.
Sulphite sodium crystals chemical, pure	2 ounces.
Hydrochinon	1 ounce.

Dissolve in the order named, using, if possible, distilled water. This solution should be kept in a yellow bottle or in a dark place. It will retain its strength for a year or more.

3378.

Water	10 ounces.
Carbonate of potash	2 ounces.
Carbonate of soda	1 ounce.

The weights are based on 437 grains to the ounce. Put in the graduate 2 drams of No. 1 and 1½ drams of No. 2, then fill up to 3 ounces with water. If the developer works too slowly, add 1 dram additional of No. 2.

This will develop several plates in succession. When through, pour the developer into a separate bottle, filtering it through cotton, and preserve for use on future plates, adding a little fresh developer to it.

Make up the following stock solutions: 1. Hydroquinone, 8 grains; distilled water, 8 drams. This must be kept well corked and in a cool, dark place. 2. Carbonate of potash (dry), 12 drams; distilled water, 3 ounces. When quite dissolved filter carefully. This will keep any time. 3. Tartaric acid, 1 dram; distilled water, 80 drams; methylated spirit (pure), 2 drams. This will keep if well corked. This No. 3 solution is 4 ounces in all, water, acid, and spirit together. To develop a quarter plate, take of these stock solutions: Hydroquinone, 30 minims; add water to make up to 1 ounce; carbonate of potash solution, 2 drams; water, 6 drams. This makes 2 ounces developer when mixed and should then be poured over the plate, while in the developing dish. Keep the solution moving. The image should appear in from 20 to 30 seconds, and when the detail appears in the shadows add tartaric acid solution, 30 minims. Put this in the developing cup, and pour the developer from the plate into the cup, and return the solution to the dish.

3379.

Carbonate of soda	4½ ounces.
Sulphite of soda	2½ ounces.
Hydrochinon	150 grains.
Water	36 ounces.

When freshly prepared the bath is too strong and should have a third of water added to it; afterward each time of using a certain quantity of new solution should be added. The solution is not filtered; the clear part is decanted off.

3380.

Citric acid	5 grains.
Bromide of potassium	10 grains.
Hydrochinon	60 grains.
Sulphite of soda	120 grains.
Water	10 ounces.

Grind the hydrochinon in a mortar with warm water, then add the rest and pass it on to the boy to be shaken until thoroughly dissolved; either filter or allow to stand till clear. The alkali to be either caustic soda (4 to 6 grains per ounce), or common crystals of soda (40 or 50 grains per ounce), or any chosen mixture of the two. Equal quantities of each for developing.

3381.

A.

Sulphite of soda	2½ ounces.
Boiled water	16 ounces.

B.

Crystal carbonate of soda	½ pound.
Water (boiled)	20 ounces.

C.

Hydrochinon	1 dram.
Rectified 90 per cent alcohol	2½ ounces.

Take ½ ounce each of A and B, and add ½ dram of C.

If over exposure occurs, add to this quantity, say, 2 or 3 drops of

Bromide of ammonium	200 grains.
Water	2 ounces.

3382.

For Chloride Plates

Hydrochinon	2 grains.
Sulphite of soda	10 grains.
Carbonate of ammonia (or pot)	10 grains.
Bromide of potassium	1/10 grain.
Water	1 ounce.

3383.

A.

Hydrochinon	120 grains.
Sulphite of soda	1 ounce.
Bromide of potassium	25 grains.
Water	15 ounces.

B.

Dry powdered pure carbonate of potash	2 ounces.
Dry powdered pure carbonate of soda	2 ounces.
Water to make up to	20 ounces.

A and B are mixed in equal parts for development, and the picture is brought out in about three minutes when ordinary bromide plates are used.

3384.

Carbutt's Hydrochinon Developer.

A.

Warm distilled water	20 ounces.
Sulphite soda crystals	4 ounces.
Sulphuric acid	1 dram.
Hydrochinon	360 grains.
Bromide potassium	30 grains.
Water to make up to	32 ounces.

B.

Carbonate potash	1 ounce.
Caustic soda in stick	½ ounce.
Water, to make	32 ounces.

C.
Accelerator.
Caustic soda.............. 1 ounce.
Water, to make........... 10 ounces.
D.
Restrainer.
Bromide potassium........ ½ ounce.
Water .... 5 ounces.

Take of A 1 ounce, B 1 ounce, water 2 to 4 ounces—the first for instantaneous and short exposures on eclipse and special plates, and the latter for time exposures, portraits and views on our B landscape and ortho. plates. For lantern transparencies, 1 ounce A, 1 ounce B, water 4 ounces; 15 to 30 drops of a 10 per cent solution bromide potassium. After using, filter into bottle for future use, and for starting development on time exposed plates and films.

3385.

Hydrochinon Developer.—J. D. Cooper communicates to the British Journal of Photography the following formula:

Hydrokinone .... 6 grains.
Bromide potassium........ 1 grain.
Citric acid................ ½ grain.
Sulphite sodium (crystals). 20 grains.
Water .... 1 ounce.

The sulphite and other ingredients are first dissolved, then the hydrokinone is added.

An alkali solution of carbonate of soda (crystals) is made, 40 grains of soda to 1 ounce of water.

Equal quantities of the hydrokinone and soda solutions make up the developer for negatives.

The formula is somewhat strong for films rich in silver. If too much density is produced, the right amount may be obtained by dilution, which will adapt the developer perfectly for the production of opals or lantern slides.

3386.

Hydrochinon Developer (Piffard).—Hydrochinon (Merck's), 50 grains; carbonate of potash, 150 grains; sulphite of soda crystals, 200 grains; water, 10 full ounces. Mix and filter. After using it may be returned to the bottle for future use.

3387.

Hydrochinon—For Lantern Slides.
A.
Hydrochinon .... 10 grains.
Sulphite soda crystals, C.
P. .... 60 grains.
Water .... 1 ounce.

B.
Carbonate of potash, C. P. 30 grains.
Water .... ½ ounce.

Add B to A, and also enough water to make the whole measure 2 fluid ounces, and pour upon the plate.

The development starts rather slower than usual, but when once commenced proceeds with remarkable uniformity.

3388.

A developer for negatives is made up as follows:

A.
Hydrochinon .... 15 grains.
Water .... 1 ounce.

B.
Carbonate of soda crystals,
C. P.................... 30 grains.
Water .... 1 ounce.

Use equal parts of each, and less of No. 2 in case over exposure is feared. After use the developer may be preserved until as high as forty plates have been developed.

3389.

Hydrochinon Developer for Lantern Slides.—At a general meeting of the North Middlesex Photographic Club, Mr. Beadle read an interesting paper on slide making, and recommended the following developer:

Hydrochinon .... 160 grains.
Sodium sulphite........... 2 ounces.
Nitric acid............... 60 grains.
Potassium bromide........ 30 grains.
Water, to make up to..... 20 ounces.
For the second solution:
Sodium hydrate........... 160 grains.
Water .... 20 ounces.

Equal parts of the two solutions form the developer. For use, take equal parts of this solution and water. The picture should come up quickly and perfect in details, with full density in the shadows.—American Journal of Photography.

3390.

Compound Hydroquinone and Eikonogen Developer.—In consideration of the fact that eikonogen, per se, tends to give flat negatives, though the energy of the developer is impaired, and that hydroquinone, per se, acts rather slowly, giving, however, great density, a combined hydroquinone and eikonogen developer is used and strongly recommended by a well-known amateur photographer. Its composition is the following:

No. 1.

Sulphite of soda cryst.....	60 grams.
Cryst. soda...............	40 grams.
Distilled water............	1000 c. c.

After solution, to be filtered; keeps any time.

No. 2.

Eikonogen	50 grams.
Hydrochinon	50 grams.

Are placed together in a porcelain mortar, rubbed down to fine powder, and then kept dry for use in a well-stoppered glass bottle. For use, take 1 gram of No. 2 and dissolve it in 100 c. c. of No. 1. The solution keeps well for several weeks. This developer is said to possess all the advantages of the hydroquinone, iron oxalate and pyro developers, without their disadvantages. The greatest advantage, however, consists of the fact that the developer, if larger quantities are to be prepared, is always ready at hand, and that larger or smaller quantities may always be prepared without any delay.—H. E. Gunther, in Photo. News.

3391.

No. 1.

Soda carbonate............	60 grains.
Water	1 ounce.

No. 2.

Hydrochinon	2 grains.
Soda sulphite.............	60 grains.
Water	1 ounce.

For use mix

No. 1.....................	1 ounce.
No. 2.....................	2 ounces.
Water	1 ounce.

The above is a modification of a formula given by C. E. Van Sothern, in which he advises the use of 12 grains hydrochinon to 1 ounce water. It is usually advisable to employ a larger quantity than I have stated when it is found that the gelatine plate used gives a thin image. For line work, negatives and transparencies, the developer may be used over and over again, and then be bottled for use as a starter on another batch of plates. Each successive exposure should be longer when the old developer is used.

3392.

Hydrochinon Developer for Bromide Prints.—Sodic sulphite, 3 ounces; water, 30 ounces; hydrochinon, 45 grains; sodic carbonate (pure but not dried) 4½ ounces; potassic carbonate, 4½ ounces; potassic bromide, 60 grains. Divide the water into two parts. Dissolve the sodic sulphite, hydrochinon and bromide in one part, and the other ingredients in the other part. Mix the solutions in equal parts for use.

3393. Paramidophenol Developer.

This new developer, introduced by Messrs. Lumiere, has now been tried also by our German authorities, and their judgments are, on the whole, favorable to this reducing agent. Professor Vogel finds that the pure paramidophenol is very insoluble, so that it was impossible to prepare with it the solution recommended by Messrs. Lumiere. Dr. Schuchardt, of Gorlitz, has, however, succeeded in producing a hydrochloric preparation of this substance, which, in the hands of Prof. Vogel, proved to be more soluble than the first one, though it is said to dissolve much less readily in cold water than hydroquinone. It is, therefore, necessary to heat the water previously. The developer thus obtained is very energetic, giving, however, somewhat thin negatives, and the mixed solution soon becomes brown. If the paramidophenol solution and the sodium sulphite solution are kept separately, they will keep clear. Also Profs. Eder and E. Valenta state that the paramidophenol forms an excellent developer, giving, according to its composition, every degree of softness or intensity. The color of the negative is grayish black, the film being free of every bluish or greenish color, even if a neutral fixing bath is used. The authors recommend the use of a dilute solution for the reason that then the paramidophenol does not crystalize out of its solution, and the developer becomes less expensive. Moreover, the diluted solutions form equally excellent developers as the concentrated ones. The formulae recommended by the authors are the following:

3394.

Paramidophenol Soda Developer.

Water	1000 c. c.
Sodium sulphite...........	80 grams.
Carbonate of soda.........	40 grams.
Paramidophenol	4 grams.

3395.

Paramidophenol Potash Developer.

Water	1000 c. c.
Sodium sulphite...........	120 grams.
Carbonate of potash.......	40 grams.
Paramidophenol	4 grams.

The latter is specially well suited for plates which tend to give thin negatives, while the soda developer yields more delicate images. With the latter, also, transparencies on gelatino bromide emulsion may be developed very successfully.—H. E. Gunther, in Photo News.

3396. Hydroxylamine Developer.

Hydroxylamine hydrochlorate, 2 grains; caustic soda, 3 grains; potassium bromide, ½ grain; water, to 1 ounce, adding citric acid, 1 grain or less, if the water used is hard, to prevent the precipitation of lime carbonate (from the carbonate always present in caustic soda) upon the face of the negative. If the citric acid is necessary the bromide of potassium may be omitted, except in cases of over exposure. Hydroxylamine is stated to have a considerable tendency to cause frilling (and therefore must be used dilute) and to be unsuitable for developing plates that have received anything less than a full exposure.

3397.

Hydroxylamine and Pyro. Developer.—In a paper read before the Photographic Society of Philadelphia, reported in the American Journal of Photography, by Dr. Charles L. Mitchell, the following formula is given:

No. 1.
Hydroxylamine chloride... 30 grains.
Pyrogallol .... 240 grains.
Water .... 16 ounces.

No. 2.
Sodium carbonate (crystals) 1¼ ty. ounces.
Sodium sulphite (crystals). 4½ ty. ounces.
Water .... 16 ounces.

To develop, take of No. 1 from 1 to 2 fl. ounces; No. 2, ½ fl. ounce; water, 4 ounces; flow over the plate, and if the image does not appear within thirty or forty seconds, add more of No. 2 solution in small portions at a time, until development commences.

I have developed a dozen lantern slides, using the same developer for all, and after the last plate was finished, the developer was but of a moderately light orange color. The mixture of the pyro and the hydroxylamine chloride seems to possess remarkable keeping qualities. As a general rule, pyro. mixtures should be stored in yellow or amber colored glass bottles, provided with rubber corks, as the amber color prevents the actinic light from penetrating to the contents of the bottle. The developer is very superior for negatives, giving clear shadows free from stain. Hydroxylamine, though a somewhat new article in photography, can be had from the largest dealers and manufacturers in photographic materials.

3398. Iron Developers.

1. For Cold Tones:
Potass citrate............. 136 grains.
Potass oxalate............ 44 grains.
Hot distilled water........ 1 ounce.

2. For Warm Tones:
Citric acid............... 120 grains.
Ammonia (carbonate)...... 88 grains.
Cold distilled water....... 1 ounce.

3. For Extra Warm Tones:
Citric acid............... 180 grains.
Ammonia (carbonate)...... 60 grains.
Cold distilled water....... 1 ounce.

In mixing the solutions Nos. 2 and 3, it is advisable to place the crystals of the salts in a deep vessel, and after adding the water to leave alone till all effervescence ceases. Make over night. To 3 parts of any of the above formulae add 1 part of the following at the time of using:

Sulphate of iron........... 140 grains.
Sulphuric acid............. 1 drop.
Distilled water............ 1 ounce.

To develop place the exposed plate in a porcelain dish, flood over with sufficient of either of the solutions just mentioned, and keep the dish rocking. The time required to complete development will vary from one to ten minutes, according to the developer used and the density required. The first formula given is the quickest and the last is the slowest developer.

3399.

Ferrous Citro-Oxalate Developer:

No. 1.
Potassium citrate......... 700 grains.
Potassium oxalate......... 200 grains.
Water .... 3½ ounces.

No. 2.
Ferrous sulphate.......... 300 grains.
Water .... 3½ ounces.

Mix in equal parts.

For black and white tones, develop with ferrous oxalate. The following is the formula:

3400.

Oxalate Solution:

No. 3.
Neutral oxalate of potash. 1 ounce.
Bromide of potassium..... 2½ grains.
Hot distilled water........ 5 ounces.

3401.

Iron Solution.
Pure proto-sulphate of iron 2 drams.
Hot distilled water........ 2 ounces.

To develop, mix together 2 parts of oxalate solution with 1 part of iron solution, and pour in 1 wave across the plate. Rock well during development, which it is advisable to continue as long as detail is visible in the high lights of the picture. Rinse well after development, and previous to fixing. The fixing solution should be of the strength of 1 ounce in 4 ounces of water. The hyposulphite of soda solution should not be mixed till required, as a trace of this salt in the developing bath is ruinous.

3402.

The following oxalate developer is said to keep well, and was proposed by Mr. Archer Clarke at a regular meeting of the London and Provincial Photographic Association:

No. 1.

Citric acid................	1 ounce.
Citrate of ammonium.....	1 ounce.
Chloride of ammonium....	1 dram.
Bromide of ammonium....	1½ drams.
Oxalate of potash.........	10 ounces.
Water	50 ounces.

No. 2.

Protosulphate of iron,	3 ounces and 60 grains.
Citric acid................	1 ounce.
Water	50 ounces.

Mix in equal proportions.

3403. Pyro (Pyrogallic Acid) Developers.

The following formula, given by Captain Abney, in his splendid treatise on photography (of the greatest service to the expert), is an excellent one, giving the very highest results, and is deservedly popular. The solutions here given will have to be made up and kept in tight-fitting stoppered bottles:

No. 1.
Pyro Solution.

Pyrogallic acid............	50 grains.
Sodium sulphite...........	150 grains.
Citric acid................	10 grains.
Water	1 ounce.

No. 2.
Bromide Solution.

Potassium bromide........	50 grains.
Water	1 ounce.

No. 3.
Ammonia Solution.

Ammonia (0.880)............	2 drams.
Water	2¼ ounces.

These are not exactly 10 per cent solutions, but for all practical purposes may be regarded as such. Ten drops of No. 1 (pyro solution) will contain 1 grain of pyrogallic acid; 10 drops of No. 2 (bromide solution) 1 minim of potassium bromide; 10 drops of No. 3 (ammonia solution) 1 minim of pure ammonia.

3404.

Beach's Potash Developer.
Pyro Solution.

Warm distilled water.....	4 fl. ounces.
Sulphite of soda (pure)....	4 ounces.

When cooled to 70° F., add

Sulphurous acid (strong)...	3½ fl. ounces.
Pyrogallic acid............	1 ounce.

3405.

Potash Solution.
A.

Carbonate potash (chem. pure)	3 ounces.
Water	4 ounces.

B.

Sulphite soda (chem. pure crystals)	2 ounces.
Water	4 ounces.

Mix a and b separately, and then combine in one solution.

3406.

Carbutt's Pyro Developer.
Pyro Stock Solution.
A.

Distilled or ice water......	10 ounces.
Sulphuric acid.............	1 dram.
Sulphite of soda, crystals..	4 ounces.

Then add Schering's pyro, 1 ounce, and water to make 16 fl. ounces.

3407.

Stock Soda Solution.
B.

Water	10 ounces.
Soda sulphite crystals.....	2 ounces.
Soda carbonate crystals (or dry gran., 1 ounce)......	2 ounces.
Potash carbonate..........	1 ounce.

Dissolve, and add water to make measure 16 fl. ounces.

Bromide Solution.
C.

3408.

Bromide of sodium or potassium	½ ounce.
Water	5 ounces.

For Developer:

Dilute 1 ounce of stock b with 7 ounces of water for cold weather and 10 to 12 ounces of water in summer. To 3 ounces of dilute b add 1½ to 2¼ drams of a. The more pyro the denser the negative, and vice versa. No yellowing or fogging need be apprehended if our directions are followed. Development should be countinued until the image seems almost buried, then wash and clear.

3409.

Cramer's Pyro Developer.—Prepare the following solutions:

Alkaline Solution.

A.

Water,	1250 c. c.
Carbonate of sodium crystals (sal soda)	50 grm.
Sulphite of sodium crystals	60 grm.

This will produce negatives of a warm tone. If the sulphite is increased to 6 ounces the negatives will be of a gray or black tone. The alkaline solution must be kept in well stoppered bottles. If the negatives show yellow stain, make a fresh solution and try another lot of sulphite crystals.

3410.

Pyro Solution.

B.

Distilled or pure ice water	300 c. c.
Oxalic acid	1 grm.
Sulphite of sodium crystals	6 grm.
Pyrogallic acid	50 grm.

All pyro solutions work best while fresh. Eight grains dry pyro may be substituted for 1 dram of this solution.

3411.

Bromide Solution.

C.

Water	300 c. c.
Bromide of potassium	30 grm.

For use:

Alkaline solution	250 c. c.
Pyro solution	10 c. c.

When the developer is quite new the addition of

Bromide solution..10 to 40 min. 1 to 3 c. c.

is necessary to make it work perfectly clear.

Keep the developer moderately warm in winter, cool in summer.

Bromide solution produces intensity, contrast and clearness. It should be added when the developer is strong in alkali and new, also when developer is warm, when plates are over-exposed, or when the plates develop without sufficient strength and brilliancy. Use Cramer's clearing solution.

In compounding developers, carbonate of potassium or of sodium in different forms may be used to answer the same purpose, if proper attention is paid to their relative strength.

Twelve parts carbonate of sodium crystals (commonly termed sal soda or washing soda) are equivalent to 5 parts carbonate of sodium, dried, or 6 parts carbonate of potassium.

The sulphite of sodium is added to prevent rapid decomposition of the pyro or eikonogen. Too much sulphite in the developer renders its action slower.

3412.

Cramer's One Solution Developer.—Stock Solution:

Sulphite of soda, crystals	3 ty. ounces
Bromide of ammonium	½ ty. ounce.
Bromide of potassium	1½ ty. ounces.
Pyrogallic acid	2 ty. ounces.
Dissolve thoroughly in distilled water	32 fl. ounces.
Add sulphuric acid, c. p	20 minims.
Finally strongest aqua ammonia	8 fl. ounces.
And water to make up bulk to	40 fl. ounces.

Measure the sulphuric acid and the aqua ammonia very exactly, and keep the latter in a cool place.

For use dilute as follows: For normal exposures, 1 ounce to 11 ounces water. For instantaneous exposures, use 1 ounce with 3 or 6 ounces water. For overexposed plates, 1 to 20 ounces. Fix in alum and hypo bath.

3413.

The pyro. and carbonate of soda developer will give softness. Dissolve in

Water	6 ounces.
Sodium sulphite	2 drams.
Sodium carbonate	2 drams.

and just before using add

Dry pyrogallic acid	3 grains.

Should the density be too weak, put in twice the quantity of pyro. The softness is regulated by the quantity of pyro. No bromide is necessary.

3414.

Hoover's Potash Developer.—1. Water, 24 fl. ounces; sulphite of soda crystals, 4 ounces; citric acid, 120 grains; bromide ammonium, 40 grains; pyrogallic acid, 2 ounces. 2. Water, 24 fl. ounces; sulphite of soda crystals, 4 ounces; carbonate of potash, 6 ounces. To develop a 5x7 plate, take water 4 ounces; No. 1, 2 drams; No. 2, 2 drams. If more intensity is required, use more of both No. 1 and No. 2. More of No. 1 will restrain, more of No. 2 accelerate.

3415.

Hoover's Potash Developer.—A. Water, 12 fl. ounces; crystals sodium sulphite, 2 ounces; citric acid, 60 grains; bromide ammonium, 20 grains; pyrogallic acid, 1 ounce.

B. Water, 12 fl. ounces; crystals sodium sulphite, 2 ounces; potassium carbonate, 3 ounces. Mix A and B in equal parts and use one dram of the mixture to each ounce of water.

TABLE SHOWING COMPARATIVE VALUE OF ALKALINE CARBONATES IN DEVELOPERS.

O. G. MASON, M. D.

COMMERCIAL NAME.	Chemical Symbol.	Molecular Weight	The Commercial Salt contains of the pure Salt about	100 parts of 36 per cent. Acetic Acid Require for Saturation.	Solubility in Water (approximate).
Soda, Caustic	NaHo	40	80 to 92%	26·66 parts of 90% soda.	1 part in 2
Sodium Carbonate } Carbonate of Soda } Sal Soda, Crystals }	$Na_2CO_3, 10H_2O$	286	96 to 98%	89·38 " 96% "	1 " 2
The same, anhydrous or in dry powder	Na_2CO_3	106	About 98 to 99%	89·38 to 99% dry Sal. Soda.	1 " 6
Sodium Bicarbonate Bicarbonate of Soda } "Sesqui-carbonate of Soda" }	$NaHCO_3$	84	98 to 100%	50·91 of 99% Bicarb. Soda.	1 " 12

Equal work is done by 80 parts of Caustic Soda, 286 parts of Sal Soda (crystals), 106 parts of Sal Soda (dry), 168 parts of Bicarbonate of Soda. These quantities must be increased to make up for any impurity contained in the sample being used; for this purpose the usual percentage of impurity given in the above table may be assumed for all ordinary photographic uses.

Potassa (Caustic Potash)	KHO	56	80 to 95%	37·33 parts of 90% Potassa.	1 part in 1
Potassium Carbonate } Carbonate of Potassa } Sal Tartar } Saleratus }	$K_2CO_3, 1\tfrac{1}{2}H_2O$	165	76 to 96% Usually about 81%	51·11 parts of 81% Carb. Potassa.	1 " 1
Potassium Carbonate, dry	K_2CO_3	140	About 95%	122·74 parts of 95% Carb. Potassa.	1 " 1
Potassium Bicarbonate } Bicarbonate of Potassa }	$KHCO_3$	100	100%	60 parts of 100% Bicarb. Potassa.	1 " 4

Equal work is done by 112 parts Caustic Potassa, 165 parts (about) Carbonate Potassa, 200 parts of Bicarbonate Potassa. These quantities must be increased in proportion to impurities, as noted in case of Soda. These two alkalies are interchangeable for doing the same amount of work when *pure*, and when the one named in a given formula cannot be obtained, the table may assist in choosing a substitute of proper strength and solubility.

Dry or anhydrous Carbonate of Potassium is not usually found in the market.

ACKLAND'S TABLE FOR THE SIMPLIFICATION OF EMULSION CALCULATIONS.

	Equivalent Weights.	Weight of AgNO₃ required to Convert One Grain of Soluble Haloid.	Weight of Soluble Haloid required to Convert One Grain AgNO₃.	Weight of Silver Haloid produced by One Grain of Soluble Haloid.	Weight of Soluble Haloid required to produce One Grain of Silver Haloid.	Weight of Silver Haloid produced from One Grain AgNO₃.
Ammonium Bromide............	98	1·734	·576	1·918	·521	⎫
Potassium "	119·1	1.427	·700	1·578	.638	⎬
Sodium " ....com.	103	1·650	·606	1·825	·548	⎬ 1·106
Cadmium "	172	·968	1·012	1 093	·915	⎬
" " ....anh.	186	1·25	·800	1·382	·728	⎭
Zinc "	112·7	1·509	·663	1·670	·660	
Ammonium chloride............	53·5	3·177	·315	2·682	·373	⎫ ·844
Sodium "	58·5	2·906	·344	2·453	·408	⎭
Ammonium iodide.............	145	1·172	·858	1·620	·617	⎫
Potassium "	166·1	1·023	·977	1·415	·707	⎬ 1·352
Sodium "	150	1·133	·882	1·566	·638	⎬
Cadmium....................	183	.929	1·076	1·284	·778	⎭

3416. Tin Types, Developer for.

Messrs. Spiller & Crook, after long experience, give the following as a good developer for ferrotype plates:

Water .... 1 ounce.
Sulphate Iron.............. 14 grains.
Saltpeter .... 10 grains.
Acetic acid, No. 8......... 30 minims.
Nitric acid................ 2 minims.

Some have added:

Sulphate of potash........ 10 grains.

A potassium collodion should be used. The tones which this developer give are of a metallic luster, resembling the daguerrotype.

3417. The Dusting on Process.

1. Saturated solution bichromate of ammonia, 10 drams; honey, 6 drams; albumen, 6 drams; distilled water, 40 to 60 drams.

2. Dextrine, 1 ounce; grape sugar, 1 ounce; bichromate, 1 ounce; water, 1 pint.

Eikonogen.—See Developers.

3418. Enameling Photo Prints.

Use very clean plates and rather larger than the prints to be enameled. Wipe them well, rub them with talc, and remove the excess with a soft brush passed lightly over the surface. In a dish, half filled with ordinary water, immerse the photographs and allow them to soak. This being done, coat one of the talcked plates with enameling collodion in the ordinary way, agitate to cause the ether to evaporate, and when the film has set—that is to say, in a few seconds—steep this plate, the collodionized surface up, in a second dish containing pure water. Now take one of the prints in the first dish and apply the printed side to the collodion, remove the plate from the dish, keeping the print in its place with the finger of the left hand, and remove the air bubbles by lightly rubbing the back of the photograph with the forefinger of the right hand. Care has been taken beforehand to prepare some very pure starch paste, passed through a cloth, and some thin cardboards, or simply thick paper, the size of the plates used. The air bubbles having completely disappeared, and the perfect adherence of the print ascertained, dry with bibulous paper, and spread over the prepared cardboard on paper a coating of the collodion by means of a flat brush. Apply this sheet on the print, pass the finger over it to obtain complete adherence, and give it twenty-four hours to dry. At the expiration of this time, cut with a penknife the cardboard or paper even with the print, and detach by one corner. If the plate has been well cleaned, the print will come off itself. We get in this manner a very brilliant surface, and as solid as that obtained by the use of gelatine, which, as it is seen, is entirely done away with in this process. The prints are afterward mounted on thick cardboard in the usual way. It is possible, by mixing with the collodion some methyl blue dissolved in alcohol (a few drops are sufficient), to obtain moonlight effects, especially if a rather strong negative has been used. For sunsets, make use of an alcoholic solution in corcinine.—F. Tarniquet, in Science en Famille.

PROF. BURTON'S TABLE OF COMPARATIVE EXPOSURES.

Apertures Calculated on the Standard System of the Photographic Society.	Sea and Sky.	Open Landscape.	Landscape with Heavy Foliage in Foreground.	Under Trees, up to	Fairly Lighted Interiors.	Badly Lighted Interiors up to	Portraits in Bright Diffused Light Out of Doors.	Portraits in Good Studio Light.	Portraits in Ordinary Room.
	Secs.	Secs.	Secs.	Mins. Secs.	Mins. Secs.	Hrs. Mins.	Secs.	Mins. Secs.	Mins. Secs.
No. 1, or f/4	1/160	1/50	1/8	0 10	0 10	0 2	1/6	0 1	0 4
No. 2, or f/5 657	1/80	1/25	1/4	0 20	0 20	0 4	1/3	0 2	0 8
No. 4, or f/8	1/40	1/12	1/2	0 40	0 40	0 8	2/3	0 4	0 16
No. 8, or f/11·314	1/20	1/6	1	1 20	1 20	0 16	1 1/3	0 8	0 32
No. 16, or f/16	1/10	1/3	2	2 40	2 40	0 32	2 2/3	0 16	1 4
No. 32, or f/22·627	1/5	2/3	4	5 20	5 20	1 4	5 1/3	0 32	2 8
No. 64, or f/32	2/5	1 1/3	8	10 40	10 40	2 8	10 2/3	1 4	4 16
No. 128, or f/45·255	4/5	2 2/3	16	21 20	21 20	4 16	21	2 8	8 32
No. 256, or f/64	1 3/5	5 1/3	32	42 40	42 40	8 32	42	4 16	17 4

3419. **Encaustic Paste.**
No. 1.

Pure wax	500 parts.
Gum elemi	10 parts.
Benzole	200 parts.
Essence of lavender	300 parts.
Oil of spike	15 parts.

3420. No. 2.

A glacé appearance may be given to prints by rubbing over the surface lightly with clean flannel the encaustic paste made by dissolving in 200 grams of benzole the following ingredients:

Gum elemi	10 grams.
Essence of lavender	300 grams.
Oil of spike	15 grams.
Filter and add	
Pure virgin wax	500 grams.

The whole should be set on a water bath, which will aid in dissolving the wax. To make the paste thinner add more of the essence of lavender.

3421. No. 3.

Dr. Eder's Cerate (Encaustic) Paste.—White wax (pure), 100 grains; dammar varnish, 40 drops; oil of turpentine, 100 drops.

3422. No. 4.

Salomon's.—Pure virgin wax, 250 parts; gum elemi, 5 parts; benzole, 100 parts; essence of lavender, 150 parts; oil of spike, 7½ parts.

3423. No. 5.

Best white wax (cut in shreds), 2 ounces; turpentine, 10 fl. ounces. Dissolve with moderate heat. If too hard, add a small quantity of turpentine.

3424. **Faded Photographs, to restore.**

The following method is simple and in most cases quite effective: Put the card in warm water until the paper print may be removed from the card backing without injury. Hang up the paper in a warm place until perfectly dry, and then immerse it in a quantity of melted white wax. As soon as it has become thoroughly impregnated with the wax it is pressed under a hot iron to remove excess of the latter, and rubbed with a tuft of cotton. This operation deepens the contrasts of the picture and brings out many minor details previously invisible, the yellowish whites being rendered more transparent, while the halftones and shadows retain their brown opaque character. The picture thus prepared may then be used in preparing a negative which may be employed for printing in the usual way.

Faded prints can be restored by means of the following solutions: A. Sodium tungstate, 100 parts; water, 5000 parts. B. Precipitated chalk, 4 parts; bleaching powder (chloride of lime), 1 part; sodium aurochloride, 4 parts; distilled water, 400 parts. Solution B is made in a well-corked yellow glass bottle, is allowed to stand twenty-four hours, and is then filtered into another yellow bottle. The faded prints are well washed, and placed in a mixture of 1 to 2 parts of B and 40 parts of A. When the intensification is sufficient, the prints are immersed in a solution of 1 part of hypo. in 10 parts of solution A until all yellowness has disappeared, and are then well washed.—(H. Laudaurek, A. Phot. B., 21, 420.)

3425. Failures.

Foggy Negatives.—Caused by over-exposure; white light entering camera or dark room; too much light during development; decomposed pyro, introduction of hypo. or nitrate of silver into the developing solution, from the fingers or from tablets used for wet plates; developer too warm or containing too much carbonate of soda or potassium.

Weak Negatives with Clear Shadows.—Under development.

Too Strong with Clear Shadows.—Under exposure.

Weak Negative with plenty of Detail in the Shadows.—Want of intensity, caused by over exposure. Shorter exposure with longer development will, in most cases, produce sufficient intensity, and an addition of more pyro. stock solution to the developer will seldom be necessary.

Fine Transparent Lines.—Using too stiff a brush in dusting off plates.

Transparent Spots.—Dust on plate or air bubbles while developing.

Crystallizations on the Negative and Fading of Image.—Imperfect elimination of the hypo.

Yellow-colored negatives are caused by not using enough sulphite of sodium in developer, or if the article used is old and decomposed.

Yellow stains are caused by using old hypo. bath which has assumed a dark color, or by not leaving plate in hypo. bath long enough.

Mottled appearance of negative is caused by precipitation from fixing bath containing alum, if the solution becomes old or if it is turbid.

3426. Films, to Strip.

M. Izards recommends the following plan of stripping photographic films from glass. Make a solution of rubber in benzol, and coat your negative with it; when dry, apply a film of collodion, yet another of rubber, and finally, another of collodion. A narrow strip of black paper is then cemented to the margin of the plate all round, and this, when the film is dry and is stripped with a penknife, makes a suitable frame.

3427. Fixing Bath.

Carbutt's New Acid Fixing and Clearing Bath.

No. 1.

Hyposulphite of soda	16 ounces.
Sulphite of soda	2 ounces.
Sulphuric acid	1 dram.
Chrome alum	½ ounce.
Warm water	64 ounces.

Dissolve the sulphite of soda in 8 ounces of the water. Mix the sulphuric acid with 2 ounces of the water, and add slowly to the solution of soda sulphite; dissolve the chrome alum in 8 ounces of the water, the hyposulphite soda in the remainder, then add the sulphite solution, and last the chrome alum. This fixing bath will not discolor until after long usage, and both clears up the shadows of the negative and hardens the film at the same time.

Let remain two or three minutes after negative is cleared of all appearance of silver bromide. Then wash in running water for not less than half an hour to free from any trace of hypo. solution. Swab the surface with wad of wet cotton, rinse, and place in rack to dry spontaneously.

No. 2.

Cramer's Fixing Bath.—After developing and rinsing, the negatives may be fixed in a plain hypo. bath, 1 part hyposulphite of soda to 4 parts of water, but the following formula is especially recommended:

Water	1 qt.	1 liter.
Sulphite of sodium crystals	4 oz.	120 grm.

After being dissolved add

Sulphuric acid	½ oz.	15 c. c.
Chrome alum, powd.	3 oz.	90 grm.

Dissolve and pour this into a solution of

Hyposulphite of soda	2 lb.	1 kilo.
Water	3 qt.	3 liters.

This bath combines the following advantages: It remains clear after frequent use; it does not discolor the negatives and forms no precipitate upon them. It also hardens the gelatine to such a degree that the negatives can be washed in warm water, provided they have been left in the bath a sufficient time. The plate should be allowed to remain in the bath five to ten minutes after the bromide of silver appears to have been dissolved. The permanency of the negative and freedom from stain as well as the hardening of the film depends upon this.

No. 3.

Fixing Bath.

Hyposulphite of soda	500 grams.
Water	4 liters.

No. 4.
Hot Weather Bath.

Hyposulphite of soda	1 kilo.
Powdered alum	1 kilo.
Bicarbonate of soda	250 grams.
Water	8 liters.

3428. Flash Light Powder, to Burn.

A square metallic spirit lamp, having a flat top, is fitted with two wicks, one in front of the other, and separated by two or three inches. Immediately behind this lamp is a short wide-mouthed bottle containing magnesium in powder. Dipping into this powder is a glass tube, the other end being carried up through the cork and bent toward the flames of the spirit lamp, which are in a line with the direction of the blowpipe. A second short piece of tube is passed through the cork, its outer end being connected with the rubber tube of a pneumatic ball. On giving this ball a quick, sharp squeeze, a small quantity of the powder is suddenly ejected from the blowpipe nozzle against the flames, this being attended by a dazzling flash. This is capable of being repeated as long as any of the magnesium powder remains in the bottle.—Br. Jour. of Photography.

3429. Flash Light Powders.

1. Magnesium powder, 6 ounces; potassium chlorate, 12 ounces; antimony sulphide, 2 ounces; 75 to 150 grains of the powder should be used. 2. 15 grains of gun cotton and 30 grains of magnesium powder are used.

No. 3.

Magnesium	40 per cent.
Permanganate of potassium	40 per cent.
Peroxide of barium	20 per cent.

4. Purchase 1 ounce of magnesium powder and 1 ounce of negative gun cotton from dealers in photographic materials. Place on a dust pan enough cotton, when pulled out, to measure about 3½ inches in diameter. Sprinkle it over with 20 grains of magnesium powder to form a thin, even film. Lay over the magnesium thus arranged a very thin layer of gun cotton. Connect to the bunch of cotton a small fuse of twisted cotton about 6 inches long, so that it will extend to the side of the dust pan. Then set the pan on a step ladder near the object, and when ready, light the gun-cotton fuse with a match, when instantly a brilliant flash will ensue. There are several ready prepared magnesium compounds now sold with special devices and lamps to fire them.

3430. To Find the Focus of a Lens.

The focus of a lens, i. e., the distance it is from the ground glass when the object to be photographed is in correct focus, differs with the distance at which the object photographed is from the camera. The focus, however, for the purpose of definition, is what is known as the equivalent focus, and is taken as that distance at which an object at a considerable distance off is found to be in focus. The simplest way to find the equivalent focus of a lens is to point the lens and camera at the sun, and focus the image of the latter on the ground glass. The distance, then, between the ground glass and the lens, if a single one, or between the ground glass and the diaphragm aperture, will be the equivalent focus of the lens. There are more exact and mathematical methods than this, but it will be found to be practically all that is desired except for purely scientific purposes.

Formaldehyde.—See Developers.

3431. Frilling.

1. The following formula of Captain Abney's is, in most cases, a sure remedy against frilling:

Tough pyroxyline	6 grains.
Alcohol (0.820)	½ ounce.
Ether (0.75.)	½ ounce.

Apply this to the film before development; the solvents must then be washed away in a dish of clean water. When all repellent action is gone, apply the developing solution.

2. No. 1. Gallic acid, 1 part; alcohol, 10 parts. No. 2. Silver nitrate, 1 part; water, 16 parts; acetic acid, ½ part. Mix 1 part No. 1 with 4 parts water and add a few drops No. 2.

3432. Frost Pictures on the Windows.

The beautiful fairyland-like forms which frost often takes on the window panes of a cold morning form a splendid and attractive subject for camera work. They are best taken when the light falls on them sideways, and not full from the front. Set the camera dead square with the window and, behind the window pane and a foot from it, put a board covered with black velvet or other dark non-actinic material. Use a slow plate, stop down until the utmost sharpness is obtained, and give an exposure of three or four seconds, calculated at f/16. Of course in most cases to secure these pictures the photographer must be up early.

3433. Glazing Gelatine Prints.

The use of highly hand-polished sheet vulcanite rubber for imparting a high gloss to the surface of gelatino-bromide prints is now well known, but, in consequence of the difficulty in obtaining good samples, and of its high cost, the general use of it has been somewhat limited. A substitute, in the shape of ferrotype plates, costing but a mere fraction of the rubber, has been recently tried with success. Upon the smooth, varnished side of the sheet is laid the moist print, film side down. It is then squeegeed by passing a rubber roller over the back, which presses out all the air bells. In an hour or so the print, when dry, can be pulled off at one corner, and will possess a high gloss. A slight heat applied on the rough side of the metal sheet will materially hasten the drying.—Scientific American.

3434. Glace Prints.

Apply the prints face down while wet to the smooth varnished side of a ferrotype plate, squeezing it by rolling a rubber roller over the back, having blotting paper between the print and paper. When dry it will have a high polish and drop off the sheet. The polish is called glace finish. To mount such prints without losing the gloss, make the following mounting solution: Soak 1 ounce refined gelatine in cold water for an hour, then drain off and squeeze out the water as much as possible; put the gelatine in a jelly pot and place the latter in a pan of hot water on the fire; when the gelatine has melted stir in slowly 2½ ounces pure alcohol, and bottle for use. This glue will keep indefinitely, and can be melted for use in a few minutes by standing the bottle in a basin of hot water. As it contains a very small percentage of water, it hardly affects the gloss of the prints and dries almost immediately.

3435. Glass Substitute, Orange.

Mr. J. B. Huffman, of Chillicothe, Mo., sends the following substitute for orange glass for dark room work to the St. Louis Photographer. It is simple and easily tried:

Asphaltum................	3 parts.
Spirits of turpentine.......	1 part.

Coat the glass plate from one to four times, as desired, flowing the same as if it were collodion.

3436. Photographic Dark Room Windows.

The following formula has been recommended as a stain for dark room windows:

Water	100 c. c.
Gelatine..................	5 grammes.
Nitrate of silver..........	1 gramme.

Glass coated with this solution is exposed to light until it assumes a reddish brown tint. It is then washed to eliminate the nitrate of silver. A surface is thus obtained through which the actinic rays do not pass. The coloration may be deepened by increasing the proportion of nitrate of silver up to 3 or even 4 grammes. Glass tinted in this way may also be used to shade the dark room lantern.

3437. Gold, Chloride of.

Dr. John H. Janeway, an amateur photographer, suggests the following method: Dissolve a $2.50 gold piece in 6 drams of chemically pure muriatic acid, 3 drams chemically pure nitric acid, and 3 drams distilled water. Put the gold in a large graduate, pour on the acids and water, cover the graduate with a piece of glass to shut off or retard the escape of fumes, and set in the sun or in a warm place. When the gold is dissolved add bicarbonate of soda very gradually, stirring with a glass rod at each addition, until effervescence has ceased and the froth subsided, and the carbonate of copper which has been formed is deposited as a green precipitate. Now add 6 ounces of water, and let the whole settle for not over thirty minutes, and then very carefully filter the solution. To the clear golden liquid which has passed through the filter add carefully enough nitric acid, chemically pure, to turn blue litmus paper decidedly red, then add enough pure water to make the solution measure 32 fluid ounces. The solution will keep for any length of time, and 1 ounce will tone 4 sheets of paper.—From Philadelphia Photographer.

3438. Halation and Its Prevention.

Halation is the term given to the halo which often surrounds windows in photographs of interiors, and blocks up the details. It is, too, often found to occur in landscapes taken in a strong light, the tops of trees and other objects which are surrounded by strong light being lost in a mist, or entirely obliterated. It is caused by reflection from the back of the plate, and occurs most strikingly in plates of the cheap class, which are thinly coated. With very thickly-coated plates it rarely occurs, except when taking brightly-lighted interiors. To prevent it, the back of the plate may be coated with a mixture of powdered burnt sienna, ½ ounce; gum arabic, ½ ounce; glycerine, 1 ounce; water, 5 ounces. This is readily washed off before development. A special ready-made preparation is sold for this purpose by Tylar, if preferred. Another way is to cut dead black needle paper, or black American cloth, to the size of the plate, coat it with glycerine and squeegee it onto the back of the plate when placing it in the slide.

No. 1.

Cornu (Compt. Rend., B. S. F. Phot.) has discussed the phenomena of halation, and points out that in order to prevent halation entirely the varnish or pigment put on the back of the plate must have the same refractive index as glass. Such a pigment is obtained by mixing lampblack with certain essential oils, a mixture of oil of cloves and oil of cinnamon answering very well.

No. 2.

Debenham (Phot. J.) has investigated the relative efficiency of various substances when applied as a backing to plates with a view to prevent halation, and finds that very good results are obtained with a mixture of gelatine and burnt sugar, or gum, burnt sugar, and Chinese ink.

No. 3.

J. Pike (B. J. Phot. A.) backs plates with a mixture of matt varnish and collodion deeply stained with rosaniline. The collodion he makes by dissolving 1 ounce pyroxylin in 12 ounces methylated spirit and 36 ounces methylated ether of sp. gr. 0.735.

No. 4.

Mr. W. E. Debenham (Jnl. of Photo. Soc. N. S., xiv) has devised an apparatus for estimating the efficiency of plate backings. He employs a paraffine lamp behind an optical lantern condenser, and a graduated screen in front of it, reflecting the light into the camera lens by a right-angled prism, on the reflecting surface of which the material to be tested is placed. He has tested a considerable number of substances, and the following list enumerates them in the order of their efficiency, and gives occasional explanatory remarks:

a. No backing.
b. Two parts of lampblack with 1 part of bitumen. Optical contact very poor when dry.
c. Carbon tissue squeegeed on after soaking it in a mixture of equal parts of glycerine and water. Practically impossible to get optical contact.
d. Burnt sienna laid on with a sponge.
e. A benzine solution of bitumen applied thickly.
f. A commercial dead black.
g. Gum and burnt sienna.
h. Gelatine, burnt sugar and China ink.
i. Gelatine and burnt sugar.
j. Gum, burnt sugar and China ink.

It seems that with backing e the exposure must be increased about 240 times to get an effect equal to that when no backing is applied. The last three give practically equal results, and are very strikingly superior to the bitumen e. Mr. Chapman Jones (Photography) holds that under theoretically perfect conditions the whole of the photographically active light that impinges upon a sensitive plate would be retained in the film, and be available for the production of the image on development, and that the film ought to be, and practically can be, so opaque that backing the plate is unnecessary in landscape work and portraiture. Some Continental savants have given much attention to the subject of halation, but they do not appear to have added anything to our knowledge of the matter.

Hydrochinon. See Developers.

Hydroxylamine. See Developers.

3439.   Hypo., to Remove.

No. 1.
Hydroxyl.

Peroxide of hydrogen (20 vol.)	1 dram.
Water	5 ounces.

After washing the negative well it is immersed for a couple of minutes in the solution and again rinsed in water, when the intensification with silver can be at once proceeded with.

No. 2.

Where peroxide of hydrogen is not obtainable the following may be used as a substitute, the solution containing that substance in combination with others:

Barium dioxide	1 ounce.
Glacial acetic acid	1 ounce.
Water	4 ounces.

Reduce the barium dioxide to a fine powder and add it gradually to the acid and water, shaking until dissolved. A few minutes' immersion in this solution will effectually remove or destroy the last traces of hypo.

3440.   Hypo., Test for.

A simple test to tell when the hypo. is eliminated is to add to the washing water in which the prints are immersed a small quantity of an alcoholic solution of iodine. This will change the white back of each print to a light blue color, which proves that hypo.

is still present in the paper. The prints are continued to be washed until the blue disappears from the back of the print. We then know that the hypo. is completely eliminated.

3441. Ink for Writing on Photographs.

The following answers very well for numbering and marking proofs, the writing being executed on a dark portion:

Iodide of potassium	10 parts.
Water	30 parts.
Iodine	1 part.
Gum	1 part.

The lines soon bleach under the strokes by the conversion of the silver into iodide.

3442. Ink, Printing Process.

By means of gelatino-bromide of silver emulsions, rapid printing paper can be successfully made, but its manufacture is attended with 'considerable bother; and as it will keep well it is advisable for the beginner to purchase it ready prepared from dealers in photographic materials. One method of preparing the paper is, first, to make a sensitive emulsion as given by Henderson on page 293 of the November 8, 1884, issue of the Scientific American, and then to coat a sheet of plain Saxe paper with it, by laying the moistened sheet upon a level plate of glass, and bending the edges up by strips of wood, to form a paper dish. The emulsion while warm is now poured on the center of the sheet until a pool is formed large enough to permit it to be spread equally over the sheet by a glass rod. It is then allowed to cool, and when sufficiently set the sheet of paper is hung up to dry. It may now be exposed, film side away from the face of the thick cardboard drawing, in an ordinary printing frame for two or three seconds to diffused daylight, or for a minute and a half to the light from a large kerosene lamp. The image is then developed by immersing the exposed sheet in a solution of ferrous oxalate of potash composed of saturated solution of neutral oxalate potash acidified with a solution of oxalic acid sufficient to turn blue litmus paper red, 6 ounces, saturated solution of sulphate of iron, 1 ounce. The iron must be poured into the oxalate. Half a dozen exposed sheets may be developed one after the other, in the same solution. The sheet is next washed by soaking in a pan of water for four or five minutes, removed and immersed in a solution of—

| Hyposulphite soda | 1 ounce. |
| Water | 6 ounces. |

for eight minutes, which fixes the print; the latter must now be washed for two or three hours in several changes of cold water, when it may be hung up to dry, which it must do spontaneously, as the application of heat will melt the gelatine film. Examination of the print will show the lines and figures non-reversed as in the original drawing, because the sensitive sheet was laid on film side away from the drawing. The operation of preparing and developing the paper must be carried on in a dark room lighted only by a deep ruby-red non-actinic lamp.

3443. Intensification. A

With correct exposure and development, intensification need never be resorted to. The following formula is, however, very effective:

1. Bichlor. mercury, 240 grains; chloride ammonia, 240 grains; distilled water, 20 ounces.
2. Chloride ammonia, 480 grains; water, 20 ounces.
3. Sulphite of soda (crys.), 1 ounce; water, 9 ounces.

Let the plate to be intensified wash for at least half an hour; then lay in alum solution for ten minutes and again wash thoroughly; this is to insure the perfect elimination of the hypo. The least trace of yellowness after intensifying shows that the washing was not sufficient.

Flow sufficient of No. 1 over the negative to cover it, and allow to either partially or entirely whiten; the longer it is allowed to act the more intense will be the result; pour off into the sink, then flow over No. 2, and allow to act one minute; wash off and pour over or immerse in No. 3, until changed entirely to a dark brown, or black. No. 3 can be returned to its bottle, but Nos. 1 and 2 had better be thrown away. Wash thoroughly and dry.

3444. Intensification. B

In the following paragraphs various methods of intensifying gelatino-bromide plates are arranged according to the amount of density producible by their means.

1. Almost Imperceptible Increase of Density.—The negative is soaked for a minute in water, then dried rapidly by taking off the surface moisture with a soft cloth or blotting paper, after which the plate is placed in a horizontal postion and exposed to a current of warm, dry air, until it is quite dry.

2. Perceptible Increase of Density.—The wet negative is wiped back and front with a

cloth, then immersed for a few minutes in a bath of methylated spirits; when taken out it is drained for a few seconds, wiped again with a dry cloth and held before the fire or over a gas flame, keeping it at a safe distance at first and in a horizontal position.

3. Slight Increase of Density.—The plate, after being washed from the hypo., is immersed in a saturated solution of bichloride of mercury in water. It should remain in this bath until it becomes white; if it refuses to bleach, it is probable that the hyposulphite has not all been removed. The bleached plate is rinsed for about 3 seconds—not more—in water, so as to remove the surplus mercury solution from the surface, then it is at once dipped into a bath consisting of a semi-saturated solution of sulphite of soda. This second bath will slowly turn the plate black, and will also, as a consequence of the insufficient washing, cover the surface of the film with a dense white deposit, which cannot be rubbed off; but this deposit will very quickly dissolve away in the final washing and leave the image perfect. The density will remain the same if the plate is dried slowly, but will be increased by drying quickly, according to No. 2.

4. Moderate Increase of Density.—The plate is treated precisely as in No. 3, except that a thorough washing is given between the bichloride of mercury and the sulphite of soda baths. This gives additional density. No white deposit will be produced, but a good final washing should be given. Extra density may also be produced by quick drying.

When the image is of a deep yellow or non-actinic color, such as is sometimes produced with pyro. development, the use of this intensifier, No. 4, will alter the color to a neutral gray of about equal printing value. If it should then prove to be too dense, the plate can be immersed for a few minutes in the hypo. bath. This will take away the extra density, and leave a gray image equal in depth to the original yellow one, but of course much quicker for printing purposes.

5. A Vigorous Intensifier.—The plate, or rather the film upon it, is bleached in a saturated solution of mercury bichloride in water, washed, dried; then, when dry, immersed in a semi-saturated solution of sulphite of soda, washed again and dried. The only difference between this process and No. 4 is in the drying of the plate between the mercury and sulphite of soda baths. This drying causes a decided increase of density.

6. A Powerful Intensifier.—This, the well-known ammonia process, is about equal in strength to the preceding. The plate is bleached as before and washed thoroughly. If the washing is too short, stains will be produced which cannot be removed. After washing, the wet plate is immersed in very weak ammonia (water, 20 parts; ammonia, 1 part). The plate instantly turns black. A fair amount of washing should then be given to secure permanence and freedom from stains. Dry slowly, if the density is sufficient.

7. In addition to the above, we recommend Monckhoven's cyanide of silver intensifier, made as follows:

No. 1.
Bichloride of mercury...... 120 grains.
Bromide of potassium...... 60 grains.
Water .... 12½ ounces.

No. 2.
Cyanide of potassium crystals (pure)................ 120 grains.
A. Water................... 6¼ ounces.
B. Nitrate of silver........ 120 grains.
Water .... 6¼ ounces.

Pour A into B, which forms cyanide of silver. A slight excess of silver will settle at the bottom of the bottle, which assists in keeping the solution up to its full strength and does no harm.

The plate should be left in No. 1 until the film appears white on the back. It is then thoroughly washed and immersed in No. 2, or the solution may be poured on quickly. Immediately the film will commence to blacken, and the plate should be kept in until there appears to be no white color on the back. If left too long, the cyanide will commence to reduce the negative.

This intensifier acts rapidly and imparts to the film a bluish black color. It is an excellent intensifier for lantern slides, imparting a desirable warm purple color.

8. To Cure Over Intensification.—There is a very simple method of reducing negatives which have been intensified by mercury solutions. It is simply to leave them in the fixing bath for a longer or shorter period, according to the amount of reduction desired. If left for half an hour, the whole of the extra density imparted by the intensifying process will be removed, and the plate will then be in its original condition. The hypo. should of course be finally freed from the film by a copious washing.

9. Cramer's Intensifying Solution. Prepare a saturated solution of bichloride of mercury in water, and of this pour a sufficient quantity gradually into a solution of—

Iodide of potassium............ 50 grammes.
Water......................... 250 c. c.

until the point is reached when the forming red precipitate will no longer dissolve by shaking; but be careful not to add more mercury than just enough to make the solution very slightly turbid. Now add—

Hyposulp. of soda.. 1 oz.   40 grammes.
Dissolve and fill up with water to make total solution ....20 ozs.   800 c. c.

For use this should be diluted with about 3 parts of water. If the plate has not been thoroughly fixed, the intensifying solution will produce yellow stains. Be careful not to overdo the intensifying. Should it have gone too far, the negative can be reduced by placing it in the fixing bath for a short time.

10. **Intensifying Solution.**—Saturated solution bichloride mercury.

Iodide potassium.......... 40 grammes.
Water .... 180 c. c.
Hypo..................... 30 grammes.
Water to make up to...... 600 c. c.

11. **Lead Intensifier.**—Lead nitrate, 20 grains; ferricyanide of potassium, 30 grains; distilled water, 1 ounce, and filter. Follow, after very thorough washing, with ammonium sulphide in 10 times its bulk of water. The washing before the ammonium sulphide should be continued until the drainings from the plate give a scarcely perceptible blue color, with ferrous sulphate solution, that is, until the ferricyanide is quite washed out, for the least trace of lead remaining will surely cause fog.

12. **Uranium Intensifier.**—Uranium nitrate, 4 grains to 1 ounce of water. After soaking the plate in this, mix the liquid with a dilute solution of potassium ferricyanide made by running water over a few crystals to wash them, and then shaking them with a dram or two of water a few seconds. Add more ferricyanide as necessary.

13. **Intensification with Cupric Bromide.**—Prepare cupric bromide solution by mixing a solution of 1 part potassium bromide in 25 parts water with a solution of 1 part cupric sulphate in 25 parts water, allow to settle, and filter or decant off the clear liquid. Wash the negative until free from hypo, and immerse in the cupric bromide solution, which will convert it into a brilliant white positive. Wash well and immerse in strong ammonia solution diluted with 12 parts of water. This intensifier gives increased contrasts.—S. R. Bottone, Y. B. Phot. 1891, 115, 116.

3445. Lantern Plates, a Use for Spoiled.

The best thing to do when lantern plates have been spoiled by over exposure or errors in development, or by the light getting at them, is to strip the films from them, and use them as cover glasses for binding up the completed slides.

3446. Leaf Photographs.

Pass the paper first through a solution of gelatin, 1 part in 20 parts of hot water, and use a strong solution of potassium bichromate; or the gelatin and bichromate may be used together. Wash with hot water. A strong blue background may be produced as follows: Dissolve in 2 ounces of pure water 120 grains of red prussiate of potash (potassium ferrocyanide), and separately 140 grains double citrate of iron and ammonium in 2 ounces of water; mix the solutions, filter, float the paper for a few minutes on the filtrate; print from the dried paper as before, and wash thoroughly in water. By adding a little phosphoric acid to the bichromate solution and exposing the print before washing to the vapor of a hot solution of aniline in alcohol, a blackish-green or red positive is obtained. Or, prepare the paper with solution of iron sesquichloride, and develop after exposure with a very dilute solution of silver nitrate. Use plain photographic paper.

3447. Light, the Safest for Dark Room Use.

Bear in mind that very rapid plates are sensitive to light of any color. The safest light is a combination of a ruby and yellow, just strong enough to enable you to judge of intensity of negative and progress of development, and the plate should not be held close to the light for examination for more than a few seconds.

The following combinations make a safe light:

Orange-colored paper with ruby glass.
Orange glass with cherry fabric.
Ruby glass with canary fabric.
Orange and ruby glass combined with ground glass.

Green is not as non-actinic as ruby and yellow combined, and it has furthermore the disadvantage that with it the intensity of negative cannot be judged so well as with the ruby light.

To make sure your light is safe, make the following test:

Cover one-half of a lightning plate with opaque paper and expose it to the light for about two minutes at the distance generally observed while developing. Develop, and if

3448. Lightning, Photographing of.

A very interesting study is lightning photography. It is a puzzling one to the beginner, yet it is, perhaps, the simplest form of photography which can be imagined. If the photographer has had much experience, he will doubtless know the point at which his camera requires to be racked out to insure the lens being in proper focus for a distant object. If this is so, he need have no further trouble than, when night comes on and the lightning commences to play, to rack out his camera to this point, fix it up, and direct it toward that portion of the sky from which the lightning appears, then place the dark slide in the back, and draw the slide, remove the cap, and wait for the flash. It being night, no harm can come to the plate by reason of this exposure during the interval of waiting. The lightning will impress itself upon the plate without any need of shutter or other contrivance. If the point at which the camera is in focus is at a distance which is not known, there will probably be a lamp somewhere or other within sight, and in this case a rough focus can be obtained upon that.

3449. Photographing on Linen or Other Fabric.

For decorating table napkins, bed room trimmings, etc., the following simple process works satisfactorily, and photographers may often do much extra business by introducing it to their customers:

Boil the fabric in water containing a little soda, so as to remove the dressing, iron smooth, and saturate with

>   Ammonium chloride......2 grammes.
>   (about 31 grains.)
>   Water ....250 cubic cents.
>   (about 9 ounces.)
>   White of two eggs.

The above are well beaten together, allowed to subside, and strained. When dry, sensitize on the usual silver bath—rather a strong bath is to be preferred—expose, tone, and fix as for an ordinary print on albumen paper.—Photo. Review.

3450. Machinery, Photographing of.

A color for coating machinery previous to photographing:

>   Dry white lead........... 5 pounds.
>   Lampblack...........2 to 5 ounces.
>   Gold size................. 1 pint.
>   Turpentine................ 1½ pints.

The amount of lampblack is varied to suit machine or lighting. This paint is easily removed with turpentine.

Matt Surface on Silver Prints.—Mount the print in the ordinary way, avoiding lumps. Roll, and afterward sift on the surface finely ground pumice powder. With a circular motion rub gently with the palm of the hand. Proceed until the surface desired is obtained. The use of plain paper is recommended.

3451. Moonlight Effects.

The so-called moonlight effect is a photographic deception. To secure this effect select a view with the sun almost in front of the camera, but itself hidden or partly obscured by clouds, and preferably a day when the sky is full and well defined, and well broken up with cloud masses. Then expose about the usual time for the view in question, and develop with a developer containing only ¼ grain of pyro. to the ounce, until the details are just out. Wash off the developer, and apply a fresh one, 4 grains of pyro. and 4 grains of bromide to the ounce, until the high lights have attained the requisite density. Another method which frequently gives good results, is, still with the sun in front and preferably shining strongly, to give a very short shutter exposure, and develop strongly. This gives brilliant lighting, and dense masses of shadow.

3452. Mounting Prints.

For a large collection of receipts for mounting photographs, see Pastes.

Prints, to Mount on Glass.—To mount prints on glass, follow the directions given by J. E. Dumont; that is, take 4 ounces gelatine and soak half an hour in cold water, then place in a glass jar, adding 16 ounces of water; put the jar in a large dish of warm water and dissolve the gelatine. When dissolved, pour into a shallow tray. Have your prints rolled on a roller, albumen side out; take the print by the corners and pass rapidly through the gelatine, taking great care to avoid air bubbles. Hang up with clips to dry; when dry, squeeze carefully on to the glass. The better the quality of glass the finer the effect.

Gelatine Mountant.

>   Gelatine .... 4 ounces.
>   Water .... 16 ounces.
>   Glycerine .... 1 ounce.
>   Alcohol, 90 per cent....... 5 ounces.

3453. Negatives.

Method for Quickly Drying Gelatine Negatives.—After the final washing, place the plate in a bath of methylated spirit for four or five minutes. On taking it out flow two or three times with common methylated sulphuric ether. After this the negative will dry in a current of air in two or three minutes.

To Take Gelatine off Disused Negatives.—Place in a hot bath, in which previously a good dose of washing soda and soap has been dissolved.

To Remove Varnish from a Negative.—Warm (cautiously) the negative before a fire or over a spirit lamp; then pour a little methylated spirit upon it, and with a tuft of cotton wool gently rub the face of the negative; drain and repeat. Then cover with the spirits, drain and let dry.

To Prevent Negatives from Frilling.—Soak the plates before development in a saturated solution of Epsom salts. Then wash, and develop as usual; or use water containing a little Epsom salts, ½ ounce or more to a pail of water.

To Fill Cracks in a Varnished Negative.—Procure some finely powdered lampblack and gently rub with a circular motion all over the negative, using the finger or a soft piece of wash leather for the purpose. This will cause all the cracks to disappear.

To Print from Cracked Negative.—Place the printing frame at the bottom of a narrow box, at least 2 feet deep, and with blackened sides: over the negative in the frame put a sheet of thin tissue paper. Another way: Suspend from a roasting jack a board upon which a printing frame can rest, the roasting jack being in motion all the time of printing. Or, in the case of a slight crack, move the frame about in the hands briskly during the process of printing.

3454. Paper.

Preparation of Paper with Arrowroot (Monkhoven).—Water, 150 parts; chloride sodium, 3 parts; citrate sodium, 3 parts; arrowroot, 3 parts. Stir the arrowroot flour and thoroughly mix in some cold water; then pour while constantly stirring into the boiling water. Coat the paper with the starch mixture by means of a brush. It should not be floated on the silver bath longer than one-half to one minute. Fuming in the ammonia box eight minutes makes the prints more intense and brilliant.

Ashman's Durable Paper.—After the paper is sensitized, float it back downward for five minutes on the following solution: Water, 50 parts; gum arabic, 1½ parts; hydrochloric acid, 1 part; citric acid, 1 part; tartaric acid, 1 part. Dry as quickly as possible after removal.

Preparation of Paper with Gelatine (Abney.)—Water, 240 parts; chloride of ammonium, 3 to 4 parts; gelatine; ½ part; citrate of sodium, 5 parts; chloride of sodium, 1 to 1½ parts.

Albumenized Paper, to Give a Matt Surface to Prints on.—Mount the print in the ordinary way, but be careful to avoid any lumps. Well roll, and then sift on finely-ground pumice powder. Rub gently with palm of the hand, using circular motion. Examine from time to time. Continue operation until the proper surface is obtained.

Albumen Paper, Sensitizing Bath for Albumenized Paper.—Thirty-five to 60 grains of silver nitrate to the ounce of water; add enough carbonate of soda to cause slight turbidity, and filter.

Durable Sensitized Paper.—Float the albumenized paper on a 10 per cent solution of nitrate of silver for four minutes, draw it over the glass rod to drain, and then float the back of the sheet for a like period upon a bath composed of

Citrate of potash.......... 1 part.
Water.................... 30 parts.

Finally wash in rain water.

Debenham's Method.—Sensitize by the usual nitrate solution, with the addition of 10 drops of perchloric acid to each ounce of the sensitizing bath.

Albumen Paper, Preservative Book for Sensitized Paper.—Soak thick blotting paper in a saturated solution of bicarbonate of soda, and when this is dry make a book of it. Keep the sensitive paper between the leaves of this book, the sheets being kept in pairs, face to face.

Fuming.—This is the process of subjecting ready sensitized paper to the fumes of ammonia. Hang the sheets separated in a box and place a saucer of ammonia in the bottom and allow the vapor to act for fifteen minutes. Ready sensitized paper is giving way to the Omega, Aristotype and other papers.

3455. Paper Negatives.

At a regular meeting of the London and Provincial Photographic Association Mr. W. Turner gave the following as his method of making paper negatives: The picture or drawing to be copied is made translucent by means of lard diluted with turpentine—1 part of lard to 3 parts of turpentine.

The mixture was then boiled for three minutes, which, he claimed, killed the grease, and it was then rubbed over the drawing. When surface dry the drawing was placed in a printing frame with sensitized silver paper, and a negative made, which was fixed in an old hypo. bath rich in silver, and washed in the usual way.

The plain paper was prepared by floating Saxe paper on the following:

Sodium chloride	200 grains.
Gelatine	30 grains.
Water	20 ounces.

Dissolve the gelatine and chloride separately and mix; float three minutes. When dry, sensitize by floating one or two minutes on the following:

Silver nitrate	1 ounce.
Citric acid	1 dram.
Water	14 ounces.

He stated that the paper would keep good for six weeks.

Pastes for Mounting.—See Pastes.

3456. Photo-Chromos.

Allow the photograph to remain in water until thoroughly soaked; then place it between blotting paper, and let it remain until just damp enough to be pliable. Then coat the face of the picture with good starch paste and lay face down on the glass. Commence in the center of the picture and rub outward toward the edges, to dispel all air and excess of paste, care being observed not to get paste on the back of the print. While rubbing, keep the paper damp with a sponge. When dry lay on a heavy coat of castor oil, and after a time, rub off the excess of oil with a cloth. After standing a day or two, it may be colored. Cover the back with a thin plate of glass and bind the edges.

Photographing.—See Clouds, Frost, Lightning, Moonlight, Snow, Sun, etc.

3457. To Prevent Pinholes.

Pinholes, or minute transparent spots on the negative, are most frequently caused by the presence of minute particles of dust on the film, which, during exposure, prevent the light getting to the film at those particular spots. To prevent pinholes therefore, steps must be taken to guard against dust. The plates should be wiped over before being placed in the slide with a camel hair brush, or, better still, with a piece of velvet stretched on a stick. The slide itself should also be dusted out first, while both it and the interior of the camera bellows should be rubbed lightly over with glycerine, to which any dust which may be flying about will stick in preference to the plate. The slides, too, should be carried in a case which is fairly dust proof.

3458. Primuline Process.

Primuline, a product of the action of sulphur on paratoluidine, discovered by A. G. Green, dyes cotton, linen, and similar fabrics without a mordant even better than it does wool or silk. The color fades somewhat rapidly when exposed to light, but the primuline itself is not sufficiently sensitive to be available for photographic purposes. If the primuline is treated with dilute nitrous acid, it forms diazoprimuline, which has the power of forming a variety of coloring matters by combination with various phenols and amines. Diazoprimuline in contact with vegetable and animal fibres is very sensitive to light, and upon exposure is decomposed, and loses its power of forming coloring matters. If, therefore, a fabric or surface dyed with primuline and converted into diazoprimuline is exposed to light behind a transparency or anything similar, and is afterward treated with a phenol or amine, an image is obtained, the color of which depends upon the nature of the developer, but which is positive from a positive, negative from a negative.

The material (cotton, linen, silk, wool, paper, wood, gelatine, celluloid, xyloidine, etc.) is dyed in a hot solution of primuline, washed, and diazotized by immersion in dilute solution (0.25 per cent) of sodium nitrite acidified with hydrochloric or some other acid. It is again washed and allowed to dry spontaneously in the dark. The sensitized material, which will keep for some time, is exposed to daylight or the electric light, the time of exposure being determined by means of some unprotected strips of the same material, which are exposed alongside the printing frame. As soon as these strips cease to give any color when touched with a drop of the particular developer that is going to be used, decomposition is complete in the high lights of the object that is being copied. The sensitive material is removed from the frame, and at once, or after some time, is developed by immersion in a dilute (about 0.25 per cent) solution of a phenol or amine; e. g., for red, an alkaline solution of beta naphthol; for maroon, an alkoline solution of beta naphthol disulphonic acid; for yellow, an alkaline solution of phenol; for orange, an alkaline solution of resorcinol; for brown, a slightly alkaline solution of pyrogallol, or a solution of phenylene diamine hydrochloride; for purple, a solution of beta naphthylamine hydrochloride; for blue, a slightly acid solution of eikonogen. If a design in different colors is desired, the different developers may be applied with a brush. After development, which requires two or three minutes, the prints are washed in water for a short time; in the case of the blue and purple developers the final washing must be done in a very weak solution of tartaric acid. Wool and silk require a longer time in exposure and development than does cotton or linen, and the maroon and blue developers are not suitable for wool or silk. In all the applications primuline may be replaced by its homologues; for silk dehydrothiotoluidine sulphonic acid may be used. Among the possible uses of the process may be mentioned the reproduction on linen of architect's drawings, etc. A. G. Green, C. F. Cross, and E. J. Bevan, Eng. Pat. No. 7,453, May 13, 1890. J. C. S. I., 9, 1001-1004. Phot. N., 34, 701, 702, 707, 708.

The Brit. Jour. Phot. 37, 657, 658, recommends the following proportions for primuline developers: Red, naphthol, 40 grains; caustic soda or potash, 60 grains; water, 10 ounces; orange resorcinol, 30 grains; water, 10 ounces; caustic potash or soda, 50 grains. Purple, naphthylamine, 60 grains; hydrochloric acid, 60 minims; water, 10 ounces. The following developers are also recommended: Ink, black., eikonogen, 60 grains; water, 10 ounces. Brown tones, pyro., 50 grains; water, 10 ounces.

After washing in plain water the ground is cleared by washing in soap and water. If the transparency printed from is not dense enough to allow complete decomposition in the high lights, the results are improved by exposing the whole of the back of the print to light for a short time.

3459. Printing Processes.

The blue process has been treated under blue paper, but an additional formula is given here, as well as formulas for blue, violet, red, and green prints.

Blue Prints.—Float the paper until it lies quite flat upon a solution prepared as follows:

No. 1.
Water.................... 2 fl. ounces.
Red prussiate of potash... 120 grains.

No. 2.
Water.................... 2 ounces.
Ammonia citrate of iron... 140 grains.

When these two are dissolved, mix them together and filter into a clean bottle.

The solution should not be exposed to a strong light, and the paper must be floated on it in a very subdued light, and in the same manner as paper is floated on a silver solution. When it no longer curls, but lies flat on the solution, take it by the corners and raise it slowly from contact, and hang it up to dry in a dark place. When dry, it can be used at once, or may be kept for future use by rolling it, prepared surface in, and placing it in a tin box or other receptacle, free from light and dampness.

To make a print on this paper, place the prepared surface in contact with the negative in a printing frame and expose to sunlight.

The time of exposure will vary according to the density of the negative and the intensity of the light. The rule is to allow the light to act long enough for the portions which first turn blue to become gray, with a slight metallic luster. At this point remove the paper from the frame and place it in a dish of clean water.

It now gradually becomes a rich blue throughout, except the parts which should remain white. Change the water from time to time, until there remains no discoloration in the whites; dry, and the picture requires no further treatment.

The blue color may be totally removed at any time by placing the print in ammonia water.

This is the standard formula.

Another Process for Blue Prints.—Float the paper for a minute in a solution of

Ferricyanide of potash.... 1 ounce.
Water..................... 5 ounces.

Dry it in a dark room, and then expose beneath a negative until the dark shades have assumed a deep blue color, then immerse the print in a solution of

Water..................... 2 ounces.
Bichloride mercury........ 1 grain.

Wash the print, and then immerse it in a hot solution of

Oxalic acid............... 4 drams.
Water..................... 4 ounces.

Wash again and dry.

Another Process—the Cyanotype.—Float the paper on a solution of the sesquichloride of iron. Dry and expose, afterward wash the prints, and then immerse them in a bath of ferricyanide of potash. The picture will appear of a blue color in all those places where the sun has acted.

Process with Salts of Uranium.—The paper, without having undergone any preceding preparation, except that of having been excluded from the light for several days, is floated on a bath of the nitrate of uranium as follows:

Nitrate of uranium	2 drams.
Distilled water	10 drams.

The paper is left on the bath for four or five minutes, it is then removed, hung up, and dried in the dark room. So prepared, it can be kept for a considerable time.

The exposure beneath a negative varies from one minute to several minutes in the rays of the sun, and from a quarter of an hour to an hour in diffused light. The image which is thus produced is not very distinct, but comes out in strong contrast when developed as follows:

Nitrate of Silver Developer.

Distilled or rain-water	2 drams.
Nitrate of silver	7 grains.
Acetic acid	a mere trace.

The development is very rapid in this solution. In about half a minute it is complete. As soon as the picture appears in perfect contrast, the print is taken out and fixed by immersion in water, in which it is thoroughly washed.

Chloride of Gold Developer.—This is a more rapid developer than the preceding. The print is fixed in like manner by water, in which it must be well washed, and afterward dried. When dried by artificial heat, the vigor of the print is increased. Prints that have been developed by the solution of nitrate of silver may be immersed in the gold bath, which improves their tone.

The picture may be developed, also, by immersing the prints in a saturated solution of bichloride of mercury and afterward in one of nitrate of silver. In this case, however, the times of exposure must be increased.

Pictures may be obtained, also, by floating the papers on a mixture of equal quantities of nitrate of silver and nitrate of uranium in about six times their weight of water.

When dry, they are exposed beneath a negative. In this case the image appears, as in the positive printing process, with chloride of silver, being effected by the decomposition of the nitrate of uranium, which, reacting on the nitrate of silver, decomposes this salt and reduces the silver. These prints require fixing in the ordinary bath of hyposulphite of soda, and then washing, as usual.

Process for Red Pictures.—Float the papers for four minutes in the preceding bath of nitrate of uranium, drain, and dry. Next expose beneath a negative for eight or ten minutes, then wash, and immerse in a bath of

Ferricyanide of potash	30 grains.
Water	3 ounces.

In a few minutes the picture will appear of a red color, which is fixed by washing thoroughly in water.

Process for Green Pictures.—Immerse the red picture, before it is dry, in a solution of

Sesquichloride of iron	30 grains.
Distilled water	3 ounces.

The tone will soon change to green; fix in water, wash, and dry before the fire.

Process for Violet Pictures.—Float the paper for three or four minutes on a bath of

Water	2 ounces.
Nitrate of uranium	2 drams.
Chloride of gold	2 grains.

Afterward take them out and dry. An exposure of ten or fifteen minutes will cause the necessary reduction; the picture has a beautiful violet color consisting of metallic gold. Wash and dry.—Estabrooke.

3460.   **Prints.**

Trimming Prints.—There is more art in print trimming than at first meets the eye. It is not sufficient merely to cut off the edges evenly, so as to include everything there was on the plate, or to place a cutting shape upon it and trim it round. There are two main considerations in print trimming. First, that the sides of the print are cut true with the horizontal or vertical lines of the picture. If your picture is a sea view, cut the top and bottom of the print parallel with the horizon line. If you have no horizon line to go by, take the side of a house, or anything else in the picture, which must of necessity be vertical. Use this as your guide, and cut the sides of your picture parallel with it. Of course in both cases the other two sides will be square with the first two treated. Secondly, trim your print down, if it can be improved thereby. In the majority of cases the appearance of a picture will be improved by cutting off a little of the foreground, reducing the amount of sky by half an inch or more, or cutting off more or less of either or both ends. Get four pieces of white cardboard and cover up different portions of your print and see whether you cannot improve its appearance by exclusion of superfluous parts.

Washing Prints.—No care can be too great to insure the thorough washing of photographic prints, especially silver prints. If it is possible, they should be washed in running water, in such a washer as Wood's or Jeffery's patent. In these washers a steady current of water is caused, which has the effect of constantly turning the prints over and over, and exposing them at all points to its washing action, while the surplus is removed by means of a siphon, or other arrangement from the bottom. Hypo. which has to be removed from the prints entirely, or fading will result, is heavier than water, and consequently sinks to the bottom, being taken off with the outflow of the surplus water. Mere soaking is not sufficient, but if a constant flow of water, such as that suggested, or a proper apparatus cannot be obtained, one of the best methods of removing the fixing agent will be to soak the prints alternately in hot and cold baths, allowing them to remain, say, five minutes in each and giving them at least half a dozen changes from one to the other. This method of washing, however, is not suitable for bromide prints, the gelatine surface of which would be destroyed by hot water.

Titles on Prints.—To print the name on the photograph, several methods may be adopted. The simplest is to write the title of the subject on a slip of paper with aniline copying ink, or with ordinary copying ink mixed with gamboge or vermilion. Then slightly dampen the surface of the negative near the bottom right or left hand corner in as unobtrusive and unimportant a portion of the picture as possible. Press down the paper with the writing upon it. Leave for a few minutes and then remove the paper, when the writing will be found to have adhered to the negative. When printed, the name will print out white. Another way is to write backward on the negative, while another and better plan is to write the name in Indian ink on the surface of the paper before it is printed on. The ink will wash off in the after operations and leave the name in white where the surface of the paper has been protected by the ink.

3461.   Proof, to Preserve.

Dip the proof in a solution of hyposulphite of soda, 20 grains, dissolved in 5 ounces of water for ten minutes, then wash in changing water for two hours.

Red Pictures.—See Photo Printing Processes.

3462.   Retouching Powder.

This powder is prepared by mixing together

Dextrine .... 2 parts.
Resin (very finely powdered) .... 1 part.

It may be employed both for application to negatives and to albumenized prints. A leather stump is the best means of application.

3463.   Sensitizing Paper.

For Blue Prints.—1. Red prussiate of potash, 5 parts; water, 50 parts.

2. Ferric oxalate of potassium, 5 parts; water, 50 parts. Mix the two solutions in the dark, and coat the paper with the mixture by means of a sponge. See also Blue Prints.

3464.   Monkhoven's Sensitizing Solution.

Nitrate of silver, 6 parts; nitrate of magnesia, 6 parts; distilled water, 50 parts. Each time, after sensitizing a sheet in this solution, 1 dram of a one-to-eight solution of nitrate of silver should be added to the bath for every 100 square inches of paper sensitized.

Sensitizing Solution for Paper.

Nitrate of silver .... 5 drams.
Distilled water .... 5 ounces.
Nitric acid .... 2 drops.
Kaolin .... 1 ounce.

3465.   Silk Photo., Printing on.

1. In the Photographische Mitarbeiter the following recipe for preparing silk for printing from is given:

No. 1.
Tannin .... 40 grams.
Water .... 1000 c. c.

No. 2.
Salt .... 40 grams.
Arrowroot .... 40 grams.
Acetic acid .... 150 c. c.
Water .... 1000 c. c.

No. 1 is mixed with No. 2, well shaken, and filtered. The older the mixture, the better it is for use. In this bath the silk is thoroughly immersed, and allowed to remain for three minutes, when it is taken out and hung up to dry.

Sensitizing solution is composed of a silver one to ten, acidified with nitric acid.

Toning Bath.
No. 1.
Chloride of gold .... 1 gram.
Water .... 200 c. c.

No. 2.

Sulphocyanide of ammonium	20 grams.
Water	500 c. c.

No. 1, after shaking, is mixed with No. 2. In a few days the mixture will become clear, when it is ready for use. It is preferable to dilute with from two to four times the quantity of water. Fixing and washing as usual.

2. To print on silk prepare the following solution:

Boiling water	20 ounces.
Chloride of ammonium	100 grains.
Iceland moss	60 grains.

When nearly cold, filter and immerse the silk for fifteen minutes. Sensitize for fifteen minutes in an acid 20 grains to ounce silver bath, and when dry stretch the fabric over cardboard. Print deeper than usual and tone in

Water	20 ounces.
Acetate of soda	2 drams.
Chloride of gold	3 grains.

Common whiting, a few grains. Fix in hypo. 1 to 20.

To Photograph on Silk.—Immerse the silk in

Water	1 ounce.
Gelatine	5 grains.
Chloride of sodium	5 grains.

Hang it up to dry; then float for half a minute on a 50-grain solution of nitrate of silver; dry print, tone and fix, as usual.

Silver Baths, to Renovate.—See Baths, Silver.

3466. **Silver Nitrate, to Make.**

To make nitrate of silver out of pure silver, place the silver in a beaker and pour into it three-quarters of a fluid ounce of strong nitric acid sp. gr. 1.4 for every ounce of metal. The beaker is heated till the whole of the silver dissolves. The solution is then poured into an evaporating basin, and the excess of acid driven off by boiling. The operations should be conducted in the open air. The salts left may be recrystallized by dissolving in the smallest possible quantity of boiling water and allowing it to cool. The crystals of pure nitrate of silver will gradually form. The salt remaining in the mother liquor can be recovered by evaporation. To prepare chloride of gold the copper in the coin must first be eliminated. The gold coin is put into a beaker, and a mixture of three parts of hydrochloric acid and one of nitric acid is poured into it and heat applied until the metal is dissolved. The excess of acid is then expelled by evaporation. The impure gold chloride, when free from acid, is dissolved in boiling water, and a cold saturated solution of protosulphate of iron added, till a dark precipitate of pure gold is no longer produced. The precipitate of gold must be poured on a filter and washed by pouring boiling water constantly over it, till the wash water no longer produces a precipitate with a solution of barium chloride, proving that the gold is free from the excess of sulphate of iron. The gold is again dissolved in nitro-hydrochloric acid, the solution evaporated to dryness, the latter part of the operation being carried on slowly to prevent spurting. The yellow crystalline chloride of gold thus prepared should be preserved in a well-stoppered bottle or a sealed tube, as the salt is very deliquescent.

Snow Scenes, Exposure for.—After the photographer has been working during the bright days of summer, and has probably put away his camera for a month or two, he naturally goes for it when the snow comes down, but the exposure will be found to be very puzzling. He knows that the light in winter—perhaps he has made a few experiments—is very dead, and that four or five times the exposure of his summer pictures is the rule. So he starts away and gets poor results. The rough and ready rule for photographing snow scenes is to give them the same exposure as would be given to the same view in summer. Really, what one has to do to get the finest effect is to photograph the snow, and leave the uncovered patches to take care of themselves. Snow being white, reflects a great deal of light, and therefore the exposure must be very short.

3467. **Sun, the Position of.**

Do not expose when the sun is either directly in front of the camera or directly behind it. If directly in front, if the whole plate escapes being fogged by the sun shining into the lens, the result will be an almost entire absence of detail in the shadows, and a flat and uninteresting picture. On the other hand, if the sun is right behind the camera, no shadows will be seen, or rather only the brightly lighted sides of every object will be seen by the lens, and a flat picture, lacking in contrast, will result. If these two extremes are avoided, pictures may be taken in almost any other direction with advantage, the shadows serving to create contrast, and give rotundity and life to the picture.

Beware of the Sun.—When the sun is brilliantly shining, be careful to keep your slides from its direct rays. A capital plan is to have what is known as a poacher's pocket made in the inside of your coat, large enough to carry a couple of dark slides. They can be carried here right up to the moment of placing them in the camera, and should be slipped from the pocket into a fold of the focusing cloth. This should also be spread right over the camera, dark slide and all, while exposure is being made. If these precautions are taken, there will be very little to fear from the light getting through the slides, unless they leak very badly. If there are any cracks or crannies whatever in the dark slide, the direct rays of a powerful sun will find them out.

3468. Tin Types, Formulas for Making.

The plate is coated with a collodion made as follows, but it can be bought at photo. dealers ready made:

No. 1.

Collodion.—Alcohol and ether, equal parts; gun cotton sufficient to make moderately thick film, say 5 or 6 grains to the ounce; put the cotton in the ether first, when it is well saturated pour in the alcohol, to which add:

Iodide of ammonium..4 grn. to the oz.
Iodide of cadmium...2 grn. to the oz.
Bromide of cadmium .1 grn. to the oz.
Bromide of copper...1 grn. to the oz.

There are 8 grains of salt to the ounce. When the collodion has set, the plate is immersed in a silver bath, made by dissolving 50 grains of nitrate of silver in 1 ounce of distilled water, and kept there from two to five minutes. It is then put into a plate holder, exposed for twenty-nine seconds in the camera, and developed with the following:

Developer.
No. 2.

Water .... 64 ounces.
Protosulphate of iron..... 4 ounces.
Acetic acid................ 4 ounces.
Alcoholic solution of tannin, 10 grains to the ounce.................. 4 ounces.

The acid and tannin solutions should be added after iron has been dissolved. The developer has to be flowed over the plate with one sweep. The picture is fixed by putting the plate into

Cyanide of potassium..... 2 ounces.
Water .... 64 ounces.

Then washed and dried.

3469. Toning Baths.

The treatment of the prints is sometimes followed by passing them into a dilute solution of sodium acetate or ordinary common salt, about 1 per cent, such as here shown, and stirring them about for five minutes, when it will be seen they have assumed a brick red color, the object of which is threefold: First, the fibres become charged with a substance which acts as a chlorine absorbent, a necessary property to be mentioned further on. Secondly, a definite color is insured to start with, thus obviating the possibility of mistaking fresh prints in the toning bath for those which have become purple by reason of the deposited gold, an important consideration when dealing with fumed paper. Thirdly, the last trace of free nitrate of silver is removed, thereby preventing a too rapid decomposition of the toning bath. This applies to all toning baths.

Theoretically considered, it is proper that the last trace of silver nitrate should be removed, but those who are engaged in the daily practice of commercial work do not insist upon the strict observance of such a rule in all cases. An especial exception is permitted and advocated when dealing with prints from a weak or under-exposed negative, this class being found to yield richer tones by not washing any of the free silver out.

The plan of soaking prints in a solution of sodium acetate was originally recommended, in lieu of a washing, by Mr. A. L. Henderson, as long ago as 1861, the following being an outline of the method suggested by him: Slightly over-printed proofs are soaked in a bath composed of

Sodium acetate............ 240 grains.
Water..................... 10 ounces.

The unwashed proofs are moved about in this solution at least ten minutes, in order to convert all the free silver nitrate into acetate of silver. After slight rinsing in clean water, the proofs are toned with

Gold terchloride.......... 4 grains.
Sodium acetate............ 240 grains.
Water..................... 10 ounces.

No. 1.

Chloride of gold.......... 1 grain.
Acetate of soda........... 30 grains.
Water..................... 8 ounces.

This must not be used till one day after preparation. It keeps well, and gives warm, rich tones.

No. 2.

Chloride of gold	1 grain.
Bicarbonate of soda	4 grains.
Water	8 ounces.

This is ready for immediate use after preparation, but it will not keep.

No. 3.

Chloride of gold	1 grain.
Phosphate of soda	20 grains.
Water	8 ounces.

This gives rich tones of a deep purple nature, but must be used soon after preparation.

No. 4.

Gold solution	10 drams.
Acetate of lime	20 grains.
Chloride of lime	1 grain.
Tepid water	20 ounces.

The gold solution before mentioned is prepared by neutralizing as much as is required of a 1 grain solution of chloride of gold by shaking it up with a little prepared chalk, then allowing it to settle, and filtering off the clear liquid. This toning bath improves by keeping. To use, add 2 ounces of it to 8 ounces of tepid water, which will prove sufficient to tone a full-sized sheet of paper.

No. 5.

| Chloride of gold | 15 grains. |
| Water | 5 ounces. |

Neutralize with lime water; make up to 15 ounces with water, and add 2 drams chloride of calcium. This stock solution will keep for a long time. For use, dilute 1 ounce with 10 ounces of water.

No. 6.

Platinum tetrachloride, sirupy solution, color of old East India sherry	5 minims.
Hydrochloric acid	150 minims.
Water	20 ounces.

Wash away with free silver thoroughly, warm the toning solution to 70° F., and fix in a 20 per cent hypo. bath.

No. 7.

Mr. A. Watt, in the second volume of the News, gives a formula which runs as follows:

Solution of platinum	30 minims.
Hypo	3 grains.
Hydrochloric acid	5 minims.
Water	5 ounces.

This bath is said to act instantly. The strength of the platinum solution here given is indefinite, but any of our experimental members can soon ascertain the amount of dilution necessary to obtain the most favorable results.

Alkaline Toning.—Owing to the bleaching action which occurs in toning silver prints with gold, which is slightly acid, certain experiments were made, and it was found that bleaching increased in proportion to the quantity of hydrochloric acid added. Now, in the action of toning chlorine is disengaged, and in order to render this powerful bleaching agent inert it has been proposed to introduce a substance capable of combining with it, and thus, in absorbing it, prevent undue loss of vigor. To obtain this a slightly alkaline toning bath became a necessity.

No. 8.

Sodium carbonate (Na_2HCO_3)	5 grains.
Auric terchloride ($AuCl_3$)	1 grain.
Water	10 ounces.

Instead of the dry bicarbonate we will use a saturated solution. In this, as well as the following formulas, 3 prints of the same subject should be toned, viz., ordinary, fumed and preserved.

No. 9.

Sesquichloride of gold	15 grains.
Phosphate of soda	300 grains.
Distilled water	1¾ pints.

And in the same communication it is mentioned that 180 grains of borax may be substituted for the phosphate with a like result. Therefore it will be seen that a borax toning bath is not of recent discovery, although it does not appear to have been quoted in many formulae for at least a dozen years after its publication.

No. 10.

Gold terchloride	1 grain.
Sodium acetate	10 grains.
Sodium chloride	10 grains.
Hot water	20 ounces.

Mix twenty-four hours before use. Neutralize with chalk or whitening (carbonate of lime).

No. 11.

Ready Sensitized Paper Bath for.

A.

| Water | 1 liter. |
| Chloride of gold | 1 gram. |

B.

Water	1 liter.
Borax	10 grams.
Tungstate of soda	40 grams.

No. 12.

Schweier's Borax Toning Bath.

Chloride of gold solution, 1:50	3 c. c.
Borax solution, 1 to 10	100 c. c.
Water, distilled	100 c. c.

Ready at once.

No. 13.
E. L. Wilson's Toning Bath.

Water	16 fl. ounces.
Acetate sodium	30 grains.
Chloride sodium	30 grains.
Chloride gold	2 grains.
Nitrate uranium	2 grains.

The gold and uranium, previously dissolved in a little water, must be neutralized with sufficient bicarbonate soda. Add gold to renew as required.

No. 14.

Terchloride of gold, 1 per cent solution	1 part.
Hyperchloride of lime (white powder)	3 parts.
Distilled water	1000 parts.

The action is complete in ten to fifteen minutes, when the prints require washing in two changes of water to free them from the chloride of lime remaining in the fibres previous to fixing in 1 to 6 of hypo. If the tone is satisfactory at the expiration of fifteen minutes, the ordinary washing could be proceeded with.

No. 15.

If not, the proofs are submitted to a final bath composed of

Gold terchloride	2 parts.
Hypo	200 parts.
Distilled water	1200 parts.

The proof ought not to be left in this bath less than 15 minutes, as that is the minimum time necessary to insure the permanency of the picture; but it may be allowed to remain in it for as much longer as is requisite for obtaining the desired tone.

No. 16.

The uranium and gold toning bath has many friends. The tones are said to be richer, and to economize gold, while it is very easy to work. The originator of the formula is unknown, but the following formula is recommended. After washing away the free silver tone in the following mixture:

No. 1.

One grain acid solution of gold terchloride	1 ounce.
Water	7 ounces.

Neutralize with sufficient of a 20 per cent solution of sodium carb. (Na2HCo3).

No. 2.

Three grains solution of uranium nitrate	1 ounce.
Water	7 ounces.

Neutralize as in No. 1. Warm each to 70° F., and mix. The bath is then ready for use. It can be used repeatedly if desired, by acidifying with citric acid and neutralizing before use; but nothing is gained by using it a second time:

3470. Miscellaneous Toning Baths.

1. **To Obtain Black Tones on Silver Prints.**—Scholzig prints on sensitized albumenized paper under green or dark yellow glass, and tones with borax, 90 grains; uranium nitrate, 4 grains; gold chloride, 3 grains; water, 24 ounces. Teape prints under green glass, and tones with gold chloride, 1 grain; saturated solution of borax, 1 ounce; water, 6 ounces. (Phot. N., xxxiv., 623). Slightly washed prints absorb more gold in toning and give more permanent images than well washed prints (ibid., 639). The effects observed when silver printing is carried on under green glass are due to the specific action of the rays transmitted by the glass. Signal green absorbs the greater part of the rays that act on silver chloride, but transmits rays that act upon silver albuminate or silver citrate. When albumenized paper is printed under green glass the image consists almost entirely of altered silver albuminate, while with gelatino-citrochloride under similar conditions the image consists of altered silver citrate.—(Abney, Phot. Il., 702-704).

No. 2.

Platinum or palladium toning can be effected by means of a slightly acidulated solution of platinic or palladic chloride mixed with sodium sulphite.

The gradual decomposition of toning baths containing platinum and silver metals can be prevented by the addition of one of the highest salts of the particular metal. For example—Platinum toning bath: Potassium chloroplatinite, 1.5 part; platinum tetrachloride, 0.05 part; acetic acid, 15 parts; water, 1000 parts.

No. 3.

Osmium Toning Bath.—Ammonium osmiochloride, 1.50 part; potassium osmate, 0.1 part; acetic acid, 15 parts; water, 1000 parts. Similar baths are used in the case of iridium toning or palladium toning. The quantity of the higher salt present in each case is not sufficient to injure the prints.—(P. Mercier, B. S. F., Phot. (2), vi., 194, 195).

No. 4.
Acetate and Bicarbonate Bath.

Acetate of soda	120 grains.
Bicarbonate of soda	10 grains.
Chloride of gold	4 grains.
Water	20 ounces.

Make up fully twenty-four hours previously to its being required. The bath keeps indefinitely, and gives rich, warm brown tones. The prints for this bath should be printed deep. The toning will be complete when all the red has disappeared from the prints, except in the shadows, when examined by reflected light.

No. 5.
Borax Bath for Warm Brown Tones.

Borax	100 grains.
Water	10 ounces.
Chloride of gold	1 grain.
Water	10 ounces.

Mix. This bath will not keep, and should only be prepared as required, and then thrown away. One grain of gold is sufficient to tone 1 sheet of paper. The borax bath will suit all the ready-sensitized papers in the market. Use powdered borax, and dissolve it in hot water. Afterward make up to 10 ounces. Next add 1 grain of chloride of gold, or 1 dram of gold solution, to 10 ounces of water, and then mix the two solutions.

No. 6.
Gastine's Platinum Toning Bath.

Chloride of platinum	15 grains.
Chloride of sodium	60 grains.
Bitartrate of soda	18 grains.
Water	3½ ounces.

First dissolve the platinum and chloride of sodium, and bring the solution to the boiling point. Add the bitartrate slowly with constant stirring. This bath will keep, but is to be diluted ten to twelve times with water for use. Purple black tones are obtained by a long immersion; for sepia, tone less.

No. 7.

Platinum Toning Bath.—To make a platinum toning bath substitute platinum chloride for gold chloride in the acetate of soda bath; thus:

Platinum chloride	1 grain.
Acetate of soda	30 grains.
Water	8 ounces.

Dip a piece of blue litmus paper into the bath; if it turns red it is acid, and a solution of carbonate of soda must be added, drop by drop, until the blue color returns.

No. 8.
Spaulding's Stock Solution.

Water	5 ounces.
Gold chloride	5 grains.

For use take

Water	4 ounces.
Soda bicarbonate	1 grain.
Common salt	2 grains.
Stock solution of gold	1 ounce.

No. 9.
Tungstate of Soda Toning Bath.
No. 1.

Water	16 ounces.
Borax	20 grains.
Tungstate of soda	75 grains.

No. 2.

Water	4 ounces.
Chloride of gold	4 grains.

Mix 8 ounces of No. 1 with 1 ounce of No. 2, and allow the mixture to stand half an hour before using.

No. 10.

Toning and Fixing in One Bath.—The operation of toning and fixing is much simplified by using the combined bath. The print coming out of the printing frame is left in the bath till the color is arrived at, then washed and dried. The bath is composed of two solutions, and will keep for a long time. Dissolve water, 24 ounces; hyposulphite of soda, 6 ounces; sulphocyanide of ammonia, 1 ounce; acetate of soda, 1½ ounces; saturated solution of alum, 2 ounces. Fill the bottle containing the solution with scraps of sensitized paper, bad prints that are not fixed, and leave it for a day. Then filter, and add the following solution: Water, 6 ounces; chloride of gold, 15 grains; chloride of ammonium, 30 grains. It is necessary to print deep enough, and to leave the prints in the bath till, in looking through them, the desired color, brown dark or bluish, is observed. Used for Omega and other paper.

No. 11
Toning and Fixing in One Bath.

Chloride of gold	1 grain.
Phosphate of soda	15 grains.
Sulphocyanide of ammonium	25 grains.
Hyposulphite of soda	240 grains.
Water	2 ounces.

Dissolve the gold separately in a small quantity of water and add it to the other solution.

No. 12.
Combined Toning and Fixing Bath.

Water	32 ounces.
Hypo	8 ounces.
Chloride of gold	15 grains.
Nitrate of lead (c. p.)	75 grains.

No. 13.

Bromide Prints, Toning with Platinum.

Potassium platino-chloride.	7 grains.
Distilled water	16 ounces.
Hydrochloric acid	1¼ drams.

For twenty minutes, wash and soak to a 15 per cent solution of copper chloride.—E. Vogel.

No. 14.

Brown Tones on Bromide Paper.—Dr. Miethe states that good brown tones may be given to bromide prints by a short treatment of the fixed and well-washed prints in

Bichloride of mercury	10 parts.
Common salt	10 parts.
Water	500 parts.

No. 15.

Black Tones on Gelatino-Chloride Paper.—The following bath gives very rich dark tones:

Chloride of gold	5 grains.
Nitrate of uranium	5 grains.
Bicarbonate of soda	75 grains.
Distilled water	4 ounces.

No. 16.

Black Tones on Matt Surface Prints.—A very good toning bath for prints on matt surface paper is:

Borax	90 grains.
Nitrate of uranium	4 grains.
Gold	3 grains.
Water	24 ounces.

The above quantity of gold is sufficient to tone at least three dozen whole plate prints. If more are to be toned the proportions of gold and uranium should be increased. The bath remains in good condition for a long time, but fresh gold must be added occasionally to keep the bath up to strength.

No. 17

Gelatino-Chloride Paper, Toning and Fixing:

Solution No. 1.

Hyposulphite of soda	200 grams.
Alum	80 grams.
Nitrate of lead (pulverized)	2 grams.
Boiling water	400 c. c.

The solution is allowed to stand for two days; then once more 400 c. c. of boiling water are added, and the solution is filtered. Meantime, the following solution is prepared in a bottle:

Solution No. 2.

Sulphocyanide of ammonia.	160 grams.
Water	1200 c. c.

Solution No. 1 is mixed with solution No. 2, and then added.

Sol. of gold chloride, 1 per ct. 10 to 20 c. c.

With this bath the prints take any desired tone within three to five minutes.

No. 18.

Toning Bromide Prints.—By M. V. Portman.—The following toning bath answers well, after fixing, if the print is at all green:

Sulphocyanide of ammonium	30 grains.
Chloride of gold	1 grain.
Water	4 ounces.

Half a minute in this bath will give the print a rich black tone; a longer time will turn the print blue, which answers very well for moonlight effects.

No. 19.

Experiments in Toning Gelatino-Chloride Paper.—From the Photographic News we take the following: The use of paper coated with a gelatino-citro-chloride emulsion in place of albumenized paper appears to be becoming daily more common. Successful toning has generally been the difficulty with such paper, the alkaline baths commonly in use with albumenized having proved unsuitable for toning this paper. On the whole the bath that has given the best results is one containing, in addition to gold, a small quantity of hypo. and a considerable quantity of sulphocyanide of ammonium. Such a bath tones very rapidly, and gives most pleasing colors. It appears, moreover, to be impossible to over-tone the citro-chloro-emulsion paper with it in the sense that it is possible to over-tone prints on albumenized paper with the ordinary alkaline bath. That is to say, it is impossible to produce a slaty gray image. The result of prolonged toning is merely an image of an engraving black color. Of this, however, we shall say more hereafter. We wish first of all to refer to an elaborate series of experiments by Lionel Clark on the effects of various toning baths used with the gelatino-citrochloride paper.

The results of these experiments we have before us at the time of writing, and we may at once say that, from the manner in which the experiments have been carried out and in which the results have been tabulated, Lionel Clark's work forms a very useful contribution to our photographic knowledge, and a contribution that will become more and more useful, the longer the results of the experiments are kept. A number of small prints have been prepared. Of these several—in most cases, three—have been toned by a certain bath, and each print has been torn in two. One-half has been treated with bichloride of mercury, so as to bleach such portion of the image as is of silver, and finally the prints—the two halves of each being brought close together—have been mounted in groups, each group containing all the prints toned by a certain formula, with full information tabulated.

The only improvement we could suggest in the arrangement is that all the prints should have been from the same negative, or from only three negatives, so that we should have prints from the same negatives in every group, and should the better be able to compare the results of the toning baths. Probably, however, the indifferent light of the present season of the year made it difficult to get a sufficiency of prints from one negative.

The following is a description of the toning baths used and of the appearance of the prints. We refer, in the meantime, only to those halves that have not been treated with bichloride of mercury.

No. 1.

Gold chloride ($AuCl_3$)	1 grain.
Sulphocyanide of potassium	10 grains.
Hyposulphite of soda	½ grain.
Water	2 ounces.

The prints are of a brilliant purple or violet color.

No. 2.

Gold chloride	1 grain.
Sulphocyanide of potassium	10 grains.
Hyposulphite of soda	½ grain.
Water	4 ounces.

There is only one print which is of a brown color, and in every way inferior to those toned with the first bath.

No. 3.

Gold chloride	1 grain.
Sulphocyanide of potassium	12 grains.
Hyposulphite of soda	½ grain.
Water	2 ounces.

The prints toned by this bath are, in our opinon, the finest of the whole. The tone is a purple of the most brilliant and pleasing shade.

No. 4.

Gold chloride	1 grain.
Sulphocyanide of potassium	20 grains.
Hyposulphite of soda	5 grains.
Water	2 ounces.

There is only one print, but it is from the same negative as one of the No. 3 group. It is very inferior to that in No. 3, the color less pleasant, and the appearance generally as if the details of the lights had been bleached by the large quantity either of hypo. or of sulphocyanide of potassium.

No. 5.

Gold chloride	1 grain.
Sulphocyanide of potassium	50 grains.
Hyposulphite of soda	½ grain.
Water	2 ounces.

Opposite to this description of formula there are no prints, but the following is written: "These prints were completely destroyed, the sulphocyanide of potassium (probably) dissolving off the gelatine."

No. 6.

Gold chloride	1 grain.
Sulphocyanide of potassium	20 grains.
Hypo	5 grains.
Carbonate of soda	10 grains.
Water	2 ounces.

This, it will be seen, is the same as 4, but that the solution is rendered alkaline with carbonate of soda. The result of the alkalinity certainly appears to be good, the color is more pleasing than that produced by No. 4, and there is less appearance of bleaching. It must be borne in mind in this connection that the paper itself is strongly acid, and that, unless special means be taken to prevent it, the toning bath is sure to be more or less acid.

No. 7.

Gold chloride	1 grain.
Acetate of soda	30 grains.
Water	2 ounces.

The color of the prints toned by this bath is not exceedingly pleasing. It is a brown tending to purple, but is not very pure or bright. The results show, however, the possibility of toning the gelatino-chloro-citrate paper with the ordinary acetate bath if it be only made concentrated enough.

No. 8.

Gold chloride	1 grain.
Carbonate of soda	3 grains.
Water	2 ounces.

Very much the same may be said of the prints toned by this bath as of those toned by No. 7. The color is not very good, nor is the toning quite even. This last remark applies to No. 7 batch as well as No. 8.

No. 9.

Gold chloride	1 grain.
Phosphate of soda	20 grains.
Water	2 ounces.

The results of this bath can best be described as purplish in color. They are decidedly more pleasing than those of 7 or 8, but are not as good as the best by the sulphocyanide bath.

No. 10.

Gold chloride	1 grain.
Hyposulphite of soda	½ ounce.
Water	2 ounces.

The result of this bath is a brilliant brown color, what might indeed, perhaps, be best described as a red. Two out of the three prints are much too dark, indicating, perhaps, that this toning bath did not have any tendency to reduce the intensity of the image.

The general lesson taught by Clark's experiments is that the sulphocyanide bath gives better results than any other. A certain proportion of the ingredients—namely, that of bath 3—gives better results than any other proportions tried, and about as good as any that could be hoped for. Any of the ordinary alkaline toning baths may be used, but they all give results inferior to those got by the sulphocyanide bath. The best of the ordinary baths is, however, the phosphate of soda.

And now a word as to those parts of the prints which have been treated with bichloride of mercury. The thing that strikes us as remarkable in connection with them is that in them the image has scarcely suffered any reduction of intensity at all. In most cases there has been a disagreeable change of color, but it is almost entirely confined to the whites and lighter tints, which are turned to a more or less dirty yellow. Even in the case of the prints toned by bath No. 10, where the image is quite red, it has suffered no appreciable reduction of intensity.

This would indicate that an unusually large proportion of the toned image consists of gold, and this idea is confirmed by the fact that to tone a sheet of gelatino-chloro-citrate paper requires several times as much gold as to tone a sheet of albumenized paper. Indeed, we believe that, with the emulsion paper, it is possible to replace the whole of the silver of the image with gold, thereby producing a permanent print. We have already said that the print may be left for any reasonable length of time in the toning bath without the destruction of its appearance, and we cannot but suppose that a very long immersion results in a complete substitution of gold for silver.

11. Toning Bath for Gelatino-Chloride Emulsion Paper.

Wash the prints in clean water and then tone in the following:

A.

Distilled water	25 ounces.
Acetate of soda (recrystallized)	1 ounce.
Into which pour a solution of 1 per cent of chloride of gold	2 ounces.

B.

In 10 ounces of distilled water dissolve 2 drams of sulpho-cyanide of ammonia, and add 1 ounce solution of 1 per cent chloride of gold.

For toning, mix in the proportion of 20 ounces of A to 6 of B, if possible the evening before using.

12. Transparencies on Silver Paper.

Print on the back of heavily-silvered paper until the picture is well printed, viewing the paper by transmitted light.

Tone and fix; make the paper translucent, when dry, with

Poppy oil	½ ounce.
Balsam fir	⅛ ounce.
Spirits of turpentine	¼ ounce.

3471. Trays, to Make.

Use wood, and smear over with 4 parts resin, 1 part gutta percha and a little boiled oil, melted together and applied hot to the perfectly dry wood. Do not use zinc.

3472. Trays and Graduates to Clean.

Wash with nitric acid and use a rag.

3473. Silver Wastes, to Recover.

I. From Nitrate Bath.—1. Add solution of caustic potash or lime, as long as there is a brown precipitate. Allow it to settle, pour off the liquid and collect silver oxide for reduction; vide III. below.

2. For 1 pound of silver add 1 ounce sulphuric acid and ½ pound zinc and allow it to stand two days. Precipitate as a chloride, wash 8 or 10 times by decantation, and dissolve gradually in nitric acid. Test the complete washing by hydrochloric acid. Wash with water till zinc nitrate is removed. If zinc clings to silver, wash with hydrochloric acid.

3. Suspend a sheet of copper in bath for two or three days.

4. Acidify as nitric acid, precipitate as silver chloride by sodium chloride or hydrochloric acid and reduce as III.

5. Immerse in bath 2 strips of copper attached to a Daniell's battery. Silver deposited on the copper as in No. 3.

6. Add sodium bicarbonate or hydrate. Reduce as in III. below, or, if pure enough, dissolve precipitate at once in nitric acid.

7. Concentrate bath made alkaline by sodium carbonate and add aqueous solution of

oxalic acid neutralized with sodium carbonate. Filter, dry and fuse with equal weight of sodium bicarbonate.

8. Deposit either with or without a battery on iron. Fuse with potassium nitrate and sodium carbonate.

II. Hyposulphite Bath.—1. Precipitate as silver sulphide by potassium sulphide. Reduce as III. or dissolve in nitric acid.

2. Precipitate with hydrosulphuric acid, and reduce as III.

3. Decompose hypo. by waste nitrosulphuric acid from manufacture of gun cotton for collodion. Have silver sulphide and sulphur with sodium nitrate and sulphate in solution. Suspend zinc in the solution, then boil two or three hours; wash on filter, dry, fuse with borax and sodium carbonate.

4. Suspend sheet copper in the solution.

5. Add hydrochloric acid, which sets free sulphur and precipitates silver chloride. Oxidize the sulphur by aqua regia and reduce silver chlorides as in III.

6. Add sodium hypochlorite to the alkaline solution. Wash, precipitate and fuse with mixed carbonates. This gives no fumes of sulphur. Sodium bisulphate and chlorides are bi-products.

III. Reduction of Silver Chloride, Oxide or Sulphide.—1. Mix with 1/3 its weight of colophony. Heat moderately in a crucible till greenish-blue flame ceases, then suddenly increase the heat, when a button of the metal is obtained.

2. Melt with alkaline carbonates enough to cover surface from air; then mix with 75 per cent chalk and 4 per cent charcoal, and heat.

3. Ignite with niter on red hot plate, carefully, and in small quantities to avoid explosions, run down to a bead with sodium carbonate and borax.

4. If a chloride, reduce to an oxide by boiling with strong potash, then reduce by glucose; or boil the chloride with glucose and sodium carbonate.

5. Add silver chloride dissolved in ammonia to a boiling solution of 1 part glucose and 3 parts sodium carbonate in 40 per cent of water, keeping up the boiling all the time.

6. Add to silver chloride sodium hydrate in solution and grape sugar, and expose to sunlight in an open dish with occasional stirring. Reduce to dark brown oxide of silver soluble in nitric acid.

7. Mix with five times its weight of sodium carbonate. Fill a Hessian crucible half full and sprinkle sodium chloride over the top. Heat slowly in anthracite fire. After half an hour increase the heat until the crucible is white hot. When complete fusion has taken place, allow to cool and break out the button of silver.

8. Fuse with 2 parts carbonate sodium and potassium mixed.

9. Add pure zinc and dilute sulphuric acid and let it stand two days. Wash silver off with water acidulated with sulphuric acid to remove all zinc; finally fuse to a button.

10. Mix one-half its weight dry sodium carbonate and one-quarter its weight of dry clean sand and ignite.

IV. a. Gold Wastes, Recovered.—1. Make just acid with hydrochloric acid, add solution containing 2 ounces pyrogallic acid, let it stand twenty-four hours; filter, dissolve in aqua regia, and product, after evaporation, will be found better for toning than that precipitated by iron.

2. Acidify toning bath, and add sulphate of iron, 2 grams, to 1 gram chloride of gold.

b. Separated from Silver.—1. Treat button obtained by fusing waste from hypo. baths, toning and fixing with dilute nitric acid. Wash insoluble part with ammonia to remove silver chloride, if present, and dissolve in aqua regia.

2. Digest 20 grams in flask with 1 fl. dram hydrochloric acid, 15 minims of nitric acid and 2 drams of water. After fifteen minutes boil, add 2 ounces water; filter. Silver chloride with organic matter left undissolved. Reduce as III. above.

V. Paper Wastes.—1. Soak paper in strong solution of saltpeter and burn.

2. Treat with nitric acid, precipitate with sodium chloride or potassium hydrate. Then put with III., above for reduction.

VI. Cyanide Solution.—1. Dilute with water, precipitate by (2) potassium sulphide. (2) sodium chloride, and reduce as III.

2. Decant bath into iron kettle, warm, add ferrous sulphate slowly, till a slight precipitate of oxide is formed. Make alkaline, and add solution of grape sugar until of a brownish yellow color. Allow to settle, siphon off the liquid. Wash sediment on filter, and ignite to recover silver.

VII. Developer.—1. See II., 3, 4, 5, 6, with hypo. bath; 1 and 2 not applicable, for iron sulphide would be formed.

2. Reduce by its own iron, if ferrous sulphate.

Reduction of Photographic Wastes.—The following recipes are the result of the experiences of many. Some of the notes are very important. If followed closely you may, as other people have done, reduce photographic wastes to 982/1000 fine.

Paper Clippings.—Burn the papers to a fine ash; then mix with 1½ its weight of the following flux:

Bicarbonate of soda.......	1 pound.
Pearlash	1 pound.
Common salt...............	4 ounces.

Silver Paper, to Reduce.—Burn all your papers and preserve the ashes thereof, then add nitric acid until all the silver is extracted, and filter through muslin cloth. Now add common salt to form silver chloride, and evaporate to dryness, and reduce to metallic silver in crucible by adding 2 parts of sodium carbonate and a modicum of borax to one of silver chloride. Mix well and heat gradually at first, and finish with white heat, then wash well until nothing but silver remains. Treat washings with salt, evaporate to dryness, and reduce as above in crucible.

Recovery of Silver from Hypo Bath.—The Photographische Wochenblatt recommends the precipitation of silver from the fixing bath with an old oxalate developer that still contains enough protoxide for this purpose. The precipitate is in a very fine state of division and difficult to filter.

Silver from Waste Solutions.—One of the simplest methods of recovering silver from waste solutions is the following: First dilute the liquid about one-third with water (double this quantity if much gum is present), heat the solution to about 180° Fah., and gradually add solution of pure sulphate of iron (iron sulphate 5 ounces, water 1 pint) until no further precipitate forms. Decant the liquid portion, throw the precipitate on a filter and wash it thoroughly with hot water. To the washed precipitate—consisting of finely divided metallic silver—add strong pure nitric acid and heat over a water bath until the silver has all been dissolved. Evaporate to dryness over the water bath (in a porcelain dish, capsule) and dissolve the residue in hot water (distilled or rain). Filter this solution and concentrate it over a water bath, then set it aside to crystallize. Remove the crystals, concentrate in a similar manner the mother liquid and obtain another crop of crystals. These crystals (of nitrate of silver) are pure enough for ordinary purposes, but if required to be used for photographic purposes they should be redissolved in water and recrystallized. Where the liquid containing the silver contains also much insoluble organic matter, it is sometimes preferable to separate the silver by evaporating the liquid to dryness and fusing the residue with an equal quantity of borax glass in a blacklead crucible.

3474.   Waxing Solution.

For carbon prints, or for removing collodion films.—Beeswax, 40 grains; benzole, (rectified), 8 ounces.

3475. Photography. Accelerator, the "Excelsior."

This accelerator is of German origin. It can be employed both with ferrous oxalate or pyrogallol. Zinc filings, 100 parts; water, 500 parts; sulphuric acid, 50 parts.

Shake well and set aside for a few days. The vial should be well corked. Add then 250 parts of sodium sulphite, set aside again for a few days, and dilute with an equal volume of: Ammonium sulphite, 250 parts; water, 500 parts. This is the stock solution. If to be used with pyrogallol, one should add 1 part of ammonium sulphocyanate to 50 parts of it, or 4 parts of ammonio-citrate of iron if employed with ferrous oxalate.

These solutions keep for a long time in well corked bottles.

For pyrogallol 2½ p. 100 are added to the developing solution and for ferrous oxalate 5 p. 100. A greater percentage produces yellow fog.

In the chemical action, which takes place in the preparation of the accelerator, sodium hyposulphite (formerly hydrosulphite) is formed, and to it is due the accelerating property.

The process is not new; it is similar to that published in 1877 by Mr. L. O. Sammann, for the development of the luminous image on collodion emulsion films.

3476. Colored Photographic Prints, Formulas for Making Different.

Mr. A. Lizzard, in Anthony's Bulletin, gives a translation from a French work on the different processes for producing prints in various colors.

"Process with nitrates of uranium and copper." By means of this process, which is as rapid as that of the salts of silver, prints of a brown tone are obtained very warm, very agreeable and of an artistic stamp.

The sensitizing bath is composed of: A. Uranium nitrate, 23 grams; distilled water, 80 c. c. B. Copper nitrate, 7 grams; distilled water, 80 c. c.

Mix these two solutions in a tray and immerse in it the gelatine sized paper, for about two minutes; then dry it in the dark. The paper thus prepared will keep for a considerable length of time, and it becomes also very leathery. The exposure to the sun requires not longer than ten minutes, a weak image showing in the printing frame. It is then developed by immersing in a solution of: Yellow prussiate of potash, 16 grams; distilled water, 700 c. c.

The image will instantly appear with a rich red brown tone, with metallic reflection and bronzed. When the immersion has been sufficient, the image will appear with a nearly equal intensity on both sides, because it is in the body of the paper. By this means very fine transparent pictures are easily obtained. As soon as the print reaches the desired tone, wash it in pure water until the whites have become clear and pure, and all soluble salts eliminated; then hang it up to dry. No other fixing will be necessary.

In place of the yellow prussiate bath, if one is used, composed of 2 parts chloride of platinum to 100 parts water, the prints will be a beautiful black.

In the same book is given a "process with nitrate of silver and uranium" which promises very fine results. Float a sheet of paper on a sensitizing bath composed of the following: A. Uranium nitrate, 60 grams; distilled water, 50 c. c. B. Silver nitrate, 8 grams; distilled water, 50 c. c.

Mix the two solutions, float the paper for two or three minutes and hang it up to dry in a dark room. Expose it under the negative and immerse in a bath composed of: Protosulphate of iron, 16 grams; tartaric acid, 8 grams; sulphuric acid, a few drops; distilled water, 200 c. c.

The development is very rapid and the print is fixed by washing in pure or rain water. The sensitiveness of this paper is so great that in diffused light a print is visible and black in eighteen seconds, and in half an hour before a kerosene light of moderate size at five inches distant from the flame. The process is very simple, and the chemicals of the ordinary kind to be found in every well conducted dark room.

3477. Faded Photographs.

Put the card in warm water until the paper print may be removed from the card backing without injury. The prints can be restored by means of the following solutions: a. Sodium tungstate, 100 parts; water, 5000 parts. b. Precipitated chalk, 4 parts; bleaching powder (chloride of lime), 1 part; sodium aurochloride, 4 parts; distilled water, 400 parts. Solution b is made in a well corked yellow glass bottle, is allowed to stand twenty-four hours, and is then filtered into another yellow bottle. The faded prints are well washed, and placed in a mixture 1 to 2 parts of b and 40 parts of a. When the intensification is sufficient, the prints are immersed in a solution of 1 part of hypo. in 10 parts of solution a until all yellowness has disappeared, and are then well washed.

3478. Lantern Slides, To Color.

Use transparent colors, namely, Prussian blue, gamboge, carmine, verdigris, madder brown, indigo, crimson lake, and ivory black, with the semi-transparent colors, raw and burnt sienna, and vandyke and copal brown, thinning oil colors with ordinary megilp to a degree just sufficient for the proper working, and using for a medium for laying on the first coat of water colors gelatine thoroughly dissolved and hot. When perfectly dry this coat can be shaded and finished with water colors mixed in the ordinary way with cold water, but the manipulation of the added colors must be gentle, so as not to disturb the layer first put on the glass. A thin coat of the best mastic varnish heightens the effect of shades painted in water colors, but oil colors require no varnish.

3479. Photographing on Wood, Using Dry Plates.

Gelatine, 2 drams; white curd soap, 2 drams; water, 16 ounces. Soak gelatine for some hours, then dissolve in a bath of hot water. Add the soap in small shavings, stir with a glass rod or slate pencil till completely mixed, then add powdered alum until the froth produced disappears; strain through muslin. The block is now coated with this mixture and a little zinc white, rubbed well into the wood, with the thinnest coating possible, and finished off smoothly and evenly all over, and left to dry. It is then brushed over with the following composition, a camel hair brush being used. It is advisable to use a wide one, to prevent streaks in the finished block; Albumen, 1 ounce; water, 6 drams; ammonium chloride, 18 grains; citric acid, 5 grains.

Beat the albumen to froth and allow to settle, using the clean portion, add the water, then the ammonium chloride, mixing well with rod; finally the acid. One coating with the brush from end to end of the block in one sweep is quite sufficient. When the block is dry pour over a small quantity of silver solution, made by dissolving nitrate of silver, 50 grains; water, distilled, 1 ounce.

Move the solution over the surface by the aid of a glass rod, and pour off the surplus into another bottle for filtering for further use. When dry, print the block under a reversed negative to just the depth you require, as there is hardly any loss in the finishing. When printed, hold the block face down in a dish of strong salt and water for three minutes. This will cause the print to fade a little. Wash under a spray of water, and fix in a saturated solution of hypo. by holding the block face down on the bath for about five minutes; this will bring back all detail; finally wash for about ten minutes, stand on end to dry; the block is then ready to be engraved. The picture may be toned, but this is not necessary. In order to make the reverse negative it is only needful to take the photograph through the film, care being taken to have the glass quite clean. Another method would be—strip and turn the film by means of a solution of hydrofluoric acid. In case you make a negative through the film, remember to turn the focusing glass round.

TABLE OF LATIN TERMS USED IN PRESCRIPTIONS.

From Scoville's Art of Compounding.

Term or Phrase.	Contraction.	Meaning.
a a		Of each.
Abdomen, inis	Abdom.	The belly.
Ablutio-ionis		A washing, cleansing.
Absente febre	Abs. feb.	In the absence of fever.
Accurate		Carefully, accurately.
Accuratissime	Accuratiss	Most carefully, most accurately.
Acerbitas-atis		Sourness.
Acerbus, a, um		Sharp, sour, harsh (to the taste).
Acetum saturninum		Solution of subacetate of lead.
Ad (prep. w. accus.)		To, up to.
Ad conciliandum gustum		To suit the taste.
Ad secundum vicem	Ad 2d. vic.	To the second time.
Adde, addatur	Add	Add (thou), let it be added.
Addantur, additus		Let them be added, adding.
Addentus, addendo		Adding, for or by adding.
Adde cum tritu	Add. c. trit.	Add with trituration.
Additis sub finem coctionis		Adding toward the end of boiling.
Ad defectionem animi	Ad. def. anim.	To fainting.
Ad gratam aciditatim		To an agreeable sourness.
Ad gratum gustum		To an agreeable taste.
Adhibendus	Adhib.	To be administered.
Adjacens		Near to.
Ad libitum	Ad. lib.	At pleasure.
Admove, admoveatur		
Admoveantur	Admov.	Apply, let it or them be applied.
Admoveatur durante dolore		Let it be applied when in severe pain.
Ad partes dolentes	Ad. part. dolent.	To the painful (or aching) parts.
Adstante febre	Adst. febre	When the fever is on.
Adversum	Adv.	Against.
AEtas, atis		Age, time of life.
Aggrediente febre	Aggred. feb.	When the fever is coming on.
Agita, agitetur	Agit.	Shake, stir, let it be shaken or stirred.
Agitato, agitando		With or by shaking, or agitation.
Agita ante sumendum		Shake before taking.
Agita donec refrigerat		Stir until it is cold.
Agitando miscentur		Let them be mixed by shaking.
Agitato vase	Agit. vas.	The vial being shaken.
Albus, a, um	Alb.	White.
Alcoholisatus, i		Alcoholized, i. e., powdered extremely fine.
Aliquot		Some, a few.
Alimentum, i		Nutrient, nourishment.
Alter alteram	Alt.	The other, the rest.
Alternis horis		Every other hour.
Aluta		Leather.
Alvo astricta (or adstricta)	Alv. ast.	For confinement of the bowels (constipation).
Alvus		The belly, the bowels.
Amplus	Amp.	Large, ample.

Term or Phrase.	Contraction.	Meaning.
Ampulla		A large vessel.
Ana	a a	Of each.
Ante		Before.
Applica, applicetur		Apply, let it be applied.
Aqua astricta	Aq. ast.	Frozen water, ice.
Aqua bulliens	Aq. bull.	Boiling water.
Aqua communis	Aq. com	Common water.
Aqua fontis (fontalis or fontana)	Aq. font.	Spring water.
Aqua gelidus		Cold water.
Aqua marina	Aq. mar.	Sea water.
Aqua phagedaenica	Aq. phaged.	Yellow wash.
Aqua pluvialis	Aq. pluv.	Rain water.
Aqua potabilis		Drinkable water.
Aqua saturni	Aq. satur.	Subacetate of lead water.
Aqua urbis	Aq. urb.	City water.
Aquila alba		Calomel.
Argilla, æ		Clay.
Aut		Or.
Bacca, ae		Berry.
Balneum		A bath.
Balneum arenae	Bal. ar.	Sand-bath.
Balneum maris	Bal. mar.	Salt (or sea) water bath.
Balneum vaporis	Bal. vap.	Steam (or vapor) bath.
Bene		Well, good.
Bibe, bibatur		Drink, let it be drank.
Biduum		Two days.
Bis		Twice.
Bis in die, bis in dies, bis intra diem	Bis in. d.	Twice a day.
Bonus, a. um		Good.
Brachium		An arm.
Brevis		Short.
Bulliat, bulliant	Bull	Let it (or them) boil.
Butyrum		Butter.
Caeruleus, i	Caerul.	Dark blue, dark green.
Calefactus, i	Calef.	Warmed.
Calido solvuntur		Let them be dissolved while hot.
Calomelas or calomelanos	Calom.	Calomel.
Calor, oris	Calor.	Heat, warmth.
Capiat	Cap.	Let the patient take.
Capiat omnes cursu hodie		Let the patient take all during this day.
Capiat quantum vis (or volueris)	Cap. quant. vis.	Let the patient take as much as he will.
Capillus, i		The hair.
Caput, capitis		The head, of the head.
Carbasus, i	Carbas.	Linen, lint.
Caro, carnis		Meat, of meat (flesh).
Cataplasma atis		A poultice.
Catharticum, i		A cathartic.
Caute		Cautiously.
Celeriter		Quickly, immediately.
Cena (or caena or coena)		Supper.
Ceratum, i		A wax salve.
Charta	Chart.	Paper.
Charta cerata	Chart. cerat.	Waxed paper.
Chartula	Chart.	A small paper.
Chininum	Chinin.	Quinine.
Cibus, i		Food, victuals.

Term or Phrase.	Contraction.	Meaning.
Circitu		Near, round, about.
Cito		Quickly.
Cito dispensetur!	Cito. disp.!	Let it be dispensed quickly.
Clarus, a, um		Bright, clear.
Clausus, a, um		Closed, inclosed.
Cochleare, cochleatim	Coch.	A spoonful, by spoonfuls.
Cochleare, amplum, or magnum	Coch. amp. Coch. mag.	A tablespoonful.
Cochleare medium or modicum	Coch. med.	A dessertspoonful.
Cochleare parvum	Coch. parv.	A teaspoonful.
Coctio		Boiling.
Cogantur		Let them be combined.
Cola, coletur, colentur		Strain, let it (or them) be strained.
Colaturae (dat.)	Colatur.	To or of the strained liquor.
Collum, i		The neck.
Collunarium, i		A nose-wash.
Collutorium	Collut.	A mouth-wash.
Collyrium	Collyr.	An eye lotion.
Coloretur		Let it be colored.
Commisce, commiscetur, commiscentur		Mix together, let it or them be mixed together.
Commode (adv.)	Commod.	Rightly, properly, suitably.
Concisus		Cut.
Concuscus, i		Shaken.
Concuti, concutiatur		Shake, let it be shaken.
Congius	Cong.	A gallon.
Conquassando		By vigorous shaking.
Conserve		A conserve; also preserve.
Consperge, conspergetur	Consperg.	Dust or sprinkle, let them be sprinkled or dusted.
Contere, conteruntus	Contere.	Rub together, let them be rubbed together.
Conterendo		With or by rubbing together.
Continuantur remedia	Cont. rem.	Let the medicines be renewed.
Contra		Against.
Contritus, a, um	Contrit.	Broken, ground, crumbled.
Contusus, a, um	Contus.	Bruised.
Coque, coquetur, coquantur	Coq.	Boil, let it (or them) be boiled.
Coquantur simul	Coq. simul.	Boil together.
Cor, cordis		The heart.
Cotula, ae		A measure.
Coxa		The hip.
Cras crastinus	Cras.	To-morrow.
Cras sumendus		To be taken to-morrow.
Cras mane		To-morrow morning.
Cras nocte		To-morrow night.
Cras vespere		To-morrow evening.
Cujus, cujus libet	Cuj., cuj. lib.	Of which, of whatever you please.
Cum	C.	With.
Cum guttis aliquot		With a few drops.
Cursu (abl.)		In the passing of, during.
Cyathus, or	Cyath.	
Cyathus vinarius	Cyath. vinar.	A wineglass.
Da, detur, dentur	Da, det., dent.	Give, let it (them) be given.
De (prep. w. abl.)		From, down.
Deaurentur		Let them be gilded.
Debitae spissitudonis	Deb. spiss.	To a proper consistence.

Term or Phrase.	Contraction.	Meaning.
Debitus, a, um....................	....	Due, proper.
Decanta	....	Decant.
Decoctum	Decoc.	A decoction.
Decoque, decoquetur, decoquentur	....	Boil down, let be boiled down.
Decubitus	Decub.	Lying down.
De die in diem...................	De d. in d......	From day to day.
Dein, deinde.....................	....	Afterward, then.
Deglutiatur (antur)..............	....	Let or may be swallowed.
Dejicerit, dejiciatur..............	....	Will purge, let it be purged.
Dexter	....	Right.
Diebus alternis...................	Dieb. alt.	Every other day.
Dies (diei, gen.).................	D.	A day.
Digere, digeretur, digerentur.....	....	Digest, let be digested.
Diluculum, i, diluculo............	....	Daybreak, at dawn.
Dilue, dilutus, a, um.............	....	Dilute, diluted.
Dimidius, a, um.................	Dim.	One-half.
Directiones	Dir.	Directions.
Directione propia................	Dir. prop.......	With proper directions.
Dispensa, dispensetur............	Disp.	Dispense, let it be dispensed.
Divide, dividatur, dividantur.....	Divid.	Divide, let it be divided.
Dolor, dolore....................	....	Pain, in pain.
Donec	....	Until.
Donec alvus dejecerit............	....	Until the bowels move.
Donec alvus commode purgetur..	....	Until the bowels are properly purged.
Donec alvus soluta fuerit.........	....	Until the bowels are loosened.
Donec habeas colaturae..........	....	Until you have of strained liquor.
Donec leinatur dolor.............	....	Until the pain is relieved (or assuaged).
Donec sint residuae..............	....	Until there is ——— of residue.
Dosis	....	A dose.
Dulcedo (idinis) dulcitas-atis.....	Dulc.	Sweetness.
Duplico	....	In duplicate.
Eadem (fem.)...................	....	The same.
Ejusdem	....	Of the same.
Electuarium	Elect.	An electuary.
Emesis	....	Vomiting.
Emplastrum epispasticum.......	{ Emp. episp. }	A blistering plaster.
Emplastrum vesicatorium.......	{ Emp. vesic. }	
Enema, enemata................	Enem.	A clyster. (Injection for the rectum.)
Epistomium	Epistom.	A stopper, bung.
Et	....	And.
Etiam	....	Also, besides.
Etiam nunc.....................	....	Yet, also, besides.
Evanuerit	....	Shall have passed away, disappeared.
Ex or E (w. abl.)................	E.	From, out of.
E qua formentur.................	....	From which are formed.
E quibus sumatur................	....	From which are given.
Exhibeatur	Exhib.	Let it be exhibited (administered).
Ex modo praescripto.............	E. m. p.........	After the manner prescribed (as directed).
Ex paululo aquae	....	From (or in) a very little water.
Experime	....	Try (thou).
Ex Parte	....	Partly
Exprime, exprimatur	....	Express, let it be expressed.
Extende, Extendatur	....	Spread, let it be spread.
Extende super alutam	Extend sup. alut.	Spread upon leather.
Extende super pannum	....	Spread upon cloth.
Extrahe, extrahatur	....	Extract (thou), let it be extracted.
Extractum	Ext.	An extract.

Term or Phrase.	Contraction.	Meaning.
Fac, fit, fiat, fiant	Ft.	Make, let be made.
Facere		To make.
Farina		Flour, meal.
Fasciculus	Fascic.	A little bundle.
Febris		Fever.
Febre durante		During the fever.
Femoris interni	Fem. inter.	To the inner thigh.
Fervens (entis)	Ferv.	Hot.
Fictilis, e		An earthen vessel.
Filtra	Filt.	Filter.
Filtrum	Filt.	A filter.
Filtrum chartae		Filter paper.
Flavus, a, um	Flav.	Yellow.
Fluidus, a, um	Fld.	Fluid.
Flores benzoes		Benzoic acid.
Florescinae		Santonica.
Flores zinci		Oxide of zinc.
Formentur	Form.	Let them be formed.
Frigor, oris	Frig.	Cold.
Frustillatim (adv.)	Frust.	In small pieces, little bits.
Fuerit		Shall have been.
Fuscus, a, um		Brown, dark.
Gargarisma	Garg.	A gargle.
Gelatina		Gelatin.
Gradatim		Gradually.
Granum, grana	Gr.	A grain, grains.
Gratus, a, um		Pleasant, agreeable.
Grossus, a, um		Large, coarse.
Gummi mimosae		Gum arabic.
Gutta, Guttae	Gtt.	A drop, drops.
Guttatim		By drops.
Harum pilularum		Of these pills.
Harum pulverum		Of these powders.
Haustus, i	Haust.	A draught.
Hebdoma, ae		A week, for a week.
Herba, ae		An herb.
Heri		Yesterday.
Hora		An hour.
Hora dicubitus	Hor. dic.	At bed-time.
Horae intermediis	Hor. interm.	In the intermediate hours.
Hora somni	Hor. som.	At bed-time.
Hora unius spatio		At the end of an hour.
Idem		The same.
Identidem		Repeatedly, often.
Idoneus, a, um		Suitable, convenient.
Idoneo vehiculo	Idon. vehic.	In a suitable vehicle.
Illico		Then, immediately.
Illico lagena obturatur		Let the bottle be stoppered immediately.
Immitatur, immitantur		Let it (them) be introduced into, placed in.
In		In, within, upon—(sometimes) not.
Imprimis		Chiefly first.
Incide, incisus		Cut, cutting.
Inde		Therefrom.
Indies		Daily.
Infunde		Put or pour in.
Ingere, ingerendus		Put or force into, forcing into.

NON-SECRET FORMULAS.

Term or Phrase.	Contraction.	Meaning.
Ingerendus capsulas gelatinosas		Putting into gelatine capsules.
Injiciatur	Injic.	Let it be injected.
In impetu effervescentiae		In the height of effervescence.
In lagena bene obturatur		In a well-stoppered bottle.
In loco frigido	In. loco. frig.	In a cold place.
In massam subigantur		Let them be kneaded into a mass.
In massam cogantur		Let them be combined in a mass.
In olla ferrea vitreata		In a glazed iron pot.
In partes aequales		Into equal parts.
In pulmento		In gruel.
Instar		The form and size of.
In vaso clauso		In a closed (covered) vessel.
In vaso leviter clauso		In a loosely closed vessel.
Inter, internus		Between, inner.
Involve, involvuntur		Cover (coat), let them be covered.
Involve gelatina		Coat with gelatin.
Invoruntur		Let them be moistened, sprinkled.
Ita		In such manner.
Iteretur, iterentur		Let it (or them) be repeated.
Jam		Now.
Jentaculum, i	Jentac.	Breakfast.
Jucunde	Jucund.	Pleasantly.
Julepum	Jul.	A julep.
Juscellum		A broth.
Jusculum		Soup.
Juxta, juxtim		Near to, nigh, close by.
Kalium	K.	Potassium.
Kali		Potassa.
Kali praeparata		Potassium carbonate.
Lac, lactis		Milk, of milk.
Lamella, ae, lamina, ae		Plate, leaf, layer, scale.
Lana, ae		Flannel, wool.
Languor, oris		Faintness, feebleness.
Lapidens, a, um	Lapid.	Of stone, stony.
Lapis infernalis		Silver nitrate, lunar caustic.
Largus, a, um		Abundant, plentiful.
Laridum, lardum		Lard.
Latus, a, um		Broad, wide.
Latus, eris (lateris)		The side, of the side.
Latere admoveatur	Lat. admov.	Let it be applied to the side.
Lateri dolenti	Lat. dol.	To the painful side.
Laxamentum ventris		Purging, evacuating.
Laxus, a, um		Loose, open (app. to astricta).
Lectus, i		A bed, couch.
Leniter		Easily, gently.
Leniter terendo		By rubbing gently.
Leviter		Lightly.
Leviter clausus		Lightly closed.
Linctus, i		A linctus or lohoch.
Linimentum, i		A liniment.
Lintum, i		Lint.
Liquor-oris	Liq.	A liquor.
Luteus, a, um	Lut.	Yellow, golden yellow.
Macera, maceratur, maceruntur	Macer.	Macerate, let it (them) be macerated.
Macera donec refrigerant		Macerate until cold.
Macera per horas tres		Macerate three hours.

Term or Phrase.	Contraction.	Meaning.
Macera per sextum horae partem		Macerate ten minutes (one-sixth part of an hour).
Magnus, a, um	Magn.	Large.
Mane (indecl.)		Morning, in the morning.
Mane bene, mane plane		} Early in the morning.
Mane primo		
Manipulus, i		A handful (bundle).
Manus, i		The hand.
Mare, maris		The sea, of the sea, also sea-water.
Massa, ae	Mass.	A mass.
Matula		A vessel, pot (for liquids).
Matutinus, a, um		In or of the morning.
Medius-a-um	Med.	Midst, middle, medium.
Mensura		By measure.
Mica, ae		A crumb, morsel.
Mica panis	Mic. pan.	Crumb of bread.
Minimum, i	M.	A minim.
Minutum, i		A minute.
Misce, miscetur, miscentur	M.	Mix, let it (them) be mixed.
Misce accuratissime	M. accur.	Mix very intimately.
Misce bene	M. bene.	Mix well.
Misce caute	M. caute.	Mix cautiously.
Miscetur fortiter conquassando		Let it be mixed (with) violent agitation.
Mistura	Mist.	A mixture.
Mitte, mittatur, mittantur		Send, let it (them) be sent.
Mitte tales		Send of such, send like this.
Modicus, a, um		Moderate (sized), middling.
Modo dictu	M. dict.	As directed in the way said.
Modo praescripto	M. p.	As directed or prescribed.
Mollis, is		Soft.
Mora, ae		A delay.
More dictu	Mor. dict.	In the manner said (as directed).
More solitu	Mor. sol.	In the accustomed manner.
Mos, moris		Manner, of manner, custom, work.
Mortarium, i	Mortar.	A mortar.
Natrium, i		Sodium.
Ne tradas sine nummo	Ne. tr. s. n.	Do not deliver unless paid.
Necnon		And also, and yet.
Niger, nigra, nigrum		Black.
Nihilum album	Nihil. alb.	Zinc oxide.
Nisi		Without, unless.
Non		Not.
Non repetatur	Non. rep.	Do not repeat.
Novus, a, um		New, fresh.
Nox, noctis		Night, of the night.
Noxa, ae, or noxia, ae		An injury, hurt.
Nucha		The nape of the neck.
Numerus, i		Number.
Numero	No.	In number.
Nunc		Now.
Nutricius (nutritus) a, um		Nourishing, nutritious.
Nutritus—us		Nourishment.
Nux—nucis		Nut, of a nut.
Obduce, obducatur		Cover or conceal, let it be covered or concealed.
Obductus, a, um		Covered, concealed, coated.
Obtritus, a, um		Crushed.
Occlusus, a, um		Enclosed.

NON-SECRET FORMULAS.

Term or Phrase.	Contraction.	Meaning.
Octarius	O.	A pint.
Octuplus, octuplo	Octup.	Eight-fold,—in eight-fold.
Oculus-i		The eye.
Odoramentum, i	Odoram.	A perfume.
Odoratus, a, um	Odorat.	Odorous, smelling, perfuming.
Odora, odoretur		Perfume, let it be perfumed.
Oleosus, a, um		Oily.
Oleum—sine igne		Cold drawn or pressed—oil.
Olla, ae		A pot, jar.
Ollicula, ae		A little pot.
Omnis		All, every.
Omni hora	Omn. hor.	Every hour.
Omni mane	Omn. man.	Every morning.
Omni nocte	Omn. noct.	Every night.
Optimus, a, um	Opt.	Best.
Opus (indecl.)		Need, necessity.
Oryza		Rice.
Os, oris		The mouth, of the mouth.
Ovi putamen (inis)		An egg-shell.
Ovum, i		An egg.
Pabulum, i		Food, nourishment.
Pallidus, i		Pale, pallid.
Panis, i		Bread.
Pannus, i, pannulus, i		A cloth, rag.
Para, parita, paretur, paratus, i		Prepare, let be prepared, prepared.
Paretur inde		Let be prepared therefrom.
Pars, partis, parti		A part, of the part, to the part.
Pars affecta fricetur		Let the affected parts be rubbed.
Parte affecta fricetur		Rub upon the affected part.
Partes aequales	P. e.	Equal parts.
Partitus, a, um		Divided.
Partitis vicibus		In divided doses.
Parvus, a, um, parvulus, a, um		Little, very little, an infant.
Pastillus, i		A pastille, lozenge.
Paucus, a, um, paucies (adv.)		Little, few, seldom.
Paulatim		Little by little, gradually.
Pectus, oris		The breast.
Penicillum, i, peniculus, i		A pencil, brush, little roll.
Per (prep. w. acc.)		Through, by means of, very.
Peractus, a, um		Finished.
Percalefactus, a, um		Thoroughly heated.
Percola, percolatur		Strain through, percolate, let be strained through.
Perge, pergetur		Proceed with, continue, let be continued.
Perinde		In the same manner, just as.
Perpurus, a, um		Very clean.
Pervesperi (adv.)		Very late in the evening.
Pes, pedis, pedi		The foot, of, to, the foot.
Pessarium, i } Pessulum, i	Pess.	A pessary.
Phiala, ae	Ph.	A phial.
Phiala prius agitata	P. P. A.	The vial having first been shaken.
Pilula, ae		A pill.
Pilus, i		The hair.
Pinguis, is	Ping.	Fat, grease.
Pistillum, i		A pestle.
Placebo		I will satisfy (will please).
Plasma, atis (n.)		A form, figure. (Glycerite of starch.)

Term or Phrase.	Contraction.	Meaning.
Plasma, plasmetur		Mould (thou), let it be moulded.
Plenus, a, um		Filled.
Poculum, i, pocillum, i		A drinking cup, a little cup.
Pondere		By weight.
Pondus, eris, ponderatus, i		A weight, weighing.
Pondus civile		Avoirdupois weight.
Pondus medicinale		Apothecaries' weight.
Post cibo	Post. cib.	After eating.
Postridie		On the next day, the following day.
Potus, us		A drink, a drinking.
Prae (prep. w. abl.)		Before, also very.
Prandium, i	Prand.	Dinner.
Pridie		On the day before.
Primus, a, um		First, earliest, beginning.
Pro (adv. and prep. w. abl.)		For, in favor of, before, according to.
Pro dose		For a dose.
Proprius, a, um		Special, particular.
Pro ratione aetatis		According to the condition of age. i. e., According to the age of the patient.
Pro re nata	P. r. n.	As occasion arises, occasionally, as needed.
Pro potu cathartico		For a cathartic drink.
Proximo	Prox.	Nearest.
Prius (adv.)		Before, former.
Pugillum, i	Pugil.	A pinch.
Pulpa, ae		Pulp.
Pulvis, eris	Pulv.	A powder.
Pulvis grossus	Pulv. gros.	A coarse powder.
Pulvis subtilis or		
Pulvis subtilissimus	Pulv. subtil.	A smooth (very smooth) powder.
Pulvis tenuis or	Pulv. tenn.	An extremely fine.
Pulvis tenuissimus		(Attenuated) powder.
Purgativus, i	Purg.	A cathartic, purging.
Purus, a, um	Pur.	Pure, clean.
Pyxis, idis.		A small box, a pill box.
Quadrans, antis		A fourth, quarter.
Quadrum, i		Square.
Quadruplo		In four-fold, quadruple.
Quam (adv.)		As much as, in what manner.
Quam libet		
Quam (or qua) vis (volueris)	q. v.	As much as you wish.
Quantum libet	q. l.	
Quantum placet	q. p.	As much as you please.
Quantum vis or volueris	q. v.	
Quantum sufficit		
Quantum sufficiat	q. s.	A sufficient quantity.
Quantum satis		
Quaqua hora		Every hour.
Quaque, quisque	q. q.	Each, every.
Quartus, i		Fourth.
Quibus		To or from which.
Qui libet		Any, whatever you please.
Quisquam or quisquis		Anything.
Quoque	q. q.	Also.
Quorum		Of which.
Quotidie		Daily.
Quoties		As often as.
Quoties requiritur		As often as is required.

Term or Phrase.	Contraction.	Meaning.
Rarus, a, um		Loose, thin, rare.
Ratio, onis		Relation, proportion, condition.
Recens, ntis	Rec.	Fresh, recent, newly.
Recipe	R.	Take (thou). A recipe.
Redactus, i	Redact.	Reduced.
Redactus in pulverem	Red. in pulv.	Reduced to powder.
Regio, onis		Region, direction, portion.
Relectus, a, um		Opened, loosened.
Reliquus, i	Reliq.	Remaining, the remainder.
enova, renovetur		Renew, let it be renewed.
Renovetur semel	Renov. semel.	Let it be renewed once only.
Repetatur, repetantur	Rept.	Let it (or them) be repeated.
Res, rei		A thing, object, substance, affair.
Residuus, a, um		Residual, remaining.
Retinetur		Let it be withheld.
Rictus, us		Wide open, distended.
Rigidus, a, um		Rigid, hard, inflexible.
Ruber, rubra, rubrum	Rub.	Red, ruddy.
Rudicula, ae		A spatula.
Rudis, is		A stirring-rod.
Rumen, inis		The throat.
Saccharum saturni		Acetate (sugar) of lead.
Saepis, saepe		Often, frequently.
Sal, salis	Sal.	Salt, also shrewdness.
Sal, amarum		Magnesium sulphate.
Sal mirabile		Sodium sulphate.
Saltem		At least.
Sanguis (inis), sanguineus		Blood, bloody.
Sapor, is		A flavor, delicacy.
Satis, is		Enough, sufficient.
Scapulae, arum		The shoulder blades.
Scatula, ae	Scat.	A box.
Scrupulum, i	Sc. or ℈	A scruple.
Scutum, scuto		Protection, for protection.
Scuto pectori		For protection to the breast.
Secundo		Secondly, in order.
Secundum artem	S. A.	According to art.
Secundum legem	S. L.	According to law.
Semel		Once, a single time.
Semi, semis	ss.	A-half, half.
Semihora		Half hour.
Sensim		Gently, gradually, slowly.
Seorsum		Sundered, apart, separate.
Separatim	Separ.	Separately.
Septimana		A week.
Sero		Late, at a late hour.
Sesuncia		An ounce and a-half.
Sesqui		Once and a-half.
Sesquihora		An hour and a-half.
Sevum, i		Suet, tallow.
Sextans (ntis) sextus		Sixth-part, sixth.
Si		If.
Sic!		So, in this manner, thus.
Sicca, Siccetur		Dry, let it be dried, or drained.
Siccus		Dry, dried.
Signa, signetur	Sig.	Mark, imprint (thou). Let it be imprinted.
Signanter		Clearly, distinctly.

Term or Phrase.	Contraction.	Meaning.
Sile hujus!		Keep (thou) silence concerning this!
Simplex, simplicis	Simp.	Simple, unmixed.
Simul		Together.
Sinapismus, i		A mustard poultice, sinapism.
Sine	s.	Without.
Sine expressione	S. expr.	Without expressing, pressing.
Singillatim, singularis		One by one, singly.
Singulorum	Sing.	Of each.
Si non valeat	Si. n. val.	If it does not answer,—be of value.
Si opus sit	Si. op. sit.	If it be best,—needed.
Si vires permittebant	Si. vir. perm.	If the strength will permit.
Sit		Let it be.
Sit in promptu		Let it be in readiness.
Sitis (is), siti		Thirst, for thirst.
Solatium, ii		Soothing, assuaging.
Solitus, a, um		Accustomed, ordinary.
Solus		Alone, only.
Solve, solvatur	Solv.	Dissolve, let it be dissolved.
Solutus, solutio-onis	Sol. or solut.	Dissolved, solution.
Soluto tandem		To or in the solution finally.
Solve cum leni calore		Dissolve with a little heat.
Somnus		Sleep.
Spiritus vini rectificatus	S. V. R.	Alcohol.
Spiritus vini tenuis	S. V. T.	Proof spirit.
Spissitudo, inis		Thickness, consistency.
Spissus, a, um	Spiss.	Dense, hard.
Statim		Immediately, at once.
Stet, stent		Let it or them stand.
Stibum, i		Antimony.
Stillatim		By drops, in small quantities.
Stilus		A stake, crayon.
Stomachus, i		The stomach, alimentary canal, gullet.
Stratum, i		Layer, stratum.
Suavis		Pleasant, agreeable.
Sub		Under somewhat.
Subactus		Subdued, sinking.
Sub finem coctionis		Toward the end of boiling.
Subigatur, subigantur		Let it (them) be subdued, overcome.
Subinde		Frequently.
Subtilis		Fine, smooth, nice.
Succus, i		Juice, sap.
Suggillationi		To the bruise.
Sume, sumat, sumantur, sumatur, sumendus	Sum.	Take or employ, or consume. Let him take, let it be taken, to be taken.
Sumat talem	Sum. talem	Let the patient take—like this.
Summo mane sumendus		To be taken very early in the morning.
Summus, a, um		Highest, summit.
Super		Above, upon, over.
Superbibe		Drink afterwards.
Suppositoria, ae	Suppos.	A suppository.
Suppositoriae rectales	Suppos. rect.	Rectal suppositories.
Suppositoriae urethrales	Suppos. ureth.	Urethral suppositories.
Tabella, ae	Tab.	A tablet, lozenge.
Talis, is		Of such, like this.
Tam		So far, in so far.
Tandem		At last, finally.
Tantum, i		So much, so many.

NON-SECRET FORMULAS.

Term or Phrase.	Contraction.	Meaning.
Tegmen, or Tegumen, inis		A cover.
Tempus, oris		Time.
Tenuis		Fine, weak, thin.
Tepidus, a, um		Tepid, lukewarm.
Ter		Thrice, three times.
Tere, teretur	Ter.	Rub, triturate. Let it be rubbed.
Teres, etis		Rubbed, smooth, polished.
Tere simul	Ter. sim	Rub (triturate) together.
Testa, ae		A shell.
Testa ovi		An egg shell.
Thion, Thionas, atis		Sulphur, sulphate.
Tinctura thebaica		Laudanum, tincture of opium.
Triplico	Trip.	Triplicate.
Tritura, trituretur	Trit.	Triturate, let it be triturated.
Trochiscus	Troch.	Troche, lozenge.
Tum		Then, next, furthermore.
Turbidus, a, um		Turbid, muddy, not clear.
Tussis, is		A cough.
Tuto		Safety.
Ubi		Where, wherever, whenever.
Ulna, ae		The arm, the elbow.
Ultime, ultima	Ult.	Lastly, at the last.
Ultimo praescriptus	Ult. praesc.	The last ordered.
Una		To one, together.
Uncia, ae		An ounce.
Unctulus, a, um, unctus, a, um		Besmeared, anointed.
Unctus, us		An anointing, anointment.
Unguentum, i	Ung.	Ointment, unguent.
Unguilla, ae		An ointment-box.
Urgens, entis		Pressing, urgent.
Ustus, a, um		Burned.
Ut or uti		That, so that, in order that.
Ut dictum	Ut dict.	As directed.
Utere, utendus, i		Make use of, to be used.
Utendus more solito	Utend. mor. sol.	To be used in the usual manner.
Vapor oris		Steam, vapor.
Vas, vasis		A vessel, utensil, bottle.
Vas vitreum	Vas. vit.	A glass vessel.
Vehiculum, i	Vehic.	A vehicle.
Vel (or ve as a suffix)		Or.
Venenosus, a, um, venenum, i		Poisonous, a poison.
Verus, a, um		True, real, genuine.
Vesper, eris		The evening.
Vesperna, ae		Supper.
Vicis, is, vices		Change, alternation, turns.
Viridis, is, viride, is		Green.
Vis, viris		Strength, vigor, life.
Vitreus, a, um		Of glass, glazed.
Vitrum, i		Glass.
Volatilis, is, volatile	Volat.	Volatile.
Vomitis, onis		Vomiting.

NUMERALS.

Cardinals.		Ordinals.	
Unus.	One.	Primus.	First.
Duo.	Two.	Secundus.	Second.
Tres.	Three.	Tertius.	Third.
Quatuor.	Four.	Quartus.	Fourth.
Quinque.	Five.	Quintus.	Fifth.
Sex.	Six.	Sextus.	Sixth.
Septem.	Seven.	Septimus.	Seventh.
Octo.	Eight.	Octavus.	Eighth.
Novem.	Nine.	Nonus.	Ninth.
Decem.	Ten.	Decimus.	Tenth.
Undecim.	Eleven.	Undecimus.	Eleventh.
Duodecim.	Twelve.	Duodecimus.	Twelfth.
Tredecim.	Thirteen.	Tertius decimus.	Thirteenth.
Quatuordecim.	Fourteen.	Quartus decimus.	Fourteenth.
Quindecim.	Fifteen.	Quintus decimus.	Fifteenth.
Sexdecim.	Sixteen.	Sextus decimus.	Sixteenth.
Septemdecim.	Seventeen.	Septimus decimus.	Seventeenth.
Octodecim or duo de viginti	Eighteen.	Octavus decimus.	Eighteenth.
Novemdecim or un de viginti	Nineteen.	Nonus decimus.	Nineteenth.
Viginti.	Twenty.	Vicesimus.	Twentieth.
Viginti unus or unus et viginti.	Twenty-one.	Vicesimus Primus.	Twenty-first.
Triginta.	Thirty.	Tricesimus.	Thirtieth.
Quadraginta.	Forty.	Quadragesimus.	Fortieth.
Quinquaginta.	Fifty.	Quinquagesimus.	Fiftieth.
Sexaginta.	Sixty.	Sexagesimus.	Sixtieth.
Septuaginta.	Seventy.	Septuagesimus.	Seventieth.
Octoginta.	Eighty.	Octogesimus.	Eightieth.
Nonaginta.	Ninety.	Nonagesimus.	Ninetieth.
Centum.	One hundred.	Centesimus.	Hundredth.

NOMENCLATURE.

(From Scoville's Art of Compounding.)

The temptation to physicians to abbreviate in writing prescriptions makes it necessary that the pharmacist should be thoroughly conversant with chemical nomenclature, particularly in regard to those bodies which are most frequently prescribed as remedies.

A salt or chemical may be known by several names,—its trade or common name, its Latin or scientific name, and in many cases also by a technical or descriptive name.

The common or trade name may have been derived from the names of those who first brought them into notice, as Glauber's or Seignette's salt, or from the place from which they were first obtained, as Epsom or Rochelle salt. The Latin or scientific names designate, in a general way, the chemical composition of the bodies, and when there are a number of salts or bodies which contain the same elements, but in different proportions, more definitely descriptive names may be applied to them to avoid confusion.

Thus, "chloride of mercury" may mean either calomel or corrosive sublimate, but the terms, mild chloride of mercury, and corrosive chloride of mercury, protochloride of mercury and bichloride of mercury are definite, and cannot be confused.

The first of these terms gives a general idea of the salt,—composed of mercury and chlorine; the second distinguishes between the medicinal and physical action of two chlorides which exist, one being "mild," and the other "corrosive;" the third of the terms also distinguishes between the two chlorides, one being the "proto" (first or lowest) chloride, and the other the "bi" (second or higher) chloride.

Unfortunately, no one system of nomenclature is satisfactory for all, and much confusion may arise unless the dispenser understands the principles which underly each system. A single body may have several trade-names, and the Latin title may be thought too long.

The third system attaches certain prefixes or suffixes to the negative (acid) term, which have a constant meaning, and thus distinguish the salt clearly from others of a similar composition. This method may be used for all definite chemical compounds, but if carried out in some cases, ridiculously long words would result, and thus it is not always practical, although very convenient in many cases.

The prefixes and terminations in general use are as follows:

PREFIXES.

Mono (Gr. monos, one). **Proto** (Gr. protos, first).

These are employed to designate a single atom or molecule of acid radical in combination with a base, or the first or lowest number of a series, when more than one proportionate combination is known. Before the names of radicals beginning with a vowel, the final o of these is generally omitted, for the sake of euphony.

Examples.—PbO, Lead monoxide. FeO, Iron monoxide, or protoxide. Fe Cl$_2$, iron protochloride (not monochloride).

Sesqui (Lat. sesqui, one-and-a-half) meaning three atoms or molecules of acid radical to two of basic (since chemistry does not admit of splitting atoms), the ratio being one to one-and-a-half.

Examples.—Fe$_2$O$_3$, Iron sesquioxide (Fe$_2$Cl$_6$ is sometimes called sesquichloride—the chloride of the sesquioxide). Al^{2}O$_3$ Aluminum sesquioxide.

Bi, or **Bin** (Lat. Bis, twice), **Di** (Gr. dis, twice), **Deuto** (Gr. deuteros, second), meaning two, or double, where two molecules of acid radical are combined, or twice as many molecules as there are of the basic radical. Di has also been used to refer to the basic radical in a similar way.

Examples.—HgCl$_2$ mercury biniodide, or deuto iodide, CS$_2$ Carbon disulphite (Pb$_2$O(C$_2$H$_3$O$_2$)$_2$ Lead diacetate).

Ter (Lat. ter, three). **Tri** (Gr. tria, three). Three atoms, or molecules of the basic radical.

Examples.—Au Cl$_3$ gold terchloride. Fe$_2$O$_3$ iron trioxide. As$_2$O$_3$ arsenic trioxide. Fe$_2$(SO$_4$)$_3$ iron tersulphate.

Quadra (Lat. quatuor, or quadrus, four). **Tetra** (Gr. tetratos, fourth), meaning four atoms, or molecules, of acid radical.

Examples.—SnCl$_4$ tetra, or quadrachloride, of tin. PtCl$_4$ tetra-chloride of platinum.

Penta (Gr. penta, five). **Quinque** (Lat. quinque, five), meaning five.

Examples.—PCl$_5$ Phosphorus pentachloride.

Hexa (Gr. hexa, six). **Sex(t)** (Lat. sex, six), meaning six.

Examples.—SI$_6$ sulphur hexaiodide.

Hepta (Gr. hepta, seven). **Sept** (Lat. septa, seven), meaning seven.

Examples.—Cl$_2$O$_7$ chlorine heptoxide.

Poly (Gr. pollos, or polu, many), meaning many equivalents—usually when the exact formula is in doubt, as poly-iodides, many atoms (above three) of iodine combined with a base, etc.

Sub (Lat. sub, under). **Hypo** (Gr. hupo, under, or Lat. hypo, after). Sub refers to the base, and is used to designate salts which are composed of an oxide and another acid radical in varying proportions, or the so-called basic salts. Thus sub-acetate of lead is a combination of lead oxide PbO and lead acetate Pb (C$_2$H$_3$O$_2$)$_2$. Sub-sulphate of iron is an oxy- or basic sulphate, approximating Fe$_2$O(SO$_4$)$_2$ + Fe$_2$(SO$_4$)$_3$ = Fe$_4$O(SO$_4$)$_5$. Bismuth subnitrate Bi O NO$_3$ (approximately). Most of these salts vary in composition, hence their formulas are not included in the Pharmacopœia.

The term hypo refers to the acid radical, and usually indicates the lowest of a series of oxyacid salts.

Examples.—KClO potassium hypochlorite.
KH$_2$PO$_2$ potassium hypophosphite.

Per (Lat. per, above). **Hyper** (Gr. hyper, above). **Super** (Lat. super, above). The contracted form per is mostly used, and indicates the highest of a series of compounds, as contrasted with sub and hypo.

It is used mostly with oxy acids; when it refers to those containing the largest number of atoms of oxygen, the culmination of a series.

Examples.—KClO$_4$ perchlorate of potassium. H$_2$O$_2$ peroxide of hydrogen. Fe$_2$Cl$_6$ perchloride of iron.

Ortho (Gr. orthos, straight). Used to distinguish substances in a normal condition from a modified form of the same, or from others which have been derived from them by heat or other causes.

Example.—H$_3$PO$_4$ Orthophosphoric acid.

Pyro (Gr. pur, fire). Used to designate that the body has been produced by heat (fire). Thus 2H$_3$PO$_4$, or H$_6$P$_2$O$_8$ + heat becomes H$_4$P$_2$O$_7$, pyrophosphoric acid, water (H$_2$O) being driven out.

C$_7$H$_6$O$_5$, gallic acid, heated, becomes C$_6$H$_6$O$_3$ pyrogallic acid, CO$_2$ being driven out.

Meta (Gr. meta, beyond). Used to designate an altered condition, as distinguished from the ortho and pyro (and para) forms.

Thus, $H_4P_2O_7$ + heat becomes $2HPO_3$ metaphosphoric acid, water being driven out.

(The terms ortho, pyro and meta, as applied to inorganic compounds, usually distinguish between forms produced by heat or similar causes.)

Para (Gr. para, from beside, near to, about, etc.). Used with organic compounds, when three bodies having the same chemical composition, but differing in physical properties (solubility, melting and boiling points, etc.) and certain chemical and medicinal properties, are to be distinguished. Such cases are differentiated by the terms ortho, meta, and para.

Examples. — $C_2H_4(OH)_2$ Ortho-dihydroxy-benzol or pyrocatechin.
$C_2H_4(OH)_2$ Meta-dihydroxy-benzol or resorcin.
$C_2H_4(OH)_2$ Para-dihydroxy-benzol or hydrochinon.

Para also designates molecular aggregations of certain organic compounds, as C_2H_4O — aldehyde and $(C_2H_4O)_3$ or $C_6H_{12}O_3$ par aldehyde.

Hydro (Gr. hudor, water), used to designate the binary acids, i. e., those composed of only two elements, the prefix referring then to the hydrogen, as HCl, hydro-chloric acid, H_2S hydro-sulphuric acid.

An (Lat. an, without). De (Lat. de, away from), meaning without or deprived of. Used to denote something which has been removed, therefore, implying that the removed substance usually exists in the body normally.

Examples.—An hydrous, without water (or moisture).
De odorized, deprived of odor.

TERMINATIONS.

Ide, Id, *Uret.—Terminations used with salts composed of a base united to a single element or with cyanogen, as an acid radical, the latter being used mostly with sulphur, phosphorus and cyanogen.

Examples.—KI, potassium iodid(e).
K_2S, potassium sulphid(e), or sulphuret, sulfid.
KCN, potassium cyanid(e), or cyanuret.
H_2S, sulphuretted hydrogen, or hydrogen sulphid(e).
H_4P, phosphuretted hydrogen.

Ous, Ite.—When a series of acids differ only in the proportion of oxygen which they contain, the lower members of the series end in ous and the salts of these in ite.

Ic, Ate.—The highest members of such a series of acids, or those which contain the most oxygen, end in ic, and the salts of these in ate.

Examples.—H_2SO_3, sulphurous acid, K_2SO_3 potassium sulphite.
H_2SO_4, sulphuric acid, K_2SO_4 potassium sulphate.

The following series well illustrates the use of some of these prefixes and terminations:

HCl, hydro-chlor-ic acid. KCl, potassium chloride.
HClO, hypo-chlor-ous acid. KClO, potassium hypo-chlor-ite.
$HClO_2$, chlor-ous acid. $KClO_2$, potassium chlorite.
$HClO_3$, chlor-ic acid. $KClO_3$, potassium chlor-ate.
$HClO_4$, per-chlor-ic acid. $KClO_4$, potassium per-chlor-ate.

Oid (Gr. eidos, resemblance), used to express similarity in character and properties (not in composition).

Examples.—Alkaloid, resembling an alkali.
Crystalloid, resembling a crystal.
Resinoid, resembling a resin.

Ine, In.—In the Pharmacopoeia these terminations are used to distinguish between alkaloids and other proximate principles. All alkaloids end in ine; Latin, ina; while glucosides, neutral principles, etc., end in in; Latin, inum.

Examples.—Morphine. Latin, Morphina.
Quinine. Latin, Quinina.
Picrotoxin. Latin, Picrotoxinum.
Santonin. Latin, Santoninum.

*The latest nomenclature prefers the termination id, and also substitutes f for ph in many cases, as sulfur, fosfate, etc.

VETERINARY REMEDIES.

3480. Condition Powders for Horses, Cattle, &c.   **A**

Ground linseed oil cake	500	pounds.
Powdered antimony	50	pounds.
Powdered fenugreek	50	pounds.
Granulated saltpetre	5	pounds.
Bicarbonate of soda	25	pounds.
Powdered nux vomica	2½	pounds.
Powdered sulphate of iron	16	pounds.
Powdered salt	25	pounds.
Sulphur	50	pounds.

Mix.

Directions.—Give mixed with wetted grain; for ordinary use one tablespoonful with each feed for horses. Horses need not stop work, but should have extra care and attention in stable. For acute diseases' double the dose. Cattle require one and one-half tablespoonfuls. Sheep and hogs, one tablespoonful daily, at night.

This powder is warranted pure. As a general tonic it will be found of benefit to animals out of condition, while in fattening stock it adds to the value of the food by improving the appetite, loosening the skin and making them thrive much faster. As a remedy for epizootic in horses it is very popular. For hog cholera it is far superior to many of the so-called specifics sold. Purifies the blood and removes all humors.

3481. Condition Powders for Horses, Cattle, &c.   **B**

Ground linseed oil cake	100	pounds.
Ground fenugreek	20	pounds.
Ground gentian	10	pounds.
Powdered rosin	10	pounds.
Powdered ginger	5	pounds.
Powdered sulphate of iron	5	pounds.
Powdered salt	10	pounds.

Mix.

Dose: Same as Formula "A."

The ground linseed oil cake in the above formulas is used as a filler or vehicle for the administration of the drugs. Formerly ground mustard hull (mustard bran) was used for this purpose, but of late years ground linseed oil cake has been obtainable at much lower figures than mustard hull; the average price of ground linseed oil cake during the last five years has been eighteen dollars a ton of two thousand pounds delivered F. O. B. on cars.

3482. Condition Food for Horses, Cattle, &c.

Sold as Stock Food.

Ground linseed oil cake	500	pounds.
Ground fenugreek	50	pounds.
Ground anise seed	10	pounds.
Ground ginger, African	5	pounds.
Powdered salt	25	pounds.
Powdered licorice root	10	pounds.

Mix.

This food is sold extensively in stock countries; it has an excellent aroma and will not become wormy.

Linseed meal from the seed would be preferable in condition powders and stock food if for quick sale after mixing, but where the goods remain in stock for a year or over the large quantity of oil in it is objectionable and causes a rancid odor to be emitted from the packages.

3483. Cattle Condiment.

Stock Food.

Ground oil cake	200	pounds.
Miller's shorts	100	pounds.
Ground St. John's bread	100	pounds.
Ground fenugreek	30	pounds.
Ground anise seed	10	pounds.
Powdered salt	20	pounds.
Powdered sulphate of iron	5	pounds.
Powdered African ginger	5	pounds.

Mix.

3484. Harvey's Condition Powders.

Powdered gentian	10	pounds.
Powdered fenugreek	20	pounds.
Powdered ginger	10	pounds.
Powdered licorice	10	pounds.
Powdered nitrate of potash	5	pounds.
Powdered salt	10	pounds.
Ground oil cake	100	pounds.

Mix.

3485. Poultry Powder.

For Chickens, Ducks, Geese, or Turkeys.

Cayenne pepper	5	pounds.
Assafoetida, powdered	2½	pounds.
Fenugreek, powdered	12½	pounds.
Willow charcoal, powdered	10	pounds.
Prepared chalk, ground	25	pounds.
Golden seal, powdered	25	pounds.

Nux vomica, powdered.... 7½ pounds.
Sulphate of iron, powdered 7½ pounds.
Mustard hull, yellow, ground .... 200 pounds.

Directions.—For grown fowls, one or two teaspoonfuls of the powder mixed in meal with a little water. Promptness is essential in administering this remedy, so that the disease does not advance too far before it is used. Give twice a day for 3 or 4 days and then once a day and finally once every other day, until a perfect cure is beyond a doubt.

For all other diseases, such as swelled head, sore throat, etc., proceed as above.

3486. Egg Producing Food.

Air slaked lime............ 100 pounds.
Oyster shells, ground...... 200 pounds.
Cayenne pepper............ 10 pounds.
Venetian red.............. 40 pounds.
Black pepper, ground...... 10 pounds.

Mix.

3487. Worm Powder for Horses.

Pink root, powdered...... 8 ounces.
Jalap, powdered........... 8 ounces.
Santonine, powdered...... 8 ounces.
Wormseed, powdered...... 8 ounces.
Dry salt, powdered........ 16 ounces.
Areca nut, powdered...... 8 ounces.
Cloves, powdered.......... 8 ounces.

Mix.

Dose: One tablespoonful in bran mash.

3488. Aperient Powder for Horses and Cattle.

Buckthorn, powdered...... 1 pound.
Fenugreek, powdered...... 1 pound.
Dried magnesia sulphate... 3 pounds.

Dose two to four ounces.

3489. Hog Powder. A

Venetian red.............. 5 pounds.
Sulphur .... 5 pounds.
Salt, in fine powder, dry.. 5 pounds.
Air slaked lime........... 35 pounds.
Magnesia carbonate....... 2 pounds.
Chalk, precipitated....... 8 pounds.
Soda, bicarbonate........ 5 pounds.

Directions for Use as a Preventive.

Give one teaspoonful in feed to each hog twice a day for three days, and afterwards once a day for a week until danger from infection is past; also give the hogs a little wood charcoal every day with feed.

Directions for Use, as a Cure.

When hogs are sick keep them in a dry, clean place and change the straw often. Give one-quarter of an ounce of this powder at each feed, well mixed with the food. Give appetizing food, but no corn; at the same time feed plenty of charcoal. Give them all the shade they require. Sprinkle their pens well with lime. Remove all manure and offal of every description. Do not allow any stagnant water to stay on the premises. Fill up all the old wallows and sprinkle them plentifully with lime.

3490. Hog Powder. B

Sulphur .... 2 pounds.
Dried sulphate of iron..... 2 pounds.
Air slaked lime........... 8 pounds.
May apple root, powdered.. 1 pound.
Cayenne, powdered........ ½ pound.
Nux vomica, powdered.... ½ pound.
Colocynth, powdered...... ½ pound.
Corn meal................. 2 pounds.

Mix.

Directions for Use as a Preventive: One teaspoonful.

As a Cure: One tablespoonful well mixed with the food. See directions on Formula A.

3491. Constipation Powder for Cattle.

Aloin .... 4 drams.
Ginger .... 1 ounce.
Gentian .... ½ ounce.
Anise .... ½ ounce.

Mix.

3492. Tonic Powder for Pigs and Horses.

Powdered gentian......... 3 drams.
Powdered caraway........ 1 dram.
Powdered licorice......... 1 dram.
Whole coriander.......... ½ dram.
Whole aniseed............ ½ dram.

This quantity for a dose.

3493. Horse Powders.

Sulphur .... 4 drams.
Potass. nitrat............ 1½ drams.
Pulv. gentian............. 1½ drams.
Pulv. fenugreek.......... 1 dram.
Pulv. zingib.............. 1 dram.

M.

This quantity (or a tablespoonful) for a dose.

3494. Pig Powders.

Pulv. pot. nit.	8 ounces.
Sulphur. nig.	8 ounces.
Antim. nig.	8 ounces.
Ferri rubigo.	4 ounces.
P. sem. carui.	2 ounces.
P. sem. anisi.	2 ounces.
P. foenugrec.	16 ounces.

M.

Dose: From a dessertspoonful to a tablespoonful twice or three times a week.

3495. Embrocation for Bruises.

Calamine	½ ounce.
Glycerini	1 ounce.
Liq. ammon.	2 drams.
Aq. rose.	1 ounce.
Aq. ad.	6 ounces.

M.

This should be used internally.

3496. Cough Balls for Horses.

Nitrate of potash, powdered	4½ ounces.
Antimony tart, powdered	2 ounces.
Camphor, powdered	1½ ounces.
Licorice, powdered	3 ounces.
Molasses	q. s.

to make into mass. Divide into 24 balls.

3497. For Insect Bites.

Liq. ammoniae fort.	4 drams.
Collodion	1 dram.
Acid. salicylic.	7 grains.

M.

Apply a few drops to each bite.

3498. Horse Blister.

Cantharides	3 ounces.
Euphorbium resin	1½ ounces.
Amyl acetate	10 ounces.
S. V. R. to	20 ounces.

Macerate for 4 days, filter, and wash the marc with spirit to 1 pint.

3499. K. K. K. Horse Liniment.

Turpentine	4 gallons.
Camphor	½ pound.
Cantharides	½ pound.
Oil cajeput	2 pounds.
Spirits ammonia	2 pounds.

3500. English Horse Liniment.

Oil cajeput	13 ounces.
Spirits ammonia	6½ ounces.
Gum camphor	2 ounces.
Barbadoes tar	1 gallon.
Spirits turpentine	1¾ gallons.
Raw linseed oil	1 gallon.

3501. Wire Fence Liniment.

Acetate lead	10 ounces.
Litharge	7 ounces.
Distilled water	48 ounces.

Boil one-half an hour and stir well; let settle and decant off clear and filter balance. Pour into 2 gallons yellow cotton seed oil, stirring constantly whilst bottling.

3502. Cattle Fattening Powder.

Opium, powdered	1 ounce.
Fenugreek, powdered	6 pounds.
Ginger, powdered	¼ pound.
Salt, powdered	¼ pound.
Gentian, powdered	⅛ pound.
Curcuma, powdered	¼ pound.
Carraway, powdered	¼ pound.

Mix.

Dose: One tablespoonful in feed twice a day.

3503. Spavin Cure.

Tincture iodine	8 ounces.
Alcohol	32 ounces.
Turpentine	32 ounces.
Gum camphor	4 ounces.
Engine oil, neutral	16 ounces.

3504. Pills for Mange in Dogs.

Arsenic	1 grain.
Ferri sulphat.	1 dram.
Ext. gentian	1½ drams.

M.

Divide in 24 pills.

3505. Dog Pills for Distemper.

Jalap, powdered	2 drams.
Soc. Aloes, powdered	2 drams.
Calomel	2 drams.
Simple syrup	q. s.

to make 24 pills.

3506. Mixture for Distemper in Dogs. A

Antim. tart.	4 grains.
Sodii sulphatis	1 ounce.
Dec. aloes co. conc.	1 ounce.
Aquae ad	8 ounces.

M.

Dose: A tablespoonful, more or less, according to the size of the dog, every morning.

3507. Mixture for Distemper in Dogs. B

Chlorate of potash......... 2 drams.
Liquor ammon acet........ 1 ounce.
Spirits of nitrous ether.... 2 drams.
Tinct. hyoscyamus .... 2 drams.
Water........q. s. to make 4 ounces.
 Mix.

Dose: One to 2 teaspoonfuls three times a day.

3508. Poultry Spice.

To act as a general tonic and to stimulate the production of eggs during cold weather:

Powdered licorice .... 6 ounces.
Powdered gentian......... 1 dram.
Powdered capsicum........ 1 dram.
Powdered fenugreek....... 2 ounces.
 Mix.

"Directions for Use: One teaspoonful for eight to ten full-grown fowls and chickens proportionally, to be given three to five times a week with the morning meal. These powders will also be found beneficial to young poultry, when wanted for the table, by giving them a keen appetite. Should an overdose be given it will not injure the birds, but the stated quantity is best. They help the fowls to produce eggs in the coldest weather, and also when kept in confinement eggs are produced in abundance."

3509. Feed for Canaries.

Dried yolk of egg.......... 2 ounces.
Bruised poppy-seed........ 1 ounce.
Cuttlefish-bone .... 1 ounce.
Powdered sugar............ 1 ounce.
Fenugreek .... 1 ounce.
Capsicum .... 4 ounces.
 Mix.

3510. Parrot Seed.

Hemp seed................ ½ pint.
Millet seed ... . ½ pint.
Oats .... ½ pint.
Grd. Indian corn.......... ½ pint.
Canary seed.............. 1 pint.

3511. Mocking Bird Food.

Lean raw beef or ox heart 5 pounds.
Hemp seed................ 4 pounds.
Corn meal (yellow)........ 2 pounds.
Baker's bread............. 2 pounds.

First. Cook the meat cut into small pieces and dry in the oven until brittle (about four hours); grind coarsely.

Second. Slice the bread thin and toast yellow and dry; grind coarsely.

Third. Grind hemp seed and mix altogether.

This makes a good food that may be eaten freely. Occasionally mix some grated raw carrot with the food.

3512. Cough Powder for Horses. A

Useful in the simple coughs of horses depending on catarrh:

Pulv. camphorae.......... 3 drams.
Potass. chlorat........... 1½ ounces.
Pulv. fol. belladon........ 1½ ounces.
Pulv. anisi............... 2 ounces.

Div. in pulv. 6.
Give one twice a day in the food.

3513. Cough Powder for Horses. B

For chronic cough in the horse the following are good:

Pulv. fol. aconiti.......... 6 drams.
Pulv. digitalis............ 4 drams.
Arsenic. alb............. 4 grains.
Pulv. anisi............... ½ ounce.

Div. in pulv. 6.
Give one every night in the food.

3514. Cough Mixture for Dogs.

Tr. belladonnae............ ½ ounce.
Syr. scillae............... ½ ounce.
Tr. camph. co............ 1 ounce.
Aq. ad................... 6 ounces.
 M.

Give two teaspoonfuls three times a day.

3515. Colic Draught for Horses. A

For Simple Colic.

Chlorodyni .... 2 ounces.
Spt. aether. nit........... 2 ounces.
Ol. lini.................. 1 pint.
 M.

Give at one dose, and repeat in two hours, if necessary.

3516. Colic Draught for Horses. B

For Flatulent Colic.

Creolin .... ½ ounce.
Ol. terebinth............. 2 ounces.
Spt. ammon. arom........ 2 ounces.
Tr. assafoetidae.......... 2 drams.
Ol. lini.................. 1½ pints.
 M.

For one dose.

3517. Draught for Hoven in Cattle.

Creolin .... 1 ounce.
Ol. terebinth.............. 4 ounces.
Spt. ammon. arom......... 4 ounces.
Ol. lini................... 1½ pints.

M.

For one dose.

3518. Influenza in Horses.

Chlorodyni .... 1 ounce.
Spt. aether. nit........... 2 ounces.
Liq. ammon. acet.......... 2 ounces.
Aq. ad.................... 15 ounces.

M.

This dose is to be given every three hours during the first stage, when much shivering is evident.

3519. Throat Liniment.

Ol. terebinth.............. 1 ounce.
Liq. ammon. fort.......... 1 ounce.
Ol. olivae................. 1 ounce.

M.

3520. Stimulating White Liniment.

Ol. terebinth.............. 16 ounces.
Camphorae .... 1 ounce.
Saponis mollis .... 2 ounces.
Aq. destil. ....2 ounces vel q. s.

Mix the soap with the water; dissolve the camphor in the turpentine; mix the two, and bring down to the desired consistency with water.

3521. Ointment for Grease and Cracked Heels.

Sulphur. subl.............. 1 ounce.
Plumbi acetat............. ½ ounce.
Creolin .... ½ ounce.
Ol. eucalypti............. ½ ounce.
Vaselini .... 4 ounces.
Lanolini .... 4 ounces.

M. Ft. ung.

Apply twice daily.

3522. Fly Blister.

Pulv. cantharidis.......... 20 ounces.
Ol. terebinth.............. 12 ounces.
Acid. acet. fort........... 9 ounces.
Lanolini .... 2½ pounds.
Vaselini .... 2½ pounds.

Mix the first three, and allow to stand for twenty-four hours; then add the lanoline and vaseline, melted on a water-bath, and mix well, stirring until cold.

3523. Healing Lotion for Horses.

Healing lotion for horses, suitable for sprains, bruises, sore throats, cuts, and wounds:

Solution of lead.......... 1 ounce.
Essential oil of camphor or
  cheap eucalyptus oil..... 4 ounces.
Vinegar .... 7 ounces.
Sesame oil to............. 20 ounces.
Yolks of two fresh eggs.

Rub the yolks in a mortar, add gradually the sesame oil mixed with essential oil, then the vinegar, and lastly the solution of lead.

The oil may be colored with alkanet if considered advisable.

3524. Remedy for Veterinary Purposes.

Remedy for veterinary purposes, suitable for horses, cattle, sheep, etc., for colic, colds, scour, pain after calving, lambing, &c.:

Tr. opii.................. 1 ounce.
Tr. hyoscyam............. 1 ounce.
Spt. aether. nit.......... 1 ounce.
Sodae bicarb............. 6 drams.
Pulv. zingiber........... 2 drams.
Aq. camph. ad........... 6 ounces.

Mix. Label "Shake the bottle."

For horses—Colic: One-half for a dose, repeat in one or two hours if necessary. For colds: One-half at night, and a hot mash some time after. For cattle—one ounce to 1½ ounces for a dose. Sheep and calves, 2 teaspoonfuls to 1 tablespoonful in the case of scour, to be given in rice and cold water stirred together twice a day.

3525. Colic Drench for Horses.

Ext. cannabis indicae..... 1 dram.
Spirit .... 1 ounce.
Ol. terebinth............. ½ ounce.
Ol. menth. pip...........20 minims.
Sol. aloes (1 in 4) ad..... 4 ounces.

Dissolve the extract in the spirit, add the oils, and make up with the aloes solution.

3526. Cough Powder for Horses.

Pulv. potass. nit......... 2 ounces.
Pulv. glycyrrhiz.......... 4 ounces.
Pulv. scillae............. 1 ounce.
Pulv. gentian............ 1 ounce.

M. et div. in pulv. 12.

A powder with breakfast and supper, and one to be mixed with the contents of the nose-bag for day use.

VETERINARY TREATISE.

From the London Chemist and Druggist's Diary.

To provide matter which should be valuable not only to the country chemist, but also to his urban brother, has been the mark kept constantly in sight during the compilation of these notes. We believe that the notes on the diseases of pets, and of the smaller domestic animals, will, to an appreciable extent, secure this object. We trust, too, that the most experienced of our readers will find here some new ideas, and we wish to warn the tyro that the mere perusal of these notes will not make him an experienced veterinarian. Like all other things worth having a sound knowledge of veterinary practice costs time and patience, and those who cannot devote weeks and months to a course of study under men who make it their business to lighten the difficulties of the road must be prepared to expend more time and energy to obtain the same results.

We should strongly advise inexperienced readers to obtain some good standard work on the diseases of the horse or of cattle, and to begin to study it with the determination first to find it intensely interesting, and then to master it. Neither object is impracticable. It is difficult and invidious to select standard works for mention, and we disclaim beforehand all thought of making the list complete or satisfactory. New and revised editions have just appeared of two works whose names have long been household words—Blaine's "Veterinary Art," and Clater's "Cattle Doctor." There is a compendium work by Woodruffe Hill, and an anonymous work on the horse has recently appeared from the house of Cassell & Co. Tegetmeier and Piper seem the leading authorities on poultry and other domestic birds. Youatt's works are classical; Finlay Dunn, and Tuson are names well-known to all our readers.

The formula given at the end of the notes are not mere untried recipes; they come from the note books of experienced and intelligent men, and we can claim for them that any failure to produce the desired results will be the fault of the manipulation, not of the formula.

The notes themselves have been compiled partly from the valuable series of articles contributed to The Chemist and Druggist some twelve years ago by Mr. W. Hunting, M. R. C. V. S., and these have been supplemented from various sources, English and foreign. The whole has been supervised by an eminent veterinary surgeon.

HORSES.

3527.

Administration of Medicines. — Powders must have no disagreeable taste, nor any marked odor, except a few vegetable aromatics like coriander, caraway, and anise. They are best mixed with damp food.

Draughts are the only possible form of administering some remedies. When the head is raised to administer them, the animal, in cases of sore throat, is apt to cough and allow part of the draught to enter the windpipe. Horses can retain fluids in the mouth a long time without swallowing, and in this way sometimes reject medicine.

Electuaries made by mixing the remedy with honey or treacle are the best form of medicine for sore throats. They should be smeared on the tongue.

Balls are the handiest form, and ensures the ingestion of the whole dose. They should be cylindrical, not more than 1 inch in diameter and 2½ inches long. In cases of sore throat they should never be given, as they irritate the part and may be coughed back into the nose, whence it is extremely difficult to remove them. Nearly all balls are thoroughly dissolved in the stomach in less than half an hour.

3528.

Apoplexy affects horses employed in agricultural labor during the heats of summer. The animal falls as if struck by lightning, it lies without any sign of life but the heaving of the flanks and copious perspiration. Death follows quickly. Treatment, to be successful, must be very prompt. Remove the patient to a cool spot; douche the head with plenty of water, very cold or mixed with a little vinegar; let blood, and repeat this if the horse is young and fat; curry it vigorously; administer drinks and an enema of nitre. When the symptoms are modified, give purgatives and diaphoretics.

3529.

Ascites, or Abdominal Dropsy, appears gradually; shows itself by the swelling of the belly and members, and above all by the fluctuation of the collected fluid. It often follows pleurisy. When accompanied by symptoms of inflammation of the bowels it demands antiphlogistic treatment, otherwise we must endeavor to increase the secretions. Diuretics should be given with ammonia and aromatic infusions, and the skin well and repeatedly curried. Puncture succeeds in very few cases.

3530.

Bleymes, bruises, and other accidents or injuries to the foot and coronet are of frequent occurrence in the horse, both in the front and hind feet. They result from treads, overreaches, being run over in crowded thoroughfares, or as in railway horses, which are frequently injured by getting entangled in the points, switches, and metal bars of the lines. The best treatment is to physic, give sloppy food, and, for a time, no corn. Remove the horse's shoe, and let it remain off, pare out the foot, well poultice the foot with warm bran, keep the animal perfectly still and quiet until the lameness disappears.

3531.

Capped Elbows occur on the point of the ulna, and are caused by the animal lying on the rough sharp heel of the shoe. Treatment: Give purging medicine, and apply friction to the parts affected, with a stimulating liniment. If the case will not yield to the treatment, it may be necessary to blister the parts. In the case of capped elbows, have the horse shod short at the heels, and the shoes made smooth and rounding.

3532.

Capped Hocks are caused by injuries to the points of the hocks in the hind legs, causing a fluctuating tumor.

3533.

Catarrh is inflammation of the mucous membrane, accompanied by excessive secretion of mucus.

3534.

Cold in the Head is inflammation of the mucous membrane of the nose, with discharge from the nostrils. The animal is at first slow and drowsy in its movements, the skin is dry, the membrane of the nose redder than usual, the mucous secretion, temporarily arrested, becomes more abundant, and is at first watery and limpid, falling in drops, then white and viscid, falling in flakes. The disease lasts 15 or 20 days; if longer there is fear that it will become chronic. In slight cases the animal should be kept from draughts, damp, and cold, frequently rubbed down, and covered with care. The food should be reduced, warm mucilaginous drinks given, and the nostrils fumigated with steam. When the inflammation is severe with fever, redness of the mouth, and injection of the conjunctiva, the horse must be bled, dieted, soothing electuaries and emollient enemas should be administered.

3535.

Corns are quite unlike those of men. They occur at the angle of the sole between the outer wall and frog, and are bruises of the sensitive structures within the hoof, the result of uneven pressure of the shoe. The discolored horn is merely a symptom like that seen in our own nails when injured. Short shoes, or shoes fitted to leave at the extremity of the heel a space without bearing, are almost sure to produce corns.

Treatment: When the bruise is so severe or old standing as to have caused the formation of matter, and never in any other case, the horn should be cut away to allow the escape of the pus. If the wound is in a healthy state a little pledget of tow, dipped in tar, should be placed over it and the shoe readjusted, care being taken to place no pressure on the wall near the injury.

If matter is not present never cut away the blood-stained horn. It will take at least six weeks to replace it. Remove the shoe, foment the foot for three or four hours, then carefully replace the shoe, taking a level bearing throughout. If possible give rest for a day or two.

3536.

Coughs arise from a variety of causes, such as irritation of the larynx, air-tubes, or lung; pneumonia, pleurisy, and some nervous derangements. The treatment must vary with the cause, and the cause must be discovered by the other symptoms.

Irritation producing cough may result from the presence of foreign bodies, or mucus, when the foreign body must be removed and expectorants may be given; or it often arises without the presence of obstructions of any kind, but simply from inflammation of the sentient respiratory nerves. Expectorants should not be given in such cases.

3537.

A. Irritation of the Larynx.—(1) Acute: Symptoms.—Cough loud and hard, soon becoming softer as the membrane is covered with purulent mucus. Swallowing is difficult; even water being returned through the nose.

Treatment: Avoid dry, hard food. Balls are nearly certain to be coughed back, and often lodge in the nose. Draughts require the head to be raised in a way favorable to choking. Electuaries are the best form of medicine. Place a roll of flannel in hot water, wrap it round the throat, and cover it with some waterproof substance. Keep the bowels open, and use one of the following electuaries:

I.

Camphor	4 drams.
Ext. belladonnae	4 drams.
Acid. acetic. dil.	2 ounces.
Mellis seu theriacae	10 ounces.

A tablespoonful twice daily to be smeared on the tongue.

II.

Tannin	2 drams.
Spirit. vini rect.	2 ounces.
Mellis	10 ounces.

To be given as above.

3538.

(2) Chronic:—Symptoms: Cough loud and hard, but not frequent, occurring chiefly when the animal is changed from the stable to the fresh air, or vice versa. No general symptoms.

Treatment: Give a cough ball, such as one of the following:

I.

Opii pulv.	½ dram.
Scillae pulv.	1 dram.
Aloes pulv.	1 dram.

Make into a ball with common mass or linseed-meal and treacle. One every day.

II.

Camphor	½ dram.
Opium	½ dram.
Digitalis	½ dram.

Made as above. One every day.

III.

Ext. belladonnae	1 dram.
Ext. hyoscyami	1 dram.
Ipecacuanhae	1 dram.

Made and given as above. A seton may be placed in the throat, and the animal allowed easy work if the weather is open.

3539.

B. Bronchitis, or Inflammation of the Lining Membrane of the Air-tube. Symptoms: Cough harsh and wheezing, accompanied by a loud, rough noise in the windpipe.

Treatment: (1) General, as in simple fevers; (2) Local. Protect the neck and chest with rugs, and in chronic cases apply a blister. Give the following:

Camphor	1 dram.
Digitalis	½ dram.
Potass. nitr.	1½ drams.

Make into a ball with linseed-meal and treacle. One to be given every day.

3540.

Pneumonia and Pleurisy are serious diseases, which require professional treatment.

3541.

Broken Wind.—Cough short, loud, hollow, with double-action of the flanks in respiration. The diet must be of the best quality. Avoid bulky, innutritious food, and, above all, mouldy or dusty hay. Linseed boiled, and given cold with the corn at night, is excellent in some cases. The two useful medicines are arsenic and creasote. Give arsenic in 3-grain doses daily, or creasote in ½-dram doses made into a ball with linseed and treacle. When they offer them for sale, horsecopers "load" broken-winded animals by giving them a mixture of shot and tallow, or a pint of olive oil half an hour before showing them.

3542.

Cracked Heels are commonest in wet weather among low-bred horses with round shanks, which are also the most liable to thrush and cracks at the back of the knee and front of the hock. The cracks of the hock, knee, and heel vary from a small split to a large wound, accompanied by swelling of the leg and lameness. For mild cases use ointment of carbonate or oxide of zinc. Bad cases, with swelling and suppuration, will require warm fomentation or a poultice for a night, followed by a lotion of zinc sulphate (½ dram to 1 ounce) with a few drops of carbolic acid. When the sore is fairly dry use zinc ointment. A few diuretic balls will help the case.

3543.

Cystitis—Inflammation of the Bladder.—Symptoms: Frequent movements of the hind legs and attempts to urinate, thirst, movements of the tail; the horse turns to look at its flanks. Bleed slightly twice; give mucilaginous drinks and clysters, and apply a poultice of boiled bran to the loins. The bladder may be emptied by carefully passing the hand into the rectum and pressing gently downwards with the whole surface of the hand. As the patient improves give bitter decoctions with nitre. When the inflammation is due to stone in the bladder, this may be removed by operation.

3544.

Diarrhoea ordinarily cures itself. If it becomes serious the horse should be put on mashes, bled, and emollient enemas administered. After a day or two give 1½ ounces of a mixture of

Juniper berries............ 4 parts.
Rhubarb................... 2 parts.
Ginger .... 1 part.

If the diarrhoea follows indigestion give some warm ale and reduce work and food for a few days.

Diarrhoea, when it results from inflammation of the intestines, is somewhat serious. The evacuations are mucous, and more or less fetid; there is much thirst and little appetite; strength and health gradually fail. The evacuations are discharged without apparent pain, and mostly while at work. Bleeding must be resorted to if the inflammation is acute; solid food must be withheld in part; emollient drinks may be given, or a drench containing opium or extract of poppies; enemas of decoction of linseed, small in bulk, should be given. As the disease diminishes the ordinary diet may be resumed.

3545.

Chronic Diarrhoea is not helped by bleeding. The skin must be kept active by grooming and covering; the food should be digestible and given in small quantities at a time; work should be light, and the water the horse drinks looked to. As the diarrhoea lessens, a little parched barley or a few beans may be mixed with the oats.

3546.

Dysentery shows itself as gripes, acute pain in the belly, and violent and frequent efforts to expel excrement, which is sometimes bloody. It should be treated like acute enteritic diarrhoea.

3547.

Eczema is of two kinds, simple and acute or malignant; the latter sometimes develop into ulcers. The first symptom is the dull, rough, discolored coat, always covered with powdery dust, which seems to renew itself as often as it is removed by the currycomb; afterwards are formed pustules of different kinds, purulent pimples, crusts, sometimes dry, sometimes moistened with an acrid, stinking discharge, finally with ulceration of the skin and itching, so violent that the horse flays itself by rubbing against surrounding objects.

It is almost always enough in simple cases to groom the horse with care, and to give a gentle purge, if necessary. In severe cases bleed the horse, purge once or twice, soften the skin by emollient lotions (decoctions of mallow or linseed) applied for two or three days; then rub the affected parts once daily with citrine ointment; immediately after give a bran mash with 2 ounces of powdered guaiacum-wood, and keep the animal warm. The ointment should be washed off with soap and water before each fresh application. If the disease is inveterate the animal should, in addition, be treated as in farcy. A lotion of equal parts of liquid arsenicalis and camphorated spirits applied twice or thrice daily is very efficacious.

3548.

Enteritis, or Inflammation of the Bowels.—When it appears suddenly it is super-acute. It is accompanied by extremely severe pain in the belly; the horse is much agitated and moves incessantly, stamps its feet, paws the ground, looks at its belly, lies down and rises suddenly; the breathing is rapid and short, the nostrils dilated, the eyes anxious; the body is covered with sweat, the pulse is full and accelerated; the bowels are confined, the urine often reddish and passed with difficulty; the pain continually increases without a moment's pause, and often causes death. If the animal is entire inguinal hernia must be looked for, and, if present, treated surgically. The animal must be bled repeatedly. Tepid mucilaginous decoctions must be given as drinks, with emollient enemas, and very scanty diet; grooming and gentle exercise are auxiliaries. Inflammation of the bowels often simulates diarrhoea, which see.

3549.

Farcy.—One of the diseases on the lists of the Contagious Diseases (Animals) Acts, 1878. Any person being in possession of an animal affected with farcy, or a disease supposed to be farcy, must give notice to the nearest police constable, or to the veterinary inspector of the district in which the animal is.

It resembles glanders in contagiousness and its fatal effects in man. There are enlarged glands fixed to the jawbone, no ulcers or discharge from the nostrils, but small swellings or "buds" down the inside of the limbs, along the side of the flanks, and on the neck, varying in size from a pea to a walnut, at first hard and painful, sometimes becoming softer, and finally discharging their purulent matter. The advent of the attack is usually attended by lameness and fever.

Treatment should consist in the administration of copper biniodide, cantharides or arsenic as tonics, to be continued for a lengthened period, as powders with the food. Giving balls is most dangerous to the operator. One of the following forms may be used once daily:

I.
Pimentae pulv	2 drams.
Cupri sulph	½ dram.
Zinci sulph	½ dram.
Canth. pulv	5 grains.

II.
Canthar. pulv	5 grains.
Ac. arsenios	10 grains.
Ferri sulph	2 drams.

III.
Gentianae pulv	2 drams.
Canthar. pulv	5 grains.
Cupri diniod	½ dram.

As soon as the "buds" contain matter they should be laid open and dressed with strong carbolic acid, which generally dries up and disperses the swelling quickly. While the buds are not discharging the animal is not dangerous as a centre of contagion, and is useful for work if the worst symptoms are subdued. According to the French, a liniment of 9 parts olive oil and 1 part liquid plumbi diacet. should be applied to the buds to accelerate the formation of matter. Meanwhile give one of the following balls, night and morning:

Calomel	1 ounce.
Ammoniacum	2 ounces.
Asafoetida	2 ounces.
Hard soap	4 ounces.
Honey	q. s.

To be made into eight balls. This should be exchanged every four days for a simple purge of calomel, aloes, and soap. Give with each ball barley-water with some powdered juniper. If the treatment causes too much irritation suspend it for a day.

3550.

Fever is indicated by increased heat, rapid pulse and breathing, with arrested secretion and excretion. It is frequently caused by cold, and is known as influenza; it then runs a definite course, and terminates in a quick return to health. When complicated by derangements of the air-tubes or of the digestive apparatus, it is known as catarrhal, gastric, or bilious fever.

In the first stages a stimulant must be given, followed shortly by a diuretic. The following combination may be used:

Etheris	1½ ounces.
Sp. pimentae	3 ounces.
Liq. ammon. acet. conc.	1½ ounces.

A wineglassful, when required, in as much water; to be repeated in two or three hours, if necessary. An ordinary dose of aloes must not be given during violent fever, as it is apt to cause superpurgation. Four ounces of linseed oil or Epsom salts are sufficient. Ammonium carbonate may be given twice daily in 2-dram doses. The body should be well clothed, fresh air and cold water allowed freely, and green food, boiled barley, and linseed given as laxative foods.

3551.

Founder, or Fever in the Feet, is a disease of the horse's foot, in which the sensitive layer immediately within the hoof is congested or even inflamed. It is commonly caused by overwork, such as a long journey on a hard road, or hard work in horses out of condition.

Symptoms: First, frequent shiftings of the feet, and signs of pain, as quickened breathing and pulse. Next, fear of raising one foot lest extra weight be thrown on the other, with swaying of the body backwards and forwards without the feet being moved. If force is used the animal moves as though his back was injured, and puts the heel most markedly on the ground. When the fore feet alone are affected, as is usually the case, the hind feet are drawn forward under the belly, so as to lighten the weight on the others. The affected feet are hotter than usual, and throbbing is felt above the coronet.

Treatment: Never bleed. Give a dose of physic, remove the animal to a smooth, hard-bottomed loose-box, with a light covering of clean straw. The shoes must be removed. Give a good broad bearing-surface with the rasp, but leave the sole untouched. If the foot is level when the shoes are removed lower the toe and heels a little, to produce a sort of rocking surface. This relieves the pressure on the front of the foot, which is the part most affected. Use warm fomentations till the acute pain subsides, but no longer. Then use hand-rubbing to the limbs, and give gentle walking exercise. When the shoes are replaced fit them to the rounded surface of the foot, and leave the sole as strong as possible. Simple cases generally recover in a week, or at most two. Some cases are very tedious, and result in "pumiced foot"—a permanent incurable deformity; careful shoeing will keep sound even such animals.

The French recommend bleeding from the jugular, repeated if necessary; removal of the shoes, bathing in running water, astringent poultices of soot and vinegar, or clay with a strong solution of iron sulphate; scarification of the coronet, and friction with oil of spike on the hocks. If the disease is long standing use emollient poultices and rasp the wall of the hoof; but this rarely succeeds.

3552.

Glanders and farcy run a slow course in horses, but are speedily fatal to man and other animals, to whom they can be communicated. Cases of glanders must be reported to the authorities. See farcy.

3553.

Glanders is distinguished by the discharge from the nose of thin sticky matter, generally from one nostril. The lining membrane of the nose is ulcerated in one or more places, sometimes to perforation of the septum. The glands inside the lower jaw on the same side as the nasal discharge, are indurated, the swelling being circumscribed and fixed to the jawbone. The presence of the discharge, ulceration, and fixed swelling prove the existence of glanders. The chances of cure are small, and the risk to human life very great, so that all well-marked cases should at once be killed. Treatment, if decided on, should consist in frequently washing out the nose with a solution of potassium permanganate or carbolic acid. Feeding must be liberal.

3554.

Grease is a skin disease affecting the legs, and commonest among heavy cart-horses. It varies in extent from a small wet-looking spot covered with short broken hairs, to a red, painful, granulating surface with a stinking discharge, covering the leg, and if not checked in its progress will form into swellings, grouped together in clusters; and when it has reached this stage it is commonly called "Grapes." It may be prevented in a great measure by having the legs washed with warm water, and well dressed with a sponge first, finishing with a towel; the legs should then be bandaged with flannel. It should be dressed daily with the following lotion: Sulphates of zinc, copper, and iron, of each 1 pound, dissolved in 1 gallon of boiling water, with the addition of 4 ounces of carbolic acid. Keep the animal at work, except during the first two or three days. If the leg swells stop the application for a day and give a purgative. The following is another treatment: Prepare the animal by dieting, enemas, bathing, and emollient poultices, and, if the pain is severe, by bleeding. Then make the legs clean, shave off the hair if necessary, and bathe the parts several times a day with Goulard's water. Towards the end of the case substitute a lotion of warm aromatic wine or camphorated spirit in which some soap is dissolved. Setons should be inserted in the chest if the fore legs, or in the buttocks if the hind legs, are attacked. Bitters and sudorifics, combined with antimonials, should be given internally, such as powdered gentian with kermes mineral, guaiacum wood with diaphoretic antimony. The cure will be completed with one or two purgations.

3555.

Gripes, or Colic.—Symptoms: The name is applied vaguely to all cases of abdominal pain, but is here limited to cases of indigestion, accompanied by pain, pulse never hard, nor exceeding 44 beats a minute; pain violent, but with periods of remission.

Treatment: Do not allow the animal to be trotted about. Tobacco, opium, and turpentine must never be given. Turn the horse into a loose-box, prevent its lying on its back or rolling over by the judicious use of the whip. Administer a draught composed of 1 ounce each of sp. aeth. nit., sp. pimentae, and tr. belladonnae, in 1 pint of warm water, and repeated in half an hour if necessary. A physic ball should be given a day or so later. Injections of clean tepid water should also be used, care being taken to introduce the fluid gently, so as not to provoke rapid expulsion.

3556.

Hoof Ointments are necessary to keep in good order the feet of all horses that are shod. They must be thick enough not to spill if upset; not sticky, dark in color, and easily washed off. There are two classes: (1) Those which are used for bad feet as a protecting agent, and contain no saponifying ingredient.

I.

Barbadoes tar............ }
Burgundy pitch.......... } Equal parts.
Russian tallow........... }

II.

Stockholm tar............ 2 pounds.
Russian tallow........... 1 pound.
Venice turpentine........ ½ pound.

In each case melt together the last two ingredients, then add and thoroughly mix the tar.

(2) Those used regularly as preventives and beautifiers.

I.

Stockholm tar............ 3 pounds.
Soft soap................ 4 pounds.
Fish oil................. ½ pint.

II.

Stockholm tar............ 4 pounds.
Soft soap................ 4 pounds.
Tallow................... 2 pounds.
Fish oil................. 1 pint.

The latter is of better consistence. Soft soap by itself tends to make the hoof brittle.

3557.

Jaundice, or the Yellows, is indicated by a marked yellow coloration of the white of the eyes, and the mucous membrane of the mouth and the nostrils; the urine is deep yellowish brown, the faeces hard and dry; the horse is constipated, dull, and heavy, and loses its appetite. Do not bleed unless you want to kill the patient; administer two or three enemas in the evening of the same day; give next day a purge, which should be repeated once or more at intervals of some days. Give as the ordinary drink a decoction of the root of asparagus or strawberry with 1 ounce of nitre and several handfuls of barley-meal; and when the purgative is not administered give, night and morning, ½ ounce to 1 ounce of powdered rhubarb, either in a ball or mixed with wine; bran or barley-meal, chopped straw, and carrots should form the bulk of the food.

3558.

Mud fever occurs in wet weather. There are simple febrile symptoms coincident with an eruption on the skin of the legs and belly, or on those parts most exposed to the splashing of the mud. This may, to a great extent, be prevented by never having the legs washed when dirty, but allowing the mud to dry on, and then carefully brushing it off. As horses that have been recently clipped are more susceptible to it than others, it is a good plan to leave the hair on all the legs. Have the animal thoroughly cleaned, and if feverishness is marked give 1 ounce each of spirit of nitrous ether and solution of ammonium acetate; if necessary repeat in 12 hours. If there are any swellings caused by the friction of the bellyband or martingale give daily for a week 2 drams each of rosin and nitre made into a ball with linseed-meal and soft soap.

3559.

Open Joints.—These are openings through the tissues which allow the escape of the joint oil or synovia. Treatment: The motion of the joint must be limited for a time by splints or otherwise. The escaping synovia must be coagulated so as to form a plug and stop the opening. For this purpose the best applications are (1) silver nitrate applied in the solid form, and (2) corrosive sublimate in solution (1 dram in 1 ounce spirits of wine) applied with a feather. Care must be taken not to introduce them into the joint, but merely to touch the escaping synovia. Never remove the plug of coagulated synovia from the opening when dressing a case. The following form for open-joint powder is not so good as the two remedies mentioned, as albumen is re-dissolved by alum in excess.

Alum.................. ⎫
Ferri sulph............. ⎬ Equal parts.
Myrrh................. ⎭

Finely powder and sprinkle on the part.

3560.

Ophthalmia begins suddenly, with an extra flow of tears, partial closure of the eyelids, and intolerance of light; the eyelids may become swollen, and the watery discharge assume a purulent form. In examining the eyeball the horse's head must not be exposed to a bright light, as he then resists any separation of the lids. In a moderate light the lids are voluntarily separated a short distance if the case be mild and the head left free. When necessary to open the lids with the finger and thumb, the globe of the eye must not be pressed, as this forces forward the haw and spoils the view. On exposing the eyeball, the white part is seen to be bloodshot, the iris may be dim or quite cloudy, the inside of the eyelids is bright red.

Treatment: First make sure that no oat-husk or hay-seed is concealed under the lid. It will generally be found at the upper and outer corner of the top lid, and must be speedily removed. The following is an effectual though rough method, which is better than the unskillful use of forceps. Cover the forefinger with a fold of a silk handkerchief, place it under the upper lid at its inner part, then pass it with a circular motion, outwards, downwards, and back to the inner corner by the lower surface of the globe.

When once the eye is bloodshot, warm fomentation should be persevered in for at least an hour, and repeated for half an hour three or four times a day. An anodyne of 1 part of laudanum to 16 parts of water may be applied with a camel's-hair brush. When the redness and pain are abated, use collyria of alum, nitrate of silver, or zinc sulphate (5 grains to 1 ounce of distilled water). Apply with a camel's-hair brush three or four times a day, and remit for a day if too irritating.

Sometimes the lash of a whip causes an abrasion of the eye; olive oil is the best application.

The eye must be cleansed of all discharge before applying collyria. If a syringe is used the injection should always be at the outer corner of the upper lid, as the fluid then follows the natural course of the tears. The horse must not be turned out to grass, as feeding from the ground causes a rush of blood to the head; also the stable windows should

3561.

Pleurisy is a common and severe disease, but not necessarily fatal if promptly treated. It generally follows a chill taken while warm from exercise. It is inflammation of the lining membrane of the chest.

Symptoms: First, a shivering fit and feverishness; the pulse is accelerated; inspiration becomes quicker and shorter than expiration; there is generally a short, painful cough, pain on pressure between the ribs, and great disinclination to move the fore limbs. There is no heaving of the flanks as in pneumonia, but the abdominal muscles are contracted to fix the chest, giving the flank a peculiar tucked-up appearance. This stage is followed by the development of "water in the chest," which has a tendency to increase so as to compress the lungs fatally. The disease terminates in six or seven days.

Treatment: Never bleed nor apply local stimulants or blisters, nor give aloes, calomel, antimony, or the like. Put the animal in an airy loose-box; clothe it well, and administer 6 ounces of linseed oil and 1 of spirits of nitre, or 4 or 5 ounces of Epsom salts. To allay the pain, dip a rug into boiling water, wring it out, and quickly apply it to the chest; keep it in position by another rug and roller, and as soon as cool replace it by another. When the acute symptoms have passed give the following twice a day:

Ammon. carb.	1 dram.
Zingib. pulv.	2 drams.
Resinae pulv.	1 dram.

Made into a ball with linseed meal and treacle. Should the pulse remain at 50 or 55 per minute, and the breathing be labored, considerable effusion in the chest is probably the cause; auscultation will detect it. If present, administer a mixture of equal parts of sp. aeth. nit. and liq. ammon. acet., in ½-ounce doses, three or four times daily. Apply blisters to the sides, and, as a last resource, try tapping. Give the animal good food—turnips, carrots, grass, with boiled linseed and barley, and a constant supply of clean cold water.

3562.

Pneumonia has much likeness to pleurisy, and frequently follows it. The cough is not so dry, the pain more deeply seated, inspiration prolonged, expiration short and painful, pulse full, accelerated, and sometimes soft and irregular. The animal complains when an attempt is made to lift the head, keeps the fore legs apart, refuses to lie down and to move. The treatment recommended for pleurisy must be actively employed. The malady terminates, favorably or no, in 12 or 15 days.

3563.

Pole Evil.—A fistulous wound at the back of the head, behind the ear. Rub together equal parts of unguentum populeum and mercury; rub the swelling well with this for three days. If it does not disappear, but breaks, open the wound thoroughly, and cleanse it with a mixture of equal parts of tinctures of myrrh and aloes twice daily till it is healed. If the pus is putrified, explore the wound with a sound and press out all matter; then fill the wound with tow steeped in the above tincture. If the wound heals before the discharge of matter has ceased it must be reopened.

3564.

Pulmonary Catarrh is indicated by difficulty of breathing, abundant discharge of mucus from the eyes, nose, and mouth, and cough, with or without fever. Give warm, sweetened mashes, with 2 or 4 drams of nitre and 4 ounces of oxymel of squills to a bucketful. Give two or three doses of the following cough balls:

Marshmallow	4 ounces.
Licorice	4 ounces.
Elecampane	2 ounces.
Kermes mineral	2 ounces.

Make into 12 balls with honey

In every case stimulating and irritating medicines must be carefully avoided.

3565.

Purgatives: The best is Barbadoes aloes, the next Cape aloes in doses 1 dram larger. The following form is from Gamgee's "Veterinarians' Vade Mecum:"

Aloes	8 parts.
Rectified spirit	1 part.
Treacle	3 parts.

Melt the aloes and treacle in a water-bath, and then add the spirit. The dose of aloes for a carriage-horse is 5 drams, for a heavy cart-horse 6 drams. For every dram of aloes take one and a half of the above mass. The addition of gentian increases the action of aloes, as does a previous course of iron. Ginger seems a useless adjunct.

3566.

Pursiness attacks animals which have too little work and a heating diet. The symptoms are difficulty of respiration, irregular heaving of the flanks (especially after trotting), a dry cough, and sometimes an emission of whitish mucus from the nose. The most characteristic symptom is the kind of expiration, best seen after exercise while the animal is eating oats. The expiration has hardly commenced when the movement of the flanks is suddenly arrested, then recommences, and is completed quietly. Confirmed pursiness is incurable, and young animals should be treated by giving no hay and feeding principally on oats and chopped straw.

3567.

Quinsey is acute inflammation of the throat, which soon causes suffocation if not treated in time. Sometimes an abscess forms in the vicinity of the throat at the back of the tongue. Do not bleed on any account. Linseed poultices should be placed on the throat; barley-water, sweetened or acidulated, should be given as a drink or a gargle. Mild diet should be provided without delay. Gangrenous quinsey is very fatal; it requires similar treatment, acidulated drinks being specially indicated.

The following is another method of treatment: Make an electuary of 1 part each of nitre and sal-ammoniac, and 2 of Glauber's salt with water and meal. Smear on the tongue five or six times daily a quantity twice the size of an egg. Rub the swollen parts three or four times daily with a mixture of 2 parts each of mercury and marsh-mallow ointment with 1 part of camphor liniment. Protect from chills, and give only warm water to drink.

3568.

Quittor.—This is an opening (properly speaking a sinus) in the coronet of a horse, discharging matter and accompanied by pain and swelling. It is the result of an injury—commonly a wound by a nail—setting up inflammation and suppuration inside the hoof. The matter, unable to escape through the horn, finds its way to the coronet, and is discharged through the skin. If the suppuration continues long either some dead tissue is lodged in the part or the wall of the sinus is thickened. Blisters, firing, and even incision have been tried. The older farriers filled a small paper cylinder with corrosive sublimate and placed it in the sinus, but the best remedy is the following solution injected by a syringe:

Corrosive sublimate....... 1 dram.
Hydrochloric acid......... 10 minims.
Rectified spirit............ 1 ounce.

To be used once a day for 2 days, then diluted to half its strength or used only once in three days. If there is much pain after a fortnight apply a smart blister. Give a purgative occasionally, and at the beginning of the treatment a dose or two of opium to allay the pain. Solutions of the sulphate of zinc, iron, or copper are of little use.

Ringworm.—See under Cattle.

3569.

Sandcrack.—This name is applied to all fissures in the wall of the hoof, extending from the coronet downwards. The fissure, at first very small, runs in the direction of the fibres, and never reunites. The cause must be removed, and the fissure prevented from opening wider. In about nine months the growth of the wall will remove the fissure. After the shoe has been carefully fitted the hoof should be bound like the handle of a cricket bat with waxed string not thicker than a crowquill. If the cracks are wide they may be previously filled with the following composition:

Composition for Repairing Horses' Hoofs: Melt 1 part of ammoniacum in an iron ladle; add 2 parts of gutta-percha previously softened in hot water and cut in small pieces. Stir till thoroughly mixed and make into rolls. When wanted it must be melted, and a few touches with a hot knife will leave it smooth and not distinguishable from the hoof.

3570.

Seedy Toe is a condition of the horse's foot in which the wall is separated from the sole and sometimes from the structures attaching it to the coffin-bone. The space cannot be seen without removing the shoe, but the hoof gives a distinctly hollow sound when tapped with some hard substance.

By good shoeing a horse may be kept tolerably sound and at work, but if valuable it can be radically cured in about three months. Remove every portion of detached horn, artificially protect the foot, and by stimulating the coronet promote the reproduction of the horn.

3571.

Sore Shoulders.—If the skin is tender but not broken smear with a mixture of glycerine, 1 ounce; fuller's earth, 2 drams, boiled together and used cold. A simple skin wound should be washed with salt and water, which is increased in money value by coloring with tinct. lavand. co. When neglected a deep circular sore results, the margins become callous, and the centre is covered by a hard scab, or sit-fast, under which is always matter. The scab must be removed, and the whole sore dressed with lunar caustic or solution of corrosive sublimate in spirit of wine (1 dram to 1 ounce). In very bad cases make an incision right through the sore to change it from a circular to an elliptical wound and start healthy granulations. Chamois-leather pads, stuffed with horsehair, should be stitched on the harness above and below the sore to relieve pressure. The following is also recommended:

Wash the place with fresh water and at times moisten it with brandy and water. If there is a water-blister puncture it in several places with the fleam or bleeding instrument and rub it three or four times daily with a mixture of 3 parts of mercurial ointment, 1 part of potashes. The sit-fast should be washed daily with decoction of camomiles mixed with Goulard's water till it separates at the margins; cut it off little by little as the wound heals. If there is matter beneath the head, cut off the hard skin and strew alum or blue vitriol on the wound and keep it clean. The sit-fast may be softened with grease, cut off, and treated as above. If matter is found, the sore must be promptly opened, as it quickly spreads. The incision must be made to the bottom of the wound and all its cavities. After the bleeding has stopped wash the wound, lay tow in it, repeat this next day, placing rosin ointment on the tow, and continue this till cured.

Chaulmoogra oil has been introduced into the medicine-chest of the British cavalry regiments, on account of its remarkable effect upon horses that have been "wrung" with the collar or have sore backs.

3572.
Sores in the Mouth.—Take 1 part of vinegar, 2 parts of water, dissolve in it a little alum and honey. Tie a cloth on the end of a stick, and mop out the mouth with this solution. Avoid hard foods, and give bran mixed with Glauber's salt.

3573.
Sprain.—Chronic or old standing must not be treated like acute or recent sprains. Even the slightest demand careful treatment.

In the first stage of recent sprains inflammation must be kept down. Foment continuously with cold water, with one of the additions subjoined, until the intense pain and heat and all violent symptoms have passed off. Spirits of wine or tincture of arnica, or a mixture of equal parts of common salt, sal-ammoniac, and nitre (dissolved to saturation), may be added to the fomentation.

If much swelling or congestion exists foment with hot water, mixed with belladonna or opium.

In either case the reaction which follows if the fomentation is intermitted, is decidedly injurious.

When the violent symptoms have disappeared apply a dry bandage, with occasional mild hand-rubbing, for a day or two. Follow this by a mild stimulating application, such as liniment of ammonia or iodine, or tincture of cantharides, or the following:

Castor oil, rape oil, and
   turpentine, of each...... 2 ounces.

Shake and add

Strong ammonia and water,
   of each................. 3 ounces.

Only after the failure of this treatment should blisters be applied, once or twice, and as a last resource firing and a run at grass. Rest for a considerable time is absolutely essential. Keep the bowels open.

3574.
Stomach Staggers, or Grass Staggers, is an affection of the brain caused by impaction of the stomach. It is commonest among young animals at grass in the autumn.

Symptoms: Dulness, disinclination to move, fulness of the abdomen, perhaps distension and constipation; breathing slow and heavy, pulse slower than usual, 30 to 35 a minute instead of 40. It comes on suddenly and soon ends in death or recovery.

3575.
Sleepy Staggers, a similar disease, comes on gradually, runs a slower course, and is not attended by the marked fulness and constipation of stomach staggers.

Treatment: As the stomach is packed with food, balls and powders can hardly be assimilated. Strong solutions should therefore be given. The horse cannot vomit, so that relief must be obtained through the bowels. Give aloes in six or eight dram doses in as little water as possible, and in bad cases add 10 to 15 drops of croton oil. To arouse the stomach to action give ½ ounce of ether and 1 ounce of tincture of ginger every three or four hours, or a wineglassful of any spirit with 2 drams of carbonate of ammonia at similar intervals. Should a change for the better take place stop all medicines for a time, and allow no food for at least 12 hours. Should the symptoms remain urgent, and the head symptoms increase to blindness, give larger doses of ammonium carbonate and repeat the croton oil. Enemas are useful as adjuncts.

3576.

Strangles.—Inflammation of the mucous membrane of the nose and back of the mouth, with swelling of the glands of the jaw, which attacks sooner or later almost all young horses, especially when they are suddenly brought from grass to dry forage. The age of the horse, the cough, the distress of the animal, the nature of the discharge distinguish this from glanders. The first symptoms, generally, are loss of appetite, slight fever, the head hangs, the cellular tissue and glands of the jaw are swollen, there is a profuse white discharge from the nostrils. Soon the animal begins to recover its appetite, and the disease terminates in about 20 days. Sometimes the discharge from the nostrils forms under the jaw a large tumor, which breaks and discharges much pus. Light diet, gentle exercise, regular grooming, demulcent drinks, such as barley-water or water mixed with honey and powdered marshmallow or licorice, make up the best treatment, and the animal soon recovers vigorous health.

The following is another treatment: Keep the animal in a warm place, and cover it with a cloth. Give no drink cold, but mix it with barley-meal and honey; for food, give clover mixed with barley-meal and moistened with water. Mix equal parts of gentian, juniper berries, galangal, and honey into an electuary, and smear a piece the size of a walnut on the tongue night and morning. If the swellings are large, poultice them with bread-crumb and milk, open them, and press out the matter.

Other forms of the disease occur less frequently, but must be treated alike.

3577.

Tetanus, or Lockjaw, can generally be traced to some injury, as nail-wounds in the foot, injuries to the joints or eyes, docking or castration, though it does not occur in more than 1 per cent of these injuries. Other cases may be traced to cold.

The symptoms once seen can never be mistaken. The rigidity of the muscular system gives the animal a stiff, jointless appearance; the muscles of the limbs stand out in relief, the belly is "tucked up," and the tail elevated. The slightest excitement, as the opening of a door or approach of an attendant, aggravates this condition. The tail is thrown out horizontally, the head spasmodically raised, and the haw of the eye protruded (a very marked symptom). The mouth, if a finger be quietly inserted, will be found firmly fixed, or just able to open, perhaps ½ inch. There is an almost constant attempt on the part of the animal to open the mouth, which is accompanied by a profuse flow of saliva. The cause of death is exhaustion from the active state of the muscles, and from the inability of the animal to take sufficient food. A fatal termination may be accelerated by the animal falling down; it cannot then rise without help, but lies constantly plunging; congestion of the lung sets in, and death speedily follows.

Treatment: Injuries should be looked for, and, if found, placed in the most favorable position. In the early stages division of the nerve which leads from the injury often gives immediate relief, but after a time the spinal-cord itself becomes so affected that this entirely fails. Wounds should be fomented with warm water. All excitement should be avoided. The stable should be darkened, other horses removed, no visitors allowed, and only one attendant. Never raise the head nor attempt to administer draughts or balls. Give food that requires no mastication, as boiled barley and linseed, oatmeal gruel, milk, etc., but never bran mashes, which are starvation in disguise.

The best medicine is prussic acid, in ¼-dram doses, twice daily, combined with perfect quiet. An ordinary India-rubber enema syringe is fastened to about 12 inches of small guttapercha-tubing; it is filled so full of water as just to admit the acid, which can then be thrown to the back of the mouth with the smallest amount of water.

A very bad case should have slings placed under it to prevent falling. About three weeks is the duration of a favorable case ending in recovery; it may be protracted to three months. A fatal case terminates in from three to four days to a fortnight. The French recommend opium in large doses (2 drams to 4 drams), fomentation of the injured part, enemas, friction with camphorated oil, nitre in the drink. If the medicines cannot be administered by the mouth they should be injected into the bowels, the dose being increased one-half.

3578.

Thrush is inflammation of the lower surface of the sensitive frog, and where there is a large space of the frog raw, the horse should be shod with leather soles to prevent injury from newly-laid granite or flint stones. Dirt is an exciting cause.

First, cleanse the foot thoroughly with warm water, removing loose portions of horn. Then apply some mild astringent and stimulant. If the discharge is dried up suddenly by a strong dressing, a swollen leg is a common sequel. The following is a good application:

Alum and common salt, of each	1 part.
Stockholm tar	4 parts.

In obstinate cases substitute zinc sulphate for the salt.

3579.

Tonics.—Iron, copper, and zinc are the most reliable mineral tonics. For horses or cattle use the following:

Ferri sulph	
Gentianae pulv	
Carui seed	
Coriander seed	
Zingiberis pulv	aa 1 ounce.

Make into balls with treacle, or give in powder with the food. The dose of iron or copper sulphates is 2 drams. In cases of chronic nasal discharge the dose should be doubled, and the copper salt is preferable to the iron.

In broken wind, chronic cough, and non-parasitic skin diseases, arsenic is a valuable tonic.

Arsenic alb	5 grains.
Cantharidis pulv	5 grains.
Ferri sulph. pulv	2 drams.

Once a day with food.

For a mild tonic for horse or ox give a mixture of equal parts of common salt and gentian—a tablespoonful twice daily.

A more powerful tonic is:

Cinchona bark	4 drams.
Quassin or gentian	2 drams.
Aniseed	2 drams.

As a powder, or made into a ball with treacle.

Quinine may be given in pills; dose 1 to 8 grains.

3580.

Vives, or Strangulous Abscess, are swellings of the parotid glands situated at the top of the jawbone, at the junction of the head and neck. They result from blows or from badly-treated strangles. They should be treated like an ordinary abscess or tumor—with poultices, enemas and light diet. Remove the hair, rub daily with a mixture of 2 parts quicksilver and 3 parts ung. populeum, and cover it with wool. If it softens, it should be opened, and kept open till the daily application of this salve completely heals it. This must be done by an experienced person, as a case of discharge of saliva from the parotid gland or duct is extremely difficult to heal. If clear water flows from the horse's mouth, mix equal parts of tinctures of aloes and cinchona, and fill the wound with tow moistened in this. It should be changed twice daily. The animal must be kept warm and allowed no cold drinks.

3581.

Weed, Shot or Grease, Humor, Monday Morning Disease, or Lymphangitis, is almost peculiar to cart-horses, most frequently attacks hard-working animals, and appears after a day or two's rest.

Symptoms: Lameness, with heat, pain, and swelling in the leg—generally a hind one—first appearing high up inside the thigh, rapidly spreading downwards even below the hock. The swelling pits like dough under pressure, the impression remaining for some time. The pain is very acute, slight violence causing the limb to be raised so as nearly to overthrow the animal. Favorable cases recover in a few days under treatment, but severe or improperly-treated cases may leave permanent thick-leg or sloughing indolent sores.

Treatment: First give a dose of physic. Foment the swelling with warm water continuously for a long time; to apply it for a few minutes and then allow the limb to cool is worse than useless. Exercise as soon as the animal is able to walk tolerably well. Give diuretics. The food must not be very nutritious; bran is best. If the swelling remains after the acute symptoms have subsided, apply hartshorn and oil as a gentle rubefacient. Should the skin slough and leave sores, dress them with a lotion of zinc sulphate (2 drams with 20 minims of carbolic acid in 1 ounce water). Nearly all cases can be prevented by occasional diuretics, with bran on Sundays and other rest days.

3582.

Worms.—Ascarides, or round-worms, are the commonest; tapeworms are exceedingly rare.

Symptoms: The presence of worms in the dung is an unmistakable symptom. Poor condition, with absence of any assignable cause for it, may indicate the presence of worms when they are not found in the dung.

Treatment: To kill the worms give a good dose of aloes on an empty stomach, and follow up with the following tonic, labeled simply "The Powders." Stablemen have an idea that powders are the only form in which worm medicine can be given.

Canthar. pulv............. 1 dram.
Arsenic................... 1 dram.
Ferri sulph............... 12 drams.

Make into 12 powders. Give one daily in the corn.

3583.

Wounds generally.—Broken Knees, Sore Backs, Etc.: If a wound will heal by first intention the less done to it the better. Dirt and foreign matter must be removed and the wound cleansed, preferably by wiping with a dry cloth. If suppuration is inevitable the best application is carbolic acid, combined with glycerine and linseed oil (1 in 20), applied night and morning with a feather. In Germany slight wounds would be washed with camphorated spirit or Goulard's water, and covered with bibulous paper soaked in the same liquid, or anointed with the drying ointment mentioned under bruises.

CATTLE.

3584.

Balls pass directly into the first stomach, and there remain undigested and unabsorbed. As the mildest illness is generally accompanied by suspended rumination balls are therefore almost useless.

3585.

Draughts are the most convenient form of medicine. They should be abundant in quantity. Twelve ounces of Epsom salts in 4 quarts of water are more efficacious than 16 ounces in 2 quarts

3586.

Cold.—The animal eats little, and the ears and legs are cold. From old animals let 1 quart of blood from the jugular vein, from young ones 1 pint; to calves give daily ¼ ounce of saltpetre dissolved in water. If the animal is benumbed, standing with its legs close together, boil four handfuls of arnica herb in beer for a quarter of an hour, strain, give half of it with ½ dram of camphor in powder; cover the animal warmly for three hours, then rub down the whole body with a wisp of straw. Next day give the other half as before, and repeat the treatment on the third day. If the stiffness persists, place an issue in the breast. If purging ensues discontinue the drink and give ½ ounce of nitre dissolved in water A little meal and honey may be mixed with the drink.

3587.

Cough results from cold or from dusty hay. Good clean food must be chosen and sprinkled with salt water. Make an electuary of black antimony, 2 ounces; elecampane, 3 ounces; fennel seed, 2 ounces; a little oil of juniper and enough honey. Rub a piece the size of a hen's egg on the tongue morning and evening. When cold is the cause dissolve 1 part of elderberry jam and 2 parts of honey in 18 parts of water, and give 1 pint of this night and morning.

3588.

Cowpox (Variola Vaccina).—An eruption on the udder. There is fever, trembling, loss of appetite, rough hair, little milk, kidneys and bowels irregular. When the eruption appears the fever goes, the milk is less in quantity, watery, with little lumps in it, and curdles easily. The udder soon swells, is tender, reddens, spots like flea-bites appear, with greyish-yellow pustules which indicate the receptacles of the lymph. The pustule is ripe on the ninth day, when it dries and falls away. It is therefore, not advisable to do anything.

3589.

Diarrhoea (Scouring) results from cold or from decomposed food such as is found on sour marshy soils. Sound dry food is the best cure. Mix 2½ ounces tormentilla root, 4 ounces chalk, and 2½ ounces juniper berries, and give ½ ounce in water thrice daily.

3590.

Eye Diseases.—If the eye runs and is swollen and closed take 2 pounds of blood from the jugular vein on the affected side. Mix white-lead ointment and camphor, and make a streak the thickness of a straw daily on the upper eyelid. Lesser complaints may be cured by fomenting the eye with cold water, and keeping the animal in the stall If they are caused by blows bleeding is unnecessary, the application of the ointment suffices. If the cause is a particle of the food raise the lid, remove the source of irritation, and wash the eye with fresh water. See also Ophthalmia, under "Horses."

3591.

Fardel-bound, or Impaction of the Third Stomach in Cattle and Sheep.—The most characteristic symptoms are the grunt at each expiration, accompanied by most obstinate constipation. There is no pain on pressure of the ribs as in pleuro-pneumonia. Give an aperient of Epsom salts or calomel, with aromatics and diluents.

3592.

Foot Disease.—The horn becomes mattery in the middle of the slit. Sand or dust gets in and the animal goes lame. Examine the foot and cleanse it carefully. Take ½ ounce of green vitriol, ½ ounce of alum, powder and dissolve in water; wash the place with this, lay tow on it, and bind it up. Cut away the horn where it is diseased and mattery. Mix 2 parts of loam and 1 part of cow-dung, make it into a paste with vinegar, spread it all over the foot finger thick, bind it up, moisten it often with vinegar, and leave it for 24 hours. Repeat the treatment from the washing onwards till the hoof is well. If the hoof separates from the coronet, cut it away to prevent an accumulation of grit and other matter, and treat as above. If water is near, drive the animal into it several times daily and let it stand therein; this makes the binding-up superfluous. Good dry straw and standing for a time in water are the best remedies for this disease.

3593.

Foot-and-mouth Disease, vide Contagious Diseases (Animals) Acts, 1878, under Farcy ("Horses").—It is a contagious eruptive fever, rarely attacking the same animal the second time, sometimes affecting man.

Symptoms: At first loss of appetite and feverishness; if at grass separation from the rest of the herd. There is an eruption of little bladders or vesicles on the lining membrane of the mouth, on the udder, and between the digits. The eruption on the mouth, produces a profuse discharge of frothy saliva, and interferes with or sometimes arrests mastication. Should the eruption spread backward to the pharynx and gullet swallowing is interfered with. The eruption on the udder, if mild, merely renders milking difficult and painful, but it may be so severe as to cause inflammation of the gland. The eruption between the digits is the most dangerous symptom. The vesicles may be followed by pustules, then by suppuration round the coronet, even to the extent of detaching the hoof. The pain aggravates the fever, and sometimes leads to death. This virulent form is now uncommon.

Treatment: (a) General, for the fever. Give for an adult—

    Magnes. sulph............. 16 ounces.
    Sulph. subl................ 2 ounces.
    Zingib. pulv............... 1 ounce.

in about 4 quarts of thin gruel.

(b) Local: Wash the mouth with a simple solution of alum. Wash the feet clean and dress with a weak solution of zinc sulphate. Milk very gently, and if this causes much pain insert teat syphons. Hard food, such as turnips, may be boiled; bran mashes and the like may be given while the mouth is sore. After the removal of the local symptoms, give as a tonic, 2 drams each of gentian and iron sulphate in 1 pint of linseed tea once a day.

3594.

Hoven.—When too much green food is eaten it ferments and causes distension of the first stomach. Mix 3 teaspoonfuls of petroleum with ½ pound of brandy, or ½ ounce of sal-ammoniac with 2 pints of water; with this cleanse the excrement from the rectum, and give every half-hour an enema made by boiling in 4 pints of water 3 handfuls each of camomiles and mallow leaves; add two handfuls of salt and 1½ ounces of linseed oil, and inject a pint luke-warm. If this gives no relief the trocar must be used. The needle and tube should be inserted in the left flank a hand's-breadth below the hip, behind the stomach, just deep enough for the ring of the tube to rest on the skin. The needle must then be drawn out. If the tube gets stopped it must be cleansed with a twig. It must be left in place some hours, or as long as more gas is formed in the stomach. If the animal is uneasy under the pricking, raise one of the fore feet to make it stand still. If it wants to lie down tie the hind legs together. The wound must be washed often.

3595.

Inflammation of the Brain.—The eyes are bright and staring, tongue slimy, mouth hot, pulse quick and strong, ears and horns, hot, appetite none, the patient stares fixedly before it, is convulsed, wild, and delirious. Generally the heat of the sun is the cause. Let 3 pounds of blood from the jugular vein promptly. Dissolve 2 pounds of nitre in water and give every four hours. Place an issue in the breast. Make an enema of camomile flowers and mallow leaves, of each 3 handfuls boiled in 4 quarts of water, strain, add 2 handfuls of salt, and inject a quart of this with 1½ ounces of linseed oil every six hours. Wrap the head in linen, and keep it moist with cold water. If there is no improvement in two days let another quart of blood, and repeat this next day if needful. Bind the animal, or it will not stand for the administration of the clyster.

3596.

Inflammation of the Kidneys.—Symptoms: Loss of appetite, quick full pulse, very scanty urine, back bent, hind legs brought forward under the belly, pain in the neighborhood of the kidneys, suppression of milk. Let a quart of blood from the jugular vein; give every six hours ¾ ounce of nitre dissolved in water; administer twice daily the clyster recommended for red water. On the back, where the kidneys are situated, place folded cloths and keep them wet with cold water.

3597.

Inflammation of the Udder, Mammitis, or Garget, may result from external injury, exposure to cold, or irregular and bad milking. It is usually confined to one of the four lobes of the udder. Symptoms: The milk decreases in quantity, becomes watery and curdy, then yellowish from the presence of pus, and may be arrested. The gland swells, feels hard and hot, is very painful, the veins running from it being much distended. There is also general fever. The case generally ends well, but may result in abscess or mortification of a quarter of the udder.

Treatment: Lessen the food and give potassium bicarbonate in 2-dram doses twice daily till the acute symptoms have passed. Apply warm fomentations to the udder, and support it by a carefully-arranged bandage, through which the teats must be allowed to protrude. Draw off the milk frequently, but quietly. After the acute pain has passed use first gentle friction and later a stimulating liniment or a mild iodine ointment. As soon as pus is present make an incision without waiting for it to point. Germans advise rubbing the udder daily with a mixture of oil of bays and marshmallow ointment. If the teats swell rub them twice daily and milk dry. If wounds or cracks appear anoint them daily, after milking, with white-lead ointment. If scurf appears apply a lotion twice daily of Goulard's water, and milk dry, even if this causes pain.

3598.

Jaundice (the Yellows).—The symptoms are loss of appetite, cessation of rumination, yellowness of the mucous membrane of the mouth and nose and the whites of the eyes, of the urine and excrement. Feed the patient with boiled potatoes, bruised cabbage, turnips, clover, crushed or ground barley, and give every third morning, fasting, ½ ounce of aloes, 2 drams jalap, 2 ounces Glauber's salt with 1 quart of water. Great thirst, heat, dryness of the mouth, and rapid pulse indicate inflammation of the liver. Take 1 quart of blood from the jugular vein and insert an issue in the breast. Give an enema twice a day, and every six hours 1 ounce of Glauber's salt, ½ ounce of nitre, and 1 dram of powdered rhubarb in 1 quart of water. If the appetite returns give daily only one clyster and two doses of the drink.

3599.

Lice.—If these appear great care is necessary. Mercurial ointment, 2 ounces should be mixed with oil of turpentine 1 ounce, and rubbed in twice daily. Every other day the ointment should be washed off with warm water.

3600.

Milk—Blue.—This is indicated by blue spots in the cream. Give a dessertspoonful of powdered caraway in water daily till the blueness disappears. The milk-pails must be kept very clean and bright or a fungus will appear on them.

3601.

Milk — Bloody.—Bloody milk is caused either by congestion or by injury to the bloodvessels of the teats through stretching them too much while milking. In the first case let 2 pounds of blood. The latter is often troublesome. Avoid dragging, but draw the milk by pressure. Keep only the milk from the sound teats, and let the milk from the others fall to the ground. Blood-letting is useful here also. If the teats swell milk them dry, even if matter should come with the milk.

3602.

Milk Fever, Dropping after Calving, or Parturient Apoplexy is commonest among the best-conditioned animals and the heaviest milkers, occurring generally three days, or more or less, after calving. It is not contagious, but once attacked a cow is liable to it at each calving.

Symptoms: The premonitory symptoms are few, and may be overlooked. Any unusual change after calving is suspicious none more so than suppression of milk. With this there is arrested rumination and appetite, a glassy staring; hot horns and ears and cold extremities. The animal often shakes its head, and if made to walk does so unwillingly; pulse full and strong, bowels constipated. Second stage: Eye insensible to light, the animal falls, and either lies in a dull sleepy way with the head thrown on the shoulder, or keeps wildly dashing it from side to side; pulse quicker and weaker; breathing slow, heavy, stertorous. As the insensibility increases we have paralysis of the muscles used in swallowing, with hoven, or distension of the large stomach by gas.

Treatment: Before the animal falls it may be bled. Apply cold water or ice to the head and neck; wrap the body and legs in rugs; draw the udder gently every four hours, and gently hand-rub it to facilitate return of its proper blood supply. To relieve the constipation give 16 ounces Epsom salts and 2 ounces each of sulphur, aloes, and ginger in at least 4 quarts of thin gruel. Should this not act within six or eight hours repeat half the dose or give 1½ pint of linseed oil with 30 or 40 drops of croton oil. Give 2-dram doses of ammonium carbonate every three or four hours. Inject warm water into the rectum, and if the bladder is not naturally emptied a catheter should be passed once a day. Medicines should be administered through a tube or probang passed into the gullet, as the muscles of deglutition are more or less paralyzed. The animal should be placed in a loose-box, and if very violent the head should be fixed. Occasionally the position of the animal should be changed to avoid congestion of the lungs, but it must never be turned on its back at the risk of instantaneous suffocation. Double up the legs before turning it over. The insensibility, or the prior wild, stupid expression distinguishes milk fever from paralysis or severe cold. It can nearly always be prevented by lessening the food a week before calving, and giving an aperient a day after.

The Germans recommend taking 1 quart of blood from the jugular vein, placing an issue in the breast for 14 days, and giving daily 6 ounces of cream of tartar dissolved in water. If the symptoms look dangerous give daily in addition to the above, ¾ ounce of nitre and as much cream of tartar mixed with a spoonful of honey; thrice daily administer enemas of soap and water and vinegar, and sprinkle the animal afterwards with cold water. If in 24 hours the pulse is not improved repeat the bleeding and the enema; otherwise give only a drink and an enema.

3603.

Over-eating.—The animal lies on the ground, breathes deeply, groans, and does not ruminate. Give a dose of purging medicine and chilled water; let the animal have walking exercise.

3604.

Pleuro-pneumonia, Epizootic, or Contagious Lung Disease.—The period of incubation is generally two or three weeks, sometimes extending to eight or nine. The fatality is about 12 per cent in cases properly treated. Vide Contagious Diseases (Animals) Acts, 1878, as under Farcy, ("Horses"). This disease is highly contagious and infectious, and cannot be treated without special consent of the Privy Council, and, as in glanders and farcy, all animals must be slaughtered when affected.

Symptoms.—If the animals are out at grass the sick ones separate themselves from the others. In the stall, dulness and loss of appetite are first noticed; next comes increased rapidity of the pulse and breathing; later there is a painful grunt at each expiration; pain is evinced on pressing the spaces between the ribs or on pulling the dewlap. The animal is almost always lying on the side of the diseased lung, to give freer play to the healthy one, or on its breast when both lungs are affected. In Fardel-bound, or impaction of the third stomach, there is a grunt, but it is accompanied by most obstinate constipation, and there is no pain on pressure of the ribs. Ordinary or non-contagious pleuro-pneumonia cannot be certainly distinguished from the more dangerous disease, so that the strictest precautions should always be used.

3605.

Quinsey.—Dulness, loss of appetite, difficult breathing, rattling in the throat, dry, hot mouth, painful swellings under the throat, inability to swallow, the water returning by the nose, pulse rapid, are among the symptoms.

Take 2 pounds of blood from the jugular vein. Mix

Marshmallow powder	3 ounces.
Glauber salt	5 ounces.
Nitre	4 ounces.
Cream of tartar	4 ounces.

Rubbed with 1 pound of juniper berries. Every four hours put a spoonful of this on the tongue, and hold the head up till the animal has swallowed.

Mix

Turpentine oil	1½ ounces.
Oil of bays	1½ ounces.
Camphor spirit	1 ounce

and rub the swelling therewith thrice daily. Should the rattling in the throat increase, repeat the bleeding on the third day, and try the effect of barley-meal mixed with the drink. Should the glands and windpipe swell so that the breathing is obstructed, dissolve ¼ ounce camphor in 2 ounces linseed oil, mix with it 2 ounces liquid ammonia, and rub the windpipe therewith daily.

3606.

Red-water.—The coloring-matter of the blood passes through the kidneys with the ordinary watery matters. There is a steady and rapid falling-off in condition. There are no blood-clots in the urine, as in cases of haematuria, but the color of the secretion varies from pale sherry to nearly black. Other symptoms are: Suppression of milk, cold ears, anxious look, loss of appetite, steady increase in the rapidity and volume of the pulse, and the characteristic urine. If aid be not soon forthcoming the disease is fatal.

Treatment: Never give diuretics or astringents nor apply stimulants to the loins. Give first:

Epsom salts .... 1 pound.
Powdered aloes........... 1 ounce.
Ginger .... 1 ounce

in not less than 3 quarts of oatmeal gruel.

Then give once or twice a day in linseed tea ½ ounce each of ether, tincture of gentian, and tincture of ginger. After the disappearance of the symptoms, continue to give a tonic. Fresh air, even temperature, and frequent changes of food should be attended to. In loss of appetite give linseed and oatmeal as gruel.

The German directions are to let promptly 1 quart of blood from the jugular vein. Give 1 ounce of nitre dissolved in water morning and evening until cured. Feed with fresh green food, and administer daily 1 pint of the following enema. Boil three handfuls of groats in 2 quarts of water. To each pint add on administration ¼ ounce nitre and 1½ ounces linseed oil.

3607.

Ringworm shows itself as one or more circular spots, almost denuded of hair, and varying in size up to that of a crown-piece. Unguentum hydrargyri biniodidi rubbed into and around the spot is a specific. One application is generally enough.

A successful application is a solution of carbolic acid in 18 times its bulk of a mixture of equal parts of spirit, glycerine, and water. Apply it daily for three days with a small brush.

3608.

Rheumatism should be treated by rubbing on the painful joints once a day a dram of the following liniment:

Tincture of aconite (Fleming) .... 1 part.
Chloroform .... 1 part.
Spirit of wine .... 3 parts.

3609.

Scab generally comes from bad or insufficient feeding. Give better nourishment. Mix 2 ounces of antimony, 4 ounces gentian, 8 ounces juniper berries, 2 pounds of salt; give daily a spoonful. Dissolve 1½ ounces in a gill of water and wash the affected parts. If no progress is made insert an issue in each haunch for 14 days. Keep the animal from the others. Calves should be treated as follows: Mix 1½ ounce nitre with 1 ounce flowers of sulphur; give the animal 1½ ounces, and make an ointment of the rest, which should be rubbed into the affected place, and washed off on the third day with soap and water. If bad food is the cause, mix ½ ounce gentian, ½ ounce juniper berries, 3¼ ounces flowers of sulphur, and as much liver of antimony, powder and mix, and give ½ ounce daily. As food give crushed barley.

3610.

Stoppages, or Constipation.—The animal loses appetite, stamps with the hind legs, lies down and rises uneasily, groans heavily, at the same time heaving up the body. Anoint the hand with oil, insert it carefully in the rectum and remove the excrement accumulated. Make an enema by boiling three handfuls each of camomiles and mallow leaves in 4 quarts of water, adding two handfuls of salt. Administer 1 quart with 1½ ounces of linseed oil, rather more than lukewarm, and repeat this every half-hour until the disease is relieved. If there is no relief take 1 pint of the decoction, ¼ pound of linseed oil, ½ ounce of potassium sulphate Administer this every half-hour. If the disease persists more than half an hour let 2 pounds of blood from the jugular vein. A quarter of an ounce of asafoetida may be rubbed up with boiling water, and administered as a drench.

3611.

Suppression of milk often accompanies indigestion. Three mornings running give fasting 4 ounces Glauber's salt dissolved in water. Mix 8 ounces powdered gentian and 6 ounces powdered caraway; divide into 24 doses, and give one night and morning in a little water.

3612.

Tail-worm.—If the tail remains too long in excrement, gangrene sets in, which eats down to the bone, and the tail falls off. When this is discovered the hair should be cut off, the place cleansed and strewed with blue vitriol. If the hair is already gone, touch with a hot iron and wash with salt water.

3613.

Tapeworm.—The animal falls away in condition, the hair is rough and bristly, the head is turned often to look at the body, the animal strikes its body with the hind legs, and lashes its tail. Take valerian root, fern root, worm seed, garlic, of each 2 ounces, powder and give daily for 12 days ¾ ounce to an ox, ½ ounce to a cow, and ¼ ounce to a calf.

3614.

Thrush in Calves shows itself in whitish sores on the tongue or gums of sucking calves, and the patient refuses to suckle. Take ½ pint of vinegar, a spoonful of honey, and a little alum; mix them together, and wash out the mouth with this thrice daily. If this fails, take ½ dram of rhubarb, 1 dram of magnesia; give this in water twice daily, and continue the mouth wash.

3615.

Tonic.—During convalescence from pleuropneumonia, or during the later stages of redwater, use

Ether sulph............... 2 ounces.
Tr. zingib................ 2 ounces.
Tr. gentianae .... 2 ounces.

Give a fourth part every six hours in a pint of gruel.

3616.

White Scour is diarrhoea in calves brought up by hand on milk. It is caused by feeding them too seldom, and then giving too much milk at once; the result is that the stomach after curdling the milk is unable to digest the curds, which set up diarrhoea. A little chalk mixture may be given at first, but the cause should be removed by giving the food at regular and short intervals.

The Germans recommend for animals under 14 days old 1 dram of rhubarb and 1 dram of magnesia twice daily in water. Older calves may have twice as much. It is well to mix some wheat-meal with the milk.

SHEEP.

Sheep may be treated like cattle, reducing the dose to one-fourth.

Red eyelids are always a sign of health; when they are white or blackish the animal is ill.

3617.

Consumption.—It may result from rot or from bad food or water. The symptoms resemble those of rot—cough, falling of the wool, and paleness, swelling of the eyes, etc. Mix juniper berries, roasted acorns, and gentian, of each ½ ounce, add ¼ ounce common salt, and give an eighth part till the animal recovers.

3618.

Cough results from cold. Mix fennel-flowers, elecampane root, flowers of sulphur, of each 2 ounces, and give two spoonfuls several times a day. If the cough results from dusty food, see that the cause is removed.

3619.

Diarrhoea lasts at most only three days. Mix ½ ounce juniper berries and as much chalk, and give a teaspoonful several times a day. If blood is present in the excreta give often 1 dram each of rhubarb and magnesia and ½ ounce of honey. For sucking lambs put a piece of chalk in the stall for them to lick, and give in ewe's milk 1 dram of magnesia twice daily. For bad cases boil 1 ounce gentian root in 1 pint of water, strain, and dissolve in the decoction 1 dram of opium. Give a teaspoonful every two hours. Calamus root does good service.

Treatment: Mix barley-meal and water, add ½ ounce of nitre to each quart, and for three days give the sheep as much of this to drink as they will take. Boil quicksilver in water and give a full pint morning and evening. At midday give ¼ ounce of soot mixed with honey. Take powdered oyster-shell, ½ ounce, camphor, 20 grains, make into a paste with almonds, and give ½ dram every two hours during the first three days. Then mix conium extract, ½ ounce; castile soap, ½ ounce; squills, 2 drams. Make into a paste with water, and give 12 grains twice or thrice daily. Give every other morning, fasting, ¼ ounce, hepatic aloes for a week. Then mix milfoil, blessed thistle, wormwood, gentian root, juniper berries, bayberries, lesser centaury, iron filings, of each, 2 ounces. Give morning and evening, an hour before food, three spoonfuls of this with two spoonfuls of common salt, a handful of oats made into an electuary with honey. Continue this till the animal recovers.

3620.

Foot-rot is a very common disease amongst sheep, especially on some soils, as it is never absent from some flocks in the wet seasons. The symptoms are lameness and local inflammation; the hoof separates from the coronet, and large ulcerating sores appear; when very frequently much harm is done by the unsparing use of the shepherd's knife. Moisten loam with vinegar, put it in a bag, stick the foot into the mass and tie it up. Repeat this several times daily, cleaning out the matter from the edge of the cleft in the hoof, and cutting away all diseased horn. Make a solution of alum ½ ounce, green vitriol, ½ ounce, in ½ pint of water; dip tow in this and place it in the wound, and cover it with dry tow.

3621.

Giddiness is said to be caused generally by worms in the brain; it is rarely curable, and as the flesh is harmless it is best to kill the animal at once. Diaphoretics may be tried, as juniper berries, 4 ounces; castile soap, ½ ounce; squill, ¼ ounce; give ¼ ounce thrice daily. If the disease is caused by the presence of worms, snuff may be blown through a tube as far up the nostrils as possible.

3622.

Hog Pock.—Symptoms.—Head and face swollen, abscesses form round the nostrils, also in the legs and joints and other parts of the body. It is contagious and very troublesome to deal with. Push up the nostrils a twig covered with wool until the animal sneezes, or blow snuff up them. Take caraway 1 ounce, camphor 1 dram, olive oil ½ ounce, rub together in a mortar, and anoint the nostrils therewith. Mix elecampane, pimpinella root, hyssop, and elder, of each 1 pound, add salt, and give 1½ ounces thrice daily.

3623.

Hoven, or Tympanitis, is generation of gas in the stomach, caused through over-feeding early in the morning, when the dew is on the clover.

The safest treatment is to puncture the rumen and give a strong dose of purging medicine, with brisk exercise and change of food. The animal is completely prostrated, and needs speedy help. Give at once ¼ ounce petroleum mixed with 1 ounce brandy. If there is no relief in two hours the trocar must be used.

3624.

Inflammation of the Brain.—Great heat is commonly the cause. The head hangs, skull and ears are hot, eyes are closed and watering, mouth dry, tongue white and slimy, body trembling or shivering. Let blood immediately. Dissolve 1 dram of nitre in water, and give this thrice daily. Put cloths on the head and keep them wet with cold water until the animal recovers.

3625.

Jaundice is caused by a diseased condition of the liver, and is sometimes the sequel or associate of other diseases. Treatment: Aperients, combined with vegetable and mineral tonics. Give pure water, and change the diet occasionally.

3626.

Lice.—Mercury, 1 pound; Venice turpentine, ½ pound; turpentine oil, ¼ ounce; rocksalt, 1 ounce; rub in a mortar till the mercury is extinguished and no lumps are visible. Part the wool on the back, sides, and legs, and rub the salve in; the lice will die.

Milk Fever.—See under Cattle.

3627.

Red-water.—Powdered caraway mixed with salt must be put where the animal can lick it. The seeds of the oxtongue are useful.

3628.

"Rot" is a disease of the liver, very fatal; in some seasons actually decimating whole flocks. It is caused by a parasite called "liver-fluke," distoma hepaticum, which infects in large numbers the biliary ducts of the liver. This disease wastes the system, the animal becomes pot-bellied, the abdomen dropsical, the wool easily separated from the skin, the mucous membranes colorless. The eyeballs have a peculiar appearance not easily described, but well understood by sheepdealers and farmers. The animals become emaciated and weak in the latter stages, and death soon follows. Mr. A. P. Thomas, of the University Museum, Oxford, has just succeeded in proving that the intermediate host of the liver-fluke (the cause of sheep-rot), is a small water snail, limnaeus truncatulus. The snail, although a water snail, lives much out of water. It may be left in immense quantities on lands by floods; and, according to Mr. Thomas' observations, will continue to live there as long as the ground is moist. The parasitic larva escapes from the snail and has a tendency to encyst itself on surrounding objects, such as the roots of grass, whence it is apparently taken up by the sheep, probably in the encysted condition, to be ultimately developed into the adult form in the liver. The epidemic was previously known to be manifested amongst sheep allowed to feed on wet pastures, and particularly on flooded ground.

3629.

Scab is due to the presence of parasitic insects, called acari. Scab is on the list of the contagious diseases.

Symptoms: Minute red spots first appear when the insects burrow into the skin. These develop into little pimples, and then into pustules, which burst about 16 days after the first appearance of the red spots, when the brood of young is ready to emerge. Intolerable itching accompanies all this, and the rubbing and scratching aggravate the pustules, destroy the wool, and make sores, while the wool left on the hurdles and trees may weeks later carry the disease to healthy animals which touch it. The insect may be discovered by gently scraping a little scurf from the affected spot, and examining it under the microscope with a ½-inch objective.

Treatment is directed to destroying the acari on the surface of the skin, with subsequent applications for the benefit of those which escaped the first, with removal of all sources of contagion. Mercurial and arsenical preparations are poisonous, and are not more efficacious than non-poisonous dips. Sulphur ointment is a good application. The following dip will not disappoint:

Size	Of each.
Sulphur	1 pound.
Tobacco	
Water	5 gallons.

Infuse the tobacco in the cold water, add the size and the sulphur, stir frequently during application, and repeat at least once in about 16 days. The size makes the dip slightly sticky, and makes the fleece retain the sulphur better.

3630.

Small-pox, or Sheep-pox, is frequently met with on the Continent, but has been rarely discovered in Great Britain. It is one of the diseases included in the contagious diseases. The symptoms are heaviness, loss of appetite, arrest of rumination, dull weeping swollen eyes, and the formation of blisters on part of the foot. The sick sheep should be separated from the sound. Give morning and evening ¼ pound bruised bayberries, and as much clover when the disease first appears. Wash the eyes carefully with milk.

3631.

Swollen Udder, or Garget.—Rub together the white of an egg, some saffron, and olive oil, and rub the udder with this thrice daily. Milk the animal so long as the disease lasts, and give internally twice daily, to remove the hardened milk, 1 dram of a mixture of potassium sulphate 4 parts and nitre 1 part. Give once 1 dram of nitre and 2 drams of common salt dissolved in water.

3632.

Wens, or Tumours, often occur in wet years and accompany rot, and must be treated like that disease. The wen should be opened and emptied of its fluid contents.

3633.

Wild-fire, or Sore Lips, is more common amongst lambs than adults; it is caused through an impure condition of the blood. Sometimes it is produced by eating large quantities of vetches, or feeding off pasture mixed largely with poisonous weeds and thistles. Pimples or blisters appear on the mouth and lips, etc. Bruise together in equal parts hyssop and salt, and rub therewith the affected places.

3634.

Worms and Obstructions of the Bowels.—When troubled with worms the animal feeds greedily but does not thrive, rubs its nose in the earth, is soon very thirsty; at times the belly is puffed. Cold ears, scraping with the foot, great uneasiness, sweating in all parts of the body, wallowing and springing up again, with gathering up the limbs, are symptoms common to worms and obstructions. A speedy cure is ½ ounce of glanzruss,[*] ½ ounce wormwood, ½ ounce broken egg-shells, mixed and given in one dose; ¼ ounce of theriaca does good service. Administer enemas of wormseed mixed with sweet milk, though quicksilver boiled in milk answers better. When improvement is visible give ½ ounce hepatic aloes or 2 ounces Glauber's salt as a purgative. Lye of wood ashes is good against worms.

---

[*] Glanzruss is a kind of reddish pitch obtained during the burning of charcoal.

GOATS.

3635.

Constipation, Colic, are caused by lumpy food of bran or groats. Symptoms: Loss of appetite, cold ears, uneasily rising and lying down, anxious glances at the flanks, and sweating on the throat, flanks, and on the hind legs. Give every three hours 1 ounce Glauber's salt in water, and every half-hour ½ ounce linseed-oil till the colic is relieved. If the disease results from cold, boil 3 handfuls of camomiles in 1 quart of water, let it clear and cool, and give ½ pint every half-hour. Two drams of asafoetida may be dissolved in this or given in an enema, when it must be mixed with a little linseed oil. Colic also results from eating too much clover. In that case add 1 ounce Glauber's salt to the camomile decoction; give it every half-hour by the mouth, and every half-hour as an enema.

3636.

Cough.—Take valerian root and arnica herb, each 1½ ounces, liver of antimony ½ ounce, and 2 ounces grated horseradish, make into an electuary with elder rob or honey, and rub ½ ounce twice daily on the tongue.

3637.

Dropsy generally results from pasturing on marshy soil, but sometimes from internal causes. The swollen belly and the emaciated body are symptoms; swellings frequently accompany these. Take water-fennel seed (sem. phellandrii), gentian root, and juniper berries, of each 1½ ounces; make into an electuary with honey, add ½ ounce Venice turpentine, and give twice daily ½ ounce rubbed on the tongue.

3638.

Exhaustion.—There is little appetite, and the best food never fattens. Take angelica root, gentian, and valerian, of each 2 ounces, powder it, make it into an electuary with honey, and give ½ ounce twice daily.

3639.

Eye Diseases often result from bad food or from too much corn as food. The eye swells and is kept closed without external hurt. First seek the cause and remove it; give the animal morning and evening, 1½ ounces of Glauber's salt dissolved in water, till purging ensues. Cool the eye often with water, or anoint it with camphor and white-lead ointment. Continue for eight days if the inflammation is not reduced. If the hurt is external, use only the external applications.

3640.

Giddiness occurs more commonly among male goats. Ears and horns are hot, eyes shining and watery, head hanging; there are loss of appetite, and senseless turnings-round. Let ½ pound of blood, and give every two hours ¼ ounce nitre dissolved in water. Wrap the head in linen cloths and drench it often with cold water, and give an enema every hour as in inflammation.

3641.

Internal Inflammation results generally through chill. The symptoms are loss of appetite, ears alternately hot and cold, breathing difficult, heaving sides, strong, rapid pulse, to be observed by placing the hand on the left side behind the shoulder-blade or the ribs. Let ½ pound of blood; take 3 ounces Glauber's salt, 2 ounces cream of tartar, 1 ounce nitre, powder it, make into an electuary with honey, and give some of it every two hours. Boil two handfuls of camomiles in 4 pints of water, mix in ½ ounce linseed oil, and give an enema of this thrice daily. In inflammation of the lungs the animal does not lie down, but the treatment is the same.

3642.

Red-water affects goats kept on marshy pasture and fed on marsh-grasses. If the urine is red, let ½ pound of blood from the jugular vein, take 1 dram of nitre, dissolve in water, and give to the animal twice daily.

3643.

Scab or Itch.—Is caused by uncleanliness, bad or decomposed food, or by contagion. Small sores, becoming covered with scabs, at last overrun the whole skin. They also appear as dry scabs when the hair falls off. The latter is "dry," the former is "moist," scab. The animal must be separated from his fellows; search for the cause and remove it. Take gentian and juniper berries, of each 1½ ounces, and sulphur 1 ounce; make it into an electuary with honey, and give twice daily, ¼ ounce, or rather more, to strong animals. Now give good nourishing food of crushed potatoes and carrots with barley, groats or meal, wheat or rye bran, with a handful of oats, care being taken to break up all lumps, which might otherwise cause fatal obstructions. After about five days take beef tallow, 3 ounces, melt and stir in 1½ ounces turpentine oil. Rub the affected places with this. In winter use hogs' lard instead of beef tallow. After a few days wash the ointment off with warm water and soft soap; repeat the anointing and washing till cured, continuing the nutritious food.

DOGS.

3644.

Medicines for dogs may be either pills or draughts. Sugar-coated pills are now used by some veterinarians. To administer them, open the dog's mouth, place the pill as far back as possible, shut the mouth, and rub or tap the place where the under-jaw meets the throat. The pill will be swallowed without difficulty. If the dog returns it after swallowing, give it again, and follow it by a piece of meat. The mouth may be safely opened by taking care to fold the upper lip over the teeth. Nearly tasteless substances may be sprinkled on the food when the appetite is good.

3645.

Chorea — St. Vitus' Dance. — Involuntary movements of the muscles, best seen when the animal is quiet, sometimes affecting the whole body; at others implicating merely a group of muscles, as of the face, neck, or a limb. It may be caused by irritation from worms, or diseased teeth, or, it is said, by injury to the head, but most commonly it is a sequel to debilitating disease, especially distemper. Ether, ammonia, valerian, asafoetida, quinine, strychnine, iron, copper, zinc, silver, and arsenic have all been strongly recommended. The following have sometimes been successful:

A

Liq. arsenicalis	1 dram.
Tr. ferri perchlor	2 drams.
Inf. gent	13 drams.

A teaspoonful twice daily.

B

Zinci sulph. seu valerianat.	6 grains.
Quiniae	1 scruple.
Conf. rosae, enough to make	12 pills.

Two every day.

3646.

Distemper is contagious, affecting principally young dogs, and rarely occurring twice in the same animal; very many escape it altogether. It is a simple fever with local complications affecting the nose and throat, and, in bad cases, the lungs also. The stomach, kidneys, intestines, and even the brain are disordered as in other fevers. Its closest analogue in human diseases is influenza.

Symptoms.—In ordinary cases the symptoms are dulness, sneezing, dryness of nose, loss of appetite, disordered stomach, with watery discharge from the eyes and nose. As the disease advances the discharge becomes purulent, the sneeze becomes a cough, sometimes of a peculiar choky kind, as if some foreign body were in the throat. From the first there is a marked debility, which rapidly increases. Frequently there are complications, such as inflammation of the lungs, violent diarrhoea, disordered liver causing jaundice and various nervous affections, paralysis or convulsions; these must be treated apart.

Treatment should be chiefly good nursing. Keep the patient in a well-ventilated dry room at an even temperature (not warm). Allow fresh air, clean water, and easily digested food, but no exercise till strength returns. Sponge the nose and eyes frequently, and force down soups or broth if food is refused.

Give at first 2 to 4 grains of tartar emetic in butter or on a small piece of meat. Keep the bowels regular by mild aperients, as a mixture of equal parts of castor oil and syrup of buckthorn; dose, 2 drams to 8 drams.

When the acute symptoms have subsided give stimulants and tonics:

Quinine	20 grains.
Ginger	60 grains.
Iron sulphate	60 grains.
Extr. gentian, enough to make	12 pills.

Give two or three every day.

Quinine	20 grains.
Ammon. carb.	120 grains.
Extr. gentian, enough to make	12 pills.

Give two or three every day.

For debility, with diarrhoea, give—

Ferri carbonatis	1 dram.
Catechu pulvis	2 drams
Opii pulvis	10 grains.
Cretae prep	2 drams.

Make 12 pills with confection of roses. Two or three every day.

3647.

Fits or Convulsions are commonest in young dogs, and may often be traced to changes in the teeth, the presence of intestinal worms or distemper. While the fit is on keep the animal in a quiet place, and prevent injury to it. Only when the fits are violent and frequent may a warm bath be tried, as it is difficult to dry the animal without exciting it. After the fits are well over search for loose teeth or worms, and remove them. After removing the cause, give the following tonic to prevent the return of the fits:

Arsenic .... 1 grain.
Iron sulphate.............. 20 grains.
Extr. gentian, enough to
    make .... 15 pills.

One to be given daily. Order exercise, good food, and a dry house.

3648.

Fractures are called "simple" when the bone is only snapped in two, "comminuted" when it is splintered, and "compound" if the skin is wounded. The bones most frequently broken are the long bones of the limbs. Fractures of ribs or skull are dangerous from the chance of injury to organs within, and should be only treated by an expert.

Where the bone is well covered with flesh, detection of fractures requires care. Besides pain and lameness, the symptoms are sometimes swelling and displacement, twitching of the muscles, and crepitus, or grating, heard on moving the bone so as to bring the broken ends into contact. The twitching of the muscles is due to irritation caused by the broken ends. Ordinary extension will reduce a fracture to its proper position, while considerable force is required to reduce a dislocation, and when reduced it remains fixed.

Treatment: Special care must be taken to replace the fractured ends in their natural position, as it will be repaired by natural processes in any position in which it is fixed. Next, the limb must be kept fixed in this position. We may use either splints of thin wood, cardboard, or guttapercha, or a long bandage saturated with glue or starch to give it requisite firmness. The starched bandage is a useful form. First roll a dry bandage carefully round the limb, beginning at toes, no matter where the fracture is, and applying it as high on the limb as possible. The joint above and below a fracture should always be fixed, if possible, as this reduces movement to a minimum. If the bandage is not applied first at the toes, the compression above is sure to cause swelling and perhaps gangrene below. Over the dry bandage apply another well-soaked in strong starch, and secure the ends. Put the dog in a small cage to limit his movements. The bandage should remain on 14 days, examined daily to see if it is too tight or too loose. Compound fractures should be treated with splints, and a simple bandage so arranged that the wound can be inspected without removing the whole apparatus. Comminuted fractures should be treated like simple ones, unless they are also compound, when splints must be applied, and any splinters of bone quite detached should be removed.

In fractures of such bones as the thigh, which cannot be bandaged, the joints below should be fixed, the hair over the fracture cut short, and a plaster applied. Except for pets, these injuries are not worth treatment.

3649.

Pleurisy.—During convalescence give the following tonic:

Syr. ferri iodidi........... 1 ounce.
Inf. gent. co............... 3 ounces.
Tr. zingib.................. 1½ ounces.

A dessertspoonful thrice daily. Tr. ferri perchlor. may be given in doses of from 10 to 30 drops in infusion of quassia.

3650.

Poisoning.—According to an Australian correspondent of The Chemist and Druggist, dogs poisoned by strychnine may be completely and rapidly relieved, even when as stiff as an iceberg, by pouring about a tablespoonful of strong watery solution of tobacco into the mouth. We have relieved a poisoned dog by administering chloroform by inhalation, until the symptoms of poisoning disappeared. It is very difficult to get the dog to inhale the drug. Pull an old woolen stocking over its head, and drop the chloroform a little at a time near the nose. Or cut away a little hair from the side, drop a little chloroform on it, and cover with the hand or a wineglass. Repeat until relief is obtained.

3651.

Rabies.—Symptoms: First, restlessness and disregard of familiar things, capricious appetite, with a partiality for tearing up and swallowing all sorts of things, as sticks or filth. The animal takes to howling, and snaps at anything approaching him; there is a peculiar wild look, the eyes steadily following anything moving in front, and also moving as if fixed on imaginary things; the nose and mouth are dry; there is intolerance of light and difficulty of swallowing, which ends in paralysis and convulsions, and death in three or four days. Dumb Rabies is more rapidly fatal, and is accompanied by a paralysis of the lower jaw and a considerable discharge of saliva.

The barking, running, and foaming at the mouth often seen in dogs subject to convulsions must not be mistaken for rabies.

Bites by doubtful dogs should be cauterized, and the animal locked up for a time, to make sure whether it was or was not affected. Solid caustic soda or caustic potash, nitric acid, or solid silver nitrate are the best caustics. Care should be taken to reach the bottom of the wound.

3652.

Tonics.—In skin diseases, chorea, or other nervous affections following distemper, use the following:

Fowler's solution	1 dram.
Syrup of ginger	3 drams.
Water	5 ounces.

A tablespoonful thrice daily.

As a strong, general tonic use

Pulv. cinchonae	4 drams.
Ext. gentianae	2 drams.

Make into 40 pills, and give two twice daily.

Nux vomica (dose, ¼ to 1 grain) and strychnine (dose, 1/20 to 1/12 grain) are rather disappointing as nervous tonics.

The best are tr. ferri perchlor. and syr. ferri iodidi.

3653.

Worms.—(a) Round-worms, or ascarides, in the faeces.

Treatment: For ordinary-sized dogs, 1 dram powdered areca nut, made into pills, to be given at night, one after another, and to be followed by 1 ounce of castor oil in the morning. Repeat the treatment a week later. Or 6 grains santonica, made into a pill, and administered as the areca.

(b) Tapeworms, detected by the miserable condition of the dog and the presence of joints of the worm in the faeces.

Treatment: For a medium-sized dog, ½ dram of oil of male fern in linseed tea, or tied up in a small piece of sausage-skin. Repeat in a week, and follow up with tonic medicines.

Or give a mixture of ol. filicis maris and turpentine. This should be tied up in a small sausage-skin, when the dog will bolt it whole, otherwise it is sure to be rejected by vomiting.

PIGS.

3654.

General.—If the nature of the disease is doubtful, bleeding at the ear and tail may always be tried, and an ounce of powdered sulphur may be given every morning in thin bran wash.

3655.

Bleeding.—The easiest plan is to turn the ear back on the poll, and press the fingers on the base of the ear; this will make one or more veins prominent which can be easily opened. When the pressure of the finger is removed the blood will cease to flow. The palate veins which run on either side of the roof of the mouth are also easily opened by making two incisions, one on each side of the palate, about half way between the centre of the roof of the mouth and the teeth.

3656.

Medicine for Pigs should be mixed with the food. Where this fails, as in total loss of appetite, the draught is used. Great care must be taken not to give fluids to these animals while they are squealing, as they are very easily choked. The following method of administration has been recommended: Tie the pig by the neck with a long rope to a post in an open space. It will run round squealing till it gets tired, and then stop to think. Meanwhile, cut off the toe of an old boot, and, when the pig stops, thrust the end into its mouth. It will begin to chew it, and the draught may be safely poured through this impromptu funnel. Another plan is as follows: Let a man get the head of the animal firmly between his knees, without, however, pinching it, while another secures the hinder parts. Then let the first take hold of the pig's head from below, raise it a little and incline it slightly towards the right, at the same time separating the lips on the left side so as to form a hole into which the fluid may be gradually poured, not more being introduced into the mouth at a time than can be swallowed at once.

3657.

Apoplexy, when it occurs, is generally rapidly fatal. There are dullness, disinclination to move, heaviness of the head, uncertain staggering gait, wildness, and inflammation of the eyes, with apparent loss of sight, loss of appetite, and general numbness. Bleed promptly from the palate, give magnesia sulphate and sulphur as purgatives, or tartar emetic in water. For some time afterwards heating diet must be avoided, and a little nitre added to the water.

3658.

Cold results from insufficient food, or from taking in too much air while being driven against the wind. The appetite is small, the animal gets stiff, readily lies down, the ears are cold. Bleed at ear and tail; administer ½ ounce juniper berries mixed with ¼ ounce gentian and 1 dram camphor once a day in water till the disease vanishes.

3659.

Constipation frequently follows farrowing, and as the mass of excrement presses on the urethra and prevents the escape of the urine, inflammation of the bladder is apt to result, often causing the death of the animal. An enema of soap and warm water, or oatmeal and water, should be given daily, with a little compulsory exercise three or four times a day until relieved. The food should be scalded beans for a few days, then oatmeal or toppings.

3660.

Cough.—Slight coughs are cured by feeding with sour milk. For cough resulting from chill, make an electuary of aniseed, 1½ ounces; licorice, 1½ ounces; honey, 4 ounces; and twice a day rub on the tongue a piece the size of a walnut. These coughs must not be neglected, or they may result in consumption or intestinal diseases. Where this has already taken place, make an electuary of equal parts of gentian, licorice, and flowers of sulphur with sufficient honey, and twice a day rub on the tongue a piece the size of a walnut.

3661.

Diarrhoea results from cold. Give a handful of juniper berries once, or ¼ ounce tormentilla root twice a day. Allow no milk. Diarrhoea, or scouring, in sucking pigs, may be treated by giving the sow a few old beans or a little bole in the food. Young pigs bred on stone floors are almost sure to have diarrhoea.

3662.

Dropsy of the Belly follows wet weather. The animal is dull and off its feed, and the belly swells. It is generally relieved by keeping it in the house. If the swelling of the belly does not diminish, give, morning and evening, for eight days, ½ ounce of the following powder in the food: Juniper berries, gentian root, and calamus root, of each equal parts. After eight days dissolve ½ pound Burgundy pitch in 1 pound linseed oil, add 1 ounce balsam of sulphur, 4 ounces herb prunella, and enough parsley seed to make an electuary. Give daily for four days a piece the size of a walnut rubbed on the tongue; then give the powders for eight days, then the electuary for four days, and so on till the cure is complete.

3663.

Epilepsy.—Symptoms: Repeated grunting, restlessness, rapid breathing, pallor of the skin, staggering gait. The pig falls suddenly, lies motionless for a time; convulsions then come on and increase rapidly, the animal remaining unconscious till the fit is over. It then gets up, and seems terrified, trying to hide.

Treatment is rarely successful and the disease frequently spreads to all the first patient's companions. Bleeding, strong purges, and cold affusion of the head are indicated. Wrap the head in a cloth and keep this wet with a mixture of 1 quart of water, 1 pint of vinegar, and 1 ounce of salammoniac.—Youatt.

3664.

Eye Diseases.—Accumulations of gluey pus round the eyes, especially in porkers. Cleanse the eyes carefully with milk, and anoint daily with camphorated white-lead ointment.

3665.

Gripes, or Colic.—The animals do not eat, and bend themselves up. Give a decoction of camomiles with olive oil. If not relieved in half an hour give another dose. Caraway is also useful. A dose of castor oil proportioned to the strength of the patient should be given with a little ginger.

3666.

Hipshot.—The animal is lame in the back, or "hipshot." The hind legs will not bear its weight, and there are generally small bladders on the tongue. Cleanse the mouth with salt-water or lye. Rub the loins with a mixture of 4 parts of cantharides ointment and 2 parts of turpentine oil. Mix 1 ounce cream of tartar, 3 drams camphor, and 1 ounce nitre; divide into 12 parts, and give one thrice daily in water.

3667.

Inflammation of the Brain.—Symptoms: At first dulness, redness of the eyes, then wild, ill-directed movements; the pig runs against obstacles, the pulse is small and quick. Bleed from the ears and wash them with warm water to hasten the flow. Give Epsom salts with ginger. Administer enemas and afterwards repeated doses of sulphur.

3668.

Inflammation of the Lungs, or Rising of the Lights.—The prominent symptoms are loss of appetite, incessant and distressing cough, and heaving at the flanks. At the very first the animal must be bled, preferably from the palate. Give 2 to 4 drams each of sulphur and Epsom salts, according to the strength of the animal. Follow with a powder of digitalis, 2 grains; antimonial powder, 6 grains; nitre, 30 grains; twice daily. Keep the animals clean, warm, and well fed.

3669.

Loss of Tail.—High-bred pigs are very apt to lose their tails when young. The disease shows itself when a day and a half old. A red spot shows itself, which gradually spreads all around the root of the tail, destroying the cuticle. If once round there is little chance of saving the tail; but if at the first all the red place be well scraped with the nail or a penknife until it bleeds, and afterwards greased, a scab will form and new skin will grow and the tail will be saved.—G. Mangles. It would be worth while to try the effect of silver nitrate.

3670.

Madness.—When it results from the bite of a rabid dog the wound must be cut out with a sharp knife, and the place often washed with salt-water. When inflammation of the brain is the cause the animal is dull, does not eat, the eyes are staring and glassy, the ears warm, mouth hot and dry, it stamps its feet, scratches itself under the ear, roots in the earth, bites at everything near, and runs against the wall. Immediately cut a piece off the tail, and make an incision in the lower surface of the ear. Give thrice daily a dram of nitre in water, wrap the head in cloths, and keep it moistened with cold water. Mix 2 drams cantharides ointment with 2 ounces lard, and rub therewith a hand's-breadth on both sides of the throat near the shoulder. Repeat this till recovery is made. Sour milk is the best food.

3671.

Maggots in the Ear.—Symptoms: Head-shaking, rubbing the ears, and scratching them with the hind legs. It results from the deposit of flies' eggs in the ear. Remove the maggots, and apply turpentine till complete relief is obtained.

3672.

Measles.—Hydatids, which affect the whole body. Symptoms: Under the tongue are found small swellings. Mix tormentilla, 2 ounces; alum, 1 ounce; gentian, 4 ounces; and give 2 spoonfuls twice daily with the food.

3673.

Pocks.—Small sores form, which break, leave a scab, and disappear. The eye is specially attacked and ulcerated. Wash the places often with lukewarm milk, and cleanse them from matter, otherwise the animal will be blinded. The disease is rapidly contagious. Feed with whey, and add to the food ½ ounce of a mixture of 2 ounces of sulphur and 4 ounces of juniper berries.

3674.

Quinsey, or Strangles.—One of the most malignant of the diseases of swine. Chill seems the chief cause, and the disease is commonest in spring and autumn. There is a loss of appetite, the ears hang, the nostrils secrete mucus, the head is shaken, the mouth is dry and hot, the ears cold, the eyes watery, ultimately the throat swells, the tongue becomes red and then brown, the voice lower. Immediately let blood at the ear and tail. Give daily in whey 1 dram saltpetre and ¼ ounce Glauber's salt. If the symptoms are already threatening, make an incision two fingers broad on the under surface of the ear where the veins lie thickest, and cut off a piece of the tail. Give whey medicated as above, as much as the animal will take. If it will not, or cannot, swallow, mix 4 ounces Glauber's salt and 2 ounces nitre with enough honey to make an electuary, and rub ½ ounce on the tongue every four hours. Youatt thus describes the disease and treatment: The glands under the throat begin to swell, respiration and swallowing are impeded, hoarseness and debility supervene; the neck swells and rapidly goes on to gangrene, the tongue hangs from the mouth and is covered with saliva. Bleeding and purgatives are indicated, with setons and punctures of the swollen glands.

3675.

Running Fire should be treated like foot disease of sheep.

3676.

Scab.—A scurf appears on the skin which causes itching, so that the pig rubs itself against anything handy. Mix 1½ ounces black antimony and 1 ounce golden sulphide of antimony, and give a little with the food thrice daily. Wash the affected places with decoction of beech leaves. If this gives no relief make an ointment of nitre, sulphur, and linseed oil; rub the affected places with this, and wash the animal often.

3677.
Snuffles, Snifles, Nasal Catarrh.—There is first a slight discharge of mucus from the nostrils, gradually increasing till it causes cough, sneezing, and difficulty of breathing. The membrane of the nose becomes thickened and the nostril swollen and deformed. Blood is often discharged from the nostril, which gives temporary relief, but the hemorrhage is apt to recur, and so undermine the animal's strength. The best treatment is the administration of copper sulphate night and morning, in doses of 3 to 5 grains, with good food and cleanliness. The disease is often fatal, as it is generally well established before it is noticed.

3678.
Splenitis.—The pig avoids companions, and buries itself in the straw; it has no appetite, but excessive thirst; the respiration is short, there is cough, vomiting, grinding of the teeth, and foaming at the mouth. The groin is wrinkled, pale brown; the skin of the throat, chest, and belly (which latter is hard and tucked up) is tinged with black. Let blood copiously, purge gently, and give cooling medicines. Give a cold shower-bath in the neighborhood of the spleen by means of a watering-pot.

3679.
Spleen.—The breathing is short, cough dry, the animal runs in circles. Immediately let blood, drench plentifully with water, and give cream of tartar in whey. Mix fennel powder, 1½ ounces; rhubarb, ½ ounce; sal-ammoniac, 2 ounces; divide into 12 powders, and give one at a time mixed with the food.

3680.
Sprains, Sores, and Bruises.—Collections of pus must be opened, washed, and anointed with turpentine oil till healed. Bad bruises, resulting from blows, rub with a mixture of 2 ounces soap and 1 dram powdered camphor. Sprains treat likewise.

3681.
Stye.—A white blister the size of a pea on the tongue, which indicates a violent and very dangerous fever. There are also loss of appetite, dull eyes, rooting with the snout, trembling, uneasy grunting. Relief is sometimes obtained by opening the blister, and rubbing the wound with salt and vinegar.

3682.
Swine Fever, Cholera, Typhoid Fever, the Purple or Soldier Disease is on the list of the Contagious Diseases. As in glanders and farcy, notice of disease must be given to the nearest police constable, or to the veterinary inspector.

As soon as the animal is pronounced affected with the disease it is slaughtered and buried by the local authority, who pays one-half of the value of all animals slaughtered.

The disease is highly contagious, and, as the owners receive compensation—which is not the case in glanders or farcy—the safest way for all parties concerned is to stamp out the disease at once.

3683.
Vomiting.—Prevent the pig from eating its vomit. Dissolve the white of two eggs in two gallons of water, and allow the animal to drink of this every two hours, or give thrice daily ½ pint of camomile tea.

3684.
Worms.—The animal never thrives, although the appetite is voracious; there is cough, restlessness, squeaks of pain, savage snapping at other animals; dull, sunken eyes, hard, high-colored excrement. Turpentine may be given with safety, but other vermifuges do not seem to have been tried.

POULTRY.

3685.
Apoplexy.—Birds, apparently in robust health, fall suddenly, and are found either dead or insensible. The only hope of cure is immediate bleeding by opening one of the largest veins on the inner side of the wings by a longitudinal incision. So long as the thumb is pressed on the vein at any point between the body and the cut, blood will flow. The disease may be prevented by carefully avoiding over-feeding.

3686.
Baldness and White Comb.—White comb is a hard scurfy condition of the organ. Give good food and exercise, and a 5-grain Plummer's pill every night for a week.

NON-SECRET FORMULAS.

3687.

Catarrh and Roup.—Catarrh shows itself by a watery or adhesive discharge from the nostrils with swelling of the eye-lids. When the discharge becomes purulent and offensive, and the other symptoms are aggravated, the disease is called Roup. A dry, warm situation and stimulating food relieve slight cases. In roup the eyes and nose should be frequently washed with warm water. Balsam of copaiba in membranous capsules is the best remedy. Composition powder has been used with good effect. As the disease is contagious, the affected bird, unless it is of great value, should be killed and carefully buried.

3688.

Crop-bound.—This name is given to distension of the crop, either by over-feeding and subsequent swelling of the grain, or by the presence of some single object too large to pass into the stomach. Cut into the upper part of the crop with a sharp penknife, loosen the mass with some blunt instrument and remove it; if very offensive, wash the crop out with warm water. Feed for a few days on soft food. If the incision is small it may be left, if large a stitch or two should be inserted.

3689.

"Douglass Mixture" for Moulting Birds.—Dissolve 1 ounce of iron sulphate in 1 quart of water, add 1 dram of dilute sulphuric acid, and put 1 teaspoonful of this mixture in each quart of drinking-water. When chickens droop and seem to suffer as the feathers on the head grow, give them once a day meat minced fine and canary-seed.

3690.

Leg-weakness should be treated by tonics and good food. Give 3 to 8 grains of ferri et ammon. citr. once a day.

Paralysis affecting either of the limbs is incurable.

3691.

Vertigo.—The birds run in circles or flutter about without control of their movements. Hold the head under a stream of cold water for a time. Give 3 grains of calomel and 10 of jalap. Keep on low diet.

TURKEYS AND HENS.

3692.

Consumption.—Sores over the tail. When ripe, open them with a penknife, and sprinkle the wound with tobacco ashes.

3693.

Diarrhoea is caused by too much green food. Give warm food, chick-peas, and powdered tormentilla. Or give 5 grains each of powdered chalk and rhubarb and 3 grains of cayenne pepper. If the flux is not checked give 1 grain of opium and 1 grain of ipecacuanha every four hours.

3694.

Epilepsy.—Give wine, and anoint the head with olive-oil. Much green food must not be given.

3695.

Lice result from uncleanliness. The birds should be washed daily with cows' urine or wormwood boiled in water, and the animal and stall often sprinkled therewith. Or, better, dust into the feathers flowers of sulphur or sawdust moistened with benzoline or carbolic acid; and lime-wash the hen-house, adding a little carbolic acid to the wash.

3696.

Mortality.—Occurs in summer. Dig up a red ant's nest, and put it in the run. The hens fall on it greedily; diarrhoea is produced, and the greater disease almost always disappears.

3697.

Pip.—This is commonest among the young ones. To prevent it, add to the drinking water thyme or pepperwort or nigella-seed, and let them often run among green food. The pip—a white, horny skin—should be cut from beneath the tongue with a sharp penknife, and taken out. Moisten the part with salt dissolved in wine vinegar, and give nothing to eat. Bread cut in cubes and soaked in vinegar is good later on.

3698.

Worms on the Head.—Hang the birds up and search the head thoroughly. If small brown worms are found, which quickly become larger and feed on the head, drench with fish-oil, and thereafter rub with this occasionally.

GEESE.

3699.
Diarrhoea.—Place the twigs and buds of a young pine tree bruised in the drinking water. Mix bruised thistles with groats as food, and once a week add some tobacco ashes.

3700.
Gnats and Flies creep into the little cavities in the ears and nostrils of young geese and kill them. Anoint the ears in June and July, with linseed or olive oil. If the disease is severe, put barley at the bottom of a deep trough filled with water. The birds in reaching for the food put their heads deep into the water and wash the vermin out. Fresh fern leaves often strewed in the run drive away the insects.

3701.
Lice generally affect the young in summer. Rub the affected places with tobacco ashes, or with a mixture of fish oil and rape oil; anoint the head and the sides under the wings. If they show themselves on the throats of young geese, which is often fatal, rub the throat with mercurial ointment.

3702.
Mortality.—As a preventive, give every other morning half a spoonful of salt. Boil bearwort (Meum athamanticum) and give the decoction as drink. Feed with grains, barley, and bruised thistles, and once a week sprinkle tobacco ashes on the food when the birds come from pasture.

3703.
Pip.—Greater pimpernel plant should be steeped in water, the herb given as food and the infusion as drink. The sore should be cut off, and the wound anointed with unsalted butter.

3704.
Swelling of the Crop results from eating too much fresh corn. Pay attention to the feeding, and if the crop swells, soak bread in brandy and give as food.

PIGEONS.

Pigeons should always be supplied with old mortar or chalk in a box, where they can peck at it; and with a lump of common salt in another vessel. It is a good plan to put some lavender-stalks about the pigeon-house occasionally, and before stocking it.

3705.
The Parasites that infest pigeons are fleas, lice, feather lice, mites, and ticks. Persian insect-powder is efficacious in all cases. Fleas may be killed by sprinkling a little snuff over the birds and into their nests.

3706.
Lice usually attack weak birds. A little powdered sulphur should be dusted among the feathers, and the birds should be kept clean and in good condition.

3707.
Mites are very small insects which inhabit the cracks and nooks in the walls of the pigeon-house, issuing at night to feed on the blood of the birds. They sometimes enter the ears of young birds and cause intense annoyance. A drop of oil on the ears, under the wings, or wherever mites are seen, will destroy them. The walls should be smoothed and all cracks stopped. Birch twigs and heath should be given for the nests instead of hay. The house may be white-washed.

3708.
Ticks are larger parasites, infesting generally the head and back. Cleanliness and sulphur are the only remedies.

3709.
Feather lice are long, flat, tough insects which cling very tightly between the fibres of the feathers. Their food is the down on the quill end of the feathers.

3710.
Canker is a cheesy stinking growth on the mucous membrane of the mouth and throat. It is very fatal to young birds and is thought to be contagious. Dissect away the cheesy growth with a bit of wood cut like a spatula. Touch the spot with lunar caustic. Give scanty diet and much exercise. If the flesh round the eyes is wounded by fighting bathe with salt water for several days, and if this does not succeed try alum and water.

3711.
Moulting.—If there are any broken stumps of feathers which the bird cannot remove, considerable suffering results. The stumps must be withdrawn one by one with a pair of pincers. Give plenty of good but not oily food.

3712.

Pouters sometimes overgorge themselves with dry food, which swells in the crop, and is apt to cause death. The crop should be opened with a sharp penknife, the mass removed, and the wound sewn up. If skillfully performed, the operation is very harmless.

3713.

Roup affects the mucous membranes of the mouth, nostrils, and air-passages. Warmth will cure slight attacks. A copaiba capsule is almost a specific. When the discharge from the nostrils is offensive and purulent, apply to the eye a lotion of nitrate of silver, 5 grains to 1 ounce. The birds must be kept warm and well nourished; hempseed should be given. Dry roup is known by the dry, husky cough. Give 3 or 4 cloves of garlic every day.

3714.

Scouring, or Diarrhoea, is caused in weak birds by want of exercise. Add a pinch of sulphate of iron to the drinking water.

3715.

Scrofula shows itself in various forms. As Wing disease it forms deposits of cheesy and scrofulous matter in and around the joints, especially of the elbow. In early stages tincture of iodine applied externally may cure; but in advanced cases the bird should be killed. When it attacks the liver scrofula causes the formation of white tubercles. The birds lose flesh and are said to "go light." They must be destroyed.

3716.

Sore Eyes are common among carriers and barbs. A lotion or ointment of silver nitrate should be applied. Among old birds there is a tendency to form spouts by the turning out of the lower eye-lid. These may be removed by being cut from below upwards with a very sharp pair of scissors.

3717.

Vertigo occurs in highly fed birds. Starve for two or three days, and reduce the food afterwards.

3718.

Wasting is said to be cured by green food, especially watercress.

CANARIES.

3719.

Asthma.—When this occurs leave off hempseed, give only rape-seed and bread soaked in water and pressed, with lettuce or watercress twice a week, and occasionally bread boiled in milk till reduced to a paste. This last must always be made fresh and must be quite cold before giving it to the birds. It is a gentle purge and sensibly relieves them.

3720.

Diarrhoea frequently results from chill. Drop a little tincture of camphor in the drinking-water or on a lump of sugar.

3721.

Egg-bound.—When the bird is egg-bound a small camel's-hair pencil should be dipped in castor oil, worked to a point, and gently inserted in the vent of the bird, applying a little round the part affected, and putting a drop or two in the beak.

3722.

Red Lice are minute, almost microscopic parasites, which infest the wings and cause gradual roughening and then shedding of the feathers, so that the pinions gradually become quite bare and red. They have been removed by washing each bird thoroughly with a lotion of white precipitate and water (a pennyworth to half a teacupful), then washing with warm soap and water, wrapping in flannel, and placing before a fire till dry. Insect powder and water would probably be more efficacious.

3723.

Sore Feet, as a rule, result from dirt and want of attention. The greatest cleanliness should be observed, and water should be supplied for a bath. If the feet become sore even with this treatment, bathe the feet for five or ten minutes in warm water three or four times a day.

RABBITS.

3724.

Liver Complaint shows itself by hard, short breathing. It does little injury to the animal's general health, and none to the flesh. It is best to fatten them and kill them for the table.

3725.

Pot-belly Dropsy is caused by wet vegetable diet, and is incurable, though it may be relieved for a month or two.

3726.

Red-water is occasioned by sour food, and must be treated by mild mucilaginous food like dandelion.

Animals that are diseased should be kept apart till the bright skin, clear eye, and dry, well-pelleted dung show that health is restored.

3727.

Rot results from feeding on decaying green stuff. The animals lose flesh, and sores appear on the nose and ears. Feed on dry absorbent food, as ground malt, biscuit, dry bread, crushed beans, oak leaves, split-peas, oatmeal, herbs like thyme and sage. Give, morning and evening, ¼ gill of water. If the sores on the ears and nose be allowed to get fast hold the disease becomes contagious; the animals affected must be destroyed, and the hutch cleansed most vigilantly.

3728.

Snuffles closely resembles cold in the head, and should be treated by keeping the animal warm and comfortable.

VETERINARY FORMULÆ.

3729. Alterative Powder.

Iron oxide................ 6 ounces.
Black sulphide of antimony 3 ounces.
Flowers of sulphur........ 4 ounces.
Nitre .... 4 ounces.
Caraway oil .... 1 dram.
Anise oil .... 1 dram.
Dose, a tablespoonful.

3730. Blister. A

Spirit of turpentine....... 2 ounces.
Sulphuric acid .... 3 drams.
Lard .... 6 ounces.
Venice turpentine .... 3 ounces.
Origanum oil .... 2 drams.
Resin (black)............. 4 drams.
Yellow wax .... 4 drams.
Cantharides powder....... 1½ ounces.
Euphorbium powder....... 1 ounce.

3731. Blister. B

Venice turpentine......... 4 ounces.
Powdered cantharides..... 1½ ounces.
Powdered euphorbium..... ½ ounce.
Turpentine .... q. s.

3732. Blister. C

Powdered cantharides..... 3 ounces.
Euphorbium .... 1 ounce.
Laurel oil (oil of bay).... 2 ounces.
Resin ointment............ 2 ounces.
Turpentine .... q. s.

3733. Liq. Blister.

Powdered cantharides..... 4 ounces.
Euphorbium .... 1 ounce.
Turpentine .... 1 pint.
Digest. Methylated spirit may be substituted for the turpentine.

3734. Calves' Cordial.

Also the best medicine for diarrhoea in pigs.

Chalk .... 1 ounce.
Catechu .... ½ ounce.
Ginger .... 2 drams.
Opium .... ½ dram.
Mix and dissolve in ½ pint of peppermint-water.

For a pig give ½ ounce to 1 ounce twice a day; a teaspoonful will be enough for sucking-pigs.

3735. Cleansing Drench.

Nitre .... 1 ounce.
Flowers of sulphur........ 1 ounce.
Iron oxide .... ½ ounce.
Diapente .... 2 ounces.
Sodium sulphate.......... 4 ounces.
Magnesium sulphate....... 4 ounces.
Mix. Divide into two doses, and administer each in a quantity of gruel.

3736. Condition Powder. A

Sublimed sulphur........ ⎫
Nitrate of potash........ ⎬ equal quantities.
Black antimony .... ⎭
Dose, ½ ounce. Or—

3737. Condition Powder. B

Sulphate of iron.......... 2 parts.
Powdered gentian......... 2 parts.
Nitrate of potash .... 1 part.
Dose, ½ ounce.

Cordial Drinks are generally composed of some warm aromatic, such as ginger or caraway, with 1 pint of strong ale.

NON-SECRET FORMULAS.

3738. Cough Balls. A
Powdered ipecacuanha .... 1 dram.
Powdered squills.......... 1 dram.
Honey and licorice powder, of each enough to make a ball.

3739. Cough Balls. B
Powdered gum ammoniac.. ½ ounce.
Powdered ginger.......... 1½ drams.
Powdered squills.......... 1 dram.
Honey and licorice powder, q. s.

3740. Diapente.
Gentian .... 4 ounces.
Turmeric .... 4 ounces.
Fenugreek .... 4 ounces.
Ginger .... 4 ounces.
Anise oil .... 1½ drams.
Clove oil................. 1½ drams.
Caraway oil............... 1½ drams.

3741. Diuretic Mass.
White resin .... 30 ounces.
Nitrate of potass......... 15 ounces.
Lard .... 6 ounces.
Linseed oil .... 6 ounces.
Oil of juniper............ 1 ounce.

Melt the resin and add the oils and lard. Next add the nitre and stir until nearly cold, when the mass should be transferred to a slab and worked with glycerine.

3742. Elliman's Embrocation.
Hager gives the subjoined formula:
Whites of two eggs........ 50 grammes.
Water .... 50 grammes.
Crude pyroligneous acid.... 50 grammes.
Spirit .... 60 grammes.
Turpentine oil............ 3 grammes.

3743. Eye Lotion.
Zinc acetate .... 2 drams.
Henbane extract........... 2 drams.
Rectified spirit .... 3 ounces.
Camphor spirit .... 1 scruple.
Water to make .... 36 ounces.

3744. Fever Balls. A
Nitrate of potash......... 2 drams.
Camphor .... 1 dram.
Tartar emetic............. 10 grains.
Honey .... q. s.

3745. Fever Balls. B
Omit the tartar emetic and substitute:
Calomel .... 15 grains.
Opium .... 15 grains.

3746. Gripe Drench.
Chloroform................ 4 ounces.
Pimento oil............... ½ ounce.
Camphor................... ½ ounce.
Opium powder.............. ½ ounce.
Rectified spirit.......... 1 pint.
Chillies.................. 1 ounce.

Macerate the opium and chillies in the spirit for seven days, filter and mix the other ingredients. Dose, 1½ ounces, with 1 ounce of spirits of nitre, in a pint of warm gruel.

3747. Lotion for Cracked Hoofs, &c.
Commonly known in Scotland as the White Bottle:
This consists of
Sulphate of zinc.......... 1 ounce.
Sugar of lead............. 1 ounce.
Water .... 1 quart.

3748. Mange Liniment.
Mange Liniment.—Mange in horses, cattle, and dogs results from the attack of minute acari, which causes much itching and heat, accompanied with scurfiness and baldness of the skin. The treatment consists first in destroying the acari, and second in absolute cleanliness of the parts affected. No better preparation for horses and cattle will be found than the following, which may be applied twice a day for a short time and afterwards once a day:

Sulphur vivum............. 4 ounces.
Powdered white hellebore.. 1 ounce.
Turpentine................ 1 to 4 ounces.
Linseed oil, add to....... 24 ounces.

When a milder treatment is required, particularly for dogs, mercurial ointment, or sulphur ointment, or a mixture of sulphur, tar, and linseed oil may be tried.

3749. Bran Mash.
Mashes.—Bran Mash: Put half a peck of bran into a pail and saturate thoroughly with boiling water. Stir well and cover it, and let stand till of the temperature of new milk. Various ingredients, such as treacle, honey, sweet ale, &c., are occasionally added.
Malt Mash is made in the same way.

3750. Oatmeal Gruel.

Oatmeal Gruel.—Put 1 pound of good oatmeal into a basin and add about 1 pint of cold water. Mix this thoroughly, and then boil it with water to form 1 gallon of gruel.

3751. Ointment for Grease.

Citrine ointment	2 ounces.
Lard	2 ounces.
Turpentine	½ ounce.
Sat. sol. nitrate of copper	2 drams.

3752. Ointment for Horses' Knees.

Mercurial ointment	1½ ounces.
Honey	1 ounce.
Camphor	2 drams.
Burned cork, powdered	¼ ounce.

3753. Physic Mass.

Physic Mass.—Probably no veterinary medicines are more in demand than physic and diuretic mass. To have these, therefore, always in good condition, whether divided into balls or in bulk, is clearly a matter of the greatest importance. Should the mass or ball get to be too hard from age or other cause it will certainly be erratic in its action, while if it be not uniform in consistence and composition it will be apt to cause more or less irritation. The physic mass should in every case be made with the finest aloes, and no excipient will be found to equal glycerine. The aloes should be melted by the aid of steam, and the glycerine added in the proportion of one to six in the winter season and one to eight in the summer. A smaller proportion of glycerine will answer the purpose if the the aloes is first melted, then poured on a slab and the glycerine worked into it while hot; but this entails more labor and attention. A good apparatus for melting the aloes may be made (of any size) on the principle of a joiner's gluepot—the outer pot for boiling the water into which the smaller pot containing the aloes and glycerine is inserted. The pots may be made of any size sufficient to melt from 1 pound to 5 pounds of aloes. For larger quantities special apparatus must be devised. The mass thus made requires no special care in keeping; it will keep uniform in softness for any length of time, and will prove more easily soluble than that prepared by any other method.

Messrs. Elliman & Co. have published the following formula for a physic mass, which is plastic, ductile, and soluble:

Best Barbados aloes	10 pounds.
Glycerine	1 pound.
Castor oil	1 pound.
Powd. unbleached ginger	½ pound.

Dissolve the aloes in the glycerine by means of a water-bath, then add the castor oil, and lastly stir in the ginger previously sifted through a coarse sieve. The balls thus made will not retain their shape, but may be wrapped in waxed paper and put up in boxes like marking-ink cases.

3754.

Treatment of Distemper.—Distemper is a typhoid inflammation of the air-passages of young dogs, and is accompanied by low fever and debility. It may be recognized by the watery inflammatory state of the eyes, the dryness and heat of the nose, accompanied by frequent sneezing and general debility. An emetic of 2 grains each of tartar emetic and ipecacuanha powder for an ordinary-sized dog ought to be given on the symptoms being first observed. This should be followed by a fever treatment of ¼ to ½ grain extract belladonna with 5 grains nitrate of potash three times a day. On the abatement of all the more acute symptoms the tonic treatment may be adapted. This may consist of 1 grain each quinine and iron, with extract of gentian to form a ball—this three times a day.

3755. White Oils.

The following is an approved formula. The oils are an excellent stock liniment for man and beast:

Eggs	12
Soft-soap	5 ounces.
Turpentine	12 ounces.
Strong solution of ammonia	6 ounces.
Camphor	5 ounces.
Methylated spirit	10 ounces.
Eucalyptus oil	2 ounces.
Water to make	5 pints.

3756. Wound Stone.

Iron sulphate	2 pounds.
Alum	2 pounds.
Zinc sulphate	4 ounces.
Copper sulphate	4 ounces.

Armenian bole enough to color it.
Put up in 2 ounce packets.

PART II.

PERFUMERY, COLOGNES, TOILET ARTICLES, &c., &c.

To Prepare Handkerchief Extracts.

In the selection of materials for the preparation of fine perfumes, always buy the best pomades, essential oils, and other necessary materials. The spirits used should always be free from the odor of fusel oil or any other contaminating ingredient. Always tell your spirit merchant to give you clean cologne spirits of a strength of 188 or 190 per cent proof government standard (94 to 95 per cent actual). The pomades should be of the highest strength made, and should be purchased from some reliable agent, handling goods of a superior quality and making his importations direct from Grasse. The pomades principally used are cassie, jasmin, orange flowers, rose, tuberose and violet. There are on the market a few other pomades, such as Lily of the Valley, reseda (mignonette), heliotrope, etc., but they are not much in demand, and the first named pomades will be ample for every purpose. The essential oils needed are allspice, almond, bitter; angelica root, German; bay, bergamot, cananga (or kananga), cassia, cinnamon, citronella, cloves, coriander, dill, fennel seed, geraniol hyacinth, geraniol reseda, lavender, lemon, lemon grass, lilac, linaloe, neroli petale, neroli bigarade, nutmeg, orange, orris root, patchouli, rose, rose geranium, sandalwood, vetivert and ylang ylang. These will be enough for ordinary wants.

The other requirements for handkerchief extracts, sachets, etc., will be ambergris, ambrette seed, angelica root, powdered; cardamom seed, carmine, chlorophyll, civet, cloves, ground; coriander seed, ground; coumarin, floral waters (orange flower and rose) gum benzoin, heliotropine, ionone, musc baur musk, in grain; orris root, patchouly leaves, sandalwood, ground; styrax, liquid; vanillin, vetivert root, besides such items as coloring, ribbons, etc., etc.

In making perfumery, as with many other lines of business, the amount of money you can afford to put into the cost of the goods will mainly determine the quality of your product. Find out the amount you can obtain for your goods; calculate the cost of selling, store expenses, etc.; add the profit required, and the amount left will be an important factor in determining the expense of your formula. This article on perfumery is written for men of small means who wish to engage in a pleasant, profitable business, and who do not desire to invest much money in the venture until assured of success.

The formulas of the first quality extracts are based on goods ordinarily sold at $3.50 to $4.00 per pound. Should better goods be desired, reduce the amount of spirits used in washing the pomades; for cheaper goods use more spirits. The formulas for making handkerchief extracts from oils and tinctures alone are published to enable anyone to compete with the low grade goods offered for ten cents an ounce, at retail. I do not recommend their use, excepting where keen competition compels the offering of something very cheap, yet dear at any price.

To Wash the Pomades.

Take any pomade, say rose.................... 6 pounds.
Cologne spirits, 188 per cent .... 14 pints.

Place eight pints of the cologne spirits in an ice cream freezer; melt the pomade gently by the heat of a water bath; pour into the spirits contained in the freezer, turning the handle of the freezer slowly, and continue turning for an hour. Let the pomade stay in the spirits for three days, agitating occasionally, the oftener the better. Pour off the tincture and set aside. Pour into the freezer (containing the pomade) the remaining six pints of cologne spirits and let it remain, with occasional agitation, for three days; carefully drain off the second washing and add to the first. Label this Tincture of Rose. This tincture will have to be filtered at a low temperature, in order to remove the grease held in solution by the strong spirit. The grease may not be visible, but it is there nevertheless. If you are churning your pomade in the winter time (the proper season for work of this kind) set your tincture out of doors until the grease in solution is frozen hard, and filter through filtering paper to remove the grease; your tincture is then bright and fit for use. Should you have to wash your pomade, in summer time, after you have finished washing your pomade, place the tincture in your freezer, with some ice and salt, and turn the handle until the fat is hardened. You should also have an ice chest and plenty of ice in it. Stand your receiving bottle with funnel and paper in the ice chest, and filter your tincture at a temperature of about 40° F. to ensure the removal of the grease. Ice cream freezers are very convenient for the washing of pomades, and can be obtained of any size for hand power up to 40 quarts, and larger if required with power attachment. But if your trade is such as to require a churn larger than a 40 quart freezer, you can afford to have a perfumery churn manufactured to order.

The terms, extract of rose, extract of musk, extract of civet, etc., are confusing. I have preferred to call them tinctures, and when they are compounded they may be then known as extracts (see also tinctures for perfumery, directions for making). Remember to keep your spirits, oils and tinctures bright, and save time, expense and waste in filtering your compounds.

3757. Ardeola Bouquet.

Oil of bergamot............	2 drams.
Oil of sandalwood........	2 drams.
Oil of lemon................	1 dram.
Tincture of rose............	12 ounces.
Tincture of jasmin........	8 ounces.
Tincture of musc baur.....	2 ounces.
Tincture of ambergris.....	⅛ ounce.
Tincture of vanillin.......	2 ounces.
Tincture of orris..........	4 ounces.

Mix and filter, if necessary.

3758. Bergamot Extract.

Oil of bergamot...........	1 ounce.
Tincture of civet	1 ounce.
Tincture of ambergris....	1 ounce.
Tincture of musc baur....	1 ounce.
Cologne spirits, 188 per cent....................	32 ounces.

Mix. Color with chlorophyll and filter if necessary.

3759. Bouquet Caroline.

Tincture of cassie.........	16 ounces.
Tincture of violet.........	16 ounces.
Tincture of jasmin	16 ounces.
Tincture of orange flowers.	16 ounces.
Tincture of musc baur.....	12 ounces.
Tincture of civet	4 ounces.
Tincture of verbena	8 ounces.
Oil of lemon...............	¼ ounce.
Oil of bergamot............	¾ ounce.
Oil of neroli Portugal.....	¼ ounce.

Mix and filter if necessary.

To make Oil of Neroli Portugal mix equal parts of oil of neroli petale and oil of neroli bigarade.

3760. Bouquet Essence.
Ess. Bouquet.

Tincture of rose	16 ounces.
Tincture of orange flowers.	16 ounces.
Tincture of ambergris	3 ounces.
Tincture of civet	1½ ounces.
Tincture of orris root....	16 ounces.
Tincture of styrax	½ ounce.
Oil of bergamot...........	¾ ounce.
Oil of lemon...............	¼ ounce.
Oil of lavender............	1 dram.

Mix and filter if necessary.

3761. Bouquet Tip Top.

Tincture of rose	16 ounces.
Tincture of tuberose	16 ounces.
Tincture of benzoin	1 ounce.
Tincture of civet	1 ounce.
Tincture of vanillin	1 ounce.
Oil of bergamot...........	1 ounce.
Oil of lemon	¼ ounce.
Oil of orange sweet........	¼ ounce.
Orange flower water.......	4 ounces.

Mix and filter.

3762. Bridal Bouquet.   A

Tincture of tuberose	16 ounces.
Tincture of cassie	8 ounces.
Tincture of orange flowers.	8 ounces.
Tincture of civet	1½ ounces.
Tincture of geranium	16 ounces.
Tincture of ambergris	4 ounces.
Oil of bergamot	½ ounce.
Oil of rose	1 dram.
Oil of neroli Portugal.....	1 dram.
Oil of orange sweet........	1 dram.
Orange flower water.......	4 ounces.
Cologne spirits, 188 per cent....................	6 ounces.

Mix and filter.

3763. Bridal Bouquet.   B

Oil of rose...............	1 dram.
Oil of neroli petale.......	1 dram.
Oil of bergamot	2 drams.
Oil of coriander	10 drops.
Oil of pimento............	5 drops.
Oil of lavender...........	5 drops.
Tincture of orris	8 ounces.
Tincture of jasmin	8 ounces.
Tincture of musc baur.....	4 ounces.
Tincture of benzoin	2 ounces.
Cologne spirits, 188 per cent....................	10 ounces.

Mix and filter if necessary.

NON-SECRET FORMULAS.

3764. Bouquet D'Amour.
Tincture of musc baur	4 ounces.
Tincture of civet	2 ounces.
Tincture of vanillin	2 ounces.
Tincture of cassie	16 ounces.
Tincture of jasmin	8 ounces.
Tincture of violet	16 ounces.
Tincture of orange flowers	4 ounces.

Mix and filter if necessary.

3765. Carthage Bouquet.
Tincture of rose	32 ounces.
Tincture of tuberose	24 ounces.
Tincture of orris	12 ounces.
Tincture of ambergris	4 ounces.
Tincture of musc baur	2 ounces.
Oil of bergamot	1 ounce.
Oil of lemon	¼ ounce.

Mix and filter if necessary.

3766. Clove Pink.
Tincture of jasmin	16 ounces.
Tincture of orris	16 ounces.
Tincture of musc baur	8 ounces.
Tincture of benzoin	1 dram.
Oil of rose geranium	1 dram.
Oil of cloves	½ dram.
Oil of neroli Portugal	1 dram.
Oil of pimento	10 drops.
Oil of patchouli	10 drops.
Oil of sandalwood	1 dram.
Cologne spirits, 188 per cent	10 ounces.
Orange flower water	2 ounces.

Mix and filter.

3767. Citronelle Rose—Cheap.
Cologne spirits, 188 per cent	1 quart.
Oil of orange sweet	2 ounces.
Oil of rose geranium	3 drams.
Oil of rose	1 dram.
Oil of citronella	1 dram.
Tincture of civet	2 ounces.
Water	4 ounces.

Mix and filter.

3768. Crab Apple.
Oil of ylang ylang	30 drops.
Oil of mace liquid	10 drops.
Oil of wintergreen	2 drops.
Oil of linaloe	20 drops.
Oil of coriander	20 drops.
Oil of hyacinth geraniol	5 drops.
Tincture of cassie	2 ounces.
Tincture of violet	4 ounces.
Tincture of musc baur	¼ ounce.
Tincture of styrax	½ dram.

Mix and filter if necessary.

3769. Cremorne Valley.
Tincture of jasmin	10 ounces.
Tincture of orange flowers	10 ounces.
Tincture of rose	20 ounces.
Tincture of violet	10 ounces.
Tincture of musc baur	1 ounce.
Tincture of ambergris	1 ounce.
Oil of bergamot	½ ounce.
Oil of hyacinth geraniol	1 dram.

Mix and filter if necessary.

3770. Enchantment Bouquet.
Oil of bergamot	7 drams.
Oil of cloves	20 drops.
Oil of rose geranium	40 drops.
Oil of neroli petale	1 dram.
Oil of orange sweet	½ dram.
Tincture of benzoin	5 drams.
Tincture of orris	8 ounces.
Tincture of vanillin	1 ounce.
Tincture of nutmegs	½ ounce.
Cologne spirits, 188 per cent	14 ounces.
Orange flower water	2½ ounces.

Mix and filter.

3771. Framlingham Bouquet.
Tincture of violet	20 ounces.
Tincture of orange flowers	20 ounces.
Tincture of tuberose	10 ounces.
Tincture of cassie	20 ounces.
Tincture of rose geranium	16 ounces.
Tincture of musc baur	4 ounces.
Tincture of ambergris	4 ounces.
Tincture of neroli Portugal	2 ounces.

Mix and filter if necessary.

3772. Frangipanni—Single Strength.
Tincture of orris	8 ounces.
Tincture of tuberose	4 ounces.
Tincture of musk	8 ounces.
Tincture of vanilla	4 ounces.
Tincture of jasmin	2 ounces.
Tincture of styrax	1 ounce.
Oil of neroli Portugal	2 drams.
Oil of rose geranium	½ ounce.
Oil of sandalwood	2 drams.
Oil of cinnamon	½ dram.
Oil of bergamot	1 dram.
Oil of lavender	15 minims.
Cologne spirits, 188 per ct.	32 ounces.
Orange flower water	4 ounces.

Mix and filter. Color with tincture of red saunders or aniline brown, q. s.

3773. Frangipanni—Double Strength.
Tincture of orange flowers	16 ounces.
Tincture of vanillin	32 ounces.
Tincture of musk	20 ounces.

Tincture of coumarin	20 ounces.
Tincture of civet	16 ounces.
Tincture of orris	32 ounces.
Oil of rose	1 ounce.
Oil of sandalwood	½ ounce.
Oil of neroli Portugal	1 dram.
Oil of coriander	½ dram.
Oil of hyacinth geraniol	½ dram.
Oil of reseda geraniol	½ dram.
Oil of vetivert	¼ dram.
Cologne spirits, 188 per cent	7 ounces.

Dissolve the oils in the seven ounces of spirits; add the tinctures and filter. Color with red saunders or aniline brown, q. s.

3774. Hedyosmia.

Tincture of rose	16 ounces.
Tincture of jasmin	8 ounces.
Tincture of orange flowers	8 ounces.
Tincture of cassie	8 ounces.
Tincture of tuberose	4 ounces.
Tincture of vanillin	2 ounces.
Tincture of ambergris	2 ounces.
Tincture of styrax	½ ounce.
Oil of bergamot	3 drams.
Oil of lemon	1 ounce.
Oil of orange sweet	½ ounce.
Cologne spirits, 188 per cent	1 pint.

Dissolve the oils in the spirits, add the tinctures and filter if necessary.

3775. Heliotrope.

Tincture of heliotrope (1 to 16)	8 ounces.
Tincture of orris	16 ounces.
Tincture of rose	8 ounces.
Tincture of jasmin	8 ounces.
Tincture of styrax	2 drams.
Tincture of vetivert	2 drams.
Tincture of coumarin	8 ounces.
Oil of bergamot	2 drams.
Oil of bitter almonds	8 drops.

Mix and filter if necessary.

3776. Honeysuckle.

Tincture of rose	16 ounces.
Tincture of jasmin	16 ounces.
Tincture of violet	16 ounces.
Tincture of civet	1 ounce.
Tincture of vanillin	3 ounces.
Tincture of musc baur	2 ounces.
Oil of rose	1 dram.
Oil of sandalwood	½ dram.
Oil of bergamot	1 dram.
Oil of angelica	5 drops.
Cologne spirits, 188 per cent	10 ounces.

Dissolve the oils in the spirits, add the tinctures and filter if necessary.

3777. Imperial Bouquet.

Tincture of rose	16 ounces.
Tincture of jasmin	8 ounces.
Tincture of violet	8 ounces.
Tincture of cassie	5 ounces.
Tincture of musc baur	2 ounces.
Tincture of civet	2 ounces.
Tincture of styrax	1 dram.
Oil of lemon	¼ ounce.
Oil of bergamot	½ ounce.
Cologne spirits	7 ounces.

Dissolve the oils in the spirits, add the tinctures and filter if necessary.

3778. Jasmin.

Tincture of jasmin	24 ounces.
Tincture of orange flowers	6 ounces.
Tincture of cassie	3 ounces.
Tincture of civet	1 ounce.
Tincture of orris	8 ounces.

Mix and filter if necessary.

3779. Jess.

Tincture of rose	16 ounces.
Tincture of cassie	8 ounces.
Tincture of orange flowers	4 ounces.
Tincture of civet	2 ounces.
Tincture of tolu	2 ounces.
Tincture of vanillin	8 ounces.
Oil of rose	1 dram.

Mix and filter if necessary.

3780. Jockey Club. A

Tincture of cassie	17 ounces.
Tincture of tuberose	20 ounces.
Tincture of jasmin	17 ounces.
Tincture of rose	8½ ounces.
Tincture of vanillin	10 ounces.
Tincture of civet	5 ounces.
Oil of bergamot	3 drams.
Oil of lemon	3 drams.
Oil of rose geranium	1 dram.

Mix and filter if necessary.

3781. Jockey Club. B

Tincture of jasmin	10 ounces.
Tincture of orange flowers	8 ounces.
Tincture of rose	8 ounces.
Tincture of cassie	8 ounces.
Tincture of coumarin	4 ounces.
Tincture of civet	2 ounces.
Tincture of musc baur	4 ounces.
Tincture of vanillin	2 ounces.
Oil of rose	1 dram.

Mix and filter if necessary.

NON-SECRET FORMULAS.

3782. Johnny-Jump-Up.
Tincture of jasmin.......... 8 ounces.
Tincture of tuberose....... 8 ounces.
Tincture of orange flowers. 12 ounces.
Tincture of vanillin........ 2½ ounces.
Tincture of ambergris...... ¾ ounce.
Tincture of musk........... 4 ounces.
Oil of bergamot............ ¾ ounce.
Oil of sandalwood.......... ¼ ounce.
Mix and filter if necessary.

3783. Kensington Bouquet.
Tincture of tuberose....... 6 ounces.
Tincture of jasmin......... 32 ounces.
Tincture of rose........... 16 ounces.
Tincture of cassie......... 6 ounces.
Tincture of orris.......... 16 ounces.
Tincture of ambergris...... 1 ounce.
Tincture of musc baur..... 1 ounce.
Oil of rose................ 1 dram.
Mix and filter if necessary.

3784. Lilac, White or Purple.
Tincture of jasmin......... 16 ounces.
Tincture of orange flowers. 1 ounce.
Tincture of civet.......... 1 ounce.
Tincture of vanillin....... 4 ounces.
Oil of reseda geraniol..... 10 minims.
Oil of muguet (lilac)...... 60 minims.
Mix and filter if necessary.
Color with purple aniline if purple lilac is desired.

3785. Lily of the Valley.
Tincture of tuberose....... 6 ounces.
Tincture of jasmin......... 8 ounces.
Tincture of civet.......... 1 ounce.
Tincture of vanillin....... 2 ounces.
Oil of sandalwood.......... 2 drops.
Oil of lily of the valley (D. & O.)................. 10 drops.
Mix and filter if necessary.

3786. Linden Bloom.
Tincture of jasmin......... 16 ounces.
Tincture of musk........... 2 ounces.
Tincture of vanillin....... 2 ounces.
Oil of bergamot............ 4 drams.
Oil of linaloe............. 2 drams.
Mix and filter if necessary.

3787. Lucca Bouquet.
Tincture of rose........... 10 ounces.
Tincture of jasmin......... 10 ounces.
Tincture of violet......... 10 ounces.
Tincture of civet.......... 5 ounces.
Oil of rose................ 15 minims.
Oil of syringa............. 5 minims.
Oil of lavender............ 10 minims.
Mix and filter if necessary.

3788. Mary Stuart.
Tincture of rose........... 16 ounces.
Tincture of jasmin......... 6 ounces.
Tincture of musk........... 4 ounces.
Tincture of orris.......... 8 ounces.
Tincture of ambergris...... 1 ounce.
Tincture of vanillin....... 4 ounces.
Oil of orange, sweet....... ½ ounce.
Oil of bergamot............ ½ ounce.
Mix and filter if necessary.

3789. May Blossom.
Tincture of jasmin......... 25 ounces.
Tincture of musk........... 5 ounces.
Tincture of rose geranium.. 5 ounces.
Oil of bergamot............ ½ ounce.
Oil of linaloe............. 1½ ounces.
Cologne spirits 188 per ct... 4 ounces.
Dissolve the oils in the cologne spirits.—add the tinctures, and filter if necessary.

3790. Mignonette.
Tincture of violet......... 16 ounces.
Tincture of rose........... 8 ounces.
Tincture of orange flowers. 8 ounces.
Tincture of cassie......... 8 ounces.
Tincture of ambergris..... 2 ounces.
Oil of reseda geraniol..... 1 dram.
Oil of bergamot............ 1 dram.
Oil of rose................ ½ dram.
Mix and filter if necessary.

3791. Millefleurs.
Tincture of jasmin......... 8 ounces.
Tincture of rose........... 4 ounces.
Tincture of tuberose....... 4 ounces.
Tincture of orange flowers.. 4 ounces.
Tincture of cassie......... 4 ounces.
Tincture of orris.......... 4 ounces.
Tincture of vanillin....... 2 ounces.
Tincture of musc baur..... 2 ounces.
Oil of bergamot............ ¼ ounce.
Oil of lavender............ 1 dram.
Oil of rose geranium....... 1 dram.
Oil of neroli petale....... 5 minims.
Mix and filter if necessary.

3792. Moss Rose.
Tincture of rose........... 18 ounces.
Tincture of orris.......... 3 ounces.
Tincture of orange flowers. 4 ounces.
Tincture of musk........... 3 ounces.
Tincture of civet.......... 1½ ounces.
Oil of rose................ 1 dram.
Oil of rose geranium...... ½ dram.
Cologne spirits 188 per ct. 3 ounces.
Dissolve the oils in the spirits, add the tinctures, and filter if necessary.

NON-SECRET FORMULAS.

3793. Musk (from Grain Musk).
Tincture of musk	16 ounces.
(1 ounce to gallon.)	
Tincture of civet	1 ounce.
Tincture of ambergris	1 ounce.
Tincture of styrax	½ dram.
Tincture of orris	2 ounces.
Tincture of ambrette seed	3½ ounces.

Mix and filter if necessary.

3794. Musk (from Musc Baur).
Tincture of musc baur	16 ounces.
(1 ounce to gallon.)	
Tincture of civet	1 ounce.
Tincture of ambergris	1 ounce.
Tincture of orris	1 ounce.
Orange flower water	5 ounces.

Mix and filter. Color with aniline brown q. s.

3795. Musk Rose.
Tincture of rose	8 ounces.
Tincture of orange flowers	7 ounces.
Tincture of musk	2 ounces.
Oil of sandalwood	2 drops.
Oil of rose	10 drops.

Mix and filter if necessary.

3796. New Mown Hay. A
Tincture of cassie	8 ounces.
Tincture of orris	16 ounces.
Tincture of coumarin	24 ounces.
Tincture of civet	2 ounces.
Tincture of orange flowers	8 ounces.
Tincture of jasmin	8 ounces.
Tincture of rose	16 ounces.
Oil of sandalwood	5 drops.
Oil of cloves	5 drops.
Oil of neroli, big	10 drops.
Oil of rose geranium	20 drops.

Mix and filter if necessary.

3797. New Mown Hay. B
Tincture of tonka	25 ounces.
Tincture of musk	6 ounces.
Tincture of vanilla	2 ounces.
Tincture of styrax	¼ ounce.
Tincture of orris	8 ounces.
Oil of bergamot	1 ounce.
Oil of lemon	½ ounce.
Oil of neroli, big	15 drops.
Oil of cloves	15 drops.
Oil of patchouly	10 drops.
Oil of sandalwood	1 dram.

Mix and filter if necessary.

3798. Night-Blooming Cereus.
Tincture of tuberose	10 ounces.
Tincture of rose	6 ounces.
Tincture of jasmin	3 ounces.
Tincture of violet	3 ounces.
Tincture of vanillin	1½ ounces.
Tincture of coumarin	1½ ounces.
Tincture of musc baur	1 ounce.
Oil of neroli Portugal	30 minims.

Mix and filter if necessary.

3799. Opopanax.
Tincture of violet	8 ounces.
Tincture of cassie	4 ounces.
Tincture of orange flowers	4 ounces.
Tincture of rose	8 ounces.
Tincture of orris	16 ounces.
Tincture of coumarin	½ ounce.
Tincture of musk	2 ounces.
Oil of rose	1 dram.
Oil of bergamot	1 dram.
Oil of rose geraniol	1 dram.
Oil of patchouli	3 minims.

Mix and filter if necessary.

3800. Orange Flowers.
Tincture of orange flowers	16 ounces.
Tincture of civet	1 ounce.
Tincture of ambergris	¼ ounce.
Tincture of musk	¼ ounce.
Tincture of orris	1 ounce.
Oil of neroli Portugal	15 minims.

Mix and filter if necessary.

3801. Our Own.
Tincture of rose	8 ounces.
Tincture of jasmin	2 ounces.
Tincture of violet	4 ounces.
Tincture of cassie	2 ounces.
Tincture of musc baur	½ ounce.
Tincture of ambergris	¼ ounce.
Tincture of vanillin	1 ounce.
Tincture of orange flowers	½ ounce.
Oil of patchouli	1 drop.

Mix and filter if necessary.

3802. Patchouli.
Tincture of musk	4 ounces.
Tincture of orris	4 ounces.
Tincture of vanilla	2 ounces.
Oil of rose	½ dram.
Oil of sandalwood	20 minims.
Oil of patchouli	40 minims.
Cologne spirits 188 per ct.	6 ounces.
Rose water	2 ounces.

Mix and filter.

3803. Pearl of Pekin.

Tincture of rose.	10 ounces.
Tincture of jasmine.	6 ounces.
Tincture of cassie.	2 ounces.
Tincture of musc baur.	1 ounce.
Oil of bergamot.	1 dram.
Oil of neroli Portugal.	½ dram.

Mix and filter if necessary.

3804. Perfection.

Tincture of rose.	8 ounces.
Tincture of orange flowers.	8 ounces.
Tincture of orris.	4 ounces.
Tincture of vanillin.	1 ounce.
Tincture of civet.	½ ounce.
Tincture of musc baur.	1 ounce.
Oil of reseda geraniol.	5 drops.
Oil of hyacinth geraniol.	5 drops.

Mix and filter if necessary.

3805. Persian Pink.

Tincture of orange flowers.	4 ounces.
Tincture of rose.	8 ounces.
Tincture of cassie.	4 ounces.
Tincture of vanillin.	2 ounces.
Tincture of musc baur.	2 ounces.
Oil of cloves.	10 drops.
Oil of sandalwood.	5 drops.

Mix and filter if necessary.

3806. Pink.

Tincture of rose.	10 ounces.
Tincture of orange flowers.	6 ounces.
Tincture of cassie.	4 ounces.
Tincture of vanillin.	2 ounces.
Tincture of ambergris.	1 dram.
Oil of cloves.	5 drops.

Mix and filter if necessary.

Pink (Clove).

See Clove Pink.

3807. Pond Lily.

Tincture of coumarin.	16 ounces.
Tincture of orange flowers.	8 ounces.
Tincture of cassie.	2 ounces.
Tincture of musc baur.	1½ ounces.
Tincture of orris.	2 ounces.
Oil of rose.	1 dram.
Oil of lily of the valley (D & O).	½ dram.

Mix and filter if necessary.

3808. Prairie Blossom.

Tincture of rose.	8 ounces.
Tincture of violet.	8 ounces.
Tincture of tuberose.	12 ounces.
Tincture of orange flowers.	2 ounces.
Tincture of musk.	3 ounces.
Tincture of civet.	2 ounces.
Oil of lemon.	1 dram.
Oil of bergamot.	2 drams.
Oil of orange, sweet.	1 dram.

Mix and filter if necessary.

3809. Rondeletia.

Tincture of orris.	10 ounces.
Tincture of jasmine.	10 ounces.
Tincture of musk.	4 ounces.
Oil of lavender.	1 dram.
Oil of bergamot.	15 minims.
Oil of cloves.	5 minims.
Oil of rose.	40 minims.

Mix and filter if necessary.

3810. Rose.

Tincture of rose.	16 ounces.
Tincture of civet.	1½ ounces.
Tincture of ambergris.	½ ounce.
Otto of rose.	½ dram.

Mix and filter if necessary.

3811. Rose of Cashmere.

Tincture of coumarin.	1 ounce.
Tincture of musk.	4 ounces.
Tincture of vanillin.	4 ounces.
Tincture of jasmine.	6 ounces.
Tincture of orris.	8 ounces.
Oil of rose.	2 drams.
Cologne spirits, 188 per ct.	10 ounces.
Rose water.	2 ounces.

Dissolve the oil in the spirits. Add the tinctures and then the rose water—add the latter very slowly, and filter.

3812. Rose Geranium.

Cologne spirits, 188 per ct.	16 ounces.
Tincture of civet.	1 ounce.
Tincture of musk.	1 ounce.
Oil of rose.	1 dram.
Oil of rose geranium.	6 drams.
Oil of bergamot.	2 drams.

Dissolve the oils in the spirits, add the tinctures, and filter if necessary.

3813. Sandalwood.

Cologne spirits, 188 per ct..	12 ounces.
Oil of sandalwood..........	2 drams.
Oil of cedar.	½ dram.
Oil of melissa (lemon balm)	15 drops.
Oil of rose.	15 drops.
Tincture of civet	1 ounce.
Tincture of musc baur.	2 ounces.
Tincture of orris.	3 ounces.

Mix and filter if necessary.

3814. Spring Flowers.

Tincture of rose.	8 ounces.
Tincture of violet.	8 ounces.
Tincture of orange.	2 ounces.
Tincture of ambergris.	½ ounce.
Tincture of civet.	¼ ounce.
Tincture of musk.	¾ ounce.
Oil of rose.	30 minims.

Mix and filter if necessary.

3815. Spring Posey.

Tincture of tuberose.	10 ounces.
Tincture of orris.	10 ounces.
Tincture of cassie.	5 ounces.
Tincture of rose.	5 ounces.
Tincture of coumarin.	5 ounces.
Tincture of civet	1 ounce.
Oil of bergamot.	1 dram.

Mix and filter if necessary.

3816. Sweet Brier.

Tincture of rose.	16 ounces.
Tincture of cassie.	3 ounces.
Tincture of orange flowers..	3 ounces.
Tincture of civet.	½ ounce.
Oil of rose.	30 minims.
Oil of neroli Portugal......	15 minims.
Oil of lemon grass.	1 drop.

Mix and filter if necessary.

3817. Sweet Clover.

Cologne spirits, 188 per ct..	16 ounces.
Tincture of vanillin.	4 ounces.
Tincture of tonka.	3 ounces.
Tincture of tuberose.	4 ounces.
Tincture of styrax.........	¼ ounce.
Tincture of civet ,.	1 ounce.
Tincture of orris.	1 ounce.
Oil of rose.	1 dram.
Oil of bergamot.	1 dram.
Oil of neroli bigarade.	1 dram.
Oil of cloves.	5 drops.

Mix and filter if necessary.

3818. Sweetheart's Garland.

Tincture of jasmine........	14 ounces.
Tincture of tuberose.	8 ounces.
Tincture of orange flowers..	2 ounces.
Tincture of rose.	2 ounces.
Tincture of vanillin.	2½ ounces.
Tincture of civet.	1½ ounces.
Oil of bergamot.	2 drams.

Mix and filter if necessary.

3819. Sweet Pea.

Tincture of rose.	4 ounces.
Tincture of orange flowers..	8 ounces.
Tincture of tuberose.	6 ounces.
Tincture of vanilla.	4 ounces.
Tincture of civet	½ ounce.
Oil of rose.	10 minims.
Oil of bitter almonds.	1 drop.

Mix and filter if necessary.

3820. Sweet Pink.

Tincture of rose.	16 ounces.
Tincture of orange flowers	8 ounces.
Tincture of cassie.	8 ounces.
Tincture of vanillin.	2 ounces.
Tincture of civet.	½ ounce.
Oil of cloves...............	10 drops..

Mix and filter if necessary.

3821. Sweet Shrub.

Tincture of vanillin.	4 ounces.
Tincture of coumarin......	4 ounces.
Tincture of rose.	8 ounces.
Tincture of tuberose.	16 ounces.
Tincture of orange flowers..	16 ounces.
Tincture of tolu.	2 ounces.
Tincture of civet.	1½ ounces.
Oil of rose.	1 dram.
Oil of rose geranium.	½ dram.
Oil of bergamot.	½ dram.
Oil of neroli petale.	10 drops.

Mix and filter if necessary.

3822. Tea Rose.

Tincture of rose.	12 ounces.
Tincture of rose geranium.	8 ounces.
Tincture of neroli Portugal	2 ounces.
Tincture of orris.	2 ounces.
Tincture of civet.	1 ounce.
Tincture of sandalwood. ..	1 ounce.
Tincture of styrax.	1 dram.
Oil of rose geraniol.	½ dram.

Mix and filter if necessary.

3823. Tuberose. A
Tincture of tuberose	16 ounces
Tincture of jasmine	2 ounces
Tincture of orange flowers	4 ounces
Tincture of civet	½ ounce
Tincture of musk	¾ ounce
Oil of neroli Portugal	20 drops
Oil of rose	40 drops

Mix and filter if necessary.

3824. Tuberose. B
Tincture of tuberose	14 ounces
Tincture of rose	2 ounces
Tincture of orris	2 ounces
Tincture of vanillin	½ ounce
Oil of bitter almonds	1 drop

Mix and filter if necessary.

3825. Union Bouquet.
Tincture of rose	8 ounces
Tincture of orange flowers	6 ounces
Tincture of violet	2 ounces
Tincture of cassie	2 ounces
Tincture of tuberose	2 ounces
Tincture of jasmine	4 ounces
Tincture of vanillin	1 ounce
Tincture of civet	½ ounce
Oil of rose	1 dram
Oil of rose geraniol	½ dram
Oil of hyacinth geraniol	½ dram

Mix and filter if necessary.

3826. Upper 10.
Tincture of orris	4 ounces
Tincture of violet	4 ounces
Tincture of jasmin	4 ounces
Tincture of rose	4 ounces
Tincture of orange flowers	6 ounces
Tincture of civet	½ ounce
Tincture of ambergris	¼ ounce
Tincture musc baur	1 ounce
Oil of rose	1 dram
Oil of rose geraniol	1 dram

Mix and filter if necessary.

3827. Vandeventer Bouquet.
Tincture of orris	12 ounces
Tincture of coumarin	8 ounces
Tincture of vanillin	16 ounces
Tincture of musk	2 ounces
Tincture of rose	10 ounces
Tincture of violet	10 ounces
Tincture of cassie	5 ounces
Oil of rose	1 dram
Oil of hyacinth geraniol	1 dram

Mix and filter if necessary.

3828. Venetian Lily.
Tincture of vanillin	4 ounces
Tincture of tuberose	8 ounces
Tincture of rose	4 ounces
Tincture of cassie	4 ounces
Tincture of jasmine	2 ounces
Tincture of orange flowers	2 ounces
Oil of lily of the valley (D & O)	30 minims

Mix and filter if necessary.

3829. Violet.
Tincture of violet	18 ounces
Tincture of cassie	4 ounces
Tincture of orris	2 ounces
Tincture of vanillin	2 ounces
Tincture of rose	4 ounces
Tincture of ionone	1 ounce
Tincture of musc baur	2 ounces

Mix and filter if necessary. Color with chlorophyll.

3830. West End.
Tincture of rose	6 ounces
Tincture of cassie	3 ounces
Tincture of jasmine	3 ounces
Tincture of civet	2½ ounces
Tincture of orris	4 ounces
Oil of rose geraniol	1 dram
Oil of cloves	5 drops

Mix and filter if necessary.

3831. White Lily.
Tincture of coumarin	8 ounces
Tincture of orange flowers	4 ounces
Tincture of cassie	1 ounce
Tincture of civet	1½ ounces
Tincture of musk	1 ounce
Oil of rose	30 minims
Oil of bitter almonds	2 drops
Cologne spirits, 188 per ct.	4 ounces

Mix and filter if necessary.

3832. White Rose.
Tincture of rose	24 ounces
Tincture of violet	12 ounces
Tincture of cassie	6 ounces
Tincture of jasmine	12 ounces
Tincture of orris	16 ounces
Tincture of musk	4 ounces
Tincture of ambergris	1 dram
Oil of rose	1½ drams
Oil of sandalwood	1 dram
Oil of patchouli	10 drops

Mix and filter if necessary. Color light green with chlorophyll.

3833. Woodbine.

Tincture of jasmine	10 ounces.
Tincture of orange flowers	4 ounces.
Tincture of tuberose	2 ounces.
Tincture of vanillin	2 ounces.
Tincture of tolu	1 ounce.
Tincture of civet	1 ounce.
Oil of neroli Portugal	30 minims.
Oil of lemon	30 minims.
Oil of bergamot	2 drams.
Oil of rose geraniol	1 dram.

Mix and filter if necessary.

3834. Wood Violet.

Tincture of violet	12 ounces.
Tincture of rose	2 ounces.
Tincture of orange flowers	1 ounce.
Tincture of civet	½ ounce.
Tincture of ambergris	½ dram.
Tincture of orris root	2 ounces.
Oil of bitter almonds	1 drop.
Oil of patchouli	2 drops.

Mix and filter if necessary.

3835. Ylang Ylang.

Tincture of cassie	8 ounces.
Tincture of jasmine	2 ounces.
Tincture of orris	4 ounces.
Tincture of orange flowers	2 ounces.
Tincture of coumarin	1½ ounce.
Oil of ylang ylang	1 dram.
Oil of orange, sweet	½ dram.

Mix and filter if necessary.

FROZEN OR SOLID PERFUMES.

The solid perfume is merely perfumed hard paraffin. The hard paraffin is melted and perfumed at as low a temperature as possible, and for a mould use the lids of 2 drm. chip boxes.

3836. White Rose Solid Perfume.

Oil of geranium	½ dram.
Oil of bergamot	½ dram.
Oil of patchouli	5 minims.

From 1 to 5 drops to each block may be used, according to the moderation or extravagance of the manufacturer.

3837. Lavender Solid Perfume.

Oil of lavender	2 ounces.
Essence of bergamot	1 ounce.
Oil of cassia	5 minims.
Oil of geranium	40 minims.
Oil of orange	5 minims.

Mix and perfume the wax as before.

3838. Bouquet Solid Perfume.

Oil of coriander	18 minims.
Oil of cloves	2 drams.
Oil of nutmeg	1 dram.
Oil of lavender	3 drams.
Oil of sandal	1 dram.
Oil of bergamot	1 ounce.
Otto of rose	½ dram.
Oil of geranium	½ dram.
Oil of orange	10 minims.

Mix.

3839. Cologne Solid Perfume.

Zieliz, in Brit. and Col. Druggist.

Essence of bergamot	1 ounce.
Essence of lemon	1 ounce.
Oil of citronella	½ ounce.
Oil of neroli	½ ounce.
Oil of rosemary	80 minims.
Oil of geranium	10 minims.

Mix.

CHEAP HANDKERCHIEF EXTRACTS.

Cheap handkerchief extracts, made from oils and tinctures, all of them should be filtered at a low temperature to prevent after precipitation and cloudiness.

3840. Alpine Bouquet.

Oil of bergamot	3 drams.
Oil of rose geranium	1 dram.
Oil of cinnamon	½ dram.
Tincture of vanillin	1 ounce.
Cologne spirits, 188 per ct.	20 ounces.
Rose water q. s. or	14 ounces.
Magnesia carbonate	1 ounce.

Mix the oils and tincture with 4 ounces of the cologne spirits; place the magnesia in a mortar, pour on the solution of oils, and triturate well; take the remaining 16 ounces of cologne spirits, mix with the 14 ounces of rose water, and slowly add to the contents of the mortar, stirring constantly and uniformly for 10 minutes. Filter through filtering paper, and at as low a temperature as possible. If weather is warm, filter in an ice chest at a temperature of about 40° F. The product should measure 2 pints.

3841. Bordentown Bouquet.

Oil of bergamot.	2 drams.
Oil of lemon.	1 dram.
Oil of pimento.	5 drops.
Oil of lemon grass.	3 drops.
Tincture of orris root.	2 ounces.
Cologne spirits, 188 per ct.	20 ounces.
Orange flower water.	14 ounces.

Proceed as directed for Alpine bouquet.

3842. Bouquet Essence.
(Ess. Bouquet.)

Oil of lavender.	30 drops.
Oil of neroli.	10 drops.
Oil of bergamot.	30 drops.
Oil of rose.	10 drops.
Cologne spirits, 188 per ct.	20 ounces.
Orange flower water.	15 ounces.
Magnesia carb.	1 ounce.

Proceed as directed for Alpine bouquet.

3843. Bouquet D'Amour.

Oil of lavender.	2 drams.
Oil of cloves.	1 dram.
Oil of bergamot.	2 drams.
Oil of rose geranium.	5 minims.
Tincture of coumarin.	1 ounce.
Cologne spirits, 188 per ct.	20 ounces.
Water, q. s. or	14 ounces.
Magnesia carbonate.	1 ounce.

Proceed as directed for Alpine bouquet.

3844. Brighton Nosegay.

Oil of bergamot.	30 drops.
Oil of lavender.	10 drops.
Oil of neroli petale.	5 drops.
Oil of patchouli.	1 drop.
Oil of rose geranium.	30 drops.
Oil of lemon grass.	2 drops.
Oil of cassia.	2 drops.
Oil of pimento.	2 drops.
Extract of jasmine.	½ ounce.
Cologne spirits, 188 per ct.	20 ounces.
Water, q. s. or	14 ounces.
Magnesia carb.	1 ounce.

Proceed as directed for Alpine bouquet.

3845. Clove Pink.

Oil of cloves.	10 drops.
Tincture of orris.	10 ounces.
Tincture of vanillin.	2 ounces.
Tincture of ambrette.	2 ounces.
Cologne spirits, 188 per ct.	6 ounces.
Orange flower water.	5 ounces.
Rose water.	9 ounces.

Dissolve the oil in the tinctures and cologne spirits; add the waters slowly, and filter through talcum at a low temperature.

3846. Everlasting Bouquet.

Tincture of civet.	2 ounces.
Tincture of coumarin.	2 ounces.
Tincture of vanillin.	2 ounces.
Tincture of orris.	14 ounces.
Rose water.	15 ounces.

Mix the tinctures; add the rose water slowly, and filter through powdered French chalk (talcum).

3847. Frangipanni.

Oil of sandalwood.	1 dram.
Oil of neroli.	1 dram.
Oil of rose geranium.	1 dram.
Tincture of musc baur.	2 ounces.
Tincture of vanillin.	2 ounces.
Tincture of orris.	8 ounces.
Cologne spirts, 188 per ct..	8 ounces.
Cinnamon water.	7 ounces.
Orange flower water.	7 ounces.

Proceed as directed for Alpine bouquet.

3848. Heliotrope.

Tincture of heliotropin.	4 ounces.
Tincture of civet …	2 ounces.
Tincture of orris.	8 ounces.
Tincture of coumarin.	1 ounce.
Tincture of ambrette.	5 ounces.
Rose water.	14 ounces.

Mix the tinctures, and slowly add the rose water; filter at a low temperature.

3849. Jockey Club.

Oil of bergamot.	1½ drams.
Oil of lavender.	½ dram.
Oil of rose.	15 minims.
Tincture of musc baur.	1 ounce.
Tincture of orris root.	8 ounces.
Tincture of vanillin.	3 ounces.
Cologne spirits, 188 per ct.	8 ounces.
Rose water.	14 ounces.

Proceed as directed for Alpine bouquet.

3850. Lilac, White or Purple.

Oil of muguet (lilac)	1 dram.
Oil of kananga	1 dram.
Tincture of musc baur	1 ounce.
Tincture of orris	7 ounces.
Cologne spirits, 188 per ct.	12 ounces.
Orange flower water	7 ounces.
Rose water	7 ounces.

Proceed as directed for Alpine bouquet.

If a purple lilac is needed, color with purple aniline, q. s.

3851. Mary Stuart.

Otto of rose	½ dram.
Oil of sandalwood	10 drops.
Oil of bergamot	1 dram.
Tincture of orris	8 ounces.
Tincture of vanillin	2 ounces.
Tincture of civet	2 ounces.
Tincture of musc baur	2 ounces.
Cologne spirits, 188 per ct.	6 ounces.
Rose water	14 ounces.

Proceed as directed for Alpine bouquet.

3852. Moss Rose.

Otto of rose	½ dram.
Oil of rose geranium	10 minims.
Tincture of musc baur	2 ounces.
Tincture of orris	6 ounces.
Cologne spirits	12 ounces.
Rose water	14 ounces.

Proceed as directed for Alpine bouquet.

3853. Musk Rose.

Oil of rose	½ dram.
Oil of rose geranium	10 minims.
Tincture of musc baur	1 ounce.
Tincture of ambrette	3 ounces.
Tincture of orris	2 ounces.
Cologne spirits	14 ounces.
Rose water	14 ounces.

Proceed as directed for Alpine bouquet.

3854. Musk. Cheap.

Tincture of ambrette	8 ounces.
Oil of angelica root	10 drops.
Tincture of civet	1 ounce.
Tincture of musc baur	2 ounces.
Cologne spirits, 188 per ct.	9 ounces.
Rose water	14 ounces.

Dissolve the oil of angelica root in the cologne spirits; add the tinctures and shake well. Then add the water slowly and filter. Color with caramel.

3855. Tea Rose.

Oil of rose	15 minims.
Oil of rose geranium	15 minims.
Oil of sandalwood	10 minims.
Cologne spirits, 188 per ct.	20 ounces.
Rose water	7 ounces.
Orange flower water	7 ounces.

Dissolve the oils in the cologne spirits; add the rose water and filter.

3856. White Rose.

Oil of rose	15 minims.
Oil of rose geranium	10 minims.
Oil of patchouli	2 minims.
Tincture of ambrette	2 ounces.
Tincture of orris	4 ounces.
Cologne spirits, 188 per ct.	12 ounces.
Rose water	16 ounces.

Dissolve the oils in the cologne spirits; add the tinctures; shake well, then slowly add the rose water and filter. Color a pale green with aniline green or prepared chlorophyll.

3857. Ylang Ylang.

Oil of kananga	2 drams.
Oil of rose geranium	10 minims.
Oil of neroli petale	5 minims.
Tincture of musc baur	1 ounce.
Cologne spirits	18 ounces.
Orange flower water	7 ounces.
Rose water	8 ounces.

Proceed as directed for Alpine bouquet.

TINCTURES FOR PERFUMERY

(Directions for Making.)

3858. Tincture (or Washings) from Pomade.

| Take any flower pomade | 6 pounds. |
| Cologne spirits, 188 per ct. | 14 pints. |

Place eight pints of the cologne spirits in a 20 quart ice cream freezer. Melt the pomade gently by the heat of a water bath, and pour into the spirits contained in the freezer, turning the handle of the freezer slowly, and continue turning for an hour. Let the pomade stay in the spirits for three days, agitating occasionally, (the oftener the better); pour off the tincture and set aside. Pour into the freezer (containing the pomade) the remaining six pints of cologne spirits, and let it remain on the pomade (with occasional agitation) for three days; carefully drain off the second washing and add to the first washing;

label this tincture of rose, orange flowers or whatever the name may be; after the second washing is carefully drained from the freezer, four more pints of spirits can be added to the pomade, and after maceration with occasional agitation, can be drained off and set aside for use in making floral waters, cheap extracts or cologne.

See also directions for washing pomade under the head of Handkerchief extracts, to prepare.

3859. Tincture of Ambergris.
Ambergris. .... 1 ounce.
Cologne spirits, 188 per ct.. 128 ounces.

Cut the ambergris into small pieces, and digest in the spirits (with occasional agitation), for at least two weeks before using. Decant the clear portion as may be needed for use; press and filter the residue.

3860. Tincture of Ambrette Seeds.
(Musk Seeds.)
Ambrette seed, ground..... 1 pound.
Cologne spirits, 188 per ct. 128 ounces.

Macerate the seed in the spirits for at least two weeks before using; agitate occasionally. Decant as needed for use; press and filter the residue.

3861. Tincture of Angelica.
Oil of angelica (German)... 2 ounces.
Cologne spirits, 188 per ct. 128 ounces.

Mix and filter if necessary.

3862. Tincture of Benzoin.
Gum benzoin, powdered. .. 2 pounds.
Cologne spirits. .... 128 ounces.

Macerate with occasional agitation for two weeks before using.

3863. Tincture of Civet.
Civet. .... 2 ounces.
Orris root, powdered. ..... 2 ounces.
Cologne spirits. .... 128 ounces.

Macerate with occasional agitation for two weeks before using.

3864. Tincture of Cloves.
Oil of cloves. .... 2 ounces.
Cologne spirits, 188 per ct.. 128 ounces.

Mix and filter if necessary.

3865. Tincture of Coumarin.
Coumarin. .... 2 ounces.
Cologne spirits. .... 128 ounces.

Dissolve the coumarin in the spirit and filter if necessary.

3866. Tincture of Curcuma.
Curcuma, powdered. ...... 8 ounces.
Cologne spirits............ 128 ounces.

Macerate the curcuma in the spirits for three days, and percolate.

3867. Tincture of Heliotrope.
Heliotropin. .... 8 ounces.
Cologne spirits. .... 128 ounces.

Dissolve the heliotropin in the spirits and filter if necessary.

3868. Tincture of Ionone.
Ionone. .... 1 ounce.
Cologne spirits, 188 per ct. 19 ounces.
Mix.

3869. Tincture of Musc Baur.
Musc baur. .... 1 ounce.
Cologne spirits, 188 per ct. 128 ounces.

Dissolve and filter if necessary.

3870. Tincture of Musk.
Grain musk. .... 1 ounce.
Carbonate of potash. ...... ½ ounce.
Hot water. .... 8 ounces.
Cologne spirits, 188 per ct. 120 ounces.

Rub the grain musk and carbonate of potash in a mortar with the hot water; pour into a bottle; add the cologne spirits. Macerate for fourteen days (agitating occasionally), before using. The older the tincture, the better the quality; therefore do not filter until all the bright portion that can be decanted off, is gone, then press the residue and filter. The marc may be washed with dilute spirit and the washing used in cheap goods. A careful perfumer, as well as a careful druggist, should always keep an eye open for economizing his by-products.

3871. Tincture of Neroli Bigarade.
Oil of neroli bigarade. .... 2 ounces.
Cologne spirits, 188 per ct. 128 ounces.
Mix and filter if necessary.

3872. Tincture of Neroli Petale.
Oil of neroli petale. .... 2 ounces.
Cologne spirits, 188 per ct. 128 ounces.
Mix and filter if necessary.

3873. Tincture of Neroli Portugal.

Oil of neroli bigarade	1 ounce.
Oil of neroli petale	1 ounce.
Cologne spirits, 188 per ct.	128 ounces

Mix and filter if necessary.

3874. Tincture of Nutmegs.

Oil of nutmegs	2 ounces.
Cologne spirits	128 ounces.

Mix and filter.

3875. Tincture of Orris (from Oil).

Oil of orris	1 ounce.
Cologne spirits, 188 per ct.	128 ounces.

Mix and filter if necessary.

3876. Tincture of Orris (from Orris Root).

Orris root, powdered	2 pounds.
Cologne spirits, 188 per ct.	128 ounces.

Macerate the orris root for fourteen days (agitating occasionally), before using. When required for use, decant from the top, the bright portion; then press the residue and filter. The marc may be dried and used as a filler for sachet powders.

3877. Tincture of Red Saunders.

Red saunders in coarse powder	8 ounces.
Cologne spirits	128 ounces.

Macerate the red saunders in the spirits for three days, and percolate.

3878. Tincture of Rose Geranium.

Oil of rose geranium	2 ounces.
Cologne spirits	128 ounces.

Mix and filter if necessary.

3879. Tincture of Sandalwood.

Oil of sandalwood, East Indian	2 ounces.
Cologne spirits, 188 per ct.	128 ounces.

Mix and filter if necessary.

3880. Tincture of Styrax.

Liquid styrax	8 ounces.
Cologne spirits, 188 per ct.	128 ounces.

Macerate the styrax in the spirits, with occasional agitation, for a week; set aside until clear; decant off the clear portion as needed, and filter the residue.

3881. Tincture of Tolu.

Balsam of tolu	12 ounces.
Cologne spirits, 188 per ct.	128 ounces.

Dissolve the tolu in the spirits by maceration and agitation; set aside until clear; decant off the clear portion as needed, and filter the residue.

3882. Tincture of Tonka.

Tonka beans, Angostura	1 pound.
Cologne spirits, 188 per ct.	128 ounces.

Cut and bruise the beans with a portion of the spirits; add the remainder of the spirits and macerate for a month before using; decant the clear portion as needed; filter the residue.

3883. Tincture of Vanilla (from the Bean).

Fine quality Mexican bean.	16 ounces.
Cologne spirits, 188 per ct.	128 ounces.

Cut the beans into small pieces (lengthwise and across the bean), bruise well in a mortar with a small portion of spirits; put them into a two-gallon bottle with the remainder of the spirits; shake occasionally, and let stand for at least a month before using; when clear, decant from the top as may be needed; press and filter the residue. The pressed marc may be macerated in dilute alcohol and used for cheap vanilla flavoring extract.

3884. Tincture of Vanillin.

Vanillin	1 ounce.
Cologne spirits, 188 per ct.	128 ounces.

Dissolve the vanillin in the spirits, and filter if necessary.

3885. Tincture of Verbena.

Oil of verbena	2 ounces.
Cologne spirits, 188 per ct.	128 ounces.

Mix and filter if necessary.

3886. Tincture of Vetivert.

Oil of vetivert	2 ounces.
Cologne spirits, 188 per ct.	128 ounces.

Mix and filter if necessary.

COLOGNE WATERS.

3887. Windsor Cologne.
Cologne spirits, 188 per ct..	64 ounces.
Oil of bergamot.	½ ounce.
Oil of cloves.	1¼ drams.
Oil of rose geranium.	5 drams.
Oil of lavender, English.	5 drams.
Oil of sandalwood.	½ dram.
Oil of patchouli.	¼ dram.
Tincture of musc baur.	4 ounces.
Tincture of benzoin.	1 ounce.
Extract of violet.	5 ounces.
Extract of white rose.	4 ounces.
Rose water.	14 ounces.

Dissolve the oils in the spirits; add the tinctures and extracts. Mix well and let stand for 2 days, then slowly add the water, and in 14 days filter, using gray filtering paper and carbonate of magnesia.

3888. Vermont Cologne.
Oil of lavender.	2 drams.
Oil of bergamot.	2 drams.
Oil of cloves.	1 dram.
Oil of rose geranium.	½ dram.
Oil of cinnamon.	2 drops.
Tincture of musc baur.	2 ounces.
Cologne spirits, 188 per ct.	32 ounces.
Rose water.	16 ounces.

Mix and filter.

3889. Lafayette Cologne.
Oil of bergamot.	2 drams.
Oil of lemon.	1 dram.
Oil of reseda geraniol.	½ dram.
Oil of rose geraniol.	15 minims.
Oil of hyacinth geraniol.	10 minims.
Tincture of vanillin.	4 ounces.
Cologne spirits, 188 per ct..	20 ounces.
Rose water.	8 ounces.

Mix and filter.

3890. Cologne, Extra Fine.
Cologne spirits, 188 per ct..	128 ounces.
Oil of lavender flowers.	½ ounce.
Oil of lemon.	1 ounce.
Oil of bergamot.	1 ounce.
Oil of rosemary.	¼ ounce.
Oil of cloves.	½ dram.
Oil of neroli Portugal.	1 dram.
Oil of rose geraniol.	1 dram.
Tincture of musc baur.	4 ounces.
Orange flower water.	32 ounces.

Mix and filter.

3891. Cologne Water, Fine.
Cologne spirits, 188 per ct.	128 ounces.
Oil of bergamot.	¾ ounce.
Oil of lavender.	½ ounce.
Oil of orange, sweet.	1 ounce.
Oil of lemon grass.	½ dram.
Orange flower water.	64 ounces.

Mix and filter.

3892. Coyt's Cologne.
Cologne spirits, 188 per ct..	24 ounces.
Oil of neroli Portugal.	2 drams.
Oil of English lavender.	3 drams.
Oil of rose geraniol.	1 dram.
Oil of vetivert.	½ dram.
Oil of sandalwood.	1 dram.
Tincture of musc baur.	8 ounces.
Orange flower water.	8 ounces.

Mix and filter.

3893. Cologne Mixture. A
(2 ounces of mixture make 4 pints of cologne water, by the addition of 48 ounces of spirits and 16 ounces of water.)
Oil of bergamot.	16 ounces.
Oil of rosemary.	8 ounces.
Oil of lavender (Eng.).	3 ounces.
Oil of lemon.	6 ounces.
Oil of orange, sweet.	6 ounces.
Oil of neroli Portugal.	1 ounce.
Oil of cloves.	½ ounce.
Cologne spirits, 188 per ct..	88 ounces.

Mix and filter if necessary.

3894. Cologne Mixture. B
Oil of bergamot.	10 ounces.
Oil of lemon.	20 ounces.
Oil of orange.	10 ounces.
Oil of rosemary.	2 ounces.
Oil of neroli, big.	1 ounce.
Oil of neroli, petale.	4 ounces.
Oil of cedrat.	1 ounce.
Oil of geraniol hyacinth.	1 ounce.
Tincture of jasmine.	32 ounces.
Tincture of musc baur.	32 ounces.
Tincture of vanillin.	8 ounces.
Tincture civet.	8 ounces.

Mix and filter if necessary.

4 ounces of this mixture added to 96 ounces of cologne spirits, 188 per cent, and 32 ounces of water, will make a very fine eau de cologne.

3895. Oil of Melisse.
Oil of bergamot.	4 ounces.
Oil of lemon.	4 ounces.
Oil of orange, sweet.	4 ounces.
Oil of rose geraniol.	1 ounce.
Oil of lemon grass.	½ ounce.
Tincture of musk.	3½ ounces.

Mix. One-half an ounce of this mixture to 22 ounces of cologne spirits, 188 per cent, and 10 ounces of water, will make Melisse water.

EAU DE COLOGNE.

Ch. & Dr. Diary.

The fifty Farinas of Cologne are more than outnumbered by recipes for the perfumes which they compound. Our difficulty is to make a choice out of the multitude, to avoid repetitions, to keep out the bad, or rather not to overlook the best. Let us begin well, however, with these two formulae which The Chemist and Druggist has immortalized.

3896.   "Sydney Gold Medal."

Oil of bergamot.	14	minims.
*Oil of citron (Citrus medica.	25	minims.
Oil of neroli petale.	20	minims.
Oil of neroli bigarade.	7	minims.
Oil of rosmarini.	14	minims.
Spts. rectif.	12½	ounces.

3897.   Paris Exhibition Prize.

Oil of bergamot.	2	drams.
Oil of limonis.	1	dram.
Oil of neroli.	20	drops.
Oil of origani.	7	drops.
Oil of rosmarini.	20	drops.
Spt. rectificat.	20	ounces.
Aq. flor. aurant.	1	ounce.

Mix in this order.

These, it will be seen, differ very materially from each other, but each has its history, and both are honorable. The first was published many years ago in The Chemist and Druggist; a subscriber in Australia made the product a stock article, pushed its sale, exhibited it at the Sydney Exhibition, and it was awarded a gold medal. The second was one of 219 sent in competition for a prize consisting of a free trip to the Paris Exhibition, which was offered by a well-known firm of distillers. An equally well-known firm of perfume distillers adjudicated, and pronounced the product of the formula to closely resemble the genuine Farina.

Neither of these is specially remarkable when first prepared; it is only by keeping six or eight months that their excellence becomes manifest.

A very good authority states that eau de Cologne, to be of first quality, must contain oil of lemon and grape spirit. We know also that the Farinas distill the perfume and keep it for a year in bulk before it is bottled. The presence of neroli is essential, that being the characteristic odor of the water; indeed, the fact is noteworthy that most of the constituents are derived from the orange family. Rosemary is a necessary accompaniment; but all other odors, such as musk, civet, and cloves, which some are apt to load it with, are injurious to the refreshing character of eau de Cologne. There is a belief, which we share, that none of the imitations of the genuine article approach it in delicacy. This is probably due to the fact that the imitations are generally more charged with essences than the original, and unquestionably distilling has a subtle influence upon the fragrance of the contained essences.

What this influence may be can only be conjectured, but that some molecular reconstruction of the essential oils takes place on distilling and keeping seems to be most probable. It becomes important, therefore, that the retail manufacturer should hasten this change through some other influence than time, and there are two simple methods which may be adopted. One of these is explained in the following formula, which is at least a century old:

3898.

Oil of neroli.	10	minims.
Oil of lemon.	40	minims.
Oil of bergamot.	50	minims.
Oil of cedrat.	15	minims.
Oil of lavender.	18	minims.
Oil of rosemary.	10	minims.
Melissa-water.	4½	ounces.
Rectified spirit.	30	ounces.

Put the oils and the spirit in a strong flask, giving the mixture a thorough shaking; then close the flask, and keep the contents just warm (120° Fahr.) for forty-eight hours, whereby perfect blending of the oils with the spirit is insured. Then place it for twenty-four hours in a cool place, after which, filter it through paper until it is obtained perfectly clear. With the filtrate mix the melissa-water.

3899.   Like "Springbrunn" Brand.

Oil of aurant. cort.	30	minims.
Oil of limonis.	30	minims.
Oil of bergamot.	12	minims.
Oil of neroli bigarade.	1	minim.
Oil of neroli petale.	2	minims.
Oil of rosmarini.	4	minims.
Spt. rectificati.	16	ounces.

M.

---

*Oil of lemon may be used.

3900. Like "Jülichs-platz No. 4."

Oil of aurant. cort.	26 minims.
Oil of limonis.	34 minims.
Oil of bergamot.	14 minims.
Oil of aurant. flor.	14 minims.
Oil of rosmarini.	14 minims.
Spt. rectificati.	16 ounces.

M.

While the use of grape spirit is undoubtedly advantageous, 1 part of this to 3 parts of treble-distilled grain spirit may be used, the product being superior to that in which grain spirit alone is employed; but it should be noted that grape spirit is an exceedingly rare commodity in the United Kingdom, just as it is on the Continent, where it is practically all absorbed in the manufacture of brandy. Doubtless, traces of the higher alcohols in this spirit have something to do with the superiority of Farina "Cologne," and it may be asked why the same should not be the case with grain spirit, also containing traces of the higher alcohols. To that we reply that we claim no special merit for the grape spirit, the superiority being obtained by the etherification—mutual between the oils and the spirit—which takes place during distillation and keeping. The same thing must take place with grain spirit under similar conditions, but these conditions seldom exist in pharmacy. What is wanted is a mixed, not a distilled, eau de Cologne, and for that the triple-distilled rectified spirit is the best. It is almost free from higher alcohols.

3901.

Oil of bergamot.	2½ drams.
Oil of lemon.	1 dram.
Oil of Portugal.	50 minims.
Oil of neroli.	20 minims.
Oil of petit-grain.	10 minims.
Oil of lavender (English).	20 minims.
Oil of rosemary.	10 minims.
Oil of melissa.	5 minims.
Spirit.	30 ounces.
Rose water.	14 drams.
Orange flower water.	14 drams.

3902.

Oil of bergamot.	100 minims.
Oil of lemon.	50 minims.
Oil of Portugal.	½ dram.
Oil of petit-grain.	10 minims.
Oil of lavender.	20 minims.
Oil of rosemary.	15 minims.
Spirit.	30 ounces.
Orange flower water.	9 drams.
Rose water.	9 drams.
Distilled water.	9 drams.

The above formulae are for preparing the perfume by the cold method. The proper plan is to add the oils to the spirit in the order in which they are set down, shake well, and set aside for a few days, shaking occasionally before adding the waters. After these are added, again set aside for a week or two, and, if not perfectly clear, filter.

3903. Formula of 1801.

Oil of bergamot.	6 drams, 15 minims.
Oil of cedrat.	1 dram.
Oil of lemon.	1 dram.
Oil of lavender.	½ dram.
Oil of Portugal.	1 dram.
Oil of thyme.	4 minims.
Oil of neroli.	1 dram 15 minims.
Oil of rosemary.	1 dram 15 minims.
Spirit.	62 ounces.

Mix and distill, then add to the distillate 2½ ounces of melissa-water and 5 ounces orange flower water, and distill again.

3904. Formula of 1813.

Oil of neroli.	10 minims.
Oil of lemon.	40 minims.
Oil of bergamot.	50 minims.
Oil of cedrat.	15 minims.
Oil of lavender.	18 minims.
Oil of rosemary.	10 minims.
Melissa water.	4½ ounces.
Spirit.	30 ounces.

Dissolve the oils in the spirit contained in a retort, giving the mixture a thorough shaking; then close the retort and keep the contents just warm for forty-eight hours. Then place it for twenty-four hours in a cool place, after which filter it through paper until it is obtained perfectly clear. With the filtrate mix the melissa-water.

3905.

Oil of bergamottae.	3 ounces.
Oil of limonis.	3 ounces.
Oil of cedrat.	3 ounces.
Oil of lavendulae.	1½ ounces.
Oil of neroli.	1½ ounces.
Oil of rosmarini.	1½ ounces.
Oil of cinnamomi.	½ ounce.
Spirit. rectificat.	355 ounces.
Eau des carmes.	48 ounces.
Spt. rosmarini.	32 ounces.

Mix, allow to stand for eight days, and distill 305 ounces of the spirit.

No. 11.
3906.

Oil of bergamottae.	2½ drams.
Oil of Portugal.	2½ drams.
Oil of limonis.	½ dram.
Oil of neroli.	¼ dram.
Oil of rosmarini.	½ dram.
Spt. rectificat.	32 ounces.

The first of the latter two formulae is that of the old French Codex, and a wonderful formula it is when we contrast it with No. 11, the recipe now officialized in France. There is no justification for cinnamon in eau de Cologne. The following are French formulae which provide very good perfumes:

No. 12.
3907.

Oil of bergamot.	2 drams.
Oil of neroli.	1 dram.
Oil of limonis.	1 dram.
Oil of myrist.	11 minims.
Oil of rosmarini.	6 minims.
Spt. vini rect.	20 ounces.

No. 13.
3908.

Oil of Portugal.	½ dram.
Oil of lemon.	½ dram.
Oil of bergamot.	12 minims.
Oil of neroli.	2 minims.
Oil of petit-grain.	3 minims.
Oil of rosmarini.	4 minims.
Spt. vini. rect.	16 ounces.

M.

The German Apotheker-Verein has endeavored to reduce to something like uniformity the many standards which are in vogue in the Fatherland for this its most famous perfume, and we have the result in No. 14. It has its peculiarities, and therein is its weakness. No. 15, also a German formula, provides a concentrated eau de Cologne, which will bear dilution with ten times its volume of fine spirit. In this case dissolve the oils in the 10 ounces of spirit, and set aside for fourteen days, shaking four times a day. Then distill the mixture twice, when the result will be 10 ounces of an exceedingly strong perfume, which improves in odor the longer it is kept, and is specially suited for exportation. It is of good odor when freshly diluted with spirit, and the dilution also improves on keeping.

No. 14.
3909.

Oil of bergamottae.	5 drams.
Oil of limonis.	5 drams.
Ess. moschi (1-50).	1 dram, 15 minims.
Oil of neroli.	½ dram.
Oil of cinnamomi.	15 minims.
Oil of caryoph.	15 minims.
Otto of rose.	15 minims.
Spt. rectificat.	56 ounces.
Aquae.	4 ounces.

Mix, allow to stand for eight days, shaking frequently, then filter.

No. 15.
3910.

Oil of Portugal.	3 drams.
Oil of bergamot.	3 drams.
Oil of cedrat.	2 drams.
Oil of lavendul.	2 drams.
Oil of neroli.	3 drams.
Oil of petit-grain.	2 drams.
Oil of rosmarini.	½ ounce.
Oil of limonis.	½ ounce.
Spt. rectif.	10 ounces.

Compound as directed above.

No. 16.
3911.

Oil of neroli.	50 minims.
Oil of rosmarin.	15 minims.
Oil of bergamot.	80 minims.
S. V. R.	16 ounces.
Aq.	5 ounces.

M.

No. 17.
3912.

Oil of bergamot.	10 drams, 40 minims.
Oil of neroli.	80 minims.
Otto of rose.	1 dram.
Musk.	10 grains.
Tincture of vanilla.	2 drams.
Jasmine extract.	10 drams, 40 minims.
Violet extract.	10 drams, 40 minims.
Spirit.	112 ounces.
Water.	10 ounces.

Mix the oils and extracts with 104 ounces of the spirit; digest the musk with the remaining 8 ounces at a gentle heat, in a closed bottle, for twenty-four hours; then add to the other liquid, add the water, cool, and filter. If convenient, set aside for some weeks before filtering.

No. 16 is "like the genuine," says our notebook, and if there be any virtue in repetition, we have that simple formula in various degrees as to quantities, but all coming to the same thing.

No. 18.
3913.

Oil of rosmar. ang.	20 minims.
Oil of bergamot, extra super.	1 ounce.
Ess. limonis.	6 drams.
Oil of lavand. ang.	2 drams.

NON-SECRET FORMULAS.

Oil of caryoph. .... 10 minims.
Oil of neroli. (Bigarade) petale................. 20 minims.
Otto rosae virgin. .... 24 minims.
Ess. cedrat. super. .... 6 drams.
Sp. vin. rect. .... 64 fl. ounces.
M.

No. 19.

3914.
Oil of bergamot. .... 3 drams.
Oil of citronell. .... ½ dram.
Oil of rosmarin. .... ½ dram.
Oil of neroli. .... 18 minims.
Ess. mosch. .... 2 drams.
Oil. lavand. ang .... 16 minims.
Oil verben. .... 12 minims.
S. V. R. .... 28 ounces.
Aq. destil. .... 2 ounces.
M.

Reference has already been made to the great variety of German formulae. The subjoined table exhibits an instructive selection. The quantities are indicated in drams, but "dp." stands for drops. It is instructive to compare with these a recipe (the first following) reputed to give a product exactly resembling that of Farina.

of the finest rosemary oil, 20 drops of otto of rose, 12 grammes (3 drs.) of acetic ether, 1,100 grammes (34oz.) of distilled orange-flower water, and 200 grammes (6 oz.) of rose water. After this mixture has stood for six months, dilute it with 5 to 7½ kilos. (8 to 12 pints) of spirit, and distil."

3916. Lily of the Valley Eau de Cologne.
Oil of bergamot. .... 4 drams.
Oil of orange flowers. ..... 45 minims.
Oil of lemon. .... 4 drams.
Oil of lavender. .... 15 minims.
Oil of rosemary. .... 15 minims.
Oil of ylang ylang. .... 15 minims.
Oil of melissa. .... 5 minims.
Rose water. .... 3 ounces.
Orange flower water. ...... 3 ounces.
Rectified spirit. .... 46 ounces.
Maiglockchen. .... 6 ounces.
Mix.

3917. Maiglöckchen.
(For use in the foregoing formula.)
Oil of linaloe. .... 2½ drams.
Oil of bergamot. .... ½ dram.

	Dieterich		Buchmeister			Askinson		Deite		Vomacka	
	I.	II.	III.	IV.	V.	VI.	VII.	VIII.	IX.	X.	XI.
Spirit.................	8,250	8,250	900	875	900	2,000	915	8,250	8,100	8,000	8,000
Water.................	1,500	1,500	.....	.....	.....	.....	80	500	.....	.....	.....
Oil of bergamot........	100	100	9	25	8	25	5	85	150	12	14
" lemon.............	50	50	12	15	8	25	10	75	135	30	33
" rosemary..........	50	50	16 dp.	48 dp.	1	25	1	5	10	4	14
" orange flowers.....	30	10	1	1	2	80	.....	.....	40	3	14
" neroli.............	10	10	.....	40 dp.	.....	.....	.....	.....	.....	.....	.....
" ylang ylang........	2	1	.....	.....	.....	.....	.....	.....	.....	.....	.....
" lavender..........	.....	10	1	4	.....	.....	1·2	10	10	.....	.....
" wintergreen.......	.....	1	.....	.....	.....	.....	.....	.....	.....	.....	.....
" peppermint.......	.....	.....	28 dp.	.....	.....	.....	.....	.....	.....	.....	.....
" thyme............	.....	.....	16 dp.	.....	.....	.....	.....	.....	.....	.....	.....
" rose..............	.....	.....	4 dp.	.....	.....	.....	.....	.....	.....	.....	.....
" melissa...........	.....	.....	trace	trace	.....	.....	.....	.....	5	.....	.....
" orange peel.......	.....	.....	.....	.....	.....	.....	.....	40	.....	80	26
" petitgrain........	.....	.....	.....	.....	.....	.....	.....	15	.....	.....	.....
Acetic ether...........	10	10	.....	.....	.....	.....	.....	.....	.....	.....	.....
Acetic acid, 80 per cent.	10	10	.....	.....	.....	.....	.....	.....	.....	.....	.....
Orange flower water...	.....	.....	80	80	.....	.....	.....	500	800	.....	.....
Rose water............	.....	.....	.....	.....	.....	.....	.....	500	800	.....	.....

3915. Gegenüber dem Jülichs-platz.

We give this in the fashion that it comes to us:—

"Mix 350 grammes (11 oz.) of lemon oil, 270 grammes (8½ oz.) of bergamot oil, 20 grammes (5 drs.) of the finest French lavender oil, 12 grammes (3 drs.) of Mitcham peppermint oil, 120 drops of the best French oil of neroli, 100 drops of French oil of white thyme, 100 drops

Oil of rose-geranium. ..... 45 minims.
Essence of musk. .... 75 minims.
Jasmine extract. .... 16 ounces.
Rectified spirit. .... 48 ounces.
Mix.

3918. Eau de Cologne.
Oil of bergamot. .... 2 drams.
Oil of lemon. .... 1 dram.

Oil of neroli.	20 drops.
Oil of origanum.	6 drops.
Oil of rosemary.	20 drops.
Cologne spirits, 188 per ct	20 ounces.
Orange flower water.	4 ounces.

Mix.

3919. Florida Water. A

Oil of lavender.	1 ounce.
Oil of bergamot.	1 ounce.
Oil of lemon.	1 ounce.
Oil of orange.	¼ ounce.
Oil of cloves.	1 dram.
Oil of cassia.	2 drams.
Cologne spirits, 188 per ct.	1½ gallons.
Rose water.	½ gallon.

Mix and filter.

3920. Florida Water. B

Oil of bergamot.	1 ounce.
Oil of rosemary.	¼ ounce.
Oil of lemon.	¼ ounce.
Oil of cassia.	⅛ ounce.
Oil of cloves.	15 minims.
Tincture of orris.	8 ounces.
Tincture of styrax.	½ ounce.
Cologne spirits, 188 per ct.	1 gallon.
Rose water.	½ gallon.

Mix and filter.

3921. Florida Water Mixture. A

Oil of lavender (French).	16 ounces.
Oil of bergamot.	16 ounces.
Oil of lemon.	16 ounces.
Oil of orange.	4 ounces.
Oil of cloves.	1 ounce.
Oil of cassia.	2 ounces.
Cologne spirits, 188 per ct.	73 ounces.

Mix and filter if necessary.

4 ounces of this mixture added to 96 ounces of cologne spirits, 188 per cent., and 32 ounces of water, will make Florida Water.

3922. Florida Water Mixture. B

Oil of bergamot.	16 ounces.
Oil of rosemary.	4 ounces.
Oil of lemon.	4 ounces.
Oil of cassia.	2 ounces.
Oil of cloves.	2 drams.
Tincture of orris.	64 ounces.
Tincture of styrax.	8 ounces.
Cologne spirits.	30 ounces.

Mix and filter if necessary.

4 ounces of this mixture added to 96 ounces of cologne spirits, 188 per cent, and 32 ounces of water, will make Florida water.

LAVENDER WATERS.

3923. Lavender Water.—Glenn's.

Oil of lavender, Mitcham.	1 ounce.
Oil of bergamot.	½ ounce.
Tincture of vanillin.	1 ounce.
Tincture of coumarin.	½ ounce.
Cologne spirits, 188 per ct.	40 ounces.
Water.	10 ounces.

Dissolve the oils in the spirits; add the tinctures, and set aside for 3 days before adding the water. Add the latter slowly and let it stand 2 weeks before filtering.

3924. Lavender Water.—English.

Oil of lavender, Mitcham.	2 ounces.
Oil of bergamot.	1 ounce.
Tincture of vanillin.	4 ounces.
Tincture of angelica.	4 ounces.
Cologne spirits, 188 per ct.	88 ounces.
Rose water.	32 ounces.

Dissolve the oils in the spirits; add the tinctures, and set aside for 3 days before adding the rose water. Let it stand 2 weeks before filtering.

3925. Lavender Water.—Barclay's.

Oil of lavender, Mitcham.	1 ounce.
Oil of bergamot.	½ ounce.
Oil of neroli petale.	15 minims.
Oil of rose geraniol.	15 minims.
Tincture of ambrette seed.	4 ounces.
Tincture of angelica.	1 ounce.
Cologne spirits, 188 per ct.	84 ounces.
Rose water.	32 ounces.

Dissolve the oils in the spirits; add the tinctures, and set aside for 3 days before adding the rose water. Let it stand 2 weeks before filtering.

3926. Lavender Water.—Amber.

Oil of lavender.	2½ ounces.
Oil of bergamot.	5 drams.
Tincture of coumarin.	4 ounces.
Tincture of vanillin.	2 ounces.
Tincture of civet.	1 ounce.
Tincture of rose.	16 ounces.
Cologne spirits, 188 per ct.	74 ounces.
Rose water.	32 ounces.

Color amber with red saunders, if preferred colored. Dissolve the oils in the spirits; add the tinctures; set aside for 3 days before adding the rose water. Let it stand for 2 weeks before filtering. The four formulas for lavender water make very nice goods; the latter is the best.

NON-SECRET FORMULAS.

3927. Lilac Water.

Extract of lilac	16 ounces.
Cologne spirits, 188 per ct.	70 ounces.
Water	44 ounces.

Mix the extract of lilac with the cologne spirits, and add the water slowly. Filter.

3928. Melisse Water.

Oil of melisse, (see oil of melisse)	2 ounces.
Cologne spirits	88 ounces.
Water	40 ounces.

Dissolve the oil in the spirit and add the water; filter.

3929. Verbena Water.

Oil of lemon grass	¾ ounce.
Oil of bergamot	¼ ounce.
Oil of neroli petale	1 dram.
Oil of cloves	10 drops.
Oil of cinnamon	20 drops.
Cologne spirits, 188 per ct.	96 ounces.
Water	32 ounces.

Dissolve the oils in the spirit; add the water, and filter.

3930. Violet Water. A

(First Quality.)

Tincture of violet	32 ounces.
Tincture of cassie	16 ounces.
Tincture of rose	16 ounces.
Tincture of orris	32 ounces.
Tincture of vanillin	16 ounces.
Oil of bergamot	¼ ounce.
Oil of bitter almonds	5 drops.
Cologne spirits, 188 per ct.	88 ounces.
Rose water	40 ounces.

Dissolve the oils in the spirit; add the tinctures, and set aside for 3 days; then add the water slowly, stirring well, and let stand for 2 weeks before filtering. Color with Chlorophyll to the tint required.

3931. Violet Water. B

Second Quality.

Tincture of cassie	32 ounces.
Tincture of orris	64 ounces.
Tincture of vanillin	16 ounces.
Tincture of ambrette seed	8 ounces.
Oil of bitter almonds	5 drops.
Oil of bergamot	¼ ounce.
Cologne spirits	64 ounces.
Rose water	72 ounces.

Proceed as directed for formula A.

3932. Violet Water. C

Third Quality.

Tincture of orris	64 ounces.
Tincture of vanillin	16 ounces.
Oil of sandalwood	½ ounce.
Oil of bergamot	1 ounce.
Oil of rose geranium	½ ounce.
Cologne spirits, 188 per ct.	80 ounces.
Rose water	96 ounces.

Dissolve the oils in the spirit; add the tinctures, and set aside for 3 days; then add the water slowly, stirring well, and let stand for 2 weeks before filtering. Color with chlorophyll or aniline green to the tint required.

BAY RUMS, ETC.

3933. Bay Rum Mixture. A

Oil of bay	1 ounce.
Oil of white thyme	1 ounce.
Oil of allspice	1 ounce.
Oil of cloves	¼ ounce.
Cologne spirits, 188 per ct.	¾ ounce.

Mix.

½ ounce of this, to one gallon of proof spirits for ordinary Bay rum. An improved article may be made by doubling the quantity of the Bay rum mixture used, and also by substituting 8 ounces of New England rum for 8 ounces of the proof spirits. Some compounders use 2 drams of salts of tartar to each gallon of Bay rum. Many customers prefer it that way.

3934. Bay Rum Mixture. B

Oil of bay	1 ounce.
Oil of cloves	1 ounce.
Oil of red thyme	2 ounces.
Oil of allspice	2 ounces.

Mix. See directions on formula A.

3935. Bay Rum Mixture. C

Oil of bay	2 ounces.
Oil of allspice	1 ounce.
Oil of orange, sweet	1 ounce.
Oil of cloves	½ ounce.
Oil of geraniol hyacinth	½ ounce.

Mix. See directions on formula A.

3936. Bay Rum Mixture. D

Oil of bay	2 ounces.
Oil of cloves	¼ ounce.
Oil of orange, sweet	½ ounce.
Oil of neroli petale	1 dram.
Oil of allspice	1 dram.
Oil of cardamom	5 drops.

Mix. See directions on formula A.

3937. Vinegar Aromatic.

Cologne spirits, 188 per ct.	16 ounces.
Oil of bergamot.	½ dram.
Oil of lemon.	20 drops.
Oil of lavender, French.	40 drops.
Oil of cloves.	15 drops.
Oil of rosemary.	10 drops.
Oil of cassia.	5 drops.
Tincture of coumarin.	8 ounces.
Tincture of orris.	2 ounces.
Acetic ether.	1¼ ounces.
Acetic acid, No. 8.	3 ounces.
Water.	5½ ounces.

Dissolve the oils in the spirit; add the tinctures and acetic ether. Mix the acid and water and add, stirring constantly for 5 minutes. Filter.

3938. Vinegar Rouge.

Cologne spirits, 188 per ct.	16 ounces.
Carmine No. 40.	3 drams.
Aqua ammonia, stronger.	2 ounces.
Water.	3 pints.

Place the carmine in a large mortar and powder it; add the ammonia and rub well; then add the spirit and lastly the water. Let it stand one week before using.

SACHET POWDERS, ETC.

3939. Sachet or Solid Perfumes.

From the London Chemist and Druggist's Diary.

The popularity of sachets is comparatively modern, but the pot-pourri jar is very old. The form of the perfumes is similar, but their uses are essentially different, and the composition also. What is popularly known as pot-pourri is a mixture of coarsely powdered aromatic drugs and resins, dried odorous leaves, especially the rose. The pot-pourri plays to the flowers the part which musk and civet play to volatile oils in liquid perfumes—it fixes and blends the perfume.

The sachet is a distinct thing. It is wanted for its individuality, to place in some handkerchief-box, drawer, or dress cupboard, and it is essential that it must be elegant in material and get-up. Custom compels us to have it in fairly fine powder, the basis by preference powdered orris, although rice-flour is, on the whole, as good and cheaper.

Solid perfumes are a quite recent variety of sachet. They are composed of solid paraffin, wherewith the essential oils of any particular bouquet have been blended while liquid; not a bad style at all, and worthy of attention where cheapness is requisite. Another kind of solid perfume is made by massing any sachet powder with tragacanth mucilage, and drying it at a heat not exceeding 80° Fahr.

3940. Pot-pourri. A

The whole of the solids are to be coarsely powdered, the liquids evenly sprinkled over the mixture, and then all well shaken together.

Orris root.	16 ounces.
Benzoin.	5 ounces.
Coriander.	4 ounces.
Cinnamon.	1 ounce.
Cloves.	1 ounce.
Pimento.	1 ounce.
Tonquin bean.	½ ounce.
Ess. bouquet.	½ ounce.

3941. Pot-pourri. B

Vanilla.	1 ounce.
Orris root.	1 ounce.
Cloves.	1 ounce.
Cinnamon bark.	1 ounce.
Oil of lavender.	10 minims.
Oil of neroli.	10 minims.

3942. Pot-pourri. C

Coriander.	4 ounces.
Orris root.	4 ounces.
Calamus.	4 ounces.
Rose-petals.	4 ounces.
Lavender flowers.	2 ounces.
Mace.	½ ounce.
Cinnamon.	½ ounce.
Cloves.	2 drams.
Essence of musk.	¼ dram.
Common salt.	2 ounces.

3943. Pot-pourri. D

Rose petals.	8 ounces.
Lavender flowers.	4 ounces.
Orris root.	2 ounces.
Vanilla.	2 drams.
Cloves.	2 drams.
Storax.	½ ounce.
Siam benzoin.	1 ounce.
Ambergris.	20 grains.
Musk.	4 grains.
Common salt.	2 ounces.
Oil of lemon.	1 dram.
Oil of vetivert.	½ dram.

3944. Pot-pourri. E

Lavender flowers.	1 pound.
Rose petals.	1 pound.
Orris root.	1 pound.
Table salt.	8 ounces.
Cloves.	4 ounces.
Cinnamon.	4 ounces.
Benzoin.	4 ounces.
Pimento.	4 ounces.
Vanilla.	3 ounces.
Musk pod.	1 ounce.
English oil of lavender.	1 dram.
Oil of sandalwood.	1 dram.
Oil of rose geranium.	1 dram.
Oil of bergamot.	2 drams.
Oil of lemon.	2 drams.
Essence of ambergris.	½ ounce.
Otto of rose.	10 minims.

Grind all the solids to coarse powder, and with the mixture intimately incorporate the oils.

Nos. C to E are good examples of complete pot-pourri; omitting the salt and flowers, we have the powder for mixing at home with these omitted articles. The plan to adopt is such as the following: Take a 2-gallon jar and fill it with rose petals, orange-blossoms, and lavender flowers, sprinkle them well with salt, and then disperse through the contents 4 oz. of any pot-pourri which does not contain the dried flowers. If lavender and orange flowers are not obtainable, the powder should contain oils of neroli and lavender. Generally speaking, rose leaves only are preserved in England.

3945. Pot-pourri. F

Vanilla.	1 ounce.
Orris root.	1 ounce.
Cloves.	1 ounce.
Cinnamon.	1 ounce.

Mix.

3946. Pot-pourri. G
Violet Odor.

Black currant leaves.	7 ounces.
Cinnamon.	8 ounces.
Rose leaves.	8 ounces.
Powdered orris root.	18 ounces.
Powdered Benzoin.	4 ounces.
Ess. oil of bitter almonds.	3 drams.
Grain musk.	1 dram.

Mix.

3947. Pot-pourri. H

Gum benzoin.	2 ounces.
Orris root.	1 ounce.
Cloves.	1 ounce.
Storax.	½ ounce.
Cinnamon.	2 drams.

Grind together and add—

Grain musk.	½ dram.
Coarse and dry salt.	2 ounces.
Oil of lavender.	20 minims.

Mix.

3948. Pot-pourri. I

Cinnamon.	½ ounce.
Cloves.	½ ounce.
Mace.	½ ounce.
Orris root.	4 ounces.
Oil of lavender.	40 minims.
Oil of lemon grass.	40 minims.
Oil of lemon.	40 minims.
Oil of bergamot.	40 minims.

Mix.

3949. Pot-pourri. J

Pimento.	2 ounces.
Cinnamon.	2 drams.
Essence of musk.	12 minims.
Essence of ambergris.	12 minims.
Oil of lavender.	12 minims.

Mix.

3950. Lord Plymouth's Pot-pourri.

Benzoin, siamensis contus.	8 ounces.
Pulv. rad. iridis.	8 ounces.
Pulv. storacis.	8 ounces.
Pulv. rad. angelicae.	8 ounces.
Gran. moschi.	1 scruple.
Fabae tonkae.	No. 4.
Macis.	½ ounce.
Caryophyll.	½ ounce.
Cort. cinnam. contus.	¼ ounce.

Mix all these when they have been bruised or powdered, and add—

Ol. lavandul. ang.	1 dram.
Otto rose.	1 dram.
Flor. rosae.	4 ounces.
Flor. lavandulae.	4 ounces.

Again mix.

3951. Sachets. A

The simplest way to make sachets extemporaneously is to take a sufficient quantity of a basis, and add to it liquid perfume in the proportion of a drachm to the ounce. The resulting compound is suited for ordinary retail sale, and if a more permanent article is desired, the ingredients of any perfume, minus spirit, may similarly be mixed with the basis. The following are suitable bases:

Bran.	7 ounces.
Powdered orris root.	1 ounce.

Mix.

3952. Sachets. B

Ground rice.	4 ounces.
Powdered orris root.	4 ounces.

Mix.

The latter may be colored with a few drops of a proof spirit solution of an aniline dye.

In compounding sachets the whole of the liquid ingredients should be mixed and triturated for five minutes with twelve times their bulk of orris root or other non-resinous basis. The resins, if any in the formula, should be separately mixed with a portion of the fibrous basis.

3953. Acacia or Cassie.

Cassie flowers.	equal parts
Powdered orris root.	of each.

Grind the flowers and mix with the orris.

3954. Bouquet de Caroline.

Powdered orris root.	2 pounds.
Grain musk.	10 grains.
Oil of bergamot.	½ ounce.
Oil of lemon.	½ ounce.
Otto of rose.	½ dram.

Mix.

3955. Chypre.

Powdered orris root.	1½ pounds.
Rasped cedarwood.	1 pound.
Rasped sandalwood.	1 pound.
Vanilla (ground).	4 ounces.
Tonka bean (ground).	2 ounces.
Essence of musk.	1 ounce.
Oil of rose geranium.	½ dram.
Otto of rose.	25 minims.
Oil of bergamot.	15 minims.

Mix.

3956. Ess. Bouquet. A

Powdered orris root.	16 ounces.
Grain musk.	1 dram.
Otto of rose.	1 dram.
Oil of bergamot.	3 drams.
Oil of lemon.	40 minims.

Mix.

3957. Ess. Bouquet. B

Powdered orris root.	2 pounds.
Powdered sandalwood.	2 pounds.
Powd. orange peel (sweet).	2 pounds.
Artificial musk.	1 grain.
Coumarin.	2 grains.
Vanillin.	2 grains.
Otto of rose.	1½ drams.
Oil of bergamot.	2 drams.
Oil of ylang ylang.	20 minims.
Oil of neroli.	20 minims.
Oil of rose geranium.	15 minims.
Oil of cinnamon.	5 minims.
Essential oil of almonds.	5 minims.
Jasmine extract.	2 ounces.

Mix.

3958. Ess. Bouquet. C

Powdered orris root.	4 pounds.
Ground cassie.	1 pound.
Rose petals.	1 pound.
Ground vanilla.	3 ounces.
Oil of bergamot.	1 ounce.
Oil of lemon.	1 ounce.
Essence of musk.	2 ounces.
Essence of ambergris.	½ ounce.
Oil of rose geranium.	1 dram.

Mix.

3959. Frangipanni. A

Powdered orris root.	16 ounces.
Powdered Tonka bean.	4 ounces.
Musk.	10 grains.
Civet.	½ dram.
Otto of rose.	10 minims.
Oil of sandalwood.	10 minims.
Oil of neroli.	10 minims.

Mix.

3960. Frangipanni. B

Powdered orris root.	16 ounces.
Powd. sweet orange peel.	16 ounces.
Powdered sassafras.	3 ounces.
Coumarin.	1 grain.
Otto of rose.	20 minims.
Oil of sandalwood.	3 minims.
Oil of rose geranium.	3 minims.
Essential oil of almonds.	2 minims.
Essence of musk.	1½ drams.
Essence of civet.	1½ drams.
Jasmine extract.	1½ ounces.

Mix.

3961. Frangipanni. C

Powdered orris root.	3 pounds.
Rasped sandalwood.	4 ounces.
Ground vanilla.	4 ounces.

NON-SECRET FORMULAS.

Ground Tonka bean. ...... 2 ounces.
Oil of neroli. .... 1 dram.
Oil of rose geranium. ..... 1 dram.
Oil of bergamot. .... 1 dram.
Oil of sandalwood. .... 40 minims.
Otto of rose. .... ½ dram.
Oil of vetivert. .... 10 minims.
Essence of musk. .... 1 ounce.
Essence of civet. .... ½ ounce.
Mix.

3962.   Heliotrope.   A
Orris root, in coarse powd 6 ounces.
Vanilla, in coarse powder.. 2 drams.
Musk. .... 3 grains.
Otto of rose. .... 1 minim.
Essential oil of almonds. .. 1 minim.
Mix.

3963.   Heliotrope.   B
Powdered orris root. ...... 16 ounces.
Powdered vanilla. .... 4 ounces.
Powdered benzoin. .... 1 ounce.
Musk. .... 5 grains.
Civet. .... 15 grains.
Essential oil of almonds. .. 10 minims.
Otto of rose. .... 10 minims.
Mix.

3964.   Heliotrope.   C
Powdered orris root. ...... 8 ounces.
Coumarin. .... 15 grains.
Vanillin. .... 10 grains.
Musk. .... 5 grains.
Essential oil of almonds. .. 1 minim.
Otto of rose. .... 1 minim.
Spirit. .... 2 drams.
Mix.

3965.   Jockey Club.   A
Powdered orris. .... 16 ounces.
Musk. .... 5 grains.
Otto of rose. .... 40 minims.
Oil of bergamot. .... 1 dram.
Oil of sandalwood. .... 1 dram.
Mix.

3966.   Jockey Club.   B
Powdered orris root. ...... 12 ounces.
Ground sandalwood. ...... 2 ounces.
Essence of musk. .... ½ ounce.
Oil of bergamot. .... 2 drams.
Essence of civet. .... 2 drams.
Otto of rose. .... 8 minims.
Mix.

3967.   Jockey Club.   C
Sweet orange peel, dried
 and ground. .... 2½ pounds.
Powdered orris root. ...... 1½ pounds.
Ground rose petals. ...... 1½ pounds.
Siam benzoin. .... 4 ounces.
Ground sandalwood. ...... 2 ounces.
Cloves. .... 1 ounce.
Coumarin. .... 10 grains.
Musk. .... 1 grain.
Civet. .... 1 grain.
Otto of rose. .... 1 dram.
Oil of bergamot. .... 1½ drams.
Oil of rose geranium. ..... ½ dram.
Oil of neroli. .... ½ dram.
Oil of cinnamon. .... 10 minims.
Oil of bitter almonds. ..... 10 minims.
Oil of ylang ylang. .... 10 minims.
Jasmine extract. .... 4 ounces.
Mix.

3968.   Lavender.   A
Lavender flowers. .... 16 ounces.
Dried thyme. .... 1 ounce.
Dried spearmint. .... 1 ounce.
Powdered cloves. .... ½ ounce.
Powdered caraway. .... ½ ounce.
Oil of lavender. .... 2 drams.
Mix.

3969.   Lavender.   B
Ground lavender flowers.. 16 ounces.
Ground benzoin. .... 1 ounce.
Oil of lavender. .... ½ ounce.
Essence of musk. .... ½ ounce.
Mix.

3970.   Lign Aloe.
Powdered orris root. ..... 3½ pounds.
Ground rose leaves. ...... 1 pound.
Ground sandalwood. ...... 8 ounces.
Ground vanilla. .... 4 ounces.
Oil of lign aloe. .... 1 ounce.
Essence of civet. .... 1 ounce.
Essence of musk. .... ½ ounce.
Oil of rose geranium. ..... 40 minims.
Otto of rose. .... 20 minims.
Mix.

3971.   Marechale.
Powdered orris root. ..... 1 pound.
Ground sandalwood. ...... 8 ounces.
Ground rose petals. ...... 4 ounces.
Ground cloves. .... 4 ounces.
Essence of musk. .... 1 ounce.
Oil of bergamot. .... 1 dram.
Oil of rose geranium. ..... 1 dram.
Oil of vetivert. .... 1 dram.
Mix.

3972. Millefleurs. A
Powdered orris root	16 ounces.
Grain musk	5 grains.
Civet	10 grains.
Otto of rose	20 minims.
Oil of neroli	20 minims.
Oil of cloves	½ dram.
Oil of bergamot	1 dram.

Mix.

3973. Millefleurs. B
Powdered orris root	2 pounds.
Ground lavender flowers	1 pound.
Ground cassie flowers	1 pound.
Ground rose flowers	1 pound.
Ground sandalwood	8 ounces.
Ground Tonka beans	4 ounces.
Ground benzoin	4 ounces.
Ground vanilla	3 ounces.
Ground cinnamon	2 ounces.
Ground cloves	2 ounces.
Essence of musk	½ ounce.
Essence of civet	½ ounce.
Oil of bergamot	½ ounce.
Oil of rose geranium	½ dram.
Oil of patchouli	10 minims.

Mix.

3974. Mousselaine.
Powdered orris root	2 pounds.
Ground rose flowers	8 ounces.
Ground cassie flowers	8 ounces.
Ground sandalwood	8 ounces.
Ground benzoin	2 ounces.
Essence of musk	2 ounces.
Oil of vetivert	1 dram.
Oil of rose geranium	35 minims.
Oil of neroli	5 minims.

Mix.

3975. Musk. A
Powdered orris root	2½ pounds.
Grain musk	½ dram.
Otto of rose	1 dram.

Mix.

3976. Musk. B
Rice flour	12 ounces.
Artificial musk	10 grains.

Stain the flour with a few drops of solution of aniline yellow, and triturate the musk intimately with it.

3977. New-mown Hay. A
Bouquet de Caroline sachet	8 ounces.
Verbena sachet (No. 1)	4 ounces.
Violet (No. 1)	4 ounces.

Mix.

3978. New-mown Hay. B
Powdered orris root	2 pounds.
Ground Tonka beans	4 ounces.
Ground vanilla	2 ounces.
Essence of musk	6 drams.
Oil of rose geranium	1 dram.
Oil of bergamot	½ dram.
Otto of rose	15 minims.
Oil of almonds	5 minims.

Mix.

3979. Opoponax.
Powdered orris root	3 pounds.
Ground rose petals	1 pound.
Ground cassie petals	1 pound.
Ground Tonka beans	4 ounces.
Ground vanilla	3 ounces.
Ground musk-pods (or essence of musk)	1 ounce.
Essence of civet	½ ounce.
Oil of bergamot	2 drams.
Oil of rose geranium	1 dram.
Oil of citron	½ dram.
Oil of patchouli	½ dram.
Oil of citronella	15 minims.
Otto of rose	5 minims.

Mix.

3980. Patchouli.
Powdered orris root	16 ounces.
Powdered patchouli leaves	8 ounces.
Otto of rose (or oil of rose geranium)	½ dram.
Oil of patchouli	1 dram.

Mix.

3981. Rondeletia.
Powdered orris root	3 pounds.
Ground lavender flowers	1½ pounds.
Ground cloves	½ ounce.
Essence of musk	1 ounce.
Essence of ambergris	1 ounce.
Oil of bergamot	2 drams.
Oil of English lavender	2 drams.
Oil of cloves	2 drams.
Oil of rose geranium	½ dram.
Otto of rose	20 minims.

Mix.

3982. Rose Geranium.
Powdered orris root	2 pounds.
Oil of rose geranium	½ ounce.
Otto of rose	10 minims.
Essence of musk	½ dram.

Mix.

NON-SECRET FORMULAS.

3983. Rose.
Ground rose petals........ 1½ pounds.
Powdered orris root....... 8 ounces.
Ground sandalwood........ 4 ounces.
Powdered patchouli leaves. 2 ounces.
Essence of civet.......... ½ ounce.
Oil of rose geranium...... ½ dram.
Otto of rose.............. 20 minims.
Mix.

3984. White Rose.
Powdered orris root....... 16 ounces.
Rice flour................ 8 ounces.
Otto of rose.............. 2 drams.
Oil of patchouli.......... 15 minims.
Mix.

3985. Red Rose.
Powdered orris root....... 16 ounces.
Rasped sandalwood......... 8 ounces.
Rasped cedarwood.......... 8 ounces.
Musk...................... 5 grains.
Otto of rose.............. 1 dram.
Color the orris powder with solution of carmine before mixing with the other ingredients.

3986. Sweet Briar.
Powdered orris root....... 4 pounds.
Ground sandalwood......... 1 pound.
Essence of ambergris...... 1 ounce.
Essence of musk........... ½ ounce.
Oil of lemon.............. 1 dram.
Oil of lemongrass......... 1 dram.
Oil of neroli............. 1 dram.
Oil of bergamot........... 40 minims.
Oil of rose geranium...... ½ dram.
Otto of rose.............. ½ dram.
Mix.

3987. Verbena. A
(1)
Powdered orris root....... 2 pounds.
Civet..................... 10 grains.
Oil of lemon grass........ 1 dram.
Otto of rose.............. 20 minims.
Mix.

3988. Verbena. B
(2)
Powdered orris root....... 3 pounds.
Essence of musk........... ½ ounce.
Oil of lemon grass........ 3 drams.
Oil of bergamot........... 2 drams.
Oil of rose geranium...... ½ dram.
Mix.

3989. Violet. A
(1)
Powdered orris root...... 2 pounds.
Powdered benzoin......... 4 ounces.
Cassie extract........... 1 ounces.
Otto of rose............. 10 minims.
Essential oil of almonds... 10 minims.
Mix.

3990. Violet. B
(2)
Powdered orris root...... 3 pounds.
Essence of musk.......... 1 ounce.
Oil of bergamot.......... ½ dram.
Essential oil of almonds.. 20 minims.
Otto of rose............. 20 minims.
Mix.

3991. West End.
Powdered orris root...... 1 pound
Grain musk............... 10 grains.
Civet.................... 20 grains.
Otto of rose............. 20 minims.
Oil of bergamot.......... 40 minims.
Mix.

3992. Ylang-Ylang. A
(1)
Powdered orris........... 1 pound
Powdered benzoin......... ½ ounce.
Civet.................... 5 grains.
Oil of ylang ylang....... 20 minims.
Essential oil bitter almonds 3 minims.
Mix.

3993. Ylang-Ylang. B
(2)
Powdered orris root...... 3 pounds.
Ground cassie flowers.... 1 pound.
Rose flowers............. 1 pound.
Ground pimento........... 4 ounces.
Ground Tonka bean........ 2 ounces.
Ground vanilla........... 2 ounces.
Ground benzoin........... 1 ounce.
Essence of musk.......... 1 ounce.
Essence of civet......... ½ ounce.
Oil of bergamot.......... 2 drams.
Oil of ylang ylang....... 2 drams.
Oil of pimento........... 1 dram.
Oil of rose geranium..... 1 dram.
Otto of rose............. 20 minims.
Mix.

FUMIGATING PERFUMES.

These are used for quickly putting down bad odors in sick-rooms and other apartments. As a rule they are not very nice, being rather balsamic than flowery; still, they are decidedly antiseptic, and fulfil their purpose admirably.

3994. Paper. A

Select good white blotting-paper, and cut each demy sheet lengthways into three equal pieces. Make a solution of 1 ounce of potassium nitrate in 12 ounces of boiling water; place this solution in a large plate, and draw each strip of paper over the solution so as to saturate it. Then dry by hanging up.

The dried paper is to be saturated in a similar manner with either of the following solutions:

(1)

Siam benzoin	1 ounce.
Storax	3 drams.
Olibanum	2 scruples.
Mastic	2 scruples.
Cascarilla	2 drams.
Vanilla	1 dram.
Rectified spirit	8 ounces.

Bruise the solids and macerate in the spirit five days, filter, and add—

Oil of cinnamon	8 minims.
Oil of cloves	8 minims.
Oil of bergamot	5 minims.
Oil of neroli	5 minims.

Mix.

3995. Paper. B

(2)

Benzoin	1½ ounces.
Sandalwood	1 ounce.
Spirit	8 ounces.

Macerate as No. 1, and add

Essence of vetivert	3 drams.
Oil of Lemon grass	40 minims.

Mix.

After the paper is dry, cut it up into suitable sized pieces to go into a commercial envelope—ten pieces for 6d.

3996. Ribbon.

Take ½-inch cotton tape and saturate it with nitre in the same manner as the paper above described; when dry saturate with the following tincture:

Benzoin	1 ounce.
Orris root	1 ounce.
Myrrh	2 drams.
Tolu balsam	2 drams.
Musk	10 grains.
Rectified spirit	10 ounces.

Macerate for a week, filter, and add 10 minims of otto of rose.

Another good formula, which may also be used for fumigating paper, is—

Olibanum	2 ounces.
Storax	1 ounce
Benzoin	6 drams.
Peruvian balsam	½ ounce.
Tolu balsam	3 drams.
Rectified spirit	10 ounces.

Macerate ten days, and filter.

3997. Pastilles. A

(1)

Vegetable charcoal	6 ounces.
Benzoin	1 ounce.
Nitrate of potash	½ ounce.
Tolu balsam	2 drams.
Sandalwood	2 drams.
Mucilage of tragacanth	q. s.

Reduce the solids to fine powder, mix, and make into a stiff paste with the mucilage. Divide this into cones 25 grains in weight, and dry with a gentle heat.

3998. Pastilles. B

(2)

Powdered willow charcoal	8 ounces.
Benzoic acid	6 ounces.
Nitrate of potash	6 drams.
Oil of thyme	½ dram.
Oil of sandalwood	½ dram.
Oil of caraway	½ dram.
Oil of cloves	½ dram.
Oil of lavender	½ dram.
Oil of rose	½ dram.
Rose water	10 ounces.

Proceed as in No. 1, but this recipe is much the better of the addition of 20 grains of powdered tragacanth.

These are nice recipes, the first being from the French Codex, and the second is said to give a product closely resembling Piesse & Lubin's pastilles.

TOILET POWDERS, ENAMELS, CREAMS, ETC.

3999. Face and Complexion Powder. A
Zinc oxide.................. 3 pounds.
Precipitated chalk......... 4 pounds.
French chalk............... 10 pounds.
Magnesia carbonate, light.. 1½ pounds.
Perfume with—
Oil of rose................. 1 dram.
Tincture of rose geranium. ½ ounce.
Tincture of musc baur..... ½ ounce.

Dissolve the oil in the tinctures and spray the powder with the solution; mix well, and run through a sifter twice.

For pink powder color with carmine.

For yellow powder color with fine yellow ochre.

4000. Face Powder. B
Oxide of zinc............... 3 pounds.
French chalk............... 7 pounds.
Perfume with—
Rose geraniol.............. 1 dram.
Tincture of rose........... ¼ ounce.
Tincture of musc baur..... ½ ounce.

Proceed as directed for formula A.

4001. Violet Powder.
Powdered starch........... 10 pounds.
Powdered orris root....... 5 pounds.
Tincture of violet......... 1 ounce.
Tincture of vanillin....... ½ ounce.
Tincture of musc baur..... ¼ ounce.

Mix the starch and orris root; spray the powder with the perfume and run through a sifter and mixer twice.

4002. Rose Powder.
Powdered starch........... 10 pounds.
Powdered orris root....... 5 pounds.
Perfume with—
Oil of rose geraniol....... 10 drops.
Tincture of rose........... 1 ounce.
Tincture of vanillin....... ½ ounce.
Tincture of musc baur..... ⅛ ounce.

Mix the starch and orris; dissolve the oil in the tinctures and spray the powder; run through a sifter and mixer twice.

4003. Invisible Face Powder.
Bismuth subcarb........... 1 pound.
Magnesia carbonate........ 1 pound.
French chalk............... 10 pounds.
Perfume the same as rose powder formula.

4004. Phantom Face Powder.
Precipitated chalk......... 5 pounds.
French chalk............... 10 pounds.
Carbonate of magnesia..... 3 pounds.
Oxy-chloride of bismuth... 3 pounds.
Perfume with—
Oil of rose geraniol....... 15 drops.
Tincture of rose........... 1 ounce.
Tincture of vanillin....... ½ ounce.
Tincture of musc baur..... ¼ ounce.

Dissolve the oil in the tinctures and spray the powder; mix well and run through a sifter and mixer twice.

4005. Borated Talcum.
Powd. French Chalk purified .... 10 pounds.
Powd. boric acid.......... 8 ounces.
Perfume with—
Tincture of violet......... 1 ounce.
Tincture of jasmine....... ½ ounce.
Tincture of vanillin....... ½ ounce.

Mix the talcum and boric acid; spray with the tinctures and run through a sifter and mixer twice.

4006. Infant Powder.
Powdered starch........... 4 pounds.
Powdered French chalk... 4 pounds.
Powdered boric acid....... ½ pound.
Powdered orris root....... 1½ pounds.
Oil of wintergreen......... ½ ounce.

Mix and run through sifter and mixer.

4007. Oriental Rouge.
French chalk, powdered... 10 pounds.
Carmine, No. 40........... 3 ounces.
Aqua ammonia, q. s. to dissolve the carmine.

Mix well and run through sifter and mixer.

4008. Cream of Roses.
Oxide of zinc, pure........ 2½ pounds.
Glycerine.................. 24 ounces.
Filtered water............. 128 ounces.
Carmine solution.......... q. s.
Cologne spirits dilute..... 64 ounces.
Extract of white rose..... 4 ounces.
Mix.

Use about 6 drams of the carmine solution to give the mixture a natural tint.

4009. Balm of Roses.
Oxychloride of bismuth.... 2½ pounds.
Glycerine.................. 24 ounces.
Filtered water............. 160 ounces.
Carmine solution.......... q. s.
Cologne spirit, 188 per cent 2 pints.
Extract of white rose..... 4 ounces.
Mix.

Use about 6 drams of the carmine solution to give the mixture a natural tint.

Should a rose-colored preparation be needed use carmine solution q. s. for the required tint.

4010. Frostilline Cream.

Gum tragacanth	3 ounces.
Hot water	144 ounces.
Chlorate of potash	6 ounces.
Glycerine	48 fl. ounces.
Oil of rosemary	½ dram.
Oil of cassia	10 drops.
Oil of rose geranium	5 drops.
Oenanthic ether	5 drops.
Cologne spirits 188 per cent	3 ounces.

Mix.

4011. Witch Hazel Cream. A

Gum tragacanth	3 ounces.
Boric acid	6 ounces.
Dist. ext. of witch hazel	144 ounces.
Glycerine	3 pints.
Tincture of rose	2 ounces.
Tincture of violet	1 ounce.

Mix.

4012. Witch Hazel Cream. B

Quince seed	4 ounces.
Hot water	16 ounces.
Glycerine	32 fl. ounces.
Dist. ext. of witch hazel	128 ounces.
Boric acid	6 ounces.
Tincture of rose	2 ounces.
Tincture of violet	1 ounce.

Macerate the quince seed in the hot water; add the glycerine and witch hazel in which the acid has been previously dissolved; let stand for two days, stirring occasionally; strain and add the perfume.

4013. Cold Cream, Glenn's.

White vaseline	16 ounces.
Beef suet, purified	4 ounces.
White wax	4 ounces.
Spermaceti	4 ounces.

Melt together and when cool perfume with

Oil of rose	1 dram.
Oil of rose geranium	1 dram.
Oil of sandalwood	½ dram.

4014. Cold Cream.
(C. & D.)

White petrolatum oil	10 ounces.
White wax, pure	12 ounces.
Spermaceti	12 ounces.
Lanoline	16 ounces.
Glycerine	8 ounces.
Borax	3 drams.
Rose water	16 ounces.

M. S. A.

4015. An Elegant Cold Cream.
(C. & D.)

Glycerine	6 ounces.
Lanoline	1½ ounces.
White petrolatum	4½ ounces.

Mix the lanoline and petrolatum, and then incorporate the glycerine; flavor with otto of rose or oil of ylang ylang, and put up in jars or collapsible tubes.

"This is the finest preparation of its kind I have ever seen," says Mr. Frank Edel in the Spatula. It is easily made and keeps perfectly."

4016. Borico-salicylic Glycerine.
C. & D.

This is an excellent antiseptic, and the addition of a small percentage of it to any glycerine-preparation for the hands and face is decidedly beneficial:

Boric acid	1 ounce.
Salicylic acid	1 ounce.
Distilled water	1 ounce.
Glycerine	3 ounces.

Put the whole of the ingredients in a flask, bring to the boil, and add 45 grains of calcined magnesia. Continue the heating until all the water has evaporated, and, when cold, make up to 5 fluid ounces with glycerine.

4017. Boro-glyceride Lanolin.

Boric acid	5 drams.
Glycerine	2½ ounces.
Distilled water	1½ ounces.

Dissolve by the aid of heat and add—

Anhydrous lanoline	11 ounces.
Olive oil	4 ounces.

Mix well.

This is put up in collapsible tubes; perfume to taste.

4018. Toilet Cream (not a jelly).

Lanoline	1 ounce.
Almond oil	1 ounce.
Oleate of zinc (powder)	3 drams.
Ext. white rose	1½ drams.
Glycerine	2 drams.
Rose water	2 drams.

Mix.

4019. Camphor Cream.

White petrolatum	3½ pounds.
Beef suet	1 pound.
White wax	1½ pounds.
Spermaceti	½ pound.
Camphor	1 pound.

Melt and pour into moulds.

4020. Camphor Ice. A
White petrolatum	2 pounds.
White wax, pure	2 pounds.
Gum camphor	4 ounces.
White rosin	4 ounces.
Glycerin	16 fl. ounces.

Melt, and stir well; when nearly cool pour into moulds.

4021. Camphor Ice. B
White petrolatum	2 pounds.
Paraffin wax, hard	2 pounds.
Gum camphor	4 ounces.
White rosin	4 ounces.
Glycerin	16 fl. ounces.

Melt, and stir well; when nearly cool pour into moulds.

4022. Lime Juice and Glycerine. A
Borax	½ ounce.
Boiling water to dissolve borax	10 ounces.

When cold add—
Oil of sweet almonds	20 ounces.
Oil of lemon	½ ounce.

4023. Lime Juice and Glycerine. B
Carbonate of potash	½ ounce.
Hot water	10 ounces.
Olive oil	20 ounces.
Stronger water of ammonia	½ ounce.
Oil of lemon	¼ ounce.

Dissolve the carbonate of potash in the water; add the oil gradually, shaking after each addition. Then add the oil of lemon and lastly, the water of ammonia.

4024. Freckle Cream.
Red iodide of mercury	40 grains.
Oleate of zinc, powdered	1¼ ounces.
Lanoline	15 ounces.
White petrolatum oil	5 ounces.
Glycerin	2 ounces.
Extract of white rose	½ ounce.

M. S. A.

4025. Remedy for Removing Freckles.
From the Scientific American Encyclopedia.
A Good Remedy for Removing Freckles.—Sulphocarbolate of zinc, 1 ounce; glycerine, 12 ounces; rose water, 12 ounces; alcohol, 3 ounces; spirits of neroli, ½ dram. Mix them. To be applied twice a day, leaving it on for half an hour to one hour.

The following is recommended by the Druggists' Circular as a preparation for this purpose which does not contain mercury: Ammonium chloride, 1 dram; distilled water, 7 ounces; cologne water, 2 drams.

4026. Remedy for Freckles.
1. The following is quoted by New Remedies from a German medical journal: Sulphocarbolate of zinc, 2 parts; glycerine, 25 parts; rose water, 25 parts; spirits, 5 parts. Dissolve and mix.

The freckled skin is to be anointed with this twice daily, and allowed to stay on from one-half to one hour, and then washed off with cold water. Anaemic persons should also take a mild ferruginous tonic. In the sunlight a dark veil should be worn.

2. Scrape horse-radish into a cup of cold sour milk, let stand twelve hours, strain, and apply two or three times a day.

4027. Hydrokinone Wash for the Skin.
Hydrokinone	48 grains.
Acid phosphoric glac	30 grains.
Glycerine	2 drams.
Aqua dest	6 ounces.

Misce.
These two lotions are stated to give excellent results, especially the latter. They are to be applied to the skin of the face, etc., in the usual way at least twice in the course of twenty-four hours, after it has been washed and dried carefully. If the skin be of the nature known as "greasy," a preliminary wash with tepid water containing a few drops sal volatile or liq. ammon. fort. is advisable.

4028. Albadermine.
Under this empirical title, a process of removing "tan" and the milder variety of "freckles," a foreign surgeon has devised the following:

Solution A.
Potass. iodid	2 drams.
Iodine pur	6 grains.
Glycerine	3 drams.
Infus. rose	4 ounces.

Dissolve the iodide of potassium in a small quantity of the infusion and a dram of the glycerine; with this fluid moisten the iodine in a glass mortar and rub it down, gradually adding more liquid until complete solution has been obtained; then stir in the remainder of the ingredients, and bottle the mixture.

4029. Albadermine.
Solution B.
Sodae hyposulph, thiosulphate	1½ ounces.
Aqua rose exot	1 pint.

Dissolve and filter.
With a small camel's hair pencil or piece of fine sponge apply a little of "Albadermine A" to the tanned or freckled surface, until a slight but tolerably uniform

brownish yellow skin has been produced. At the expiration of fifteen or twenty minutes moisten a piece of cambric, lint, or soft rag with "B," and lay it upon the affected part, removing, squeezing away the liquid, soaking it afresh, and again applying until the iodine stain has disappeared. Repeat the entire process thrice daily, but diminish the frequency of the application if tenderness be produced. In the course of three to four days to as many weeks, the freckles will either have disappeared entirely or their intensity will be greatly diminished. "Summer freckles" yield very speedily to this treatment.

4030. Anti-Freckle Lotion.

Hydrarg. bichlor.	12 grains.
Acid hydrochlor. pure	3 drams.
Fruct. amygd. amar.	1½ ounces.
Glycerina, Price's	1 ounce.
Tinct. benzoin	2 drams.
Aqua flor. aurant.	q. s.

Dissolve the corrosive sublimate in 3 ounces of the orange flower water, add the hydrochloric acid, and set aside. Blanch the bitter almonds, and bruise them in a Wedgwood mortar, adding thereto the glycerine and using the pestile vigorously; a smooth paste is thus obtained. Then add gradually about 9 ounces of the orange flower water, stirring constantly, continuing this operation until a fine, creamy emulsion is the result. Subject this to violent agitation—preferably with the aid of a mechanical egg whisk—and allow the tincture of benzoin to fall into it the while drop by drop. Then add the mercurial solution, filter, and make up the whole to the measure of 1 imperial pint, with more orange flower water.

This preparation is recommended to us by an eminent dermatologist as being invariably efficacious in the treatment of ephelis, and always greatly ameliorating lentigo, even if it does not entirely decolorize the patches in the latter case. A general whitening of the skin is produced by this lotion without any irritation. It is as well, however, not to apply it to any abraded surfaces. It has been found far superior in practice to a preparation—which it somewhat resembles—sold at a high price in Paris under the name of Lait Antiphelique.

4031. Bismuth Ointment for Freckles.

Bismuthi subnit.	3 drams.
Ung. simp.	2 ounces.

Fiat ung.

Apply to the face, etc., at night, and remove in the morning with a little cold cream previous to washing. This is from a private American source.

4032. Copper Oleate for Freckles, etc.

This is a much more effective and reliable ointment for the purpose than the preceding which is really only suited for the milder form of sunburn, while the oleate of copper will remove the more persistent and obstinate lentigo. It is thus prepared:

Cupri oleas, ver.	1 ounce.
Petrogell. alb. Burgoyne's.	3 ounces.

Incorporate thoroughly without heat.

This is to be applied in the same manner as the preceding, washing the surface of the skin, however (after the cold cream), about every third morning, with a little weak ammonia water in order to prevent any inadvertent accumulation of copper.

4033. Cosmetic Gloves.

Mock kid or lamb-skin gloves rubbed over, on the inside, with a composition of the following kind: Spermaceti cerate (hardest, melted), 5 ounces; balsam of Peru, 1 dram; stir for five minutes, pour off the clear portion, add of oil of nutmeg, ½ dram; oil of cassia, 12 to 15 drops; essence of ambergris, 12 to 15 drops; and stir the whole until cold. Worn by ladies in bed, at night, to soften and blanch the hands, and to prevent and cure chaps and chilblains.

4034. Solidified Glycerine for Toilet Use.

Transparent soap, 1½ ounces; water, 6 ounces; inodorous glycerine, 36 ounces. Dissolve the soap in the water by heat, add an equal weight of glycerine. When dissolved, add the rest of the glycerine, water q. s. to make up the weight. When nearly cold add any perfume desired. Put in glass jars. It is of a pale amber color, and is transparent.

LOTIONS.

These preparations, popularly called "washes," are local external applications consisting of water, or some simple aqueous vehicle, holding in solution medicinal or cosmetic substances. Medicinal lotions are usually applied by wetting a piece of linen with them, and keeping it on the part affected; cosmetic lotions, by simply moistening the skin with them.

4035. Acetic Lotion.

Acetic Lotion—Take of good strong vinegar, 1 part; water, 2 or 3 parts; mix. In bruises, contusions, sprains, etc., and as a general refrigerant wash or lotion to sound parts; also to remove freckles.

4036. Lotion of Acetate of Lead.

Lotion of Acetate of Lead.—Take of sugar of lead, ¼ ounce; distilled or soft water, 1 pint; dissolve. Sometimes a little vinegar is added, a like quantity of water being omitted. Used in excoriations, burns, sprains, contusions, etc.; also as an occasional cosmetic wash by persons troubled with eruptions.

4037. Acetic Acid Lotion for Baldness.

Lotion of Acetic Acid for Baldness.—The following lotion is superior for a shampooing liquid, for removing dandruff, and as a useful and pleasant application for baldness. It is, of course, moderately stimulating, and in those cases in which the hair follicles are not destroyed, but have become merely inactive, it is likely to prove efficacious. Take of acetic acid, 1 dram; cologne water, 1 ounce; water, to make in all 6 ounces.

4038. Alum Lotion.

Alum Lotion.—Take of alum (crushed), 1½ drams; distilled or soft water, 1 pint; dissolve. A little rose water may be introduced to scent it.

4039. Arsenical Cosmetic Lotion. A

Arsenical Cosmetic Lotion.—1. Take of arsenious acid (solid or crystallized), 3 to 5 grains; crush it to a fine powder, place it in a jug or basin; pour on it of distilled or soft water (boiling), ¾ pint; and promote solution by constantly stirring the liquid for some time with a small glass rod or a clean piece of wood. After repose, and when cold, pour off the clear solution into a clean bottle, carefully observing not to disturb the sediment or any undissolved portion, which must be entirely rejected. To the clear liquid add, of eau de rose (foreign), 1 ounce; glycerine (Price's), 1 ounce; and after mixture, by agitation, further add enough cold distilled water or pure soft water to make the whole measure exactly one pint. It should then be poured into 5-ounce or 6-ounce bottles, only one of which, for safety, should be kept out for use.

4040. Arsenical Cosmetic Lotion. B

2. As the last, but adding, with the arsenious acid, an equal weight of carbonate of potassium. This addition facilitates the solution of the former, but the product is said to be slightly less effective as a cosmetic wash.

4041. Arsenical Cosmetic Lotion. C

3. Solution of arsenite of potassa, 1 fl. ounce; eau de rose, 1 fl. ounce; glycerine (Price's), ½ ounce; distilled or pure soft water (cold), 1 pint; mix. A convenient formula, but less esteemed than No. 1.

4042. Bichloride of Mercury Lotion.

Lotion of Bichloride of Mercury.—Corrosive sublimate (in coarse powder), 10 grains; distilled water, 1 pint; agitate them together until solution is complete. The addition of 5 or 6 grains of pure sal ammoniac or 5 or 6 drops (not more) of hydrochloric acid, increases the solvent action of the water, and renders the preparation less liable to suffer change, but it is not otherwise advantageous. When absolutely pure distilled water is not used, this addition of acid should be made to prevent decomposition. Some persons dissolve the sublimate in 2 or 3 fluid drams of rectified spirit before adding the water, to facilitate the process; but this also, though convenient, is unnecessary. This is a deadly poison.

4043. Borax Lotion. A

Lotion of Borax.—1. Borax (powdered), 2½ drams; distilled water, ½ pint. Mix. An effective wash for sore gums, sore nipples, excoriations, etc.; applied twice or thrice daily, or oftener.

4044. Borax Lotion. B

2. Borax (powdered), 3 drams; glycerine, ¾ ounce; rose water or elder flower water, 12 ounces. Mix.

4045. Cherry Laurel Lotion.

Cherry Laurel Lotion, Cherry Laurel Shaving Wash.—Cherry laurel water (genuine, distilled), 2 fluid ounces; rectified spirits, 1 fluid ounce; glycerine, ½ ounce; distilled water, 7½ fluid ounces. Mix. Used to allay irritation of the skin, particularly after shaving, the part being moistened with it by means of the tips of the fingers; also used as a wash for freckles and acne, and to remove excessive moistness or greasiness of the hair.

4046. Lotion of Chlorate of Potassium.

Lotion of Chlorate of Potassium.—Take of chlorate of potassium (powdered) ½ ounce; distilled water, ½ pint; rose water, 4 ounces; glycerine, 1 ounce. Dissolve.

NON-SECRET FORMULAS.

4047. Face Lotion.
Face Lotion.—As a face lotion, oatmeal made into a paste with glycerine 2 parts, water, 1 part, and applied to the face at night, with a mask worn over, will give in a short time, if faithfully pursued, a youthful appearance to the skin.

4048. Lotion to Remove Freckles.
Freckles, Lotion to Remove.—Alum and lemon juice, of each, 1 ounce; rose water, 1 pint. Bathe the face three or four times daily.

4049. Glycerine Lotion. A
Glycerine Lotion.—1. Glycerine (pure), 1 ounce; distilled or pure soft water, 19 ounces. Mix. A good strength for daily use as a cosmetic wash, or as a vehicle for other ingredients, for which purpose it is greatly preferable to milk of almonds; also as a lotion to allay itching and irritation of the skin, prevent chaps, excoriation the effects of weather, climate, etc. It is likewise applied to the hair instead of oil.

4050. Glycerine Lotion. B
2. Glycerine, 1 ounce; distilled water, 9 ounces. Mix. A proper strength when more marked effects are desired; as in chapped hands, lips, nipples, obstinate excoriations, abrasions, chafings, sun-burns, persistent roughness or hardness of the skin, etc.

4051. Emollient Glycerine Lotion.
Lotion, Emollient Glycerine.—Take of mucilage of quince seeds, 6 fl. ounces; glycerine, 1 fl. ounce; orange flower water, 1 fl. ounce. Make a lotion.

4052. Gowland's Lotion.
Gowland's Lotion.—Jordan almonds (blanched), 1 ounce; bitter almonds (do.: say 7 to 9), 2 to 3 drams; distilled water, ½ pint; form them into an emulsion. To the strained emulsion, with agitation, gradually add of bichloride of mercury (in coarse powder), 15 grains, previously dissolved in distilled water, ½ pint; after which further add enough distilled water (2 or 3 teaspoonfuls) to make the whole measure exactly 1 pint.

4053. Horse Radish Lotion.
Horse Radish Lotion (for the skin).—Horse radish root, 1½ ounces; boiling water, 1½ pints; borax, 3 drams. Used for freckles, tan, etc.

4054. Lotion of Iodide of Potassium.
Lotion of Iodide of Potassium.—Iodide of potassium, 1 to 2 drams; distilled water, 1 pint; dissolve.

4055. Glycerine Lotion.
Glycerine Lotion for Irritation of the Skin.—Mix 1½ ounces glycerine with 1½ pints water. Allays itching, removes dryness, etc. For chapped hands or lips, add 3 or 4½ drams borax.

4056. Lemon Juice Solution.
Lemon Juice Solution.—Fresh lemon juice, 2 ounces; glycerine, 1 ounce; rose water or rain water, with 3 or 4 drops otto of roses added, 1 pint. Anoint the hands and face 3 or 4 times daily, and allow to remain on several minutes before wiping. For clearing the complexion, and making the skin white and soft.

4057. Mosquito Lotion.
Mosquito Lotion.—Aqua ammonia, 2 ounces; glycerine, 1 ounce; rose water, 8 ounces.

4058. Sulphureted Lotion. A
Sulphureted Lotion.—1. Sulphuret of potassium, 1 dram; distilled water, 1 pint; dissolve. Used to render the skin soft, white, and smooth, particularly when there is a tendency to slight eruptions of a pustular or vesicular character. One-half to 1 ounce glycerine improves it for present use.

4059. Sulphureted Lotion. B
2. Sulphide of potassium, 1½ drams; water, ½ pint; dissolve. A cleanly and effective remedy for itch, used twice or thrice daily. It does not soil the linen and leaves very little smell.

4060. Sulphureted Lotion. C
3. (Cazenave.) Sulphuret of potassium, 1 dram; white soft soap, 2 drams; water, 8 ounces; dissolve. Used as the last; also to destroy pediculi.

4061. Sun Burn Lotion. A
Sun-burn Lotion.—1. Two drams tincture of benzoin and 2 ounces rose water. Mix and shake well. This is an excellent recipe for sun-burns.

4062. Sun Burn Lotion. B

Acid citric	1 dram.
Ferri sulphas pur	18 grains.
Camphora	q. s.
Aq. flor. sambu	3 ounces.

The sulphate of iron must be in clear green crystals, unless the granulated form, which is preferable, be available, and in either case the salt should be fresh and free from oxidized portions, or "rustiness;" it should be dissolved in half the elder flower water (all of which is better, if not quite recently distilled, for being quickly raised to the boiling point and cooled out of contact of air before use), the citric acid being also in solution in the other half, and the two fluids mixed, filtered if necessary, and bottled immediately; a lump of camphor about the size of a small peppercorn to be added to the contents of each bottle.

4063. Milk of Roses. A

English Milk of Roses.—1. Almonds (blanched), 1½ ounces; oil of almonds, 1½ ounces; white soft soap, 1 dram; rose water, ¾ pint; make an emulsion; to the strained emulsion add a mixture of essence or spirit of roses, ½ fluid dram; rectified spirit, 2½ fl. ounces; and, subsequently, of rose water, q. s. to make the whole measure 1 pint. More spirit is often ordered and used; but much of it is apt to cause the separation of the ingredients. In many samples, and in the inferior ones generally, it is omitted altogether. Some makers add a few drops of oil of bergamot, with 2 or 3 drops each of oil of lavender and otto of roses, dissolved in the spirit.

4064. Milk of Roses. B

2. Oil of almonds, 1 ounce; white soft soap, 1 ounce; salt of tartar, ½ dram; boiling water, ⅓ pint; triturate and subsequently agitate until perfectly united. When cold, further add, of rectified spirit, 2 fl. ounces; spirit of roses, a few drops; rose water, q. s. to make the whole measure a pint.

4065. Eczema Ointment.

| Creolin | 1 ounce. |
| Yellow petrolatum | 3 ounces. |

4066. Eczema of the Hands. A

| Creasoti | 10 minims. |
| Glycerini | 1 ounce. |

M.
Apply with a feather, and wear a glove over the hand.

4067. Eczema of the Hands. B

Dr. Frank H. Barendt, writing in the Provincial Medical Journal, recommends two applications for the treatment of localized eczema, viz.:

Adepis benzoati	⎫
Adepis lanae	⎬ Equal parts.
Amyli	⎪
Zinci oxidi	⎭

M. Fiat pasta.
This is a modification of Lassar's paste.

Oxidi zinci	⎫
Amyli	⎬ Equal parts.
Talci veneti	⎭

Tere bene. Fiat pulvis aspersorius.

The paste is to be spread thickly over the affected area, then covered with bandages. If the patient avoid all wetting of the dressings it will expedite cure. Gloving of the hands is imperative, and, except when the paste is being renewed, the gloves, which should be two or three sizes too large, are to be worn continuously. The hands should be dressed after the day's work is done. As the eczema improves, the paste may be discarded and the dusting-powder copiously dredged into the fingers of the gloves.

4068. Startin's Remedy for Eczema Rubrum.

Magnes. sulph	½ ounce.
Tr. ferri mur	2 drams.
Tr. zingib	1 dram.
Tr. colchici	1 dram.
Aq. ad	8 ounces.

M. Ft. mist.
One ounce bis terve in die.

Ung. hyd. fort	½ dram.
P. hyd. nit. ox	10 grains.
Adeps recent	1 ounce.

M. Ft. ung.
Omne mane utend.

4069. Sea Foam.

Cologne spirits, 188 per cent	4 ounces.
Castor oil	1 ounce.
Oil of lavender	15 minims.
Stronger water of ammonia	½ ounce.
Water q. s. to measure	16 ounces.

Mix the oils and spirit; add the ammonia and enough water to make up to 16 ounces.

4070. Ammonia Dry Shampoo.

Powdered castile soap	2 ounces.
Cologne spirits, 188 per cent	16 ounces.
Carbonate of potash	½ ounce.
Oil of bergamot	10 drops.

Oil of lemon................ 5 drops.
Water .... 3 ounces.
Aqua ammonia............ 5 ounces.

Dissolve the oils and soap in the cologne spirits; add the potash and the water; let stand with occasional agitation for 3 days; filter, then add the ammonia.

4071.   Shampoo Liquid.   A
            Ch. & Dr.

Below we give a number of formulae from which a suitable one may be selected:

Tinct. arnica.............. 1 dram.
Tinct. cantharides........ 2 drams.
Water of ammonia........ 3 drams.
Alcohol .... 8 fl. ounces.
Soft water................ 8 fl. ounces.

4072.   Shampoo Liquid.   B

Aqua ammonia............ 2 fl. ounces.
Tinct. cantharides........ 1 fl. ounce.
Tinct. capsicum........... 1 ounce
Alcohol .... 32 fl. ounces.
Water .... 32 ounces.
Carbonate of potash...... 1 ounce.

4073.   Shampoo Liquid.   C

Ammonia carbonate....... 4 drams.
Borax .... 1 ounce.
Dissolve in water.......... 2 pints.
Add:
Glycerin .... 2 ounces.
Jamaica rum.............. 6 pints.
Bay rum.................. 2 pints.

4074.   Shampoo Liquid.   D

Alcohol .... 8 fl. ounces.
Water .... 8 fl. ounces.
Soap .... 2 fl. ounces.
Carbonate of potash...... 4 drams.
Oil of lavender............ 20 minims.
Tinct. quillaia............. 2 fl. ounces.

4075.   Shampoo Liquid.   E

Glycerin .... 1 fl. ounce.
Aqua ammonia............ 2 fl. ounces.
Alcohol .... 16 fl. ounces.
Water........q. s. to make 32 fl. ounces.

4076.   Shampoo Liquid.   F

Carbonate of potash...... 1½ drams.
Tinct. cantharides........ 2 drams.
Water of ammonia........ ½ ounce.
Bay rum.................. 1½ ounces.
Alcohol .... 1½ ounces.
Water .... 1½ ounces.

4077.   Dandruff Pomade.

Pilocarpine .... ½ dram.
Quinine hydrochlorate..... 1 dram.
Precipitated sulphur....... 2½ drams.
Peruvian balsam.......... 5 drams.
Ox-bone marrow.......... 3 ounces.

Make a pomade.

This is rather an expensive, but seemingly effective, article, proposed by the Pharm. Zeitung.

4078.   Pomade for Scurf.

Ung. hydrarg. nitratis..... 3 drams.
Cera alb.................. ½ dram.
Vaselin .... 1 oz. 1 drm.
M.

4079. Brilliantine Clear and Inseperable.

Castor oil, clear white..... 1 ounce.
Cologne spirits, 188 per cent .... 4 ounces.
Tincture of rose .... 30 minims.
Tincture of jasmin........ 15 minims.

4080.   Lip Salve Rose.

White petrolatum......... 3 pounds.
Purified beef suet......... 1½ pounds.
White wax, pure.......... 1 pound.
Spermaceti .... 6 ounces.
Vermilion, to color........ q. s.

Perfume with:
Oil of bergamot........... 1 ounce.
Oil of rose geranium...... 3 ounces.
Oil of sandalwood......... ¾ ounce.

Melt the wax and the fats together; when nearly cold add the perfume and stir in enough Chinese vermilion to give the salve a rose color.

4081.   Chapped Hands and Face.
            Ch. & Dr.

An excellent remedy for chapped hands and face, and one that, if properly used, will cure the most painful cases in from twelve to twenty-four hours, is compounded as follows:

Tr. benzoin. co............ 10 minims.
Spt. vini. rect............. 2 drams.
Aquae rosae.............. 30 minims.
Glycerini ad.............. 1 ounce.
M.

Sig: Apply to chapped surfaces at night, after they have been washed with soap and warm water, and thoroughly dried. A second application is rarely required. This remedy is equally efficacious in the treatment of fissured, bleeding, and sore lips.—Med. Times.

4082. Plain Shaving Cream.

Mutton suet	85 pounds.
Coca nut oil	15 pounds.
Potash, lye	50 pounds.

4083. Stick Pomade.—Coudray's.
Cosmetiques.

Beef suet	4½ pounds.
Paraffin wax	1¼ pounds.

Perfume with:

Oil of lavender	1 ounce.
Oil of red thyme	½ ounce.
Oil of myrbane	1 dram.

Color with lamp black or burnt umber, as required. For pink color use vermilion q. s.

4084. Stick Pomade.—Black. A.

Orange flower pomade	2 pounds.
Cassie flower pomade	½ pound.
Petrolatum	4½ pounds.
Yellow wax	8 pounds.
Oil of cloves	1 ounce.
Oil of white thyme	1 ounce.
Oil of bergamot	2 ounces.
Oil of orange	2 ounces.
Oil of nutmegs	¼ ounce.
Lamp black, to color	q. s.

4085. Stick Pomade.—Black. B

Suet	1½ pounds.
Wax	½ pound.
Germantown lampblack	½ ounce.
Venice turpentine	16 drams.
Oil citronelle	5 1/3 drams.
Oil of lemongrass	5½ drams.
Oil of lavender	2 2/3 drams.
Oil of cinnamon	1 1/3 drams.
Oil of cloves	1 1/3 drams.

4086. Stick Pomade.—White. A

Suet, or washed pomade	1½ pounds.
Wax, best white	½ to 1 lb.
Venice turpentine	16 drams.
Bergamot oil	½ dram.
Cinnamon oil	1 1/3 drams.
Lavender oil	20 drops.
Cloves oil	40 drops.
Citronelle oil	¼ dram.
Lemongrass oil	½ dram.

4087. Stick Pomade.—Black. C

Petrolatum, yellow	2 pounds.
Paraffine, hard	4 pounds.
Rosin, brown	½ pound.
Lamp black	q. s.

4088. Stick Pomade.—White. B

Petrolatum, white	2 pounds.
Paraffine, hard	4 pounds.
Rosin, pale yellow	½ pound.
Oil of lavender	1 dram.
Oil of bergamot	1 dram.
Oil of lemongrass	¼ dram.
Oil of cassia	½ dram.

4089. Cocoa Nut Cream for the Hair.

Castor oil, E. I. white	64 ounces.
Cocoa nut oil, white	32 ounces.
Cologne spirits, 188 per cent	64 ounces.

Perfume with

Oil of lavender	1 ounce.
Oil of cloves	½ ounce.
Oil of cassia	½ ounce.
Oil of bergamot	1 ounce.

Mix the cologne spirit with the castor oil, add the perfume, melt the cocoa nut and add to the other ingredients.

HAIR PREPARATIONS.

4090. Hair Oil, Perfume for.

Oil of lavender	2 ounces.
Oil of bergamot	2 ounces.
Oil of lemon	2 ounces.
Oil of cinnamon	1 dram.
Oil of rosemary	2 drams.
Oil of rose geranium	1 ounce.
Oil of cloves	1 dram.

Mix.

4091. Hair Renewer.

Lac. sulphur	3 ounces.
Acetate of lead	1 ounce.
Water, distilled	56 ounces.
Glycerine	4 ounces.
Tincture of rose or eau de cologne, farina	4 ounces.

Triturate the lac. sulphur and glycerine together in a mortar; dissolve the lead in the water and add to the sulphur and glycerine; then add the perfume. Stir well when bottling, so as to equalize the amount of sulphur in each bottle.

4092. Quinine and Jaborandi Tonic for the Hair.

Quinine sulphate	1 ounce.
Cologne spirits, 188 per ct.	48 ounces.
Fluid extract of jaborandi.	6 ounces.
Glycerine	48 ounces.
Bay rum	24 ounces.
Water	48 ounces.
Rose water	84 ounces.
Vinegar of cantharides	6 ounces.

Triturate the quinine in a mortar with the vinegar of cantharides; add the water and enough acetic acid to entirely dissolve the quinine; add the glycerine, cologne spirits, bay rum, jaborandi and rose water; add color, either red or brown, as may be desired, and filter. This is an excellent hair tonic.

4093. Jaborandi Hair Tonic.

Fluid extract of jarborandi	1 ounce.
Spirits of ammonia aromatic	4 ounces.
Rose water	3 ounces.
Glycerin	½ ounce.

Mix the fluid extract with the spirits of ammonia; add the glycerin and rose water.

4094. Hair Dye.

Black or Brown.

No. 1.

Pyrogallic acid	2 ounces.
Water, distilled	80 ounces.
Cologne spirits, 188 per cent	16 ounces.

Mix (for the large bottle).

No. 2.

Silver nitrate	4 ounces.
Water, distilled	24 ounces.
Ammonia water, 16°.q. s. or	8 ounces

(for the small bottle).

Dissolve the silver in the distilled water; add the ammonia water slowly with frequent shaking, until the precipitate first formed is dissolved. For small size hair dye use ¼-ounce French squares for the No. 1, and ⅛-ounce French squares for No. 2.

Directions.—First clean the hair from all oil or grease, by washing well with soap and water—and well rinsing the hair to remove the soap, then when dry, apply the contents of large bottle thoroughly (with a small brush is best), then when again dry, use contents small bottle—with another brush—tooth brush will be found most convenient. If a brown color is desired, add a few drops of soft water to contents of small bottle. When the dye is well set, wash with clean water. If the skin is soiled, wipe it off with a wet cloth immediately. This hair dye is instaneous in its effect—and is not injurious to the hair. Use in day-light.

4095. Hair Dye.

(One Solution Brown.)

Nitrate of silver crystals	70 grains.
Stronger water of ammonia	q. s.
Orange flower water	½ ounce.
Glycerin	¼ ounce.
Distilled water, to make	4 ounces.

Dissolve the silver in 2 ounces of the water and add water of ammonia q. s. to dissolve the precipitate first formed. Then add the other ingredients, making up to 4 ounces with distilled water.

Put up in dark glass bottles.

Directions for Use: After the hair has been well washed with a little borax and water, apply the dye evenly with a soft brush night and morning until the proper tint is obtained. It is advisable to prevent, as far as possible, the skin coming into contact with the dye. Pomatum and oil must not be used whilst the dyeing process is being done.

4096. Hair Colorer. A

Nitrate of silver	6 grains.
Nitrate of copper	6 grains.
Water of ammonia	q. s.
Water, q. s. to make	1 ounce.

Dissolve the nitrates in ½ ounce of distilled water, and add water of ammonia until the precipitate is dissolved.

4097. Hair Colorer. B

Permanganate of potash	60 grains.
Rose water	3 ounces.

4098. Hair Colorer. C

Pyrogallic acid	30 grains.
Spirits, proof	1 ounce.
Soda hyposulphite	½ ounce.
Water	3 ounces.

Dissolve the pyro in the spirit, the soda in the water and mix them.

4099. Hair Colorer. D

Pyrogallic acid	60 grains.
Chloride of copper	4 grains.
Cologne spirits, 188 per ct	½ ounce.
Water, q. s. to make up to	4 ounces.

4100. Bismuth Hair Dye.
No. 1.

H. F. Meier gives the Druggists' Bulletin the following formula for a bismuth hair dye to produce either brown or No. 1.

Bismuth subnitrate	200 grains.
Water	2 ounces.
Nitric acid, U. S. P. q. s. or	420 grains.

Use heat to effect solution.

No. 2.

Tartaric acid	150 grains.
Sodium bicarbonate	168 grains.
Water	32 ounces.

When effervescence of the latter has ceased, mix the cold liquids by pouring No. 1 into No. 2, with constant stirring. Allow the precipitate to subside, transfer it to a filter or strainer, and wash with water until free from the sodium nitrate formed, as this salt would be an unnecessary impediment to the operation of the dye. The completeness of the washing can readily be determined by evaporating a few drops on a watch glass. If pure water has been used, no greater amount of residue should remain than the water itself will produce. Now allow the magma to drain until its weight is reduced to at least 4 ounces. This can be readily determined without removing it from the filter and funnel if both have been previously weighed. Now transfer the magma, which consists of bismuth tartrate, to a dish, and dissolve it by the addition of sufficient aqua ammoniae. (About 90 to 100 minims of stronger water of ammonia, U. S. P., will be required.) Now dissolve 100 grains of sodium hypospulphite in 3 ounces of water, and mix the two liquids. The total volume of the product should be 7 or 8 fluid ounces, which would make the solution contain about 10 per cent of bismuth tartrate, the product from the above quantities being nearly 300 grains. The author advises the addition of 1 ounce of glycerin as calculated to make it more effective in coloring the hair, as this ingredient prevents entire drying out of the constituents, and thus favors a continuation of the decomposition. Should it be desired to produce a jet black, this may be accomplished (after the dye given above has first been applied and allowed to dry) by the application of a solution of an alkaline sulphide. It is not necessary that the latter salt should be absolutely pure, as the commercial sulphide of potassium answers quite well if fresh or undecomposed. The application of the dye and mordant is usually made by means of a tooth brush and comb, so as to avoid staining the scalp. The author points out that this dye is presumably harmless, while silver and lead dyes are known to be dangerous.

DENTAL PREPARATIONS.

4101. Cherry Tooth Paste.

Precipitated chalk	6¼ pounds.
Rose pink, powdered	3 pounds.
Orris root, powdered	10 ounces.
Gum myrrh, powdered	1 ounce.
Oil of bitter almonds, sine Prussic acid	60 minims.
Oil of cloves	15 minims.
Saccharin	60 grains.
Tincture of jasmine	4 ounces.
Glycerine	} of each
Clear water	} equal parts

to make a paste.

Place the chalk, rose pink, orris root and myrrh in a large mortar (having first sifted them to remove grit). Dissolve the oils and saccharin in the tincture of jasmine and mix with 1 quart of glycerin and 1 quart of clear water; triturate the powders with this and continue adding water and glycerine, mixed, in equal parts, until the paste is of the right consistence.

4102. Rose Tooth Paste.

Precipitated chalk	6¼ pounds.
Rose pink, powdered	3 pounds.
Orris root, powdered	10 ounces.
Oil of rose	30 minims.
Oil of rose geranium	15 minims.
Saccharin	60 grains.
Tincture of rose	4 ounces.
Glycerine	} of each
Clear water	} equal parts

to make a paste.

Proceed as directed for Cherry Tooth Paste.

4103. Charcoal Tooth Paste.

Willow charcoal, powdered	6¼ pounds.
Orris root, powdered	1¼ pounds.
Saccharin	50 grains.
Oil of rose geraniol	30 minims.
Oil of wintergreen	5 minims.
Tincture of cassie	3 ounces.
Glycerine	} of each
Clear water	} equal parts

to make a paste.

Proceed as directed for Cherry Tooth Paste.

4104. Fragrant Tooth Powder.

Precipitated chalk	2 pounds.
Cream of tartar	2 ounces.
Powdered gum myrrh	2 ounces.
Powdered orris root	4 ounces.
Powdered sugar	4 ounces.
Powdered rose pink	8 ounces.

Mix and run through sifter and mixer twice.

4105. Saponaceous Tooth Powder.

Precipitated chalk	3½ pounds.
Powdered orris root	8 ounces.
Powdered castile soap	8 ounces.
Oil of wintergreen	1 dram.
Oil of cloves	1 dram.
Oil of peppermint	2 drops.

Mix and run through sifter and mixer twice.

4106. Quinine Tooth Powder.

Precipitated chalk	16 ounces.
Quinine sulphate	30 grains.
Powdered borax	½ ounce.
Powdered soda bicarb	½ ounce.
Powdered saccharin	30 grains.
Powdered orris root	2 ounces.
Oil of rose geraniol	15 minims.
Oil of cloves	5 minims.

Mix and run through sifter and mixer twice.

4107. Carbolic Tooth Powder.

Precipitated chalk	16 ounces.
Boric acid	½ ounce.
Powdered cinchona bark	½ ounce.
Powdered pumice	1 ounce.
Powdered soda bicarb	½ ounce.
Powdered saccharin	30 grains.
Powdered orris root	2 ounces.
Carbolic acid	1 dram.
Oil of rose geranium	1 dram.
Oil of cloves	10 drops.
Oil of peppermint	5 drops.

Mix and run through sifter and mixer twice.

4108. Saponaceous Tooth Wash.—Antiseptic.

Castile soap, white	2 ounces.
Cologne spirits, 188 per ct.	48 ounces.
Water	56 ounces.
Menthol	20 grains.
Boric acid	½ ounce.
Simple syrup	8 ounces.
Glycerine	2 ounces.
Oil of wintergreen	60 minims.
Oil of peppermint	60 minims.
Oil of cloves	15 minims.
Oil of cassia	10 minims.
Carmine solution, ammoniated	q. s.
Caramel	q. s.

Dissolve the oils, menthol and boric acid in the cologne spirits; dissolve the soap in the water; add the glycerin and syrup; mix the two solutions by pouring the spirituous solution into the watery solution, stirring slowly the while; add the coloring and filter at a low temperature.

4109. Fragrant Tooth Wash.

Cologne spirits, 188 per ct.	48 ounces.
Boric acid	½ ounce.
Thymol	60 grains.
Glycerine	5 ounces.
Syrup	4 ounces.
Glycerine	2 ounces.
Water	56 ounces.
Oil of eucalyptus	40 minims.
Oil of wintergreen	60 minims.

Dissolve the oils, thymol and boric acid in the cologne spirits; add the water, glycerin and syrup. Filter.

4110. Depilatory.
(C. & D.)

Sodium sulphide	3 drams.
Quicklime	1¼ ounces.
Powdered starch	1¼ ounces.

Mix.

To be made into a paste with water and applied to the hairy part. In three or four minutes wipe it off with the back of a knife.

4111. Bust Developer.

Ferri sulphat	8 grains.
Acid. sulph. aromat.	½ dram.
S. V. R.	1 ounce.
Syrupi	4 ounces.
Syr. rhoeados	½ ounce.
Aq. ad.	8 ounces.

M.

The directions for using the preparation reveal the cause of any improvement which may follow the use of the medicine. They are to the following effect:

A teaspoonful is to be taken in a little cold water three times a day—once after breakfast, once after dinner, and once again just before retiring to rest; also the breasts should be gently rubbed at least twice a day—say, morning and night—in a circular and upward direction, and as the rubbing assists greatly the elixir in its effects, it should be continued each time for at least fifteen minutes; in fact, the longer it is continued the better.

Obviously the massage for fifteen minutes is sufficient in itself to effect the purpose.

4112. Removal of Warts.

Dr. Morison, of Baltimore, prescribes the following as an application:

Hydrarg. bichlor.	5 grains.
Ac. salicyl.	1 dram.
Collodii	1 ounce.

To be applied once a day, the upper crust of a previous application being removed before a fresh one is made. Four such applications generally soften the wart to such a degree that gentle traction removes it painlessly, the further dressing being any simple ointment.

4113. Wart Powder.

The following is effective for removing warts:

Salicylic acid	5 parts.
Boric acid	15 parts.
Calomel	30 parts.

Mix and make into a fine powder. Put up in small glass tubes, with the direction to rub a small portion on the wart thrice daily.

4114. Lotion for Removing Wrinkles.

And improving the complexion.

Pulv. sapon. castil. alb.	2 drams.
Pulv. boracis.	1 dram.
Lanolin	7 drams.
Ol. cocos.	3 drams.
Aq	7 drams.

Rub together for a quarter of an hour, then add gradually and with constant stirring:

Aq. rose (at 104 F.)....... 10 ounces.

Shake well and perfume.

This makes a nice milky lotion.

4115. Table for Diluting Alcohol or Cologne Spirits.

85% alcohol = 17 vol. of alcohol + 2 of water.
80% alcohol = 16 vol. of alcohol + 3 of water.
75% alcohol = 15 vol. of alcohol + 4 of water.
70% alcohol = 14 vol. of alcohol + 5 of water.
65% alcohol = 13 vol. of alcohol + 6 of water.
60% alcohol = 12 vol. of alcohol + 7 of water.
55% alcohol = 11 vol. of alcohol + 8 of water.
50% alcohol = 10 vol. of alcohol + 9 of water.
45% alcohol = 9 vol. of alcohol + 10 of water.
40% alcohol = 8 vol. of alcohol + 11 of water.
35% alcohol = 7 vol. of alcohol + 12 of water.
30% alcohol = 6 vol. of alcohol + 13 of water.
25% alcohol = 5 vol. of alcohol + 14 of water.
20% alcohol = 4 vol. of alcohol + 15 of water.
15% alcohol = 3 vol. of alcohol + 16 of water.
10% alcohol = 2 vol. of alcohol + 17 of water.
5% alcohol = 1 vol. of alcohol + 18 of water.

INDEX.

Acid Phosphate Solution—988, 2820.
Acid Stains, To Remove—2107-2110.
Acid Tonic Mixture—50.
Acne—890-891.
Adams Cough Cure—575.
Agueine—710.
Ague Preparations—710-714.
Alabaster, To Clean—2111, 2112.
Ale, Ginger Extract—2623.
Ale, Ginger Syrup—2624.
Alizarine Ink—2323.
Alkali Stains—2113, 2363.
Alkaline Mixture, N. Y. Hospital—1241, 1242.
Alkaline Tar Water—1207.
Alkaline Tonic Mixture—51, 52, 1884.
Allii Syrup—2652.
Aloes and Iron Pills—1287.
Alteratives—1-25.
Alterative, Indian—4.
Alterative Juice—21.
Alum Eye Water—857.
Ambrosia Powder—739.
Ammonia, Acetate of, Solution—1267.
Ammonia, Acetate of, Solution, Conc.—1266.
Ammonia, Household—1795.
Ammonol—823.
Anaemia, Tonic For—75.
Anaesthetic Solution—1827.
Anatomical Specimens, To Preserve—1842-1849.
Aniline Stains, To Remove—2114.
Animals, Stuffed, To Clean—2115.
Anise Seed Cordial—992.
Anodyne Cement—1961.
Anodyne Cream, For Catarrh—644.
Anodyne For Dentists—1828, 1829.
Antacid Draught—1865.
Antibilious Pills—1749.
Anti-Cholera Mixture—834.
Anti-Cholera Mixture, N. Y. Sun—842.
Antikamnia—824.
Anti-Malarial Pills—1768.
Anti-Pain Powder—826.
Anti-Periodic Pills—1288.
Antipyretics and Antiseptics—822-829.
Anti-Rheumatic Mixture—1259.
Antisepticina—829.
Antiseptic Mixture—829.
Antiseptics and Antipyretics—822-829.
Antiseptic Snuff—1859.
Antiseptic Solutions—1200.
Antiseptic Wound Mixture—827, 828.
Ants, To Destroy—1944.
Aperient Lozenge—744.
Aperient Medicines—183-197, 361-366, 539-541.

Aperient Powder, For Horses—3488.
Apormorphine Hyd. Syrup—2653.
Apple, Extract Of—2616.
Aqua Anethi—2860.
    Anisi—2861.
    Aurantii Flor—2862.
    Camphora—2863.
    Carui—2864.
    Chloroformi—2865.
    Cinnamomi—2866.
    Creasoti—2867.
    Foeniculi—2868.
    Lauro-Cerasi—2869.
    Menth. Pip—2870.
    Menth. Virid.—2871.
    Pimentae—2872.
    Rosae—2873.
Aristol—825.
Arnica Jelly—2637.
    Liniment—745, 747.
    Opodeldoc—764.
    Salve—778.
Aromatic Cascara—57.
Aromatic Cod Liver Oil—1807, 1809.
Aromatic Ginger Ale, Essence—955.
Aromatic Wine—74.
Arsenical Pills—1751.
Arsenical Solution, Clemen's—1771.
Artificial Sea Water—1950.
Artistic Enamel, Black—2543.
Asafetida Syrup—2654.
Asthma Cigarettes—634.
Asthma Cures—630-637.
Asthma Cure, Dick's—629.
Asthma Inhalant—633.
Asthma Mixture—632.
Asthma Mixture, (Potter)—631.
Asthma Powders—635-637.
Asthma Syrup—630.
Ayer's Formula For Sarsaparilla—1860.
Baby Dusting Powder—907.
Baby Powder—1222, 1853-1858.
Baby Quinine, A—711.
Baby Quinine, B—712.
Baking Powder, Cream Tartar—2590.
Baking Powder, General Directions For Mixing—2594.
Baking Powder, Phosphate, 1 Spoon—2588.
Baking Powder, Phosphate, 2 spoons—2589.
Baking Powder, Quick Rising—2591.
Baking Powder, Salt Rising—2592.
Baking Powder, Straight Alum, 1 spoon—2586.
Baking Powder, Straight Alum, 2 spoon—2587.
Ball Camphor—800.
Balls, Scouring—2116, 2117.

(487)

Balm of Roses—4000.
Balsam Aniseed—586.
Balsam Cream, For Catarrh—645.
Balsam, Honey and Aniseed—579.
Banana, Extract Of—2612.
Barbers' Itch Ointment—785.
Barometer Tubes, To Clean—2118.
Barrels, To Cleanse—2119.
Barsaloux Sauce—2585.
Bartholow, Cholera Cure—838.
Bateman's Drops—1837.
Baths, Toning—3469, 3470.
Bay Rum, A—3933.
Bay Rum, B—3934.
Bay Rum, C—3935.
Bay Rum, D—3936.
Beading, For Spirit—1015.
Bed Bug Exterminator—1930.
Bed Bug Poison—1892.
Bed Wetting In Children—524.
Beef, Celery and Sarsaparilla—23.
Beef, Iron and Wine—68, 69, 1871, 1872.
Beef and Malt Wine—945.
Beef Wine—67-69.
Beer, Ginger—960-962.
   Ginger, Powders—963, 964.
   Herb Extract—951.
   Hop—965.
   Hop, Bitter—941.
   Lemon—966, 967.
   Maple—968-970.
   Molasses—971.
   Ottawa—972.
   Peruvian—973.
   Root—974-977, 987.
   Spruce—978-984.
   Table—985.
   Tonic—986.
Benzine, Deodorized—2506.
Benzine Jelly—2502.
Beverages—940-1199.
Bergoline Oil Spray, For Catarrh—646.
Beverages, Preservative For—940.
Bicycle Cement For Tires—1962.
Bijou Cleaning Fluid—2505.
Biliousness, Mixtures For—132-138.
Bismuth Hair Dye—4100.
Bismuth Mixture—568.
Bismuth Mixture Co.—701.
Bitters, Aromatic—46.
   German Herb—30.
   Hop—40.
   Iron Tonic—26-29, 43, 44.
   Orange—37, 38, 997.
   Roback's—31.
   Samson's—33.
   Stoughton—35.
   Walton's—32.
   Wild Cherry—36.

Bitters, Wood's—34.
   Wormwood—998.
Bitter Wine of Iron—71, 1262.
Bitter Wine of Iron, Mitchell's—72.
Blackberry, Arom. Syr. N. F.—2656.
Blackberry Cordial—39.
Blackberry Brandy—39.
Black Currant Lozenges—1346.
Blacking Paste For Shoes—2544.
Blackboard, To Remove Grease From—2120.
Blackboard Paint—1952.
Blankets, To Clean—2121, 2122.
Blaud's Pills—1286.
Blistering Ointment, For Horses—790.
Blood Cleanser—9.
   Herbs—18.
   And Kidney Tea—723.
   And Liver Syrup—25.
   Mixture—10.
   Mixture, Clark's—14.
   Purifier, Robson's—11.
   Purifiers—1-25.
   Purifying Mixture—17, 19.
   Remedy—12.
   Renovator—48.
   Stains, To Remove—2123-2125.
   Tonic—47.
Blue Prints—3273-3277.
Bluing Disinfectant—2515.
   Indigo, Wash—2513.
   Liquid—2516.
   Prussian Wash—2514.
   Wash—2512.
Boils, Ointment For—794, 795.
Bones and Ivory, To Clean—2126-2133.
Books, To Clean—2137-2143.
Boracic Acid Powders—571.
Boracic Acid Salve—780.
Borated Talcum—4005.
Borosalicylat—871.
Bottle Capping—1958-1960.
Bottles, To Clean—2147, 2148.
Brandy—Blackberry—39.
   British—1014.
   Cherry—1001.
   Coloring—1012.
   Jersey—947.
Brass, To Clean—2149-2160.
   Instruments—2157-2161.
   Paste For—2518, 2519, 2525.
Breast Tea—721.
Breath, Offensive—1850.
Brilliantine—4079.
British Brandy—1014.
   Cordial—1861.
   Oil—751-753.
Britannia Metal, To Clean—2170.
Broadcloth, To Remove Stains From—2171.
Bromides, Solution Of, Co.—1791.

INDEX.

Bromidia—1791.
Bromidrosis Zinc Cream For—888.
Brompton Hospital Cough Specific—577.
Bronchelixir—578.
Bronchial Lozenges—1348, 1349.
Bronchitis, Infantile—542-545.
Bronchitis Mixture—404-412, 588, 626, 627.
Bronchitis, Pills For—628.
Bronze, To Clean—2172.
Bronze Statuary, To Clean—2173.
Brown Chlorodyne—1825.
Brown Leather, Paste For—2545.
    Liquid Shoe Polish—2548.
    Ointment—1218.
    Shoe Polish, A—2546.
    Shoe Polish, B—2547.
Brunswick Black, For Grates—2541.
Brushes, To Wash—2174.
Buchu Elix. Comp.—716.
    Wayne's—715.
Buckthorn Bark Syrup—2657.
Bust Developer—4111.
Butter Coloring—2006.
Butter Phosphorus—1816.
Caffeine Citrate Effervescing Gran.—1297.
    Hydro-Bromate Effervescing Gran.—1305.
    Pyro. Comp.—1306.
    Seidlitz Powders—1875.
Calcium Lactophosphates Syr.—2658.
Calcium Phosphate—2660.
Calcium Phosphate, Wiegand's—2659.
Calculation of Equivalent Weights—1204.
Calico and Linen, To Clean—2175.
Calisaya Tonic—42, 53, 1870.
Calves Cordial—3734.
Camphor Ball—800.
Canaries, Diseases of, Treatment—3719-3723.
    Asthma—3719.
    Diarrhoea—3720.
    Egg-Bound—3721.
    Red Lice—3722.
    Sore Feet—3723.
Canary Food—3509.
Canvas, To Renovate—2178.
Capillaire—1000.
Capping For Bottles—1958-1960.
Carbolic Ointment—779.
    Salve—779.
    Sponge—1951.
    Spray—1201.
Carbolized Vaseline Ointment—1216.
Carbutt's Hydrochinon Developer—3384.
Carbutt's Pyro. Developer—3400.
Carmalt's Pills—1281.
Carminatives—509, 830-843, 1258.
Carpets, To Clean—2179-2184, 2350.
Carraway Cordial—903.
Carriages, To Preserve—2185.
Cascara Cordial—57.

Cascara Syrup—2661.
Castanea Syrup—2662.
Castorina—727.
Castor Oil Emulsion—1820, 1821.
Castrollina—727.
Catarrh Cream Anodyne—644.
    Balsam—645.
    Cures—638-646.
    Cure Spray—638-641.
    Snuff—642.
    Sage's—643.
Catechol—3349.
Caterpillars, To Destroy—1949.
Catsup, Tomato—2566, 2567.
Cattle Condiment—3483.
Cattle, Diseases of, Treatment—3584-3616.
    Balls—3584.
    Cold—3586.
    Cough—3587.
    Cowpox—3588.
    Diarrhoea—3589.
    Draughts—3585.
    Draught for Hoven—3517.
    Eye Diseases—3590.
    Fardel-Bound—3591.
    Fattening Powder—3502.
    Foot Disease—3592.
    Foot and Mouth Disease—3593.
    Foot Hoven—3594.
    Inflammation of Brain—3595.
    Inflammation of Kidneys—3596.
    Inflammation of Udder—3597.
    Jaundice—3598.
    Lice—3599.
    Milk, Bloody—3601.
    Milk, Blue—3600.
    Milk Fever—3602.
    Over-Eating—3603.
    Pleuro-Pneumonia—3604.
    Quinsey—3605.
    Red-Water—3606.
    Rheumatism—3608.
    Ringworm—3607.
    Scab—3609.
    Stoppage—3610.
    Suppression of Milk—3611.
    Tail Worm—3612.
    Tapeworm—3613.
    Thrush in Calves—3614.
    Tonic—3615.
    White Scour—3616.
Celery, Beef and Sarsaparilla—53.
Celery Compound—70.
Celery, Ext. of—2617.
Celery Salt—2570.
Celluloid, To W…
Cement, Ano…
    For Bi…
    Casei…

Cement, For China and Glass—2071, 2072.
    For Metals—1985-2000.
        Metallic—1982, 1983.
    For Mica—2001.
    For Microscopes—2002.
    For Minerals—2003, 2004.
    For Mohr's—2005.
    For Porcelain—2075.
    Roman—1963.
        For Roofs—1964, 1965.
    For Rubber—1966-1980, 2076.
    For Rust—1981.
Cerate, Indian—813.
Chairs, Cane Seated, Renovating—2176, 2177.
Chamois Skin, To Cleanse—2358, 2359.
Champagne Kola Essence—956.
Chandler's Chlorodyne—1822.
Chapped Hands and Face—4081.
Chapped Hands, Ointment For—792.
Chartreuse—959.
Cheap Blood Mixture—20.
Cheltenham Salts—1302.
Cheltenham Salts, Efferv.—1304.
Chemicals and Drugs, To Pack for Export—1841.
Chemical Food—1851, 2694.
Chemical Guano—1957.
Cherry Brandy—1001.
Cherry Cough Cure—593.
Cherry and Horehound—592.
Chest Colds—445-460.
Chilblain Cream, Vance's—872.
    Cures—860-878.
    Lints—860-866.
    Ointments—867-870, 873, 878.
Children's Cough Syrup—1832.
Children's Hospital Formulas—567-574.
Children's Remedies—517-574.
Chill Pills—1765.
Chill Powder, Tasteless—714.
Chill Tonic, Tasteless—713.
China, To Clean—2188.
Chloral Hydrate Syr. Br—2663.
Chlorate Of Potash Mixture—1231.
Chloride Of Gold—3437.
Chlorides, Elixirs of—1778-1782.
Chlorides Four, Taylor's—2557.
Chlorodynes—1822-1826.
Chloroform Cough Mixture—1234.
Choleraic Diarrhoea—843.
Cholera Cramps—838.
    Drops, Thielman's —841.
    Mixture, Sun—842.
Chromos, To Clean—2189.
Chronic Constipation Pills—1750.
Chronic Headache—700.
Chrysophanic Acid Oint. Conc.—1217.
Cinchona and Iron Mixture—1240.
Cinchona Wine—1883.

Cinnamon Cordial—1002.
Cinnamon, Extract of—2609.
Citrate of Magnesia—1208, 1290, 1794.
Clark's Anodyne Cement—1961.
    (Sir Andrew) Cholera Cure—843.
    Pills—1283.
    (Sir Andrew) Pills—1748.
    (Sir Andrew) Rheumatism Mixture—664.
Cleaning Fluid, Bijou—2505.
Cleaning Powders—2107, 2453.
Cleansing and Renovating—2107, 2453.
Clear Chlorodyne—1823.
Clemen's Solution of Arsenic—1771.
Clocks and Watches, To Clean—2190.
Cloth, Black, To Clean—2191.
Cloth, Black, To Revive—2198.
Cloth Cleaning Compound—2192.
Clothes To Brush—2193.
Clouds, To Photograph—3297.
Clove Cordial—960.
Clove, Extract Of—2610.
Coca Kola Syrup—1882.
Coca Kola Wine—61.
Coca Leaves Cordial—54.
Coca Wine—55, 62, 1881.
Cocaine, Solution Of—1793.
Cochineal Coloring—1777.
Cockroach Exterminator—1931.
Codeine Cough Syrup—580.
Cod Liver Oil, Aromatic—1807, 1809.
Cod Liver Oil Emulsion—1802-1805, 1810.
Cod Liver Oil, Iodo Ferrated—1808, 1811.
Cod Liver Oil and Malt—1806.
Cod Liver Oil, Mixture Of—1814.
Cod Liver Oil with Rock and Rye—1812.
Cod Liver Oil, Tasteless—1819.
Cod Liver Oil, Wine Of—1813.
Coins and Metals, To Clean—2194-2196.
Colic Draught, For Horses, A—3515.
Colic Draught, For Horses, B—3516.
    Drench, For Horses—3525.
    Liniment—757.
Colic Mixture, For Infants—1831.
Collodio Bromide Emulsion—3298.
Collodion Styptic—1786.
Cologne, Coyt's—3892.
    Extra Fine—3890.
    Fine—3891.
    Lafayette—3889.
    Mixture A—3893.
    Mixture B—3894.
    Vermont—3888.
    Waters—3887-3894.
    Windsor—3887.
Colored Fires—2081-2094.
Colored Fires, Caution—2095.
Coloring for Brandy—1012.
Coloring for Butter and Cheese—2096.
    For Cochineal—1777.

INDEX.   491

Coloring for Extracts—2614.
   For Liqueurs—1005-1013.
Colorless Hydrastis—1772.
Color, To Restore—2197.
Colors For Show Bottles—1886.
Coltsfoot Lozenges—1345.
Coltsfoot Rock Candy—617.
Combs, To Clean—2199.
Compound Lobelia Mixture—607.
Compound Syrup of Flaxseed—587.
Compound Viburnum—58.
Compressed Tablets—1422-1507.
Compressed Tablets, To Make—1307, 1308.
Compressed Tablets, Materials to Prepare—1309-1339.
Condition Food—3482.
Condition Powders—3480, 3481.
Congested Liver, Mixtures for—127-130.
Constipation Powder For Cattle—3491.
Constipation Remedy For Females—367.
Consumption Cure, Piso's—613.
Consumption Cure, Shiloh's—612.
Consumption, Inhalant For—611.
Cooling Mixture—525, 256, 546-549.
Cooling and Teething Powders—901, 904.
Copaiba, Cubeb and Buchu—847.
   Liquor, Soluble—846.
   Mixture—845.
   Solidified—849.
Copper, To Clean—2200-2202.
Copying Ink, Hektograph—2100.
Copying Pad, Hektograph—2099.
Cordial, Aniseed—992.
   Capillaire—1000.
   Carraway—993.
   Cascara—57.
   Cherry Brandy—1001.
   Cinnamon—1002.
   Cloves—900.
   Coca—54.
   Gingeretta—996.
   Godfrey's—1834-1836.
   Lemonade—909.
   Lovage—1003.
   Neutralizing—1876.
   Noyeau—994.
   Peppermint—989.
   Raspberry—995.
   Rum Shrub—991.
   Usquebaugh—1004.
Coral, To Clean and Bleach—2203, 2204.
Corn Cures—879, 884.
Corn Salve—883.
   Solvent—881.
   And Wart Eradicator—884.
Cough Balls For Horses—3496.
Cough Balsam—591.
Cough, Cold, Influenza—404-460.
   Cure, Adams—575.

Cough Drops—619, 620.
   Linctus—368-380.
   Lozenges—618.
   Mixtures—381, 396, 1233-1236.
   Mixture For Adults—596.
   Mixture For Children—573, 598-616.
   For Dogs—3514.
   Mixture, Palatable—602, 603.
   No More Lozenges—1344.
   Powder For Horses—3512, 3513, 3526.
   Remedies—368-460, 573-621.
   Remedy Without Opium—595.
   Syrup, Children's—397-403.
   Syrup, Standard—576.
Cramer's Pyro. Solution—3409.
Cramps, A and B—1867, 1868.
Crape, To Clean—2206.
Crape, To Restore—2205.
Cream Anodyne For Catarrh—644.
   Balsam—645.
   Camphor Lint.—759.
   Furniture—2555, 2556.
Cream Soda Powder—742.
Cream of Roses—4008.
Creasote, Emulsion of—708, 709.
   Gargle—702.
   Oint. of—812.
   Pills—704-706.
   Preparations—702-709.
   For Ringworm—703.
Crimson Marking Ink—2102.
Crocks and Jars, To Remove Grease From—2316.
Croft's Table Sauce—2579.
Cross Tea—724.
Cubeb Cough Syrup—616.
Cubeb Paste—850.
Curacoa Liqueur—943.
Cure For Morphinomania—1863.
Currant Lozenges—1346.
Curry Powder—2562.
Curtains, To Clean—2207-2209.
Custard Powder—2561.
Cyclists Universal Oil—763.
Daguerrotypes, To Restore—3337.
Damiana, Wine of—65.
Damiana, Wine of, Co.—66.
Death on Rats—1893.
Decoctions, To Prepare—1839.
Delmonico Sauce—2580.
Dental Obtundent—1830.
Dental Preparations—4101-4109.
   Tooth Paste, Charcoal—4103.
   Tooth Paste, Cherry—4101.
   Tooth Paste, Rose—4102.
   Tooth Powder, Carbolic—4107.
   Tooth Powder, Fragrant—4104.
   Tooth Powder, Quinine—4106.
   Tooth Powder, Saponaceous—4105.

Dental Tooth Wash, Fragrant—4109.
    Tooth Wash, Saponaceous—4108.
Dentists, Anodyne For—1829.
Deodorized Benzine—2506.
Depilatory—4110.
Developers, Cramer's One Solution—3412, 3413.
    Eikonogen—3350, 3351.
    Eikonogen, For Bromide Paper—3375.
    Eikonogen, Himly's—3355.
    Eikonogen, Hubert's—3356.
    Hoover's Potash—3414, 3415.
    Hydrochinon—3377-3392.
    Hydrochinon and Eikonogen Comb.—3365.
    Hydroxlamine—3396.
    Iron—3398-3401.
    Paramidophenol—3393-3395.
    Potash—3404-3405.
    Pyro.—3403-3406, 3410.
Development, With Separate Solutions—3357.
Development With Single Solutions—3358-3359.
Diabetics, Lemonade for—1862.
Diamonds, To Clean—2210.
Diarrhoea—500-507.
Diarrhoea In Children—529-538, 550-557, 566.
Diarrhoea Cordial—830.
Diarrhoea Mixture For Children—835, 837, 840-843.
    Mixture, Loomis'—836.
    Mixture, Squibb's—831.
    Mixture, Thieleman's—832.
    Mixture, Velpearl's—833.
Dick's Asthma Cure—629.
Digestive Mixtures—698, 699, 701.
Digestive Pastilles—698.
    Pastilles, (Borivent)—699.
    Pills—1753.
    Powder—657-658.
    Relish—2581.
    Syrup—647.
    Tonic—648-649.
Dioviburnum Mixture—59.
Diuretic Mixture—497-498.
Diuretic Pills—1285.
Disinfectant, Taylor's Four Chlorides—2557.
Distemper Mixture For Dogs, A—3506.
Distemper Mixture For Dogs, B—3507.
Dog Cough Mixture—3514.
    Diseases Of, Treatment—3644-3653.
    Chorea—3645.
    Distemper—3646.
    Fits—3647.
    Fractures—3648.
    Medicines—3644.
    Pills—3504-3505.
    Pleurisy—3649.
    Poisoning—3650.
    Rabies—3651.

Dog Tonics—3652.
    Worms—3653.
Donovan's Solution—1801.
Dover's Powder, Syrup—2693.
Draught, Antacid—1865.
    For Hoven in Cattle—3517.
    For Hysteria—1864.
Drawing Instruments, To Clean—2211.
Drops, Bateman's—1837.
Drunkenness Cures, Miscellaneous—3235-3239.
Dusting Powder, For Sores—1222.
Dusting On Process—3417.
Dyspepsia Flatulent—652.
Dyspepsia Mixtures—183-262, 647-650.
Dyspepsia Mixtures, Alkaline—146-154.
Dyspepsia Mixtures, Bismuthic—155-182.
Dyspepsia Remedy—650.
Earache—499.
    Inflammatory—1866.
East India Sauce—2582.
Eastoni Liquor—1774.
Eastoni Syrup—1774.
Eau de Cologne—3896-3918.
    Formula 1801—3903.
    Formula 1813—3904.
    Formula No. 6—3901.
    Formula No. 7—3902.
    Formula No. 10—3905.
    Formula No. 11—3906.
    Formula No. 12—3907.
    Formula No. 13—3908.
    Formula No. 14—3909.
    Formula No. 15—3910.
    Formula No. 16—3911.
    Formula No. 17—3912.
    Formula No. 18—3913.
    Formula No. 19—3914.
    Gegenüber dem Julich's Platz—3915.
    (like) Julich's Platz—3900.
    Lily of Valley—3916.
    Maiglöckchen—3917.
    Paris Ex. Prize—3897, 3898.
    (like) Springbrunn brand—3899.
    Sydney Gold Medal—3896.
Eczema Mixture—15, 4066-4068.
Eczema Drying Salve—1229, 4065.
Effects, Moonlight in Photography—3451.
Effervescing Mixtures—1252, 1253.
Effervescent Powders—736-742.
    Salts, Base—1296.
    Salts—1296-1306.
    Salts, To Prepare—1295.
Egg Producing Food—3486.
Elixir of Acid Salicylic. N. F.—3119.
    Adjuvans, N. F.—3120.
    Aletris—2894.
    Ammonii Bromide, N. F.—3121.
    Ammon. Valerianatis. N. F.—3122.
    Ammonium Chloride—2895.

INDEX.

Elixir of Ammonium Chloride and Licorice Co. —2896.
    Ammonium Quinine and Strychnine Valerianates—2897.
    Ammonium Valerianate with Cinchonidine, Iron Phosphate, Quinine and Strychnine—2901.
    Ammonium Valerianate, Iron Pyrophosphate and Quinine—2900.
    Ammonium Valerianate with Cinchonidine and Quinine—2902.
    Ammonium Valerianate with Cinchonidine, Quinine and Strychnine—2903.
    Ammonium Valerianate with Cinchonidine and Strychnine—2904.
    Ammonium Valerianate and Iron—2905.
    Ammonium Valerianate, I., Q., and S.,—2906.
    Ammonium Valerianate and Quinine, N. F.—3123.
    Ammonium Valerianate with Strychnine —2899.
    Ammonium Valerianate with Sumbul—2898.
    Anisi, N. F.—3124.
    Antifebrin—2907.
    Antipyrin—2908.
    Apii Graveolentis, N. F.—3125.
    Aromaticum, N. F.—3126.
    Arsenic and Quinine—2909.
    Arsenic and Strychnine—2910.
    Aurantii, U. S. P.—2912.
    Beef—2911.
    Beef and Iron—2913.
    Beef, Iron and Malt—2914.
    Berberine—2915.
    Berberine and Iron—2916.
    Bismuth—2917.
    Bismuth and Cinchona—2918.
    Bismuth, Cinchona, Iron and Pepsin —2919.
    Bismuth, Cinchona, Iron, Pepsin and Strychnine—2920.
    Bismuth, Cinchona and Pepsin—2921.
    Bismuth and Gentian—2922.
    Bismuth, Gentian and Iron—2923.
    Bismuth, Gentian, Iron and Strychnine—2924.
    Bismuth, Gentian and Strychnine—2925.
    Bismuth, Golden Seal and Iron—2926.
    Bismuth and Golden Seal—2927.
    Bismuth and Iron—2928.
    Bismuth, Iron and Pepsin—2929.
    Bismuth, Iron, Pepsin and Quinine—2930.
    Bismuth, Iron and Strychnine—2931.
    Bismuth, Nux Vomica and Pepsin—2932.
    Bismuth and Pancreatin—2933.
    Bismuth, Pepsin and Quinine—2934.
    Bismuth and Quinine—2935.

Elixir of Bismuth and Strychnine—2936.
    Bismuthi, N. F.—3127.
    Bitter—2937.
    Blackberry—2938.
    Black Cohosh—2940.
    Black Haw—2939.
    Black Haw Co.—2941.
    Blue Flag—2942.
    Blue Flag and Wahoo—2943.
    Bromides 3—2944.
    Bromides 6—2945.
    Bromide of Zinc—2946.
    Buchu, N. F.—3128.
    Buchu Co., N. F.—3129.
    Buchu and Juniper Co.—2947.
    Buchu, Juniper and Potash Acet.—2948.
    Buchu, Juniper, Uva Ursi and Potassium Acet.—2949.
    Buchu and Pareira Brava—2950.
    Buchu and Pareira Brava Co.—2951.
    Buchu and Potassium Acet., N. F.—3130.
    Buckthorn and Senna—2952.
    Caffeinae, N. F.—3131.
    Calcii Bromide, N. F.—3132.
    Calcii Hypophosphitis, N. F.—3133.
    Calcii Lactophosphatis, N. F.—3134.
    Calcium Iodide—2955.
    Calcium Lactophosphate and Cinchona—2957.
    Calcium Phosphate—2958.
    Calcium and Sodium Hypophosphites with Malt—2953.
    Calcium and Sodium Hypophosphites with Tar—2954.
    Cascara Sagrada with Sodium Salicylate —2959.
    Castillon's—2960.
    Catharticum, N. F.—3135.
    Celery and Guarana—2961.
    Cherries—2962.
    Cherries with Calcium and Sodium Hypophosphites—2963.
    Chirata—2965.
    Chloral Hydrate—2964.
    Chloral Hydrate and Ammonium Valerianate—2966.
    Chlorides of Arsenic and Iron—2967.
    Chlorides of Arsenic, Iron and Mercury—2968.
    Chlorides (Four)—2969.
    Chloroform—2970.
    Chloroformi Co., N. F.—3136.
    Cinchona Co.—2972.
    Cinchona, Detannated—2971-3139.
    Cinchona, Gentian and Iron Malate—2973.
    Cinchona, Iron and Phosphorus—2975.
    Cinchona and Protoxide of Iron—2974-3140.
    Cinchona and Pepsin—2976-2977.

Elixir of Cinchona with Phosphates—2978-2979.
    Cinchona and Strychnine—2980.
    Cinchonae, N. F.—3137.
    Cinchonae, Ferri and Bismuthi, N. F.—3142.
    Cinchonae, Ferri, Bismuthi et Stry., N. F.—3141.
    Cinchonae, Ferri et Calcii Lactophosphatis N. F.—3143.
    Cinchonae et Hypophosphitum, N. F.—3138.
    Cinchonae, Ferri et Pepsini—3144.
    Cinchonae, Ferri et Strychninae—3145.
    Cinchonae, Pepsini et Strychninae, N. F.—3146.
    Cinchonidine—2981.
    Cinchonidine and Iron—2982.
    Cinchonidine, Iron and Strychnine—2983.
    Coca and Phosphorus—2984.
    Codeine—2985.
    Codeine and Terpin Hydrate—2987.
    Corydalis—2986.
    Corydalis Co., N. F.—3147.
    Crampbark, Co.—2988.
    Croton, Chloral Hydrate—2989.
    Croton, Chloral Hydrate and Quinine—2990.
    Curacoa—3148.
    Damiana, Iron, Nux Vomica and Phosphorus—2991.
    Damiana, Iron and Phosphorus—2992.
    Damiana, Nux Vomica and Phosphorus—2993.
    Damiana and Phosphorus—2994.
    Damiana, Phosphorus and Strychnine—2995.
    Dandelion—2997.
    Dandelion Co., A—2998.
    Dandelion Co., B—2999.
    Dandelion Co., C—3000.
    Dewberry Root Co.—2996.
    Emmenagogue—3001.
    Eriodictyi Arom., N. F.—3149.
    Erythroxyli, N. F.—3150.
    Erythroxyli et Guaranae, N. F.—3151.
    Eucalypti, N. F.—3152.
    Euonymi, N. F.—3153.
    Ferri Hypophosphitis—3154.
    Ferri Lactatis, N. F.—3155.
    Ferri Phosphatis, N. F.—3156.
    Ferri Phosphatis, Cinchonidinae et Stry., N. F.—3157.
    Ferri Phosphatis, Quininae et Stry., N. F.—3158.
    Ferri Pyrophosphatis, N. F.—3159.
    Ferri Quininae et Stry., N. F.—3160.
    Flavoring—3002.
    Frangulae, N. F.—3161.
    Galls, Aromatic—3003.

Elixir de Garus, A.—3004.
    de Garus, B.—3005.
    Gentian—3006, 3162.
    Gentian Co., A—3007.
    Gentian Co., B—3008.
    Gentian Co., C—3009.
    Gentian and Iron Phosphate, Nux Vomica and Quassia—3011.
    Gentian and Phosphorus—3012.
    Gentian and Iron Pyrophosphate—3010.
    Gentianae et Ferri Phosphatis—3163.
    Gentianae cum Tr. Ferri, N. F.—3164.
    Glycyrrhizae, N. F.—3165.
    Glycyrrhizae Arom., N. F.—3166.
    Golden Seal—3014.
    Grindelia, N. F.—3167.
    Guaiac—3013.
    Guarana Br.—3015.
    Guaranae, N. F.—3168.
    Helonias—3016.
    Helonias Co.—3017.
    Humuli—3169.
    Hypophosphites of Iron and Quinine, A—3018.
    Hypophosphites of Iron and Quinine, B—3019.
    Hypophosphites of Iron, Quinine and Strychnine—3020.
    Hypophosphites with Malt—3021.
    Hypophosphitum, N. F.—3170.
    Hypophosphitum cum Ferro, N. F.—3171.
    Iodide Potassium—3024.
    Iodide Potassium Co.—3023.
    Iodides, Six—3022.
    Iodo-Bromides Calcium—2956.
    Iron, Pepsin and Quinine—3025.
    Iron, Quinine and Stry. Phosphates—3035.
    Iron Peptonate, A—3029.
    Iron Peptonate, B—3030.
    Iron Phosphate, Quinine and Stry., A—3031.
    Iron Phosphate, Quin. and Stry., B—3032.
    Iron Phosphate, Quin. and Stry., C—3033.
    Iron Phosphate, Quin. and Stry., D—3034.
    Iron Protoxide—3036.
    Iron Pyrophosphate, Quin. and Stry., A—3037.
    Iron Pyrophosphate, Quin. and Stry., B—3038.
    Iron Pyrophosphate, Quin. and Stry., C—3039.
    Iron Pyrophosphate and Strychnine—3040.
    Iron, Quinine and Arsenic—3026.
    Iron, Quinine, Citrate—3028.
    Iron, Quinine and Strych. Phosphates—3035.

INDEX.

Elixir of Iron Salicylate—3041.
    Iron Salicylate Co.—3042.
    Iron Valerianate—3043.
    Iron and Wild Cherry—3027.
    Kola—3044.
    Licorice, Aromatic, A—3045.
    Licorice, Aromatic, B—3046.
    Licorice Co.—3047.
    Lithii Bromidi, N. F.—3172.
    Lithii Citratis, N. F.—3173.
    Lithii Salicylatis, N. F.—3174.
    Long Life—3048.
    Lupulin—3049.
    Lupulin and Soda Bromide—3050.
    Malt—3051.
    Malt and Pepsin—3052.
    Malti et Ferri, N. F.—3175.
    Manaca and Salicylate—3053.
    Matico Co.—3054.
    Morphine Valerianate—3055.
    Orange—3056.
    Orange Co.—3057.
    Pancreas—3058.
    Pancreatin—3059.
    Pancreatin, Bismuth and Pepsin—3060.
    Pancreatin and Pepsin—3061.
    Papain—3062.
    Paraldehyde—3063.
    Pareira Brava—3064.
    Pepsin—3065-3176.
    Pepsin Compound, A—3066.
    Pepsin Compound, B—3067.
    Pepsin, Bismuth and Stry, N. F.—3177.
    Pepsin et. Bismuthi, N. F.—3178.
    Pepsin et Ferri, N. F.—3179.
    Pepsin and Quinine—3068.
    Pepsin, Quinine and Strych.—3069.
    Pepsin and Strychnine—3070.
    Pepsin and Wafer Ash—3071.
    Phosphori—3180.
    Phosphori et Nucis Vomicae, N. F.—3181.
    Phosphorus, A—3072.
    Phosphorus, B—3073.
    Phosphorus Co.—3074.
    Phosphorus, Quinine and Stry.—3075.
    Phosphorus and Strychnine—3076.
    Picis Co., N. F.—3182.
    Pilocarpi, N. F.—3183.
    Potassii Acet., N. F.—3184.
    Potassii Acet. and Juniper. N. F.—3185.
    Potassii Bromidi, N. F.—3186.
    Pulmonic—3077.
    Quininae Valerianatis et Strychninae, N. F.—3189.
    Quinine Bisulphate—3078.
    Quinine Co., N. F.—3187.
    Quinine and Phosphate Co., N. F.—3188.
    Quinine and Strychnine—3079.

Elixir of Quinine and Strychnine Valerianates—3081.
    Quinine Valerianate—3080.
    Rhamni Purshianae, N. F.—3090.
    Rhamni Purshianae Co., N. F.—3091.
    Rhei, N. F.—3192.
    Rhei et Mag. Acet., N. F.—3193.
    Rhubarb Aromatic—3082.
    Rhubarb, Magnesia and Senna—3085.
    Rhubarb and Potassium—3084.
    Rhubarb and Potassium with Pancreatin—3083.
    Rhubarb and Senna—3086.
    Rubi Co., N. F.—3194.
    Salicylic Acid Co.—3087.
    Saw Palmetto and Pichi—3091.
    Saw Palmetto and Sandal Wood Co.—3092.
    Senna, A—3088.
    Senna, B—3089.
    Senna Co.—3090.
    Simple, A—3093.
    Simple, B—3094.
    Simple, C—3095.
    Simple, D—3096.
    Simple, E—3097.
    Simple, F—3098.
    Simple, G—3099.
    Simple, H—3100.
    Simple, I—3101.
    Simple, J—3102.
    Sodii Bromidi, N. F.—3195.
    Sodii Hypophosphitis, N. F.—3196.
    Sodii Salicylatis, N. F.—3197.
    Stillingia, A—3103.
    Stillingia, B—3104.
    Stillingae Co., N. F.—3198.
    Strych. Valerianatis, N. F.—3199.
    Sumbul—3105.
    Sumbul Co.—3106.
    Tar Co., N. F.—3107.
    Taraxaci Co., N. F.—3200.
    Terpin Hydrate—3108.
    Triple Valerianate—3109.
    Turnerae, N. F.—3201.
    Viburni Opuli Co., N. F.—3202.
    Viburnum Prunifolium, N. F.—3203.
    Wafer Ash—3110.
    Wahoo, N. F.—3111.
    White Pine Co.—3112.
    Wild Cherry—3113.
    Yerba Santa, A—3114.
    Yerba Santa Arom., B—3115.
    Yerba Santa Arom., C—3116.
    Yerba Santa Arom., D—3117.
    Yerba Santa Co.—3118.
    Zinci Valerianatis, N. F.—3204.
Elixirs of Chlorides—1778 to 1782.
Embrocations—491 to 496—3495.

Emery, to Cleanse after Using—2220-2221.
Emulsion of Castor Oil—1820-1821.
    Of Cod Liver Oil—1802-1805.
    Of Cod Liver Oil and Saccharated Lime—1230.
    Of Petroleum—1815-1817-1818.
    Of Sandal Wood—855.
    For Tapeworm—920.
Enamel for Grates, Artistic—2543.
    For Grates and Stoves—2542.
Enameling, Photo Prints—3418.
Encaustic, Paste—3419-3423.
Engravings, to Clean—2212-2219.
Epilating Stick—1211.
Equivalent Weights, to Calculate—1204.
Errhine Powder—1203.
Essence of Linseed—609.
Evaporating Lotion—1213.
Excelsior Cough Syrup—610.
Expectorant Mixture—608.
Extract, Apple—2616.
    Banana—2612.
    Beef, Celery and Sarsaparilla—23.
    Celery—2617.
    Cinnamon—2609.
    Clove—2610.
    Coloring For—2614.
    Ginger—2619.
    Ginger Ale—2623.
    Ale Aromatic—2620.
    Ale Aromatic, Soluble—2622.
    Ale, Soluble—2621.
    Lemon—2596.
    Lemon, Soluble—2597.
    Malt, Factitious—2629.
    Malt, Genuine—2628.
    Mead, Soluble—2625.
    Orange—2598.
    Peach—2618.
    Peppermint—2611.
    Pineapple—2613.
    Raspberry—2607.
    Red Clover Co.—6.
    Rose—2615.
    Sarsaparilla—5.
    Soap Bark—2627.
    Strawberry—2608.
    Tolu, Soluble—2632.
    Vanilla—2599.
    Vanilla, Cheap—2600.
    Vanilla, From Vanilline—2601.
    Vanilla From Vanilline and Coumarin—2602.
Eye Salves—797-798.
Eyes, Care Of—850.
Eye Water—856-858.
Face Powders—3999-4007.
Faded Photographs—3477.
    Photographs, To Restore—3424.

Failures in Photography—3425.
Feathers, to Clean—2223-2230.
Feed, for Canaries—3509.
    For Mocking birds—3511.
Feet, Tender—516.
Female Pills—1758.
    Tonic—692.
Ferri Peptonate—1798.
Ferric Salicylate, Solution of—1785.
Ferro. Mang. Pepsin—1797.
Fertilizers for Lawns and Flowers—1953-1956.
Fever in Children—525-526, 546-549.
Fig Syrup—726.
Films, To Strip—3426.
Fining For Ale and Porter—1020.
    For Gin—1021.
    For Port—1018.
    For Sherry—1017.
    For Whiskey—1021.
Fixing Bath, Dr. Andresen's—3366-3374.
    Bath, Carbutt's—3427.
Flannels, To Clean—2231-2235.
Flash Light Powder—3241-3242, 3428-3429.
Flatulency, Cure for—652, 655, 656.
Flavor, Pork—2578.
    Sausage, A—2573.
    Sausage, B—2574.
    Sausage, C—2575.
    Sausage, D—2576.
Flavoring For Gin—1016.
Flaxseed Co., Syr. Of—587.
Fleckenwasser—2236-2237.
Floors, To Scour—2238.
Flour, Self Raising—2593.
Fluid, Lightning, For Inhalation—646.
Fly Blister—3522.
Fly Lotion—1937.
Fly Paint—1935.
Fly Paper, Sizing For—1934.
    Paper, Sticky—1933.
Fly Poisons—1895-1898.
Fly Specks, To Remove from Brass—2239.
    To Remove from Bronze—2240.
    To Remove from Gilding—2241.
Foam, For Aerated Waters—952.
    Extract of Soap Bark, For,—2627.
Focus of a Lens, To Find—3430.
Food, Chemical—1851-2604.
    Condition—3482.
    Egg Producing—3486.
    Infants, A—2007.
    Infants, B—2008.
Foot Cream—888.
    Powder—516, 885, 887, 1885.
Foreign Liqueurs, To Make—1025.
Formaldehyde—3376.
Formula of Children's Hospital—567-574.
Formula for Lantern Slides, Dr. Mitchell's—3361.

INDEX.

Formula for Lantern Slides, Dr. Piffard's.—3362.
Formula for Lantern Slides, by Von Gothard—3304.
Formula for Lantern Slides, Warnerke—3363.
Formulae of the N. Y. Hospital—1200-1290.
Formulas for Making Tin-types—3468.
Four Chlorides, Taylor's—2557.
Fothergill's Pills—1282.
Fowler's Solution—1800.
Frames, To Renovate—2242, 2253-2257.
Freckle Remedies—4025, 4026, 4030-4032, 4048.
French Polish, A—2552.
    Polish, B—2553.
Frey's Vermifuge—908.
Frilling in Photographs—3431.
Frost Pictures—3432.
Fruit Juices—2505.
    Preservative—2630.
    Saline—731-734.
    And Wine Stains, To Remove—2243-2248.
Fumigating Paper—3994-3995.
Fumigating Pastilles—3997-3998.
    Pastilles, Insecticide—1940-1941.
    Perfumes—3994-3998.
    Ribbon—3996.
Fungicides—1920-1924.
Furniture, Appearance, To Improve—2249.
    Cream, A—2554.
    Cream, B—2555.
    Paste—2556.
    Polish—2549.
    Polish, French, A—2552.
    Polish, French, B—2553.
    Stains, To Remove—2250.
Furs, To Clean—2251-2252.
Gargles For Throat—461, to 477, 702, 1204.
Geese, Diseases Of, Treatment—3699 to 3704.
    Diarrhoea—3699.
    Gnats and Flies—3700.
    Lice—3701.
    Mortality—3702.
    Pip—3703.
    Swelling Crop—3704.
Gelatine Bromide, Clearing Solution—3290.
General Cleaning Powder—2504.
German Herb Bitters—30.
    Herb Tea—725.
    Oil Lint—746.
Gilding Powder—2520.
Gile's Iodide Ammonia Lint—748.
Gilt Frames, To Clean—2253-2258.
Gin—1022-1023.
    Finings For—1022.
    Flavoring—1016.
Ginger Ale Essence—954-955.
    Ale, Extract for—2623.
    Ale Syrup—2624.
    Beer—960-962.

Ginger Beer Powder—963-964.
Ginger Extract—2619.
    Extract Arom.—2620.
    Extract Arom., Soluble—2622.
    Extract, Soluble—2621.
    Lozenges—1343.
    Wine—942.
Gingeretta—906.
Glace Prints—3434.
Glass Bottles, To Clean—2261-2268.
Glass, Cleaning—2259-2268.
    Invisible Writing On—1943.
    Laboratory, To Clean—2269-2270.
    Substitute Orange—3435.
Glazing Gelatine Prints—3433.
Gleet, Injection For—851.
Gloss, For Starch, A—2507.
    For Starch, B—2508.
Glove, Reviving Cream For—2503.
Gloves, To Clean—2271-2285.
Glue—2006.
    Bank Note—2008.
    Bookbinder's—2009.
    Caseine—2010.
    Compound—2011.
    Cracking, To Prevent—2012.
    For Damp Wood—2013-2014.
    Dressing—2070.
    Dry Pocket—2050.
    Elastic—2015.
    Ether—2016.
    Fire-proof—2017.
    Flower Pots, Cementing Labels on—2018.
    Frozen—2019.
    Glass and Wood Joining—2020.
    Glass Repairing—2021.
    Hardening—2022.
    Hints About—2007-2046.
    Isinglass—2023.
    Ivory and Bone—2024.
    Labels on Iron—2025.
    Labels on Tinned Plate—2026.
    For Leather Goods—2028.
    Leather to Iron—2027.
    Leather, Etc., to Metals—2029.
    Liquid—2030, 2041, 2073, 2074.
    Marine—2042-2045.
    Moisture and Heat to Resist—2047-2048.
    Parchment—2049.
    Portable—2051.
    Rice—2052.
    Spaulding's—2053.
    Standing Moisture—2069.
    Tablets—2054.
    Tungstic—2055.
    Veneering—2056.
    Waterproof—2057, 2061, 2063, 2068, 2077, 2078.
    White—2062.

Glycerine and Honey Jelly—2636.
    Ioduretted—1787.
    Jelly, A—2634.
    Jelly, B—2635.
    Ointment—782.
Glycerites—3205-3220.
Glycerite of Alum, Br.—3205.
    Bismuth, N. F.—3206.
    Borax, U. S. P.—3207.
    Boric and Tannic Acids—3208.
    Boroglycerin, N. F.—3209.
    Carbolic Acid, U. S. P.—3210.
    Creasote—3211.
    Chloroform—3212.
    Gallic Acid, Br.—3214.
    Guaiac, N. F.—3213.
    Lead Subacetate, Br.—3215.
    Pepsin, N. F.—3216.
    Starch—3217.
    Tannin, U. S. P.—3218.
    Tar, N. F.—3219.
    Tragacanth, N. F.—3220.
Glycyrrhizin Syrup—2664.
Goat Diseases, Treatment of—3635-3643.
    Constipation—3635.
    Cough—3636.
    Dropsy—3637.
    Exhaustion—3638.
    Eye Diseases—3639.
    Giddiness—3640.
    Internal Inflammation—3641.
    Red Water—3642.
    Scab or Itch—3643.
Godfrey's Cordial—1834-1836.
Gold Bronze, To Clean—2286.
Gold, Chloride of—3437.
Gold, Cleaning, Dull—2288.
Gold Detergent—2287.
Gold Lace, To Wash—2290.
Gold and Silver, Removing Stains From—2289.
Gonorrhoea Mixtures—508-510, 844-855.
Gout Pills—670.
Gout and Rheumatic Remedies—478-490, 660-675.
Granite, To Remove Stains From—2291-2294.
Granular Effervescent Salts, Base—1296.
    Cheltenham Salts—1302, 1304.
    Citrate of Caffeine—1297.
    Citrate of Magnesia—1298, 1299.
    Hydrobromate of Caffeine—1305.
    Lemon, Kali—1300.
    Pyro. Caffeine—1306.
    Salts—1296-1306.
    Summer Saline—1301.
    Summer Saline, Eno's—1303.
Granular Effervescing Preparations, To Make—1295.
Grass Stains, To Remove—2295.
Grates, Enamel For—2542.

Grates, Enamel, Artistic—2543.
Gravel, Pills For—1752.
Gravity Specific—1840.
Grease Extractor—2314, 2315.
Grease Spots, To Remove—2146.
Green Soap Co., Tincture of—1208.
Gripe, Mixture For—521, 522.
Guano—1953, 1957.
Gutta Percha, To Clean—2317.
Hair Preparations—4089-4100.
    Bismuth Hair Dye—4100.
    Colorer—4096-4099.
    Cream, Cocoa Nut Oil—4089.
    Dye—4094, 4095.
    Oil, Perfume For—4090.
    Renewer—4091.
    Tonic, Jaborandi—4093.
    Tonic, Jaborandi and Quinine—4092.
Halation and Its Prevention—3438.
Hall's Solution of Strychnine—1788.
Hamburg Breast Tea—721.
Hamilton's Tonic Mixture—1251.
Ham Sausage Seasoning—2576.
Handkerchief Extracts, Cheap—3840-3857.
    To prepare—page 445.
Hands, To Cleanse From Silver and Iron Stains—3286.
Harrogate Salts—730.
Hats, To Clean—2318-2322.
Headache Capsules—694.
    Chronic, Pills For—700.
    Mixtures—342-360, 693-697, 700.
    Powder—695-697.
Healing Lotion For Horses—3523.
Healing Ointment—791.
Hektograph Copying Ink—2100.
Hektograph Copying Pad—2099.
Herb Beer Extract—951.
    Bitters, German—30
    Tea, German—725.
Hive Mixture—16.
Hoarhound Candy—621.
Hoffman's Red Drops—1783.
Hog Powders—3489, 3490.
Homeopathic Tinctures—1773.
Home Treatment, Keely Cure—3240.
Honey of Borax, U. S. P.—3221.
    Borax, Br.—3222.
Honey, Medicated—3221-3226.
Honey of Rose, U. S. P.—3224.
    With Borax—3223.
    SalicylicAcid—3225.
    Tannic Acid—3226.
Hop Beer—965.
Hop Bitter Beer—941.
    Bitters—40.
    Stout—948, 949.
Horse Blister—3498.
Horse, Blistering Ointment for—790.

INDEX.

Horse and Cattle Food—3482.
    And Cattle Powders—3480, 3481.
    Colic Draught, A—3515.
    Colic Draught, B—3516.
    Colic Drench—3525.
    Cough Balls—3496.
    Cough Powder, A—3512, 3526.
    Cough Powder, B—3513.
    Diseases of, Treatment—3527-3583.
    Administration of Medicines—3527.
    Apoplexy—3528.
    Ascites—3529.
    Bleymes and Bruises—3530.
    Broken Wind—3541.
    Capped Elbows—3531.
    Capped Hocks—3532.
    Catarrh—3533.
    Cold in Head—3534.
    Corns—3535.
    Coughs—3536-3539.
    Cracked Heels—3542.
    Cystitis—3543.
    Diarrhoea—3544, 3545.
    Dysentery—3546.
    Eczema—3547.
    Enteritis—3548.
    Farcy—3549.
    Fever—3550.
    Founder—3551.
    Glanders—3552, 3553.
    Grease—3554.
    Gripes or Colic—3555.
    Hoof Ointments—3556.
    Influenza—3518.
    Jaundice—3557.
    Liniment, English—3500.
    Liniment, K. K. K.—3499.
    Liniment, Wire Fence—3501.
    Mud Fever—3558.
    Open Joints—3559.
    Ophthalmia—3560.
    Pleurisy—3561.
    Pneumonia—3540, 3562.
    Pole Evil—3563.
    Powder—3493.
    Pulmonary Catarrh—3564.
    Purgatives—3565.
    Pursiness—3566.
    Quinsey—3567.
    Quittor—3568.
    Sandcrack—3569.
    Seedy Toe—3570.
    Sore Shoulders—3571.
    Sores in Mouth—3572.
    Sprain—3573.
    Stomach Staggers—3574.
    Sleepy Staggers—3575.
    Strangles—3576.
    Tetanus or Lockjaw—3577.

Horse and Cattle Thrush—3578.
    Tonics—3579.
    Vives—3580.
    Weed, etc.—3581.
    Worms—3582.
    Wounds, General—3583.
Household Ammonia—1795.
Hydrarg. Colocynth and Ipecac Pills—1289.
Hydrarg. and Iod. Pot. Mixtures—1244-1246.
Hydrangea, Lithiated—1792.
Hydrastis, Colorless—1772.
Hydride of Amyl Liniment—771.
Hydriodic Acid—1293.
Hydrobromic Acid—1292.
    And Hydriodic Acids, Preparation of—1291.
Hydrocyanic Mixture (for Cough)—1235.
Hydromel—3227.
Hypo., To Remove—3439.
    Test For—3440.
Hypodermic Solution Apomorphia Muriate—1273.
    of Carbolized Dist. Water—1268.
    Ext. Ergot—1269.
    Lente's Quinia—1271.
    Magendie's Morphin—1270.
    Pilocarpia Muriate—1272.
Hypophosphites, Syrup of—1261.
Hysteria, Draught For—1864.
Incense For Churches—1890.
Indelible Ink, Black—2101.
    Crimson—2102.
Indian Liniment—749.
Indigestion, Remedies—647-659.
Inebriety, Treatment of—page 326.
Infants' Colic Mixture, Hall's—1831.
    Food, A—2097.
    Food, B—2098.
    Powder—4006.
Inflammatory Earache—1866.
Influenza—594, 622-625.
Influenza in Horses—3518.
Inhalant For Consumption—611.
Injection, Brou—852.
    Gleet—851.
    Gonorrhoea—854.
    Red Wash—853.
Ink, Black Marking—2101.
    Bottles, To Clean—2147.
    Cheap, Blue Black—2104.
    Copying, Aniline—2105.
    Crimson Marking—2102.
    Powder—2106.
    Hektograph, Copying—2100.
    Printing Process—3442.
    Stains, To Remove—2144, 2145, 2324-2335.
    Violet, Stamp—2103.
    For Writing on Photographs—3441.
Insecticide, Nursery—1939.

Insecticide, Pastilles—1929-1932, 3997, 3998.
Insecticides—1899-1932.
Insect Bites, Cure For—1911, 3407.
Insect Powder Patent—1891.
Intensification—3443, 3444.
Invisible Face Powder—4003.
Invisible Writing on Glass—1043.
Iodide of Iron, Ointment—784.
    Solution for Syrup, N. F.—2649.
    Solution for Syrup Br.—2650.
    Syrup, U. S.—2646.
    Syrup, Rapid Method for Making—2648.
    Syrup, Tasteless—2647.
Iodide of Potash Liniment—770.
    Potash Ointment—788.
    Potassium and Hydrarg.—1244-1246.
Iodine, Ointment of—783.
    Tincture, Churchill's—1209.
Iodoform Cylinders—1210.
    Ointment—1220.
    Ointment Co. —1224.
Ioduretted Glycerine—1787.
Iron, Bitter Wine of—20, 71, 72, 1262.
    And Calisaya—53.
    And Cinchona Mixture—1240.
    Pots, To Clean—2441.
    And Quinine—43, 44.
    And Sarsaparilla—25.
Itch Ointments—772-774.
    Remedy—513, 514.
    Salve—786.
Ivory, To Clean—2126-2133.
Jaborandi Hair Tonic—4093.
Jaborandi and Quinine, Hair Tonic—4092.
Jackson's Ammonia Lozenges—1403.
Jackson's Pectoral Lozenges—1404.
Jelly, Arnica—2637.
    Benzine—2502.
    Glycerine, A—2634.
    Glycerine, B—2635.
    Glycerine and Honey—2636.
    Oxide of Zinc—2638.
Jersey Brandy—947.
Jet, To Clean—2349.
Kamnafuga—822.
Keeley Cure, Home Treatment—3240.
Kelly's Tonic Mixture—1249.
Kid Reviving Cream—2503.
Kidney and Blood Tea—723.
Kidney and Liver Cure—710.
Kidney and Liver Medicines—715-725.
Kitchener's Soup Herb Powder—2572.
Knapp's Tonic Mixture—1250.
Knives, To Remove Stains From—2351.
Knot Filler, Patent—2551.
Kola Champagne Essence—956.
    Coca—1882.
    Coca Wine—61.
    Elixir—957.

Kola Wine—1880.
Kreuz, The—724.
Labarraque's Solution—2509.
Lace, To Clean—2352, 2353, 2356, 2357.
    Gold and Silver—2354, 2355.
Lacquers, Not Requiring Heat, A—2521.
    B—2522.
    C—2523.
    D—2524.
LaFayette Mixture—1260.
Lantern Plates, A use for Spoiled—3445.
Lantern Slides, To Color—3478.
Laxative Digestive Powder—658.
Laxative Mixture—131.
Laxative Pills—1278.
Laxatives and Aperients—726-744.
Lead and Opium Pills—1284.
Lead and Opium Wash—1206.
Lead and Zinc Ointment—1226.
Leaf Photographs—3446.
Leather, To Clean—2360.
    Wash (Chamois Skin)—2358.
Lemon Beer—966, 967.
    Extract—2596.
    Extract, Soluble—2597.
    Kali—1300.
    Sherbet—741.
    Squash—953.
    Sugar—2560.
    Syrup, With Acid—2606.
    Syrup, Without Acid—2605.
Lemonade—999.
    For Diabetics—1862.
Lenses, To Clean—2362.
    Removing Rust From—2361.
Light, Safest for Dark Room—3447.
Lightning Eradicator—2222.
    Photographing of—3448.
    Renovator—2442.
Lime, Lyes, Alkalies—2363.
Linctus Infantilus—567.
Linen, Blistering, To Prevent—2364.
    Photographing on—3449.
    To Polish—2366.
    Scorched, Whiteness, To Restore—2365.
Liniments, Arnica—745.
    Arnica, Magic—747.
    For Colic—757.
    Cream of Camphor—750.
    Cyclists Universal—763.
    German Oil—746.
    Horse, English—3500.
    Horse, K. K. K.—3499.
    Horse, Wire Fence—3501.
    Hydride of Amyl—771.
    Iodide of Ammonia—748.
    Indian—749.
    Nerve and Bone—767, 768.
    Neuralgic—765.

INDEX.

Liniment, Red Nose—756.
    Rheumatic—671-673.
    Ringworm—760.
    Roberts'—758.
    Soap and Iodide of Potash—770.
    For Sprains—750.
    Stimulating—1878, 3520.
    Stokes'—761, 762.
    Throat—3519.
    White Oils—754, 755, 766.
    Wizard Oil—769.
Lip Salve, Rose—4080.
Liqueur Alkermes, Italian—1039, 1155.
    Amer. d'Angleterre—1082.
    Amiable Vainqueur—1157.
    Amour Sans Fin—1163.
    Anisette—1100.
    Aqua Bianca—1070.
    Barathier—1188.
    Baume Consolateur—1189.
    Baume des Grecs—1190, 1191.
    Chartreuse—959.
    Chevalier de Saint Louis—1192.
    China-China—1175.
    Christophelet—1093.
    Citronat—1053.
    Citronelle—1159.
    Columbat—1158.
    Coquette Flatteuse—1177.
    Creme des Barbadoes—1121, 1146.
    Creme de Chocolat—1129.
    Creme de Framboises—1141.
    Creme de Macaron—1131.
    Creme de Roses—1130, 1134.
    Creme Romantique—1045.
    Creme Mojon—1069.
    Creme Viozot—1068.
    Curacao—943, 1184.
    D'Amour—1080.
    D'Angelique—1128.
    D'Argent—1097.
    D'Or—1096.
    D'Orange—1126.
    D'Oranges—1098.
    D'Menthe—1127.
    des Abbes—1099.
    des Amis—1138.
    des Anges—1124.
    des Cannelle—1110.
    de Capucins—1114.
    de Celeste—1115.
    des Chevaliers de la Legion d'Honneur—1144.
    de Citron—1136.
    de Cumin—1091, 1109.
    des Dieux—1147.
    des Eveques—1084.
    de Felchmeier—1113.
    de Garus—1149.

Liqueur de Genievre—1185.
    des Grecs—1151.
    de Girofle—1086, 1133.
    de J. Saint Aure—1056.
    de Legitimite 1031.
    de Lisette—1087.
    de Manheim—1112.
    des Muscades—1107.
    des Musetier—1092.
    de Pologne—1125.
    des Princesses—1088.
    de Punch—1090.
    de Romarin—1108.
    de Scubac—1119.
Liqueur Eau Alkermes—1039.
    Americaine—1063.
    Archiepiscopale—1199.
    Carminative—1094.
    Cordiale—1075.
    Cordiale de Caladon—1050.
    Creme Romantique—1045.
    Divine—1058.
    Forcifere—1102.
    Miraculeuse—1074.
    Nuptiale—1041.
    Royale—1061.
    D'Absinthe—1038.
    D'Amour—1042.
    D'Ardelle—1049.
    D'Argent—1054.
    D'Or—1051.
    D'Orient—1072.
    de Baal—1077.
    des Barbadoes—1040.
    de Batave—1037.
    de Chypre—1036.
    de Cote—1035, 1140.
    de Didon—1065.
    des Epicuriens—1066.
    de Fantasie—1033.
    des Favorites—1081.
    des Financiers—1198.
    de Florence—1047.
    de Jacques—1034.
    de Legitimite—1031.
    de Mille Fleurs—1055.
    de Montpellier—1052.
    de Napoleon—1067.
    des Nobles—1029.
    de Paix—1060.
    des Prelats—1080.
    de Princesses—1027.
    de Pucelle—1059.
    de Rebecca—1028.
    de Rosolis de Turin—1048.
    de Sultane Zoralde—1026.
    de Sante—1062.
    de Selia—1073.
    de Sorcier Comte—1044.

INDEX.

Liqueur de Templiers—1032.
    de Tubinge—1046.
    de Vertu—1043.
    de Vie d'Andaye—1130.
    de Vie Danzick—1103, 1107.
    de Yalpa—1057.
    du Dauphin—1064.
Liqueur Elixir Monpon—1071.
    Elixir Vital de Fanchon—1030.
    Espoir des Grecs—1182.
    Gaite Francaise—1162.
    Goutte Nationale—1180.
    Guignolet d'Anges—1174.
Liqueur Huile d'Anis—1142.
    de Jasmin—1193.
    des Jeunes Maries—1194.
    de Rhum—1195.
    de Roses—1143.
    de Vanille—1145.
    de Venus—1118.
    Krambambuli—1076.
    La Felicite—1160.
    Larmes de Missolonghy—1154.
    La Valeureuse—1176.
    Limonade—1085.
    Luft Wasser—1078.
    Marasquin—1122, 1123.
Liqueur Missilimackinac—1156.
    Nectar de La Beaute—1148.
    Nectar des Dieux—1147.
    Nectar des Grecs—1151.
    Nectar du General Foy—1150.
    Persicot—1083, 1111, 1178.
    Plaisir des Dames—1161.
    Ratafia Benzoin—1106.
    Ratafia D'Absinthe—1169.
    Ratafia D'Angelique—1170.
    Ratafia D'Anis et de Carvi—1167-1171.
    Ratafia des Cassis—1168.
    Ratafia de Cerises—1164.
    Ratafia de Celery—1172.
    Ratafia de Noyeau—1165, 1196.
    Ratafia des Quatre Graines—1166.
    Ratafia de Violette—1104.
    dit Escubac—1173-1183.
    Rosolis—1079, 1135, 1153.
    de Turin—1048-1186.
Liqueur Stomachique—1116, 1120, 1132, 1137, 1187.
    Souvenir d'un Brave—1181.
    Usquebaugh—1005.
    Vespetro—1105, 1179.
    Vital—1117.
    Vital de Fanchon—1030.
Liqueurs, Coloring for—1005-1013.
    Foreign—1025-1199.
Liquor, Eastoni—1774.
    Potassa—1796.
    Sedative—1784.

Listerine—829.
Lithia and Potash Powders—1873.
Lithiated Hydrangea—1792.
Liver Disorder, Mixtures for—112-145.
Liver Invigorators—717, 718.
Liver and Kidney Cure—719.
    Mixture—720.
    Pills—140, 141.
    Pills, Little—1763, 1764.
    Syrup with Iron—25.
    Tonics—139-145.
Lobelia Mixture—607.
Lotion, Calamine—1214.
    Evaporating—1213.
    Stimulating—1215.
Lovage—1003.
Lozenge, Aperient—744.
Lozenges, Bath—1345.
    Black Currant—1346.
    Bronchial—1348, 1349.
    Coltsfoot—1345.
    Cough No More—1344.
    Ginger—1343.
    Jackson's Ammonia—1403.
    Jackson's Pectoral—1404.
    To Make—1341-1421.
    Peppermint—1342.
    Pepsin—1407-1410.
    Potassium Chlorate and Cubeb—1411.
    Potassium and Guaiac—1412.
    Practical Suggestions—1341.
    Rose—1347.
    U. S., Br. and London Hospital—1350-1421.
    Wild Cherry—1420.
    Wistar's—1421.
Lumbago, Pills for—1752.
Machinery, To Clean—2367.
    Photographing—3450.
Magic Neuralgic Drops—676.
    Toothache Drops—921.
Magnesia Citrate, Gran.—1298, 1299.
    Citrate, Solution of—1794.
Magnesian Lemonade Pow.—736.
    Orgeat Powder—737.
Mahogany, Spots on—2368.
    Stain—2550.
Malarial, anti, Pills—1768.
Malate of Iron, Solution of—1790.
Malt and Cod Liver Oil—1806.
Malt Extract, Factitious—2629.
    Extract, Genuine—2628.
Maple Beer—968-970.
Marble, To Clean—2371-2382.
    Remove Grease from—2369, 2370.
Marmalade, Scotch—2568.
Matches, To Remove Marks Made by—2383.
Matting, To Clean—2384.
Mayer's Ointment—801.

INDEX.

Mead Extract, Soluble—2625.
Mead Syrup—2626.
Meat Preservative Powder—2559.
Mendelson's Tonic Mixture—1248.
Menthol Pastilles—1757.
Mercurial Ointment—781.
Mercury and Iod. Potassa Oint.—1227.
Mercury, Oleate of—787.
Metal, Lacquers for—2521-2524.
Mexican Extract of Sarsaparilla—24.
Migraine Powder—693.
Mildew, To Prevent—2389-2399.
    Stains, To Remove—2385 to 2388, 2401, 2404.
Milk of Roses—4063, 4064.
Mist, Gonorrhoea—844.
Mixed Spices—2563, 2564.
    Spices for Pickles—2565.
Mixture, Alkaline—1241, 1242.
    Anti-Rheumatic—1259.
    Carminative—1258.
    Chlorate of Potash—1231.
    Chloroform, Cough—1234.
    Copaiba—845.
    Copaiba, Soluble—846.
    Copaiba, Cubebs and Buchu—847.
    For Cough—1233.
    Dioviburnum—59.
    Effervescing—1252, 1253.
    Hamilton's Tonic—1251.
    Hydrarg. and Iod. Potas—1244-1246.
    Hydrocyanic—1235.
    Iodide of Potash and Hoffman's Anodyne—1232.
    Iron and Cinchona—1240.
    Iron and Quinine—60.
    Kelly's Tonic—1249.
    Knapp's Tonic—1250.
    Lafayette—1260.
    For Liver Disorders—112-145.
    Mendelson's Tonic—1248.
    Nitrous Acid—1243.
    Quinine Co.—1257.
    Rhubarb and Soda—1254.
    Rochelle Salts—1255.
    Squills, Dr. Kelly's—1256.
    Sulph. Magnesia and Iron—1237-1239.
    Townsend's—1247.
    Ward, Cough—1236.
Mocking Bird Food—3511.
Molasses Beer—971.
Monocarbonate of Ammonia for Smelling Salts—1888, 1889.
Moonlight Effects in Photographs—3451.
Mounting Prints—3452.
Morphinomania, Cure for—1863.
Mosquito Lotion—4057.
Mosquito Oil—1938.
Moths, Cupboards and Trunks, to Rid of—1928.

Moth Pastilles—1929.
Mucilage, Acacia—2080.
    Stick—2079.
Muriate of Ammonia Wash—1205.
Muslins, To Cleanse—2430.
Negatives—3453.
    Paper—3455.
Nerve and Bone Liniment—767, 768.
Nerve Pills—691.
    Tonic—41, 45, 49, 76 to 84, 688-692.
Nervina—689.
Nervousness, Female, Tonic for—692.
Nervousness, Remedies for—687-692.
Nervo-Valeria—690.
Nets, To Prevent Rotting—2400.
Neuralgic Liniment—765.
    Mixtures—263-341.
    Ointment—803.
    Pills—1754.
    Pills, Brown-Sequard's—1769.
    Powder—683-686.
    Remedies—676-686.
    And Toothache Powder—685, 686.
Neurasthenia, Remedy for—687.
Neutralizing Cordial—1876, 2695.
New York Hospital, Formula of—1200-1290.
Nitrous Acid Mixture, Kelly's—1243.
Nits, Ointment for—793.
Nomenclature—page 404.
North of England Cough Syr.—597.
North of England Sauce—2584.
Noyeau Cordial—904.
    Powder—740.
Numerals—page 404.
Nursery Insecticide—1939.
Nux Vomica Pills—1290.
Obtundent, Dental—1830.
Odontodol, for Toothache—936.
Offensive Breath, Prescription for—1850.
Oil Cloths, To Renovate—2409-2414.
Oil of Cade Co. Ointment—1223.
Oil of Melisse—3895.
Oil for Mosquitos—1938.
Ointment, Barber's Itch—785.
    Blistering Horses, for—790.
    Boils, for—794, 795.
    Brown—1218.
    Carbolic—779.
    Carbolized—1216.
    Chapped Hands—792.
    Chrysophanic Acid—1217.
    Compound Pile—776, 777.
    Creasote—812.
    Eczema—1229, 4065.
    Glycerine—782.
    Grease or Cracked Heels, for—3521.
    Healing—791.
    Indian Cerate—813.

Ointment, Iodide of Iron—784.
    Iodide of Potassium—788.
    Iodine—783.
    Iodoform—1220, 1224.
    Itch—772-774.
    Kraemer's Pile—775.
    Lead and Zinc—1226.
    Mayer's—801.
    Mercurial—781.
    Mercury and Iodide of Potash—1227.
    Neuralgic—803.
    Nits, for—793.
    Oleate of Mercury—787.
    Oil of Cade Co.—1223.
    Peruvian Balsam—1221.
    Salicylic Acid—1219.
    Screw Worm—802.
    Simple—804-806.
    Sulphur—807-808.
    Tannic Acid—1228.
    Tar and Oxide of Zinc—1225.
    White Wax—809-811.
    Witch Hazel—789.
Oleate of Mercury—787.
Old Times Cough Syrup—606.
Opodeldoc Arnica—764.
    Steer's—799.
Orange Bitters—37-38-908.
    Extract, Soluble—2598.
    Wine, 56, 944, 1879.
Oriental Rouge—4007.
Ottawa Beer—972.
Oxide of Zinc Jelly—2638.
Packing Drugs for Export—1841.
Painless Tooth Extraction—930.
Paint Brushes, To Clean—2415, 2416.
    To Clean—2417-2431.
    For Flies—1935.
Paintings, To Clean—2432, 2433.
Palatable Cough Mixture—602, 603.
Paper—3454.
    Negatives—3455.
    Sensitizing—3463.
Papier Mache, To Renovate—2434, 2435.
Paraffin Oil, To Extract From Floors—2436.
Parasiticide—1212.
Parchment, To Clean—2437.
Paregoric—1838.
Parrot Seed—3510.
Paste, Blacking for Shoes—2544.
Paste, Blacking for Stoves—2530-2537.
    Encaustic—3419-3423.
    Furniture—2556.
    Polishing for Brass—2518, 2519, 2325, 2527, 2528.
    Polishing for Windows—1942.
    For Silver Plating—2526.
Pastilles—1929, 3997, 3998.
Peach, Extract of—2618.

Pearls, To Clean—2438.
Pectoral Elixir—590.
Peppermint Cordial—980.
Peppermint, Extract of—2611.
    Lozenges—1342.
Pepsin Ferro. Maug.—1797.
    Lactated—3066.
    Lozenges—1407-1410.
    Mixture for Indigestion—651.
    Wine, A—63.
    Wine, B—64.
Peptonated Iron—1798.
    Iron Solution—1799.
Percentage Solutions—1770.
Perfume for Hair Oil—4090.
Perfumery Extracts—3756A-3886.
    Ardeola Bouquet—3757.
    Bergamot Ext.—3758.
    Bouquet Caroline—3759.
    Bouquet Essence—3760, 3842.
    Bouquet Tip Top—3761.
    Bouquet Bridal Boq., A—3762.
    Bouquet Bridal Boq., B—3763.
    Bouquet D'Amour—3764, 3843.
    Carthage Bouquet—3765.
    Clove Pink—3766, 3845.
    Citronelle Rose, Cheap—3767.
    Crab Apple—3768.
    Cremorne Valley—3769.
    Enchantment Boq.—3770.
    Framlingham Boq.—3771.
    Frangipanni—3772, 3773, 3847.
    Hedyosmia—3774.
    Heliotrope—3775, 3848.
    Honeysuckle—3776.
    Imperial Boq.—3777.
    Jasmin—3778.
    Jess—3779.
    Jockey Club, A—3780, 3849.
    Jockey Club, B—3781.
    Johnny Jump-Up—3782.
    Kensington Boq.—3783.
    Lilac, White or Purple—3784, 3850.
    Lily of Valley—3785.
    Linden Bloom—3786.
    Lucca Bouquet—3787.
    Mary Stuart—3788, 3851.
    May Blossom—3789.
    Mignonette—3790.
    Millefleurs—3791.
    Moss Rose—3792, 3852.
    Musk—3793, 3794, 3854.
    Musk Rose—3795, 3853.
    New Mown Hay, A—3796.
    New Mown Hay, B—3797.
    Night Blooming Cereus—3798.
    Opopanax—3799.
    Orange Flowers—3800.
    Our Own—3801.

INDEX.

Perfumery, Patchouli—3802.
    Pearl of Pekin—3803.
    Perfection—3804.
    Persian Pink—3805.
    Pink—3806.
    Pond Lily—3809.
    Prairie Blossom—3808.
    Rondeletia—3809.
    Rose—3810.
    Rose of Cashmere—3811.
    Rose Geranium—3812.
    Sandalwood—3813.
    Spring Flowers—3814.
    Spring Posey—3815.
    Sweet Brier—3816.
    Sweet Clover—3817.
    Sweetheart's Garland—3818.
    Sweet Pea—3819.
    Sweet Pink—3820.
    Sweet Shrub—3821.
    Tea Rose—3822, 3855.
    Tuberose, A—3823.
    Tuberose, B—3824.
    Union Bouquet—3825.
    Upper Ten—3826.
    Vandeventer Boq.—3827.
    Venetian Lily—3828.
    Violet—3829.
    West End—3830.
    White Lily—3831.
    White Rose—3832, 3856.
    Woodbine—3833.
    Wood Violet—3834.
    Ylang Ylang—3835, 3857.
Perfumery Tinctures—3858-3886.
    From Pomade—3858.
    Ambergris—3859.
    Ambrette Seeds—3860.
    Angelica—3861.
    Benzoin—3862.
    Civet—3863.
    Cloves—3864.
    Coumarin—3865.
    Curcuma—3866.
    Heliotrope—3867.
    Ionone—3868.
    Musc Baur—3869.
    Musk—3870.
    Neroli Big—3871.
    Neroli Petale—3872.
    Neroli Portugal—3873.
    Nutmegs—3874.
    Orris—3875, 3876.
    Red Saunders—3877.
    Rose Geranium—3878.
    Sandalwood—3879.
    Styrax—3880.
    Tolu—3881.
    Tonka—3882.

Perfumery Tinctures, Vanilla—3883.
    Vanillin—3884.
    Verbena—3885.
    Vetivert—3886.
Perfumes, Cheap—3840-3857.
    Extract Alpine Bouquet—3840.
    Bordentown Bouquet—3841.
    Brighton Nosegay—3844.
    Clove Pink—3845.
    Everlasting Boq.—3845.
    Frangipanni—3847.
    Heliotrope—3848.
    Jockey Club—3849.
    Lilac, White or Purple—3850.
    Mary Stuart—3851.
    Moss Rose—3852.
    Musk Rose—3853.
    Musk, Cheap—3854.
    Tea Rose—3855.
    White Rose—3856.
    Ylang Ylang—3857.
Perfumes, Frozen or Solid—3836-3839.
    Bouquet—3838.
    Cologne—3839.
    Lavender—3837.
    White Rose—3836.
Peruvian Balsam Ointment—1221.
    Beer, Carbonated—073.
Petroleum Emulsion—1815, 1817, 1818.
Phantom Face Powder—4004.
Phenacetine in Rheumatism—674.
Phosphate Acid Solution—988.
Phosphorus Butter—1816.
    Pills—1766-1767.
    Rat Paste—1936.
Photo Chromos—3456.
Photographic Dark Room, Windows—3436.
    Prints, Colored—3476.
    Trade, How to do—3240A-3263.
Photographing of Lightning—3448.
    On Linen—3449.
    Of Machinery—3450.
    On Wood—3479.
Photographs, Faded—3477.
    Faded, To Restore—3424.
Photography—3264-3479.
    Accelerator—3475.
Photo Prints, Enameling—3418.
Pickle, Spice for—2565.
Pigs, Diseases of, Treatment—3654-3684.
    Apoplexy—3657.
    Bleeding—3655.
    Cold—3658.
    Constipation—3659.
    Cough—3660.
    Diarrhoea—3661.
    Dropsy—3662.
    Epilepsy—3663.
    Eye Diseases—3664.

Pigs, General—3654.
    Gripes—3665.
    Hipshot—3666.
    Inflammation of Brain—3667.
    Inflammation of Lungs—3668.
    Loss of Tail—3669.
    Madness—3670.
    Maggots in Ear—3671.
    Measles—3672.
    Pocks—3673.
    Powders—3494.
    Quinsey—3674.
    Running Fire—3675.
    Scab—3676.
    Snuffles, Sniffles, Nasal Catarrh—3677.
    Spleen—3679.
    Splenitis—3678.
    Sprains, Sores—3680.
    Stye—3681.
    Swine Fever—3682.
    Vomiting—3683.
    Worms—3684.
Pigeons, Diseases of, Treatment—3705-3718.
    Canker—3710.
    Feather Lice—3709.
    Lice—3706.
    Mites—3707.
    Moulting—3711.
    Parasites—3705.
    Pouters—3712.
    Roup—3713.
    Scouring—3714.
    Scrofula—3715.
    Sore Eyes—3716.
    Ticks—3708.
    Vertigo—3717.
    Wasting—3718.
Pile Ointments—775-777, 814-817.
    Suppositories—818-821.
Pills, Antibilious—1749.
    Antimalarial—1768.
    Arsenical—1751.
    Chill—1765.
    Chronic Constipation—1750.
    Creasote—704, 706.
    Digestive—1753.
    Dog—3504.
    Gravel and Lumbago—1752.
    Female—1758.
    Little Liver—1763, 1764.
    Menthol—1757.
    Neuralgic—1754.
    Neuralgic, Brown Sequard's—1769.
    N. Y. Hospital F.—1277-1290.
    Phosphorus—1767.
    Phosphorus, Martindale's—1766.
        For Pruritus Ani—1759, 1760.
    Roback's—1747.
    Sir Andrew Clark's—1748.

Pills, For Spermatorrhoea—1755.
    For Toothache—1756.
Pimples—889-891.
Pine Apple, Extract of—2613.
Pinholes, To Prevent—3457.
Piso's Consumption Cure—613.
Plate Glass, To Clean—2260.
Pleasant Cough Syrup—604.
Plush, To Renovate—2440.
Polish, Brown Shoe, A—2546.
    Brown Shoe, B—2547.
Podophyllin Pills—1279.
Polish, Furniture—2549.
    Furniture, French, A—2552.
    Furniture, B—2553.
    Liquid, Shoe—2548.
    Paste, Brown—2545.
    Stain Removing—2250.
Polishing Paste for Brass—2518, 2519, 2525, 2527, 2528.
    Paste for Silver—2526.
Pomade—Dandruff—4077.
    Scurf—4078.
    Stick—4084-4088.
    Stick, Coudray—4083.
Pork Flavor—2578.
Porous Plasters—1852.
Portraiture, Formula for—3360.
Position of Sun—3467.
Potassa Liquor—1706.
Potassium, Chlorate and Cubeb Lozenges—1411.
    Chlorate and Guaiac—1412.
Pots, Iron, To Clean—2441.
Poultry, Diseases of, Treatment—3685-3698.
    Apoplexy—3685.
    Baldness and White Comb—3686.
    Catarrh and Roup—3687.
    Consumption—3692.
    Crop-bound—3688.
    Diarrhoea—3693.
    Douglass Mixture—3689.
    Epilepsy—3694.
    Leg Weakness—3690.
    Lice—3695.
    Mortality—3696.
    Pip—3697.
    Powder—3485.
    Spice—3508.
    Vertigo—3691.
    Worms on Head—3698.
Powder Alterative—3720.
    Aperient for Horses—3488.
    Baby—907, 1222, 1853, 1858.
    Baking Alum, 1 Spoon—2586.
        Alum, 2 Spoon—2587.
        Cream of Tartar—2590.
        General Directions—2594.
        Phosphate, 1 Spoon—2588.

INDEX.

Powder, Baking, Phosphate, 2 Spoon—2589.
    Quick Rising—2591.
    Salt Rising—2592.
    Cattle Fattening—3502.
    Constipation, for Cattle—3491.
    Curry—2562.
    Custard—2561.
    Effervescent—736-742.
    Errhine—1263.
    For General Cleaning—2504.
    Gilding—2520.
    Hog—3489, 3490.
    Horse—3493.
    Lithia and Potash—1873.
    Meat Preservative—2550.
    Miscellaneous—1274-1276.
    Pig—3494.
    Retouching—3462.
    Sweet Seidlitz—1874.
    Teething—561-564, 806, 900-905.
    Tonic for Pigs and Horses—3492.
    Washing—2495-2501.
    Whooping Cough—907.
    Worm—572.
    For Horses—3487.
Prefixes, Chemical—page 405.
Preservative for Fruit—2630.
    For Vegetables—2631.
Preston Salts—1887.
Prevention of Halation—3438.
Primuline Process—3458.
Printing Processes, Photography—3459.
    On Silk, Photo—3465.
Prints—3460.
    Glace—3434.
    Glazing Gelatine—3433.
    Mounting—3452.
Proper Time to Give Medicine—1877.
Pruritus Ani—1759-1762.
Punch—958.
Purgative Effervescing Salt—720.
    Sarsaparilla—22.
    Tablets—728.
Purifiers, Blood—1-25.
Pyro Caffeine Comp—1306.
Quinia Mixture Co.—1257.
Quinine, Baby, A—711.
    Baby, B—712.
    And Iron Mixture—60.
    And Jaborandi Hair Tonic—4092.
    Tasteless Syrup of, 2 gr.—2644.
    Tasteless Syrup of, 5 gr.—2645.
Rabbits, Diseases of, Treatment—3724-3728.
    Liver Complaint—3724.
    Pot Belly Dropsy—3725.
    Red Water—3726.
    Rot—3727.
    Snuffles—3728.
Raspberry Cordial—995.

Raspberry, Extract of—2607.
    Vinegar—946.
    Wine Essence—950.
Raspberryade Powder—738.
Rat Poison—1932.
    Arsenic—1893.
    Phosphorus Paste—1936.
Red Clover, Ext. of—6.
Red Drops, Hoffman's—1783.
Red Nose Liniment—756.
Red Wash Injection—853-1203.
Remedy for Veterinary Purposes—3524.
Removal of Stains and Grease Spots—2449.
Renovator, Blood—48.
Retouching Powder—3462.
Rheumatic and Gout Cure, Thomas'—660.
    And Gout Remedies—478-490, 660-675.
    Liniment—671-673.
    Liniment, Stokes'—762.
    Mixture—1259.
    Mixture, Sir Andrew Clark—664.
    Pills—669.
    Powder—668.
Rhubarb and Soda Mixture—1254.
    And Soda Pills—1280.
    Wine of—73.
Ringworm—511, 512, 703, 760.
Roback's Bitters—31.
    Pills—1747.
Roberts' Ready Relief—758.
Rochelle Salts Mixture—1255.
Rock Candy, Horehound and Tolu—580.
Root Beer—974-977.
    Beer Extract—987.
Ropes, Preservation of—2402.
    To Prevent Rotting—2403.
Rose, Extract of Flavoring—2615.
Rose Eye Water—856.
    Face Powder—4002.
    Lozenges—1347.
Rugs, To Clean—2443.
Rum, To Improve—1024.
    Shrub—991.
Rust, Black Ink, To Remove—2445.
    Spots, To Remove—2444.
Saccharin Solution—1775, 1776.
Sachet—3951, 3952.
    Powder—3939-3993.
    Or Solid Perfumes—3939.
    Acacia or Cassie—3953.
    Bouquet de Caroline—3954.
    Chypre—3955.
    Ess. Bouquet—3956-3958.
    Frangipanni—3959-3961.
    Heliotrope—3962-3964.
    Jockey Club—3965-3967.
    Lavender—3968, 3969.
    Lign Aloe—3970.
    Marechale—3971.

Sachet Millefleurs—3972, 3973.
    Mousseláine—3974.
    Musk—3975, 3976.
    New Mown Hay—3977, 3978.
    Opoponax—3979.
    Patchouli—3980.
    Pot-pourri—3940-3950.
    Red Rose—3985.
    Rondeletia—3981.
    Rose—3983.
    Rose Geranium—3982.
    Sweet Briar—3986.
    Verbena—3987, 3988.
    Violet—3989, 3990.
    West End—3991.
    White Rose—3984.
    Ylang Ylang—3992, 3993.
Safest Light for Dark Room—3447.
Saffron, Syrup of, A—2641.
    Syrup of, B—2642.
Sage's Catarrh Snuff—643.
Saint Germain Laxative Tea—722.
Salicylic Acid Ointment—1219.
    Preservative Powder—2558.
    Mixture for Rheumatism—665.
    Solution for Preserving Fruit—2630.
Saline, Eno's—1303.
    Fruit—731-734.
    Summer—1301.
Sal Rochelle Mixture—1255.
Salt, Brown Gravy—2571.
    Celery—2570.
    Effervescent Purgative—729.
    Harrogate—730.
    Preston—1887.
Salves, Arnica—778.
    Boracic Acid—780.
    Carbolic—779.
    Eye—797, 798.
    Stick—796.
Santal with Cubeb and Buchu—848.
    Wood, Emulsion of—855.
Santonine Comp. Powder—572.
    Lozenges, 1362, 1363.
Sarsaparilla, Ayer's—1860.
    Beef and Celery—23.
    Extract—5.
    Extract, Mexican—24.
    Purgative—22.
    Syrup of—1, 2, 3, 8.
Satins, To Clean—2446, 2447.
Sauce, Barsaloux—2585.
    Croft's—2579.
    Delmonico—2580.
    Digestive Relish—2581.
    East India—2582.
    North of England—2584.
    Yorkshire Relish—2583.
Sausage Flavor, A—2573.

Sausage Flavor, B—2574.
    Flavor, C—2575.
    Flavor, D—2576.
Savory Spices—2577.
Sciatica Mixture—675.
Scotch Marmalade—2568.
Scouring Balls—2116, 2117.
    Bricks—2452.
    Liquid—2448-2450.
Screw Worm Ointment—802.
Sea Foam—4069.
Seasoning, Ham Sausage—2576.
Seasoning, Universal—2569.
Sea Sickness, Remedy for—1809.
Sedative Cough Syrup—615.
    Liquor—1784.
Seidlitz Powders, Caffeine—1875.
    Sweet—1874.
Self Raising Flour—2593.
Samson's Bitters—33.
Seed for Parrots—3510.
Senna Cough Mixture—1264.
Sensitizing Paper—3463.
    Solution, Monkhoven's—3464.
Shampoo, Dry—4070.
    Liquid—4071-4076.
Shaving Cream—4082.
Shawls, To Clean—2453.
Sheep, Diseases of, Treatment—3617-3634.
    Consumption—3617.
    Cough—3618.
    Diarrhoea—3619.
    Foot Rot—3620.
    Giddiness—3621.
    Hog Pock—3622.
    Hoven—3623.
    Inflammation of Brain—3624.
    Jaundice—3625.
    Lice—3626.
    Red-water—3627.
    Rot—3628.
    Scab—3629.
    Small-pox—3630.
    Swollen Udder—3631.
    Wens or Tumors—3632.
    Wild Fire or Sore Lips—3633.
    Worms—3634.
Sherbet, Lemon—741.
Shiloh's Consumption Cure—612.
Shirts, Laundrying of—2454-2458.
Shoe Blacking—2544.
    Blacking, Liquid Black—2548.
Shoe Polish, Brown, A—2546.
    Polish, Brown, B—2547.
Shoes, To Clean, Kid—2459.
    To Clean, White Satin—2460.
Show Bottle Colors—1886.
Show Windows, To Clean—2461.
Shrub, Rum—991.

INDEX.

Silk Cleaner—2462-2466.
    Photo, Printing on—3465.
Silver Bromide Emulsion—3279.
Silver, To Clean—2467-2478.
    Nitrate, To Make—3466.
    Nitrate, Stains, To Remove—2480-2485.
    Wastes, To Recover—3473.
Silverine, Solution for—2517, 2529.
Simple Ointments—804-806.
    Syrup—2639.
Sir Andrew Clark's Pills—1748.
Sizing for Fly Paper—1934.
Skeletons, To Prepare and Bleach—2479.
Sleeplessness, Mixture for—515.
Smelling Salts—1887-1889.
Snuff, Antiseptic—1850.
Soap Bark, Extract for Foam—2627.
    Liniment—770.
    For Removing Stains—2486.
Soap and Soap Making—2510.
Soda Powder—742.
    And Rhubarb Mixture—1254.
    Solution, Labarraques—2509.
Solidified Copaiba—849.
Solution of Acid Phosphates, N. F.—988, 2820.
    Acetate of Ammonium—1266, 1267, 2823.
    Acetate of Ammonium, Strong—2824.
    Aloes and Soda—2821.
    Antiseptic—1200.
    Arsenious Acid—2822.
    Bismuth, Citrate and Ammon.—2825.
    Bromides Co.—1791.
    Citrate of Magnesia—2826, 2827.
    Cocaine, 4 per cent.—1793.
    Dieterich's Peptonated Iron—1799.
    Donovan's—1801, 2837.
    Ferric Salicylate—1785.
    Four Chlorides—2828.
    Fowler's—1800.
    Hydrastis, Colorless—2829.
    Hypodermic—1268-1273.
    Iod. of Iron, Br.—2650.
    Iod. of Iron, N. F.—2649.
    Iodine Co.—2834.
    Iron Acetate—2830.
    Iron Chloride, U. S.—2831.
    Iron Citrate, U. S.—2832.
    Iron Perchloride—2833.
    Lead, Sub-acetate, U. S.—2841.
    Lime—2835.
    Lime, Chlorinated, Br.—2836.
    Magnesia Citrate—1794.
    Malate of Iron—1790.
    Mercury and Arsenic Iodides—2837.
    Morphine Acetate, Br.—2838.
    Morphine Hydrochlorate, Br.—2839.
    Pepsin, U. S.—2840.
    Potash, Br.—2842.
    Potash, U. S. P.—2843.
    Potassium Arsenite—2844.

Solution of Saccharin—1775, 1776.
    Salicylic Acid for Fruit Preserving—2630.
    For Silvering—2517.
    Soda, U. S.—2845.
    Soda, Arseniate—2847.
    Soda, Chlorinated—2846.
    For Storm Glass—1789.
    Strychnia—1788.
Solutions, Percentage Table for—1770.
Soothing Powder, Children's—903, 904.
    Powder for Children, when Relaxed—905.
    Syrup, 517-520, 565, 892-899.
    Syrup, with Morphine—893.
    Syrup, Non-poisonous—894, 897, 903.
    Syrup, without Opium—892.
Sore Throat Mixture—469-477.
Soup Herb Powder, Kitchener's—2572.
Spavin Cure—3503.
Specific Gravity—1840.
Spermaceti Ointment—811.
Spermatorrhoea Pills—1755.
Spices, Mixed—2563, 2564.
    For Pickle—2565.
    Savory, 2577.
Spirit Beading—1015.
Spiritus Acidi Formici, N. F.—2848.
    Amygdalae Amarae—2849.
    Aromaticus, N. F.—2850.
    Aurantii Co., N. F.—2851.
    Cardamomi Co., N. F.—2852.
    Curassao, N. F.—2853.
    Glonoini—2854.
    Olei Volatilis, N. F.—2855.
    Ophthalmicus, N. F.—2856.
    Phosphori, N. F.—2857.
    Saponatus, N. F.—2858.
    Sinapis, N. F.—2859.
Sponges, To Clean—2487.
Spots and Stains, To Remove—2488.
Sprains, Liniment for—759.
Spray, Bergoline Oil—640.
    Carbolic—1201.
Spring Blood Renovator—48.
Spruce Beer—978-983.
    Beer, White—984.
Squill Mixture Co.—1256.
Squills, Syrup—2640.
Stain, Mahogany—2550.
Stains and Grease Spots, To Remove—2440.
    To Remove—2323-2335, 2405-2408.
    Soap for Removing—2486.
Standard Cough Syrup—576.
Starch, Gloss for—2507, 2508.
Steer's Opodeldoc—799.
Stick Salve—796.
Sticky Fly Paper—1933.
Stimulating Liniment—1878.
    Lotion—1215.
Stokes' Liniments—761, 762.

INDEX.

Stomachic Mixture—570.
    Powder—659.
Storm Glass, Solution for—1789.
Stoughton Bitters—35.
Stove, Artistic Enamel for—2543.
    Blacking—2530-2536.
    Paste—2542.
Straw, To Clean and finish—2134-2136.
Strawberry, Extract of—2608.
Strychnine, Solution of, Hall's—1788.
Styptic Colloid—1786.
Sugar, Lemon—2560.
    Vanilla—2603.
Sulphate of Magnesia and Iron Mixtures—1237-1239.
Sulpho Saline with Iron—735.
Sulpho Saline Salt—735.
Sun Cholera Mixture—842.
Suppositories—818-821, 1265.
Sweet Seidlitz Powders—1874.
Syrup of Acacia Gum—2651.
    Allii—2652.
    Apormorphine Hyd.—2653.
    Asafetida—2654.
    Aurantii—2655.
    Blackberry, N. F.—2656.
    For Blood and Liver—25.
    Buckhorn Bark—2657.
    Calcium Lactophosphate—2658.
    Calcium Phosphate—2660.
    Calcium Phosphate, Wiegand's—2659.
    Cascara—2661.
    Castanea—2662.
    Chloral Hydrate, Br.—2663.
    Dover's Powder—2693.
    Figs—726.
    Ginger Ale—2624.
    Glycyrrhizin—2664.
    Hypophosphite of Calcium, N. F.—2669.
    Hypophosphites of Calcium, Manganese Potassium—2670.
    Hypophosphite of Calcium and Soda—2671.
    Hypophosphites, U. S., Churchill's—2665.
    Hypophosphites Co., N. F.—1261, 2666.
    Hypophosphites Co., with Iron, Nonprecipitating—2668.
    Hypophosphite with Iron—2672.
    Hypophosphite of Iron, N. F.—2673.
    Hypophosphite of Manganese, N. F.—2674.
    Hypophosphites, Parrish's—2667.
    Hypophosphites of Sodium, N. F.—2675.
    Iodide of Iron—2646-2648.
    Iodide of Iron, Rapid Method for—2648.
    Iodide of Iron, Solution for, Br.—2650.
    Iodide of Iron, Solution for, N. F.—2649.
    Iodide of Iron, Tasteless—2647.
    Iodide of Iron and Ammonium Phosphate—2679.

Syrup of Iodide of Iron and Ammonium Tartrate. Codex—2680.
    Iron Citrate Codex—2683.
    Iron Ferric Chloride Codex—2677.
    Iron Ferric Chloride, B—2678.
    Iron and Potassium Tartrate Codex—2681.
    Iron Pyrophosphate Codex—2685.
    Iron and Quinine Iodides, A—2682.
    Iron and Quinine Iodides, B—2684.
    Iron and Sodium Albuminate—2676.
    Lemon with Acid—2606.
    Lemon, without Acid—2605.
    Lobelia, Eclectic—2686.
    Lobelia, Thompsonian—2687.
    Manganese Iodide—2688.
    Manganese Phosphate—2689.
    Mead—2626.
    Mercury, Iodide, Gibert's—2690.
    Mitchella Co., Eclectic—2691.
    Opiated Codex—2692.
    Opium and Ipecac, N. F.—2693.
    Phosphates Co.—2694.
    Quinine, Tasteless, 2 Gr.—2644.
    Quinine, Tasteless, 5 Gr.—2645.
    Rhubarb, Arom.—2697.
    And Potassium—2695.
    Saccharin—2698.
    Saffron—2641, 2642.
    Sarsaparilla—1, 2, 3, 8.
    Senna with Manna—2699.
    Simple—2639.
    Squills—2640.
    Squills Co.—2700.
    Tar, U. S.—2643.
    Tolu—2633, 2696.
    Trifolium—7.
    Vanilla—2604.
    Violets—2701.
    White Pine—583, 584.
    Wild Cherry—2702.
    Yerba Santa, Arom., N. F.—2703.
Table, Ackland's—page 365.
    Alkaline Carbonates in Developers—page 364.
    Beer—985.
    Burton's—page 366.
    For Diluting Alcohol or Cologne Spirits—4115.
    of Latin Terms Used in Prescriptions—page 392.
Tablets, Compressed—1422-1507.
    To make—1307, 1308.
    Materials to Prepare—1309-1339.
Tablet Triturates—1508-1746.
    Triturates, To Make—1340.
    Purgative—728.
Tallow, To Bleach—2494.
Tannic Acid Ointment—1228.
Tapeworm Emulsion—920.
Taraxacum Mixture—743.

INDEX. 511

Tar and Oxide of Zinc Ointment—1225.
Tar Syrup—2643.
    Water, Alkaline—1207.
    Tolu and Wild Cherry—581.
    and Wild Cherry—582.
Tasteless Chill Powder—714.
    Chill Tonic—713.
    Cod Liver Oil—1819.
    Quinine Syr., 2 Gr.—2644.
    Quinine Syr., 5 Gr.—2645.
    Worm Powder—916.
Taylor's Solution of 4 Chlorides—2557.
Teas, Medicinal—721-725.
Teething Powders—561-564, 896, 900-904.
Terminations—page 406.
Thielman's Cholera Drops—841.
Thomas' Rheumatic and Gout Cure—660.
Thread-worms—527, 528.
Throat Liniment—3519.
Thrush in Children—523.
Tincture of Aconite Root—2704.
    Aloes, U. S.—2705.
    Aloes and Myrrh—2706.
    Arnica Flowers—2707.
    Arnica Root—2708.
    Asafetida Co.—2709.
    Avena Sativa—2710.
    Aurantii Amara—2711.
    Aurantii Dulcis—2712.
    Belladonna—2713.
    Benzoin—2714.
    Benzoin Co.—2715.
    Black Cohosh Co.—2716.
    Bloodroot Co., Eclectic—2717.
    Blue Cohosh—2718.
    Blue Cohosh Co.—2719.
    Blue Flag—2720.
    Buchu—2721.
    Burdock Seed—2722.
    Bryony—2723.
    Cacao—2724.
    Cactus, Grand—2725.
    Calamus—2726.
    Calendula—2727.
    Calumba—2728.
    Cannabis Indica—2729.
    Capsicum—2730.
    Cardamom Co.—2731.
    Carduus Mariana—2732.
    Carminative, Br.—2733.
    Cascara Sagrada Codex—2734.
    Castor—2735.
    Castor Ammoniated—2736.
    Catechu—2737.
    Celandine, Rademacher's—2738.
    Chloroform Co., Br.—2739.
    Cimicifuga—2740.
    Cinnamon Co.—2741.
    Cochineal, Br.—2742.

Tincture of Cochineal, Rademacher's—2743.
    Colchicum Co., Eclectic—2744.
    Colchicum—2745.
    Colocynth, Ger. Phar.—2746.
    Colocynth Seed, Rademacher's—2747.
    Conium, U. S. P.—2748.
    Convallaria, Brit.—2749.
    Copper Acetate, A—2750.
    Copper Acetate, B—2751.
    Corydalis, Eclectic—2752.
    Cubeb—2753.
    Culver's Root.—2754.
    Digitalis, Ethereal—2755.
    Ergot, Br. Phar.—2756.
    Eucalyptus—2757.
    Gelsemium—2758.
    Gentian—2759.
    Gentian Co.—2760.
    Ginger, U. S. P.—2761.
    Golden Seal Co., Eclectic—2762.
    Green Soap Co.—1208.
    Henbane—2763.
    Hips, Rademacher's—2764.
    Iodine—2765.
    Iodine, Churchill's—1209.
    Iodine Co.—2766.
    Iron Co.—2767.
    Iron—2768.
    Iron Acetate, A—2769.
    Iron Acetate, B—2771.
    Iron Chloride—2770.
    Jaborandi, Br.—2772.
    Kalmia—2773.
    Kino—2774.
    Lobelia Co., Eclectic—2775.
    Lobelia and Capsicum Co.—2776.
    Lupulin—2777.
    Myrrh—2778.
    Opium Ammon—2779.
    Opium Camphd.—2780.
    Opium Camphd, U. S.—2781.
    Opium and Saffron—2789.
    Poke Root Co.—2782.
    Poke Root, Eclectic—2794.
    Prickly Ash Berries, Eclectic—2783.
    Pulsatilla—2784.
    Quinine, Br.—2785.
    Quinine, Ammoniated—2786.
    Rhubarb, Arom.—2787.
    Phosphorus Co., Br.—2790.
    Poison Oak—2791.
    Podophyllum, Eclectic—2792.
    Quillaia—2793.
    Rhubarb, Sweet—2788.
    Rhubarb Co., Eclectic—2795.
    Rhubarb, Kohlrenter's—2796.
    Saffron—2797.
    Savin, Br.—2798.
    Savin Co., Eclectic—2799.

Tincture of Senna Co., Eclectic—2800.
 Serpentaria Co., Eclectic—2801.
 Shepherd's Purse, Rademacher's—2802.
 Skunk Cabbage, Eclectic—2803.
 Stavesacre, Eclectic—2804.
 Stillingia, Eclectic—2805.
 Strychnine, British—2806.
 Strychnine Co., Eclectic—2807.
 Sulphur, Hager—2808.
 Sulphur, Homeopathic—2809.
 Tolu, U. S. P.—2810.
 Vanilla—2811.
 Valerian Ethersol, Ger.—2812.
 Veratrum Viride—2813.
 Viburnum Co.—2814.
 Wahoo, Br.—2815.
 Warburg's, Modified—2816.
 Witch Hazel Bark, Br.—2817.
 Wormwood, Ger.—2818.
 Wormwood Co.—2819.
Tinctures, Homeopathic—1773.
Tintypes, Developer for—3416.
 Formula for Making—3468.
Toilet Lotions—4035-4062.
 Acetic—4035.
 Acetic Acid—4037.
 Acetate of Lead—4036.
 Alum—4038.
 Arsenical Cosmetic—4039-4041.
 Bichloride of Mercury—4042.
 Borax—4043, 4044.
 Cherry Laurel—4045.
 Chlorate of Potash—4046.
 Face—4047.
 Glycerine—4049-4051-4055.
 Gowland's—4052.
 Horse Radish—4053.
 Iodide of Potash—4054.
 Lemon Juice—4056.
 Sulphuretted—4058-4060.
 Sun Burn—4061, 4062.
Toilet Preparations—3990-4034.
 Vinegars—3937, 3938.
Toilet Waters—3919-3932.
 Florida, A—3919.
 B—3920.
 Mixture, A—3921.
 B—3922.
 Lavender—3923-3926.
 Lilac—3927.
 Melisse—3928.
 Verbena—3929.
 Violet, A—3930.
  B—3931.
  C—3932.
Tolu Extract, Soluble—2632.
 Syrup of—2633.
Tomato Catsup, A—2566.
 B—2567.

Tonic, Acid Mixture—50.
 Acidulous—104, 105.
 Alkaline—106-108.
 Alkaline Mixture—51, 52.
 Alterative—1884.
 Aromatic Bitters—46.
 Beer—986.
 Blood Mixture—47.
 Calisaya—42, 53, 1870.
 General Ferruginous—75-84, 109-111.
 Hop—40.
 Iron Bitters—26-29, 34, 43, 44.
 Iron and Quinine—43, 44.
 Laxative—85-90.
 Nerve—41, 688-692.
 For Nervous Debility—45, 49.
 Pick Me Ups—91-103.
 Powder for Pigs and Horses—3492.
Toning Baths—3469, 3470.
Toothache Anodyne—925.
 Ball and Stopping—934.
 Balsam—924.
 Cordial, Roback's—939.
 Drops—927.
 Essence—937, 938.
 Extraction, Painless—930.
 Gum—929.
 Odontodol—936.
 Paint—926.
 Pills—1756.
 Remedies—921-939.
 Tincture—928, 931-933, 935.
Tooth Paste, Charcoal—4103.
 Cherry—4101.
 Rose—4102.
Tooth Powder, Carbolic—4107.
 Fragrant—4104.
 Quinine—4106.
 Saponaceous—4105.
Tooth Wash, Antiseptic—4108.
 Fragrant—4109.
 Saponaceous—4108.
Townsend's Mixture—1247.
Trays and Graduates, To Clean—3472.
 To Make—3471.
Trifolium, Syrup of—7.
Triplex Pills—1277.
Triturates, Tablet—1508-1746.
Turkey, Diseases of, Treatment—3692-3698.
 Consumption—3692.
 Diarrhoea—3693.
 Epilepsy—3694.
 Lice—3695.
 Mortality—3696.
 Pip—3697.
 Worms on Head—3698.
Universal Seasoning—2569.
Usquebaugh Cordial—1004.
Vance's Chilblain Cream—872.

Vanilla Extract—2599.
  Cheap—2600.
  From Coumarin and Vanilline—2602.
  From Vanilline—2601.
Vanilla Sugar—2603.
  Syrup—2604.
Vegetable Cough Syrup—585.
  Preservative—2631.
Vermifuges—908-920.
  Frey's—908.
  Oil, Old Style—908.
Vermin Killer—1932.
Veterinary Formulae—3729-3756.
  Alterative Powder—3729.
  Blister—3730-3732.
  Bran Mash—3749.
  Calves' Cordial—3734.
  Cleansing Drench—3735.
  Condition Powders—3480, 3481, 3736, 3737
  Cough Balls—3738, 3739.
  Diapente—3740.
  Diuretic Mass—3741.
  Embrocation, Elliman's—3742.
  Eye Lotion—3743.
  Fever Balls—3444, 3445.
  Gripe Drench—3746.
  Liquid Blister—3733.
  Lotion for Cracked Hoofs—3747.
  Mange Liniment—3748.
  Oatmeal Gruel—3750.
  Ointment for Grease—3751.
  Ointment for Horses' Knees—3752.
  Physic Mass—3753.
  Treatment for Distemper—3754.
  White Oils—3755.
  Wound Stone—3756.
Veterinary Remedies—3480-3526.
  Treatise—3526A-3728.
Viburnum Compound—58.
Vin Mariani—62.
Violet Face Powder—4001.
Walton's Bitters—32.
Ward Cough Mixture—1236.
  Gargle—1204.
  Powders—1274-1276.
Warnerke's Formula for Copying Line Drawings and Engravings—3363.
Wart and Corn Eradicator—884.
Wart Powder—4113.
  Remover—4112.
Wash Bluing—2512-2516.
  Lead and Opium—1206.
  Muriate of Ammonia—1205.
  Red—1203.
  White—1202.
Washing Powder Compound—2496-2501, 2511.
  Jackman's—2495.
Water, Aerated, Foam for—952.
  Alkaline Tar—1207.
Waxing Solution—3474.
Weights, Equivalent, To Calculate—1204.

Whayne's Buchu—715.
Wheelock's Cough Mixture—605.
White Oils Liniment—754, 755.
White Pine Expectorant—583, 584.
White Wash—1202.
  Wax, Ointment of—809, 810.
Whooping Cough—558-560, 574.
  Powders—906.
Wild Cherry Bitters—86.
  Lozenges—1420.
Window Polishing Paste—1942.
Windows, Photographic, Dark Room—3436.
Windsor Toothache Drops—922, 923.
Wine of Aloes, U. S. P.—2874.
  Aromatic—74.
  Beef—67-69.
  Beef and Iron—1871, 1872, 2875.
  Beef, Iron and Cinchona—2876.
  Beef, Iron and Coca—2877.
  Beef and Malt—945.
  Cinchona, Ger. Phar.—2878.
  Cinchona Co., Codex—1883, 2879.
  Cinchona and Coca—2880.
  Coca—55, 62.
  Coca Kola—61.
  Cod Liver Oil—1813.
  Creasote—2881.
  Creasote Co.—2882.
  Damiana—65, 2883.
  Damiana Co.—66.
  Ginger—942.
  Golden Seal Co.—2884.
  Iron Bitters—29, 71, 72, 1262, 2885.
  Iron Citrate, U. S. P.—2889.
  Iron and Potassium Tartrate—2888.
  Iron and Quinine Citrate—2887.
  Iron, Sweet—2886.
  Orange—56, 944, 1879, 2890.
  Pancreatin—2891.
  Pepsin—63, 64.
  Quinine, Br. Phar.—2892.
  Raspberry—950.
  Rhubarb—73.
  Wormwood, Codex—2893.
Wire Fence Liniment—3501.
Wistar's Lozenges—1421.
Witch Hazel Eye Water—858.
  Ointment—789.
Wizard Oil, Hamlin's—769.
Wood's Bitters—34.
Worcestershire Sauces—2579-2585.
Worm Cakes—919.
  Lozenges—917, 918.
  Medicines—908-920.
  Powders—572, 913-916.
    for Horses—3487.
  Tasteless—916.
  Syrup—909-912.
Wormwood Bitters—698.
Wrinkle Lotion—4114.
Yorkshire Relish—2583.

LANE MEDICAL LIBRARY

To avoid fine, this book should be returned on or before the date last stamped below.